Provided through an unrestricted educational grant from

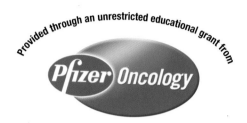

Jean-Marc Maheu, H.B.P.H.E., CCPE
Specialty Market Representative

 Oncology

AROMASIN™
PHARMORUBICIN™
SUTENT™
FRAGMIN™

Pfizer Global Pharmaceuticals
Pfizer Canada Inc.
17300 Trans-Canada Highway
Kirkland, Quebec H9J 2M5
Voice Mail: 1-800-267-2553, Ext. 1430
Fax: 905-257-9532
Email: jean-marc.maheu@pfizer.com

Breast Cancer Imaging

A Multidisciplinary, Multimodality Approach

Marie Tartar, MD
Radiologist, Scripps Green Hospital
Assistant Clinical Professor of Radiology
University of California, San Diego
La Jolla, California

Christopher E. Comstock, MD
Director of Breast Imaging
Associate Clinical Professor of Radiology
University of California, San Diego
La Jolla, California

Michael S. Kipper, MD
Clinical Professor of Radiology
University of California, San Diego
La Jolla, California

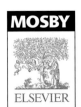

MOSBY

ELSEVIER

1600 John F. Kennedy Blvd.
Ste 1800
Philadelphia, PA 19103-2899

BREAST CANCER IMAGING ISBN: 978-0-323-04677-0
Copyright © 2008 by Mosby, Inc., an affiliate of Elsevier Inc.

Library of Congress Cataloging-in-Publication Data
Tartar, Marie.
  Breast cancer imaging : a multidisciplinary, multimodality approach / Marie Tartar, Christopher E. Comstock, Michael S. Kipper.—1st ed.
    p. ; cm.
Includes bibliographical references.
ISBN 978-0-323-04677-0
  1. Breast—Cancer—Imaging. 2. Breast—Cancer—Diagnosis. I. Comstock, Christopher E. II. Kipper, Michael S. III. Title.
  [DNLM: 1. Breast Neoplasms—diagnosis. 2. Breast Neoplasms—therapy. 3. Diagnostic Imaging. WP 870 T194b 2008]
RC280.B8T373 2008
616.99′4490757—dc22   20070452

Acquisitions Editor: Rebecca Gaertner
Developmental Editor: Joanie Milnes
Publishing Services Manager: Linda Van Pelt
Project Manager: Sharon Lee
Design Direction: Louis Forgione
Illustrations Manager: Kari Wszolek

Printed in China

Last digit is the print number: 9 8 7 6 5 4 3 2 1

Dedication

For Mary Eilenberg, my mother-in-law—a 30-year breast cancer survivor—who gave me the precious gift of her son, Steve.

MT

For Monique, my wife, whose constant support is a great strength in my life.

CC

For my parents, Aaron and Lorrayne, both of whom passed away after bouts of cancer, never experiencing the benefit of PET; and my two brothers, David and Stuart, who are both physicians, and constant sources of pleasure and pride. I hope they are able to integrate PET into their practices to help the patients they both care for so unselfishly. For my daughter, Valerie, who has always made me so proud to be her father. I hope she can someday look back and say that her dad contributed a little to the fantastic world of medicine. Finally, for my wife Chris, who has shared me with my work for yet another two years. Her ongoing support and understanding have enabled me to complete this project with my sense of humor and much of my sanity still intact.

MSK

Contributors

Christopher E. Comstock, MD
Director of Breast Imaging
Associate Clinical Professor of Radiology
University of California, San Diego
La Jolla, California

Steven S. Eilenberg, MD
Radiologist, Director of CT and MRI
Scripps Green Hospital
La Jolla, California

Michael S. Kipper, MD
Clinical Professor of Radiology
University of California, San Diego
La Jolla, California

Joan F. Kroener, MD
Medical Oncologist
Scripps Green Hospital
La Jolla, California

Eva Lean, MD
Radiation Oncologist
Oncology Therapies of Vista
Vista, California

Ray Lin, MD
Radiation Oncologist
Scripps Green Hospital
La Jolla, California

Marie Tartar, MD
Radiologist, Scripps Green Hospital
Assistant Clinical Professor of Radiology
University of California, San Diego
La Jolla, California

Preface

The idea for this text sprang unbidden into my head while traveling back from a family reunion on the East Coast in June of 2005. My first impulse was firm rejection: "Oh, no—I don't want to write another book." After all, it had only been just over a year since I had reclaimed my life after coauthoring *Clinical Atlas of PET: With Imaging Correlation* with Dr. Mike Kipper.

But the idea refused to be dismissed. I finally acknowledged to myself, "OK, intriguing idea, but it's probably been done"—which, if true, would have absolved me of any need to pursue it. Finally, I broke down and looked on the websites of the major medical publishers, expecting to find such a text already in print. To my surprise (and dismay), I didn't find anything along these lines.

A few other events and observations conspired around this time to convince me that this might be useful. I had noticed, as undoubtedly have all breast imaging specialists, that breast imaging has become dramatically more complex in recent years. This realization coincided with the increasing use of breast MRI for locally staging newly diagnosed breast cancer, and for problem solving in difficult-to-image patients. Suddenly, there was much more information, requiring correlation with multiple other modalities and frequently, additional image-guided biopsies. At the same time, breast cancer conferences evolved from relatively simple affairs, at which mammograms and breast ultrasounds were presented along with patients' histories and pathology, to much more complex working conferences in which CT, MRI, and PET/CT scans began figuring prominently.

Around this time, I did a second-look breast ultrasound on a patient with a prior history of lumpectomy and radiation for breast cancer, whose surveillance breast MRI study had shown a small enhancing mass on the opposite side. Fortunately, we found a benign-appearing correlate on the ultrasound. In reviewing the case, I noticed that the original report by the breast MRI interpreter (an exclusive breast imager) mentioned "abnormal right apical signal intensity...of uncertain significance" and recommended a chest CT. I recognized the case, having previously interpreted a PET scan on this patient, and knew the characteristic findings were due to prior radiation. When I mentioned this, she responded that she had thought of this possibility, but not being a cross-sectional imager, she wasn't sure, and so had shown it to two of our cross-sectional imaging partners (who don't do breast diagnostic work), who also weren't sure! I was surprised by this impasse. Was this a case of too much subspecialization, with well-trained and dedicated breast and cross-sectional imaging specialists each familiar with only their segment of the proverbial elephant? If so, surely more dialogue and training are needed.

Breast cancer is somewhat unusual in how many subspecialty lines it crosses. Depending on the manifestation and stage of disease, breast cancer imaging today can fall into the provinces of breast imaging specialists, cross-sectional imaging specialists, neuroradiologists, and nuclear medicine physicians. In some practices, these are separate people, with well-defined subspecialty areas. In many practices, generalists practice multiple subspecialties. I am such a practitioner, fellowship trained in cross-sectional imaging and MRI particularly, with subspecialty interests in breast and cancer imaging and in nuclear medicine and PET. In this capacity, I see breast cancer in all of its many guises, from initial diagnosis and local staging, to initial systemic staging of higher-risk patients, to surveillance and monitoring of patients with suspected or proven local or systemic metastases. A variety of tools are used to address these issues, including bone scans, CT, MRI, and PET. Along the way, I have come to appreciate how complex the imaging landscape has become, and how difficult it is for our clinician colleagues to navigate these choices without expert guidance. My hope is that by pulling together material heretofore found in disparate sources (ranging from breast imaging texts to cross-sectional imaging tomes to nuclear medicine and PET volumes), we can improve the cross-subspecialty dialogue and knowledge about breast cancer and its many and at times unique imaging manifestations. Although the examples presented in this book are either breast cancer manifestations, mimics of breast cancer, or the sequelae of treatment for breast cancer, much of the material on systemic disease is applicable to cancer imaging in general.

In developing this idea with my then-editor at Elsevier, Meghan McAteer, I quickly recognized that a project of this scope is too big and ambitious for one person. For collaborators, I sought "super-specialists" to round out my generalist-subspecialist approach. Christopher Comstock, MD, is an academic breast imager and the head of breast imaging at the University of California, San Diego. Michael Kipper, MD, with whom I had formerly worked and collaborated, is an internal medicine–trained nuclear medicine physician in San Diego. Between the three of us, we represent the variety of imaging practitioners dealing with the current spectrum of breast cancer imaging. We also sought input from oncologists specializing in breast cancer, and thanks are due to Joan Kroener, MD (medical oncology) and Ray Lin, MD (radiation oncology) of Scripps Clinic for their help. Special thanks go to Eva Lean, MD, a radiation oncologist specializing in breast cancer treatment and my friend and former colleague at Tri-City Medical Center in Oceanside, California, who agreed without hesitation to tackle the radiation therapy chapter of this book. It is our hope that we have succeeded in presenting this material in an organized and user-friendly format.

This text should not be construed as a comprehensive breast imaging resource, of which many excellent examples already exist. Accordingly, benign breast disease is not comprehensively covered. This book assumes a basic working level of breast imaging sophistication. For example, no attempt is made to teach differentiation of benign from malignant microcalcifications. Nevertheless, because one of the best ways to learn is by reviewing proven cases, ample opportunity for learning is provided through the examples of malignant microcalcifications that are presented in case histories. The major focus of the breast imaging portion of the book is on the workup and image-guided biopsy staging of complex, proven breast cancer cases, presented as they developed, with all of the twists and turns of evolving clinical cases.

Similarly, although this book does not purport to be a comprehensive breast MRI atlas, because breast MRI and MRI-guided biopsy have become so integral and useful to our breast imaging practices, many examples of these techniques are presented, again in the context of proven breast cancer and breast cancer mimic cases. Of course, along the way, many benign diagnoses were made as well, and these are presented when appropriate to the discussion of the decision-making process.

In looking for systemic manifestations of breast cancer, the clinician has a variety of choices today, including bone scans, PET, PET/CT, CT, and MRI. One goal of this book is to provide insight for imagers into the clinical scenarios prompting oncologists to request imaging studies in specific patients. Conversely, it is hoped that this work will help unravel for breast cancer clinicians some of the intricacies of the imaging choices available. How best to evaluate symptoms that may herald metastatic disease? What is the most efficient and cost-effective approach to evaluating the patient with rising tumor markers? How best to assess treatment responses in patients with known metastases? These are some of the questions oncologists grapple with in managing their patients, ideally with knowledgeable breast cancer imagers serving as their guides and consultants. It is my hope that this work will serve as a practical resource for breast cancer imaging and clinical specialists, tying together material from a variety of sources, with the aim of improving cross-specialty dialogue and elucidating the complex issues inherent in breast cancer imaging today.

Marie Tartar, MD

Acknowledgments

Thanks are due to many who helped make this project a reality: First and foremost for me, my husband, Steve Eilenberg, MD, whose moral, logistical, and culinary support and good humor have been (mostly) unwavering. Thanks also go to Les Sherman, Scripps Clinic radiology executive assistant extraordinaire, for tracking down an endless series of articles and otherwise helping me manage the minutiae of practice, and of this project. I am fortunate to be part of a very progressive and cohesive multispecialty group and breast cancer care team, which made this project possible. Finally, thanks are due to our editorial team at Elsevier, and we are grateful in particular for the diligence and oversight of Joanie Milnes and the attention to detail of Sharon Lee on this project.

MT

Thanks to Dr. Marie Tartar. Without her dedication, hard work, and diligence, this book would not have been possible. Marie, thank you for asking me to collaborate on this book with you and for all of your time and help.

CC

When Dr. Tartar approached me about collaborating on this, our second book, I remember having two thoughts. First, thank goodness it would be with Marie. Second, could I possibly keep up with her? Although the answer to that question proved to be "barely," I was ultimately reminded of what a wonderful person and teacher she has been. So, to Marie, thank you so much for all of your hard work, your incredible dedication, and most of all, your friendship.

MSK

Contents

CHAPTER 3

Local Staging: Imaging Options and Core Biopsy Strategies *76*

Christopher Comstock, MD, and Marie Tartar, MD

CASE

CHAPTER 4

Unusual and Problematic Types of Breast Cancers: DCIS, Intracystic Papillary Carcinoma, Benign-appearing Breast Cancers, ILC, Inflammatory Breast Cancer, and Breast Cancer in Implant Patients *163*

Christopher Comstock, MD, and Marie Tartar, MD

CASE

CHAPTER 5

Locally Advanced Breast Cancer (LABC) and Neoadjuvant Chemotherapy *224*

Marie Tartar, MD, Christopher Comstock, MD, and Michael S. Kipper, MD

CASE

CHAPTER 6

Imaging Surveillance for Locally Recurrent Disease *302*

Christopher Comstock, MD, Marie Tartar, and Michael S. Kipper, MD

CASE

CHAPTER 7

Breast Cancer Mimics   *349*

Christopher Comstock, MD, and Marie Tartar, MD

CASE

CHAPTER 8

Identifying Bone Metastases   *368*

Michael S. Kipper, MD, Marie Tartar, MD, and Joan F. Kroener, MD

CASE

CHAPTER 9

Liver Metastases   *435*

Marie Tartar, MD

CASE

CHAPTER 10

Thoracic Metastases, Mimics, and Treatment Effects   *467*

Marie Tartar, MD, and Michael S. Kipper, MD

CASE

CHAPTER 11

Breast Cancer Metastases to the Neural Axis   514

Marie Tartar, MD, and Steven S. Eilenberg, MD

CASE

CHAPTER 12

Multisystem Metastases and Assessment of Treatment Efficacy   554

Michael S. Kipper, MD, Marie Tartar, MD, and
Joan F. Kroener, MD

CASE

CHAPTER 13

Radiation Therapy Effects and Considerations   570

Eva Lean, MD, Ray Lin, MD, and Marie Tartar, MD

CASE

Frequently Used Abbreviations

AC PET: attenuation-corrected positron emission tomography

AC: Adriamycin (doxorubicin) and Cytoxan (cyclophosphamide); commonly used chemotherapy regimen

ADH: atypical ductal hyperplasia

ALH: atypical lobular hyperplasia

BCT: breast conservation therapy; usually lumpectomy and radiation therapy

BI-RADS: breast imaging reporting and data system

CC: cranial-caudal; mammographic view

CI: conventional imaging; in breast imaging, refers to mammography and sonography; also used to signify anatomic imaging, as opposed to molecular imaging

CMF: commonly used adjuvant chemotherapy regimen: Cytoxan (cyclophosphamide), methotrexate, 5-fluorouracil

CNS: central nervous system

CSF: cerebrospinal fluid

CT: computed tomography

DCE-MRI: dynamic contrast-enhanced magnetic resonance imaging

DCIS: ductal carcinoma in situ

ER: estrogen receptor

FDG: ^{18}F-flourodeoxyglucose; glucose analog

FDG-PET: ^{18}F-flourodeoxyglucose positron emission tomography

FLAIR: fluid-attenuated inversion recovery; fluid-sensitive brain MRI sequence

FNA: fine needle aspiration

FSE: fast spin echo

G-CSF: granulocyte colony-stimulating factor

HASTE: half-Fourier single shot turbo spin echo; also half Fourier acquisition turbo spin echo

HD: Hodgkin's disease

HU: Hounsfield unit; measure of density on CT

IDC: infiltrating ductal carcinoma

IBC: inflammatory breast cancer

ILC: infiltrating lobular carcinoma

IV: intravenous

LABC: locally advanced breast cancer

LCIS: lobular carcinoma in situ

LIQ: lower inner quadrant

LOQ: lower outer quadrant

MIP: maximum intensity projection

MLO: mediolateral oblique; mammographic view

MRI: magnetic resonance imaging

NaF: sodium fluoride

NAC PET: non–attenuation-corrected positron emission tomography

PAB: posterior axillary boost; radiation field

PEM: positron emission mammography

PET: positron emission tomography

PET/CT: positron emission tomography/computed tomography

PBR: partial breast radiation

PR: progesterone receptor

RT: radiation therapy

SCF: supraclavicular field; radiation field

SRS: stereotactic radiosurgery

STIR: short tau inversion recovery; fluid-sensitive MRI sequence

SUV: standardized uptake value; a quantitative measure of the uptake of FDG on PET, which essentially compares concentration of FDG at a suspected tumor site to the average uptake in the body

TRAM (flap): transverse rectus abdominis musculocutaneous (or myocutaneous)

TSE: turbo spin echo; also fast spin echo

TSTC: too small to characterize; used in reference to volume-averaged, hypodense, indeterminate liver lesions on CT

UIQ: upper inner quadrant

UOQ: upper outer quadrant

US: ultrasonography; also ultrasound (imaging)

WBRT: whole-brain radiation therapy

XRT: radiation therapy

CHAPTER 1

Detection of Breast Cancer: Screening of Asymptomatic Patients

Breast cancer is the most common malignancy and the second leading cause of cancer deaths among American women. In 2005, it is estimated that more than 211,000 new cases will be diagnosed, and more than 40,000 women will die of the disease.[1] Breast carcinoma mortality in the United States has declined substantially over the past 30 years, from 31.4 deaths per 100,000 women per year in 1975 to 25.9 deaths per 100,000 women per year in 2001.[2] More recent analysis by the CDC of 1999–2003 data from the National Cancer Institute (NCI) Surveillance, Epidemiology, and End Results (SEER) study and the CDC National Program of Cancer Registries (NPCR) indicated that age-adjusted incidence rates for invasive breast cancer decreased each year from 1999 to 2003, with the greatest decrease (6.1%) occurring from 2002 to 2003. For in situ cancers, rates increased each year from 1999 to 2002 and then decreased from 2002 to 2003, although the percentage decrease (2.7%) was smaller than that for invasive cancers (6.1%). In addition to advances in treatment options, the combination of increasing utilization of screening mammography and improved mammographic quality, allowing detection of cancers at an earlier stage, is likely to account for the reduction in breast cancer mortality.[3-4]

Mammography is currently the only screening test proven to reduce mortality from breast cancer in women of average risk. Other modalities, including ultrasound and dynamic contrast enhanced MRI (DCE-MRI), have demonstrated improved cancer detection in select subgroups of women. They have not been examined in women of low risk. In addition, in contrast to screening mammography, studies of these newer modalities have not evaluated mortality as an end point. Therefore, it has been assumed that improved detection rates for ultrasound and MRI will translate to a reduction in mortality.

SCREENING MAMMOGRAPHY

To date, the benefits from screening mammography for women 40 to 70 years of age have been proven in eight randomized controlled trials (RCTs) conducted in Europe and the United States during the past 40 years.[5-11] Reported reductions in breast cancer mortality range from 20% to 45%. Because of the relatively small numbers of women aged 40 to 49 years in the individual trials, the benefit from screening in this age range has been controversial. However, in 1997, a meta-analysis of women aged 40 to 49 years in all five Swedish trials found a 30% reduction in breast cancer deaths.[12] In addition, long-term follow-up of three trials (Health Insurance Plan Project [HIP], Gothenburg, and Malmö) each found statistically significant reductions in breast cancer mortality.[13-15] Therefore, for average risk women, most professional organizations in the United States recommend screening mammography beginning at the age of 40 years. For screening women younger than the age of 40 years, there are few RCT data. Therefore, decisions concerning screening practice in this age group must be based on less rigorous evidence and on a more individual basis. Given that younger women have a longer life expectancy and that cancers tend to grow more rapidly in younger women, earlier detection of these cancers may theoretically be advantageous. However, this must be balanced by the limitations of screening mammography in younger women, which include a lower frequency of breast cancer, reduced sensitivity of mammography, slightly increased radiation risk, and higher recall rates. Screening of younger women will be of most benefit in women at high risk, especially those known to carry the *BRCA1* or *BRCA2* gene mutation. Methods for estimating risk based on medical and family history include the Gail, Claus, and BRCAPRO mathematical models. Observational studies of high-risk women aged 30 to 39 years show a cancer detection rate similar to that for women aged 40 to 49 years.[16-17] In general, screening of women aged less than 40 years is restricted to high-risk subgroups (women with a 20% lifetime breast cancer risk at or before the age of 30 years or breast cancer risk at a given age equivalent to that of the average woman at the age of 40 years). These include *BRCA1* or *BRCA2* gene mutation carriers, women with a personal history of breast cancer, women with a prior diagnosis of atypical ductal or lobular hyperplasia, women with previous radiation therapy to the chest before the age of 30 years, and women with a strong family history of breast cancer (usually involving one or more first-degree relatives with premenopausal breast cancer or breast cancer before the age of 50 years).

LIMITATIONS OF MAMMOGRAPHY

Although there have been significant improvements in mammographic technique over the past 50 years, fundamental limitations remain. These include the low inherent contrast differences between tissue structures in the breast and the fact that mammographic detection of breast cancer (sensitivity) relies on the ability to visualize cancer through the background of overlying normal tissue (Figure 1). Mammographic specificity relies on the ability to distinguish benign from malignant breast lesions based on their margins and morphologic features.[18-19] However, malignant and benign lesions may have similar appearances, thereby reducing specificity. Data from the Breast Cancer Surveillance Consortium demonstrated that on average, screening mammography programs had a callback rate of 6.4% to 13.3% and a positive predictive value of 3.4% to 6.2%.[20] The mean cancer detection rate was 4.7 per 1000, and the

mean size of invasive cancers was 13 mm. The main mammographic signs of breast cancer include clustered microcalcifications, masses, architectural distortions, and asymmetrical densities. Comparison to prior mammograms is essential because some cancers may only be detected by perceiving them as a subtle change from prior studies. In addition, the availability of prior mammograms for comparison can reduce the number of unnecessary callbacks for stable benign findings.[21]

DIGITAL MAMMOGRAPHY AND COMPUTER-AIDED DETECTION

Screen-film mammography (SFM) has been the standard method used for breast cancer screening since the end of xeromammography some 20 years ago. Advances in screen-film technology and film-processing techniques have contributed to major improvements in the quality of mammographic images. In addition to high contrast, the strength of SFM lies in its extremely high spatial resolution, often greater than 10 line pairs per millimeter (lp/mm). This allows the detection of exceedingly small clusters of microcalcifications, one of the earliest signs of breast cancer. The limitations of SFM include the detection of subtle soft tissue lesions, especially in the presence of dense glandular

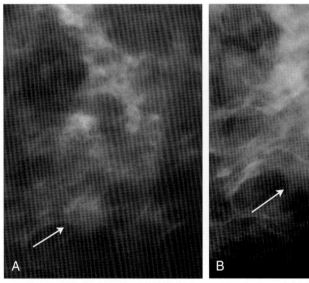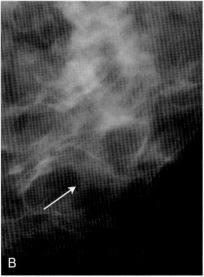

FIGURE 1.   A 58-year-old asymptomatic woman undergoing yearly screening mammography. **A,** A spiculated mass is seen in the medial left breast on the CC view, isodense to breast parenchyma. On biopsy, this proved to be an invasive ductal carcinoma. **B,** In retrospect, the mass is evident on the study 2 years before, but is difficult to differentiate from glandular tissue.

tissues, and the fact that the film serves simultaneously as the image receptor, display medium, and long-term storage medium. Recent technologic advances have led to the development of full-field digital mammography (FFDM). One of the initial concerns of FFDM is its inherent lower spatial resolution of 5 to 10 lp/mm. However, several studies have demonstrated that despite the limited spatial resolution, the visibility of calcifications on FFDM is not significantly different from that on SFM.[22–24] The higher contrast resolution of FFDM may account for its comparable detection rates. In a recent multicenter trial of 49,528 women, Pisano and colleagues[24] reported that the overall diagnostic accuracy of FFDM was comparable to SFM as a means of screening for breast cancer. The study also found that digital mammography was more accurate in women younger than 50 years, women with radiographically dense breasts, and premenopausal or perimenopausal women.

Digital mammography has the potential to overcome the inherent limitations of SFM. By directly converting the detected x-ray photons to numerical values, the process of x-ray photon detection is decoupled from the image display. The digital images can be processed by a computer, displayed in multiple formats, and fed directly to computer-aided detection (CAD) software programs. In addition, there are logistical and financial advantages of FFDM, including faster patient throughput, no film or processing costs, the ability to transmit images, and the ability to perform telemammography.

CAD programs were developed to assist a radiologist in the interpretation of screening mammograms, so that cancer detection rates could be improved. These programs rely on neural networks to analyze the images and highlight potentially suspicious findings that may have been overlooked by the radiologist. Several studies have shown improved cancer detection by radiologists using CAD versus radiologists alone, without significantly increasing callback rates.[24–27] However, other studies have shown less promising results.[28–29] A recent study by Fenton and colleagues[29] reported that CAD decreased the accuracy of screening mammogram interpretation. This was not due to a decrease in cancer detection, but rather to an increase in false-positive results. To be effective, CAD programs should not increase callback rates and should not significantly prolong interpretation times for screening mammograms. It is important to remember that CAD programs are tools that must be used in an appropriate manner. They should not be used to override a suspicious finding detected by a radiologist. In general, these systems tend to be more helpful for low-volume or inexperienced readers.

MAGNETIC RESONANCE IMAGING

Dynamic, contrast-enhanced MRI of the breast has been shown to be extremely sensitive in the detection of invasive breast cancer and is not limited by the density of the breast tissue. However, because the reported sensitivity of MRI for ductal carcinoma in situ (DCIS) ranges between 45% and 100%, MRI is currently not recommended as a replacement for mammography.[30] A more recent single institution study suggests that MRI may have a higher sensitivity than mammography for DCIS than previously thought, particularly for high-grade DCIS.[31] The use of MRI in the general population has been limited by its moderate specificity. Therefore, its use has been focused on studying patients in whom the yield from MRI is likely to be higher. Multiple studies have shown that MRI is a useful tool as an adjuvant to screening mammography in women at high risk for breast cancer.[32–34] The American Cancer Society (ACS) recommends annual screening MRI for women with a 20% to 25% lifetime risk for breast cancer.[35] This includes women with the *BRCA1* or *BRCA2* breast cancer genes, as well as women with multiple family members with breast or ovarian cancer, and women who have undergone mediastinal irradiation for Hodgkin's disease. Women whose benefit from screening MRI was considered questionable by the ACS because of insufficient data included women with a personal history of breast cancer, prior biopsy yielding atypia, or extremely dense breasts on mammography. The decision to perform screening MRI in these women should be made on a case-by-case basis. Several models may be used to calculate lifetime risk for breast cancer, including the Gail, Claus, and Tyrer-Cusick models.

ULTRASOUND

Early studies of breast ultrasound for cancer screening were disappointing because of its poor detection of small cancers and excessively high false-positive rates.[36–40] With the advent in the early 1990s of technical improvements in ultrasound, including improved spatial and contrast resolution utilizing higher-megahertz (MHz) transducers, the potential of whole-breast ultrasound as a screening tool has been revisited. Several recent single-institution studies have demonstrated a prevalence detection rate of 3 to 4 mammographically occult cancers per 1000 women screened.[41-50] However, the biopsy positive predictive values were less than 20%, lower than accepted for mammography.[51] These initial studies have focused mainly on women with mammographically higher-density breasts. Screening ultrasound appears to be more sensitive in detecting early invasive cancer, whereas mammography is more sensitive in the detection of DCIS. Of the invasive cancers, ultrasound found a higher percentage of invasive lobular carcinomas than that usually found on mammography. Therefore, whole-breast ultrasound should supplement mammographic screening, rather than replace it.

Despite these promising early results, the use of screening ultrasound in general has not been recommend by professional organizations because of concerns regarding the scientific validity of these initial studies and the lack of randomized controlled trials.

The initial studies were performed mostly by radiologists with a high ultrasound skill level and in some studies were not blinded to the mammographic findings. Therefore, the initial results of screening ultrasound may not extrapolate to its use in general clinical practice.[52] Other concerns include the lack of standardized exam techniques, interpretation criteria, false-positive results, and unnecessary biopsies. In addition, most of the initial studies on whole-breast ultrasound have evaluated prevalence (initial) detection rates, rather than incidence (subsequent) detection rates. The benefit from subsequent yearly screening ultrasound is uncertain, but likely to be less. The American College of Radiology Imaging Network (ACRIN) is currently conducting a randomized multicenter trial evaluating whole-breast bilateral screening ultrasound in high-risk, asymptomatic women with dense breasts. The study will evaluate both prevalence (year 1) and incidence (years 2 and 3) screening ultrasound detection rates as compared with mammography. Interpretation of the examinations will be performed by radiologists trained in mammographic and ultrasound interpretation, using standardized interpretive criteria.

Although ultrasound is less sensitive than MRI, because of its lower cost and availability, it is likely that whole-breast ultrasound will play an increasing role as a supplemental screening modality in women with dense breasts. Current postprocessing algorithms, including spatial compounding and harmonic imaging, as well as newer techniques such as elastography, may help to improve the specificity of breast ultrasound and decrease the number of false-positive results and unnecessary biopsies. In addition, automated whole-breast ultrasound systems, currently being developed by several manufacturers, may help to standardize and streamline whole-breast ultrasound.

MOLECULAR IMAGING

Previous attempts of breast imaging using ^{99m}Tc sestamibi and ^{18}F fluorodeoxyglucose (FDG) positron emission tomography (PET) were limited by the use of relatively low-resolution whole-body systems. However, newer high-resolution dedicated breast imaging systems have been developed. Breast-specific gamma imaging (BSGI) and positron emission mammography (PEM) allow high-resolution imaging of the breast based on metabolism, rather than anatomic changes. Their use as screening tests has not been established. Variability of uptake in primary breast tumors, as well as moderate specificities, has limited their potential. Randomized control trials are needed to evaluate their possible role as an adjuvant screening tool in certain subgroups of women.

REFERENCES

1. Jemal A, Murray T, Ward E, et al. Cancer statistics, 2005. *CA Cancer J Clin* 2005; 55:10–30.
2. Ries LAG, Eisner MP, Kosary CL, et al. SEER cancer statistics review, 1975–2001. Bethesda, MD, National Cancer Institute, 2004.
3. Elkin EB, Hudis C, Begg CB, Schrag D. The effect of changes in tumor size on breast carcinoma survival in the U.S.: 1975–1999. *Cancer* 2005; 104(6):1149–1157.
4. Berry DA, Cronin KA, Plevritis SK, et al. Effect of screening and adjuvant therapy on mortality from breast cancer. *N Engl J Med* 2005; 353:1784–1792.
5. Smith RA, Duffy SW, Gabe R, et al. The randomized trials of breast cancer screening: what have we learned? *Radiol Clin North Am* 2004; 42(5):793–806, v.
6. Shapiro S, Venet W, Strax P, Venet L. Periodic screening for breast cancer: the Health Insurance Plan Project and its Sequelae, 1963–1986. Baltimore, Johns Hopkins University Press, 1988.
7. Tabar L, Vitak B, Chen HH, et al. The Swedish Two-County Trial twenty years later. *Radiol Clin North Am* 2000; 38:625–652.
8. Alexander FE, Anderson TJ, Brown HK, et al. 14 years of follow-up from Edinburgh randomized trial of breast cancer screening. *Lancet* 1999; 353: 1903–1908.
9. Andersson I, Aspegren K, Janzon L, et al. Mammographic screening and mortality from breast cancer:

the Malmo mammographic screening trial. *BMJ* 1988; 297:943–948.

10. Frisell J, Lidbrink E, Hellstrom L, Rutqvist LE. Follow-up after 11 years: update of mortality results in the Stockholm mammographic screening trial. *Breast Cancer Res Treat* 1997; 45:263–270.

11. Bjurstam N, Bjorneld L, Duffy SW. The Gothenburg Breast Screening Trial: first results on mortality, incidence, and mode of detection for women ages 39–49 years at randomization. *Cancer* 1997; 80: 2091–2099.

12. Hendrick RE, Smith RA, Rutledge JH 3rd, Smart CR. Benefit of screening mammography in women aged 40–49: a new meta-analysis of randomized controlled trials. *J Natl Cancer Inst Monogr* 1997; 22:87–92.

13. Chu KC, Smart CR, Tarone RE. Analysis of breast cancer mortality and stage distribution by age for the Health Insurance Plan clinical trial. *J Natl Cancer Inst* 1988; 80:1125–1132.

14. Bjurstam N, Bjorneld L, Warwick J, et al. The Gothenburg Breast Screening Trial. *Cancer* 2003; 97:2387–2396.

15. Andersson I, Janzon L. Reduced breast cancer mortality in women under 50: updated results from the Malmo Mammographic Screening Program. *J Natl Cancer Inst Monogr* 1997; 22:63–68.

16. Liberman L, Dershaw DD, Deutch BM, et al. Screening mammography: value in women 35–39 years old. *AJR Am J Roentgenol* 1993; 161:53–56.

17. Curpen BN, Sickles EA, Sollitto RA, et al. The comparative value of mammographic screening for women 40–49 years old versus women 50–64 years old. *AJR Am J Roentgenol* 1995; 164:1099–1103.

18. Sickles EA. Breast masses: mammographic evaluation. *Radiology* 1989; 173(2):297–303. Review.

19. Sickles EA. Mammographic features of malignancy found during screening. *Recent Results Cancer Res* 1990; 119:88–93. Review.

20. Rosenberg RD, Yankaskas BC, Abraham LA, et al. Performance benchmarks for screening mammography. *Radiology* 2006; 241:55–66.

21. Frankel SD, Sickles EA, Curpen BN, et al. Initial versus subsequent screening mammography: comparison of findings and their prognostic significance. *AJR Am J Roentgenol* 1995; 164:1107–1109.

22. Fischer U, Baum F, Obenauer S, et al. Comparative study in patients with microcalcifications: full-field digital mammography vs screen-film mammography. *Eur Radiol* 2002; 12:2679–2683

23. Lewin JM, Hendrick RE, D'Orsi CJ, et al. Comparison of full-field digital mammography to screen-film mammography for cancer detection: results of 4945 paired examinations. *Radiology* 2001; 218: 873–880.

24. Pisano ED, Gatsonis C, Hendrick E, et al. Diagnostic performance of digital versus film mammography for breast-cancer screening. *N Engl J Med* 2005; 353:1773–1783.

25. Freer TW, Ulissey MJ. Screening mammography with computer-aided detection: prospective study of 12,860 patients in a community breast center. *Radiology* 2001; 220(3):781–786.

26. Birdwell RL, Bandodkar P, Ikeda DM. Computer-aided detection with screening mammography in a university hospital setting. *Radiology* 2005; 236(2): 451–457.

27. Morton MJ, Whaley DH, Brandt KR, Amrami KK. Screening mammograms: interpretation with computer-aided detection—prospective evaluation. *Radiology* 2006; 239(2):375–383.

28. Gur D, Sumkin JH, Rockette HE, et al. Changes in breast cancer detection and mammography recall rates after the introduction of a computer-aided detection system. *J Natl Cancer Inst* 2004; 96(3): 185–190.

29. Fenton JJ, Taplin SH, Carney PA, et al. Influence of computer-aided detection on performance of screening mammography. *N Engl J Med* 2007; 356(14):1399–1409.

30. Bazzocchi M, Zuiani C, Panizza P, et al. Contrast-enhanced breast MRI in patients with suspicious microcalcifications on mammography: results of a multicenter trial. *AJR Am J Roentgenol* 2006; 186:1723–1732.

31. Kuhl CK, Schrading S, Bieling HB, et al. MRI for diagnosis of pure ductal carcinoma in situ: a prospective observational study. *Lancet* 2007; 370(9586):485–492.

32. Kriege M, Brekelmans CT, Boetes C, et al. Efficacy of MRI and mammography for breast-cancer screening in women with a familial or genetic predisposition. *N Engl J Med* 2004; 351(5): 427–437.

33. Lehman CD, Blume JD, Weatherall P, et al. Screening women at high risk for breast cancer with mammography and magnetic resonance imaging. *Cancer* 2005; 103:1898–1905.

34. Kuhl CK, Schrading S, Leutner CC, et al. Mammography, breast ultrasound, and magnetic resonance imaging for surveillance of women at high familial risk for breast cancer. *J Clin Oncol* 2005; 23(33): 8469–8476.

35. Saslow D, Boetes C, Burke W, et al. American Cancer Society guidelines for breast screening with MRI as an adjunct to mammography. *CA Cancer J Clin* 2007; 57(2):75–89.

36. Cole-Beuglet C, Goldberg BB, Kurtz AB, et al. Clinical experience with a prototype realtime dedicated breast scanner. *AJR Am J Roentgenol* 1982; 139: 905–911.

37. Sickles EA, Filly RA, Callen PW. Breast cancer detection with sonography and mammography: comparison using state-of-the-art equipment. *AJR Am J Roentgenol* 1983; 140:843–845.

38. Egan RL, Egan KL. Automated water-path full-breast sonography: correlation with histology of 176 solid lesions. *AJR Am J Roentgenol* 1984; 143:499–507.

39. Egan RL, McSweeney MB, Murphy FB. Breast sonography and the detection of breast cancer. *Recent Results Cancer Res* 1984; 90:90–100.

40. Kopans DB, Meyer JE, Lindfors KK. Whole-breast US imaging: four-year follow-up. *Radiology* 1985; 157: 505–507.

41. Gordon PB, Goldenberg SL. Malignant breast masses detected only by ultrasound. *Cancer* 1995; 76: 626–630.

42. Kolb TM, Lichy J, Newhouse JH. Occult cancer in women with dense breasts: detection with screening US—diagnostic yield and tumor characteristics. *Radiology* 1998; 207:191–199.

43. Buchberger W, DeKoekkoek-Doll P, Springer P, et al. Incidental findings on sonography of the breast: clinical significance and diagnostic workup. *AJR Am J Roentgenol* 1999; 173:921–927.

44. Buchberger W, Niehoff A, Obrist A, et al. Clinically and mammographically occult breast lesions: detection and classification with high-resolution sonography. *Semin Ultrasound CT MR* 2000; 21:325–336.

45. Kaplan SS. Clinical utility of bilateral whole-breast US in the evaluation of women with dense breast tissue. *Radiology* 2001; 221:641–649.

46. Kolb TM, Lichy J, Newhouse JH: Comparison of the performance of screening mammography, physical examination, and breast US and evaluation of factors that influence them: an analysis of 27,825 patient evaluations. *Radiology* 2002; 225:165–175.

47. Leconte I, Feger C, Galant C, et al. Mammography and subsequent whole-breast sonography of non-palpable breast cancers: the importance of radiologic breast density. *AJR Am J Roentgenol* 2003; 180:1675–1679.

48. Crystal P, Strano S, Shcharynski S, Koretz MJ. Using sonography to screen women with mammographically dense breasts. *AJR Am J Roentgenol* 2003; 181:177–182.

49. Cortesi L, Turchetti D, Marchi I, et al. Breast cancer screening in women at increased risk according to different family histories: an update of the Modena Study Group experience. *BMC Cancer* 2006; 6:210.

50. Corsetti V, Ferrari A, Ghirardi M, et al. Role of ultrasonography in detecting mammographically occult breast carcinoma in women with dense breasts. *Radiol Med* (Torino) 2006; 111(3):440–448.

51. Quality Determinants of Mammography Guideline Panel. Quality determinants of mammography. AHCPR Publication no. 95–0632. Rockville, MD, U.S. Department of Health and Human Services, Public Health Service, 1994.

52. Berg WA, Blume JD, Cormack JB, Mendelson EB. Operator dependence of physician-performed whole-breast US: lesion detection and characterization. *Radiology* 2006; 241(2):355–365.

CASE 1

Breast cancer presenting as a small new mass on mammography

An asymptomatic 57-year-old woman underwent screening mammography, which showed a new finding of a 6-mm round mass in the anterior upper outer quadrant (UOQ) of the left breast (Figures 1 and 2). The patient had undergone a prior benign left breast needle biopsy with placement of a marker clip in the posterior upper outer left breast. Ultrasound confirmed the presence of a somewhat ill-defined 6-mm solid mass (Figure 3). Ultrasound-guided core needle biopsy yielded a diagnosis of low-grade ductal carcinoma in situ.

The patient was treated surgically with lumpectomy alone. Final histologic diagnosis was a 6-mm low- to intermediate-grade ductal carcinoma in situ with negative margins.

TEACHING POINTS

Mammographic signs of breast cancer may manifest as subtle new findings. The ability to compare to prior mammograms can facilitate the detection of subtle changes. Because the finding in this case represented a new mass, workup proceeded directly to ultrasound for evaluation. This could have represented a benign cyst. Any new solid mass requires tissue biopsy. Therefore, mammographic magnification views to analyze the margin features of this mass would not have changed clinical management.

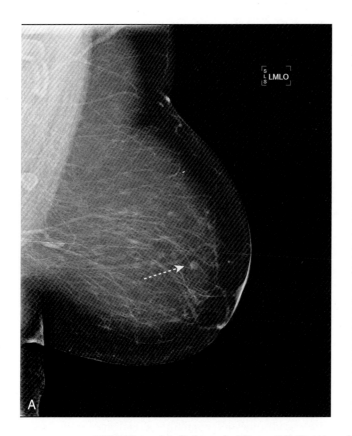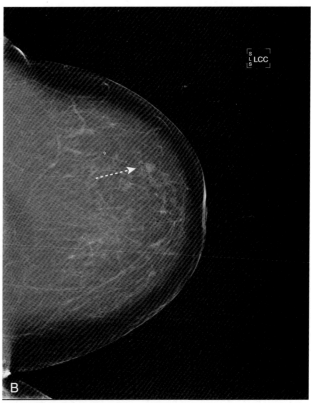

FIGURE 1. Mediolateral oblique (MLO) (**A**) and cranial-caudal (CC) (**B**) views show a small, 6-mm, low-density round mass in the anterior upper outer quadrant (*arrows*).

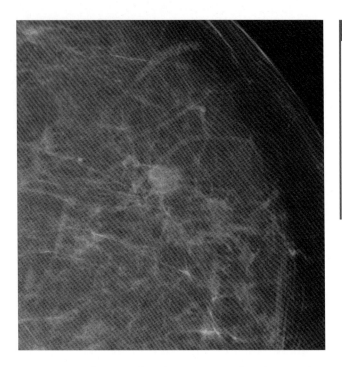

FIGURE 2. Close-up view demonstrates that the margins of the mass are ill defined.

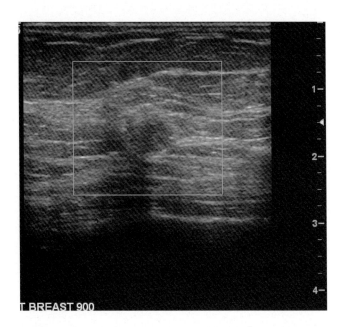

FIGURE 3. Ultrasound confirms a hypoechoic mass with internal echoes. Although this could represent a cyst with debris or thick fluid, it does not meet the criteria for a simple cyst. Therefore, it must be considered solid until proved otherwise.

CASE 2

Breast cancer presenting as a new mass on mammography

A new left lower inner quadrant mass with ill-defined margins was identified on a screening mammogram performed on an asymptomatic 67-year-old woman (Figure 1). Sonography confirmed

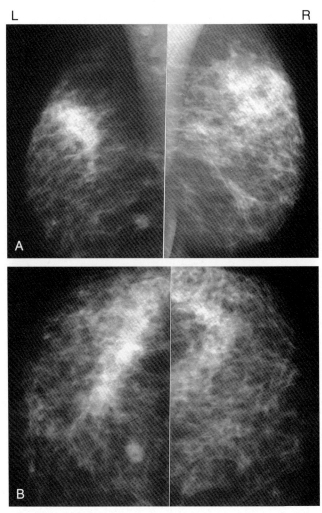

FIGURE 1. MLO (**A**) and CC (**B**) mammograms show heterogeneous increased breast parenchymal density. There is a mass with indistinct margins in the lower inner quadrant of the left breast. Although the mass is of similar density to the breast tissue, it is readily visualized in an area where the breast is relatively fatty. Mammography also raised a question of architectural distortion in the left upper breast at 12 o'clock, where more locally increased parenchymal density can be seen.

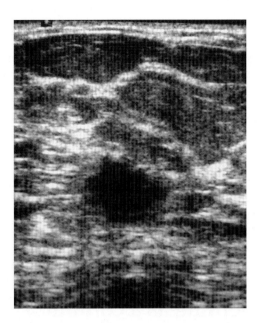

FIGURE 2. The mass is highly suspicious on ultrasound. It is solid, very hypoechoic, and taller than wide, and it has irregular, angular margins. No sonographic correlate for the questioned left upper breast architectural distortion was found.

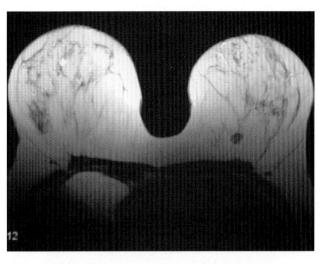

FIGURE 3. T2-weighted axial MRI shows the mass to be posterior and surrounded by fatty tissue, with an irregular margin and relatively hypointense signal intensity. Most breast cancers are hypointense on T2-weighted MRI. A fluid signal, round, cystic structure in the right chest represented a known pericardial cyst.

a suspicious, 1 cm, irregularly marginated, hypoechoic, solid mass, which was taller than wide (Figure 2). A mammographically questioned second abnormality, architectural distortion in the left upper breast, had no sonographic confirmation. MRI was recommended to further assess the question of possible multicentric disease. The suspected cancer mass was highly suspicious by MRI criteria, showing irregular margination (Figures 3 and 4) and a washout pattern of enhancement (Figure 5). No correlate was found on MRI for the questioned left upper architectural distortion. There was no evidence of multicentricity by MRI.

Subsequent image-guided biopsy of the mass confirmed invasive ductal carcinoma (IDC). Clinical and imaging evaluation suggested stage 1 disease, and the patient was treated surgically with partial mastectomy. The pathology showed a 1.5-cm invasive ductal carcinoma, estrogen receptor and progesterone receptor positive and *HER-2/neu* positive, with clear margins. Two sentinel lymph nodes were negative for malignancy.

Radiation therapy was administered after surgery, and hormonal therapy (initially tamoxifen, subsequently switched to anastrozole [Arimidex]) was begun afterward.

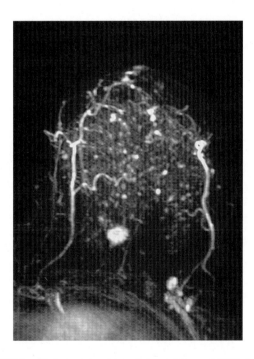

FIGURE 4. Enhanced subtracted axial breast MRI shows the mass to enhance intensely heterogeneously. The margin is irregular. Scattered, tiny punctate foci of enhancement are also noted throughout both breasts.

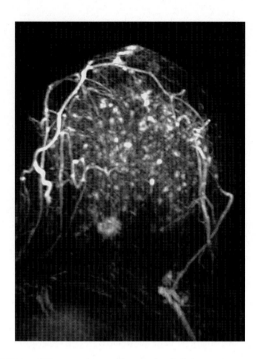

FIGURE 5. Three minutes later, the left breast mass enhancement has markedly declined. This washout suggests malignancy.

TEACHING POINTS

Mammographic detection of the new mass in the posterior lower inner quadrant of the left breast was greatly aided by the fact that it arose in a region where the patient's breast is relatively fatty. The mass is similar in density to the breast parenchyma and would have been more difficult to identify if it occurred in an area of greater breast density. The question raised on mammography of a second abnormality, with possible architectural distortion in the upper left breast, needed to be settled before a decision could be made regarding suitable surgical treatment for this patient. The lack of an ultrasound correlate was somewhat reassuring, but greater reassurance is provided by the absence of a corresponding abnormality on MRI, with its high sensitivity for invasive neoplasia. The background pattern of tiny scattered enhancing foci is commonly encountered, especially in premenopausal women, and is presumed related to hormonal effects. These findings are minimized by imaging, when possible, in the second week of the menstrual cycle. Even when they cannot be eliminated, it is generally possible to "read around"

these findings when they are fairly diffuse and symmetric.

The use of breast MRI in this case increases the confidence level that this patient's tumor is unifocal and that she is a suitable candidate for breast conservation surgery.

CASE 3

Small growing breast cancer presenting as a contour change on mammography

Routine digital screening mammography in an asymptomatic 62-year-old woman suggested an interval change compared with prior years' studies, with a 1-cm upper outer quadrant mass suggested (Figure 1). This persisted on spot compression, and ultrasound identified a corresponding suspicious 9-mm hypoechoic, solid mass, with irregular margins (Figure 2).

Ultrasound-guided core needle biopsy proved the lesion was an infiltrating ductal carcinoma (IDC). Ultrasound-guided needle localization was performed before lumpectomy. The pathology showed a 1.1-cm IDC, estrogen receptor and progesterone receptor positive, with negative margins and negative sentinel node sampling. Chemotherapy and radiation were administered subsequently.

TEACHING POINTS

Interval change can be the only sign of malignancy on screening mammograms and can be very subtle. This growing mass was largely concealed by adjacent parenchymal density, with only a subtle contour bulge suggesting its presence. Little increased density, architectural distortion, or other visual clue to the presence of this mass was seen. In this case, only systematic comparison, density for density, between current and prior mammograms enabled this IDC to be picked up at a small size and early stage (stage 1, T1N0).

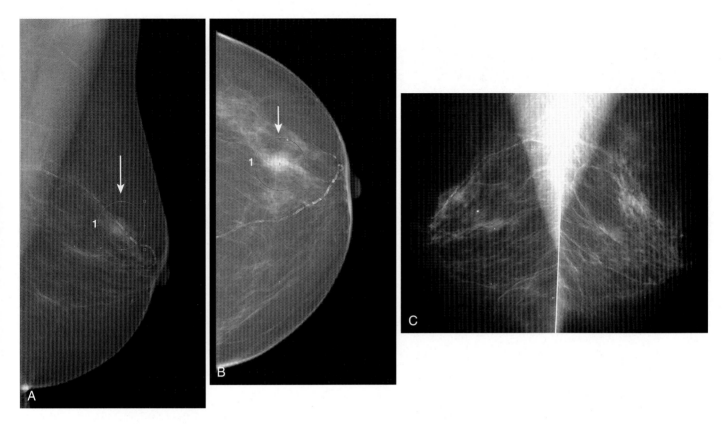

FIGURE 1. MLO (**A**) and CC (**B**) right digital mammograms show scattered fibroglandular density. A subtle contour change on the MLO view in the right upper breast tissue suggested the possibility of a developing mass (*arrows*). **C,** For comparison, a prior year's MLO mammograms.

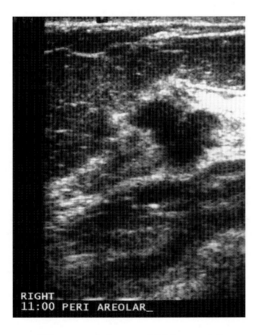

FIGURE 2. Ultrasound shows a highly suspicious corresponding mass that is taller than wide and very hypoechoic, with irregular and lobular margins. The mass is surrounded by echogenic fibrous tissue, as on mammography.

CASE 4

Slow-growing microlobulated colloid carcinoma

An asymptomatic 65-year-old female underwent screening mammography, which showed an enlarging circumscribed mass in the central right breast (Figures 1 and 2). Ultrasound demonstrated a corresponding hypoechoic solid mass (Figure 3). Subsequent ultrasound-guided core needle biopsy was performed and yielded a diagnosis of invasive colloid carcinoma.

TEACHING POINTS

This case illustrates the importance of prior mammograms in the evaluation of subtle change. A new

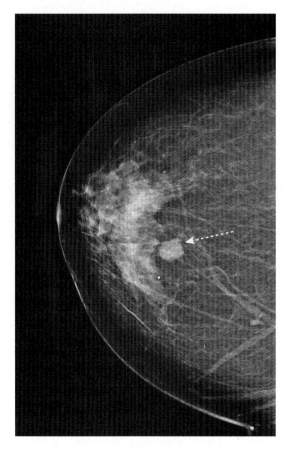

FIGURE 1.   Right CC mammographic view shows a mass in the central right breast (*arrow*).

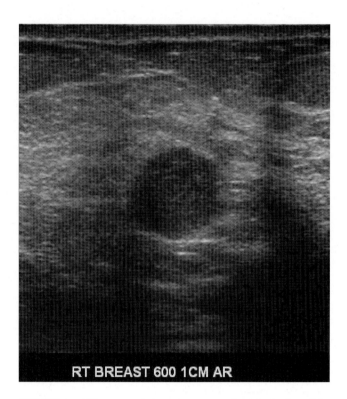

FIGURE 3.   Ultrasound demonstrates a hypoechoic solid mass with mildly irregular margins, corresponding to the mammographic mass.

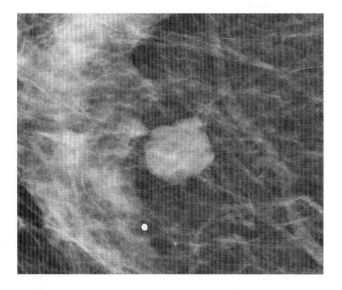

FIGURE 2.   Close-up view of the mass demonstrates partially circumscribed margins and microlobulations.

or enlarging mass should prompt further workup. In this case, because this is an enlarging mammographic mass, the workup can proceed directly to ultrasound. Evaluation of the margins of the mass on magnification mammographic views would not change clinical management. Any new or enlarging solid mass should prompt a biopsy, regardless of its appearance mammographically. The role of ultrasound in this instance is to determine whether the finding represents a cyst or solid mass. In this case, the mass was solid and demonstrated a relatively benign appearance. Some cancers, including colloid carcinoma, papillary carcinoma, and medullary carcinoma, may have relatively smooth margins.

Breast cancer presenting as a new posterior mass on mammography: Importance of inclusion of posterior breast tissue on mammography

A 70-year-old woman with a prior history of stage II ovarian carcinoma was noted on a routine screening mammogram to have a partially visualized, asymmetric density in the posterior right breast, seen only on the MLO view (Figure 1). She was recalled for additional evaluation. On spot compression, a mass was confirmed, with ill-defined margins (Figure 2). The mass was sufficiently far posterior that it was difficult to visualize entirely by mammography. Ultrasound showed highly suspicious characteristics, including being taller than wide, with irregular, angular margins (Figure 3). Ultrasound-guided core needle biopsy of the mass proved that the lesion was infiltrating mammary carcinoma. MRI confirmed that the lesion was solitary, without evidence of additional disease sites (Figure 4). Surgical therapy consisted of partial mastectomy and sentinel lymph node sampling. Final pathology showed a 1.8-cm infiltrating ductal carcinoma, with clear margins and one negative sentinel lymph node.

TEACHING POINT

This case illustrates graphically the answer to the perennial patient question about the mammogram: "Why do they pull so hard?" Inclusion of as much of the breast tissue as possible is critical to optimal breast cancer screening with mammography. Abnormalities in unimaged breast tissue cannot be identified on screening. Abnormalities such as this, in a far posterior position, which may be difficult to image entirely with mammography, may be readily visualized on other modalities, if seen even partially at screening. Critique of image quality, regarding positioning and complete inclusion of the breast tissue, is an ongoing process at both the technologist and physician review levels and should include comparison with the coverage achieved on prior studies in the same patient.

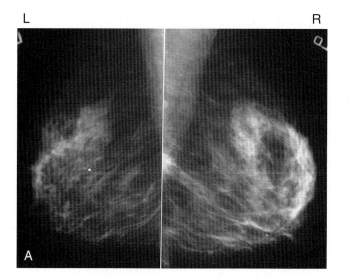
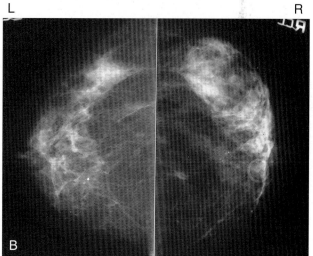

FIGURE 1. Screening mammographic views show breast parenchyma of heterogeneous increased density. On the right MLO view (**A**), overlying the inferior pectoral muscle, is a new, partially visualized density. No corresponding abnormality is seen on the craniocaudal view (**B**), probably because of the far posterior position of the lesion. Visualized margins appear indistinct and spiculated. The patient was recalled for additional views.

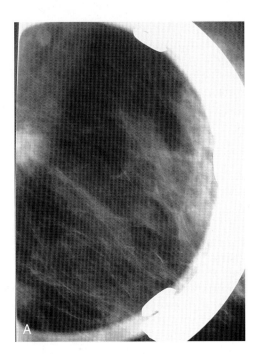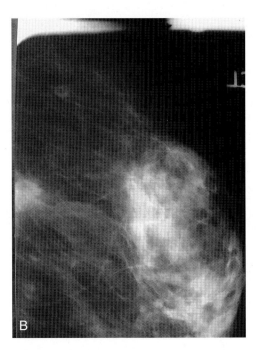

FIGURE 2. Spot compression [MLO (**A**) and exaggerated CC (**B**)] confirms the abnormality, but the far posterior position precludes complete visualization of the posterior margins. The visualized margins are irregular, with spiculation.

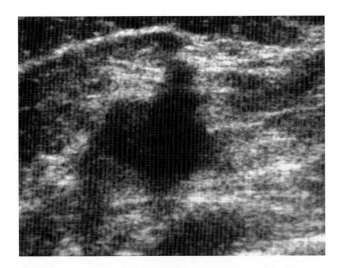

FIGURE 3. Ultrasound demonstrates the corresponding lesion well and displays multiple malignant features. The mass is intensely hypoechoic and taller than wide, and the margins are irregular and angular. The lesion is readily visualized and more accessible than with mammography; thus, ultrasound guidance was selected for histologic sampling.

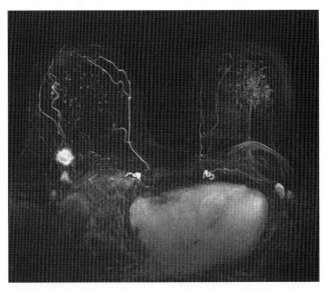

FIGURE 4. Maximum intensity projection (MIP) of a subtracted data set from the enhanced dynamic breast MRI shows the tumor to enhance intensely and early. It displays features of malignancy on MRI, including spiculated margins and rim enhancement. Both breasts show a fairly symmetric pattern of lower-level fibrocystic-type enhancement, consisting of innumerable scattered tiny foci of enhancement. Enhancement of normal-sized lymph nodes (including one projecting posterior to the mass) and internal mammary vessels is also demonstrated bilaterally here.

CASE 6

DCIS presenting as a microcalcification cluster

A new microcalcification cluster was identified on screening mammography in this 82-year-old woman. Magnification views showed pleomorphic forms (Figure 1), and stereotactic biopsy was recommended. Specimen radiography confirmed that

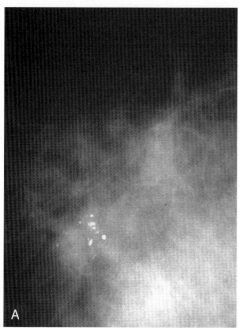

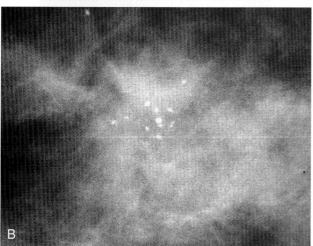

FIGURE 1. **A** and **B,** Magnification views of the calcifications in question show pleomorphism, with the clustered calcifications varying from one another in size, shape, and density.

the calcifications were sampled, and histology identified infiltrating ductal carcinoma and comedo ductal carcinoma in situ (DCIS). The patient opted for surgical therapy with mastectomy and was treated with tamoxifen for 5 years thereafter.

TEACHING POINTS

Quality control in performance of image-guided biopsies takes place at many levels. Two essential quality assurance components of stereotactic-guided biopsy programs are specimen radiography and pathology correlation. Specimen radiographs should routinely be obtained when performing stereotactic biopsy for microcalcifications and may occasionally be useful after biopsy of masses. It can be difficult, because of the presence of lidocaine and particularly if bleeding develops, to be certain with stereotactic images that microcalcifications have been obtained. This is particularly true when sampling small microcalcification clusters, especially with larger (e.g., 8-gauge Mammotome) vacuum-assisted devices.

Correlation of the pathology results with the imaging features of the biopsied lesion is also critical. For any sampled lesion, there is an acceptable range of possible pathologic results, and insistence on internal consistency between the histologic diagnosis and the imaging features of the abnormality is a basic safeguard against sampling error.

CASE 7

DCIS presenting as multiple microcalcification clusters along a ductal ray

New microcalcification clusters were noted in the medial left breast on routine mammographic screening of a 61-year-old asymptomatic woman. The most recent comparison mammogram was 3 years earlier. A suspicious, segmental distribution of the microcalcifications was noted, and magnification was performed to better visualize them.

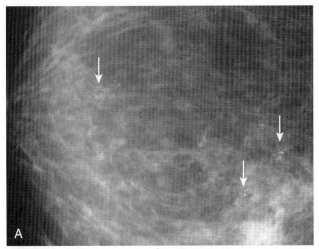

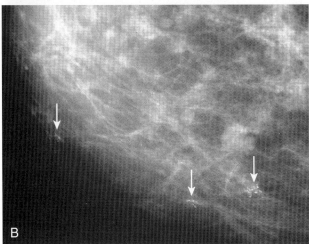

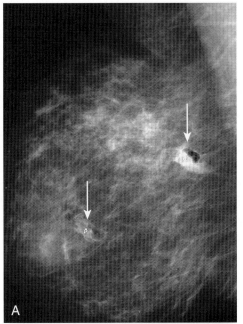

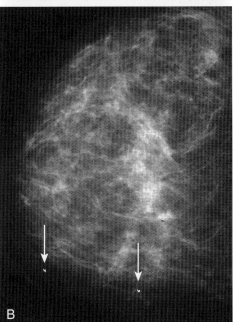

FIGURE 1.   Magnification views in 90-degree lateral (**A**) and CC (**B**) projections show three clusters of microcalcifications (*arrows*) in the medial breast, aligned in an axis toward the nipple. The morphology of the calcifications is irregular, variable, and pleomorphic. The findings were new compared with a mammogram performed 3 years earlier. The benign-appearing mass also noted in these views was proved by ultrasound to be a simple cyst.

FIGURE 2.   Post–stereotactic biopsy films [90-degree lateral (**A**) and CC (**B**)] show clips at the two sampled sites (*arrows*), corresponding to the most anterior and posterior of the three clusters. The measured distance between the sampled sites, both of which yielded DCIS, is at least 4 cm.

Magnification views of the medial breast confirmed three separate, suspicious clusters of pleomorphic microcalcifications, aligned along an axis toward the nipple (Figure 1). Stereotactic biopsy was performed on two of the three clusters, including the most anterior and posterior (Figure 2). Intermediate- to high-grade ductal carcinoma in situ (DCIS), with necrosis, was obtained from both sites. Pathology commented that the DCIS obtained from the posterior site was variably associated with microcalcifications. Based on the distance between the sampled sites (4 cm), it seemed likely that there was extensive intraductal disease, suggesting the

patient was not a suitable candidate for breast-conserving surgery. Breast MRI was performed to assess for additional, mammographically occult disease (Figure 3). No MRI findings particularly suggestive of unsuspected or occult invasive disease were seen.

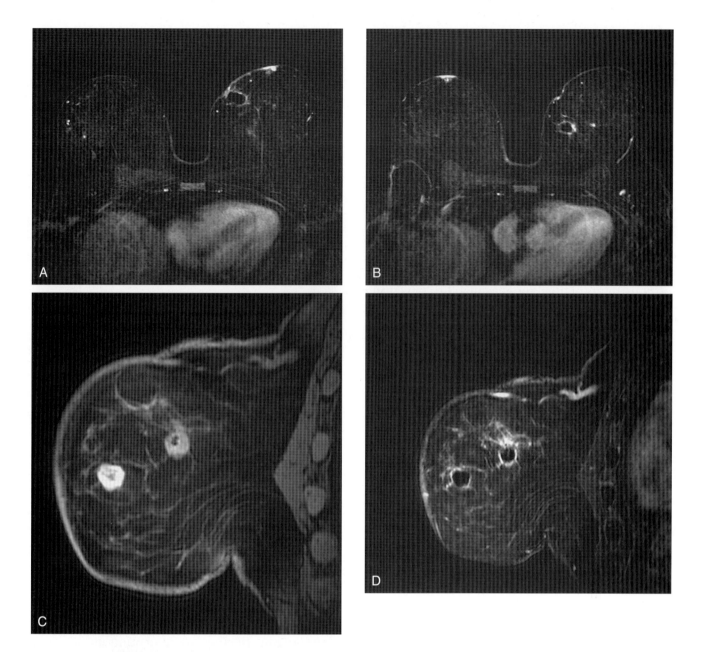

FIGURE 3. **A,** Enhanced subtracted bilateral breast MRI shows a thin rim of enhancement corresponding to the anterior biopsy site from which DCIS was obtained in the medial left breast. Nipple enhancement is also noted, which is a frequently seen normal finding. **B,** At another level, the second, more posterior biopsy site is seen. The rim enhancement at the lateral aspect of the biopsy cavity is less smooth, with slightly nodular foci of enhancement. **C,** Fat-saturated, unenhanced T1-weighted gradient echo sagittal view shows hyperintense blood products within the two small postbiopsy cavities. **D,** A delayed (about 5 minutes after injection) enhanced subtracted sagittal image shows rim enhancement of the two postbiopsy cavities. Parenchymal enhancement is now seen above the posterior biopsy cavity.

The patient underwent mastectomy and sentinel lymph node sampling. The mastectomy specimen pathology showed residual foci of intermediate-grade cribriform DCIS with central necrosis, including four foci (ranging in size from < 1 mm to 4 mm) adjacent to the anterior biopsy site and one 2-mm residual focus adjacent to the posterior biopsy site. Four sentinel lymph nodes were negative for malignancy.

TEACHING POINTS

This case provides many interesting lines of inquiry for discussion. In an ideal world (in which there are no constraints of time, room availability, or waiting patients), all three of these suspicious microcalcification clusters might have been sampled. In the real world, in which many patients are not able to tolerate the prone position required for stereotactic sampling long enough to perform three biopsies, the next best option is to choose sites for biopsy with the greatest potential yield in terms of decision making. In this case, the clusters were equally suspicious, but the most anterior and posterior clusters were larger and likelier to yield a higher number of calcifications in the sampling. In addition, the smaller, middle cluster was fairly close to the most posterior cluster. Sampling the farthest apart clusters is the most efficient approach when histologic confirmation of suspected multifocal disease is desired. The similar-appearing middle cluster would be presumed to be the same histology.

Breast MRI can be very helpful in the assessment of the breast for additional or occult invasive disease. In this particular case, breast MRI did not show any separate or unsuspected sites of disease, indicating that the calcifications seen on mammography were the best imaging "map" of the extent of disease. Unfortunately, even that cannot be depended on to demonstrate the full disease extent, because the histologic sample from the posterior cluster noted that not all of the identified DCIS was associated with microcalcifications. The negative breast MRI result is not surprising in this case because the volume of residual disease found at mastectomy was small (although multiple foci of DCIS were found, the largest focus was 4 mm). In addition, DCIS as a histology can be variable in enhancement, the process on which MRI visualization depends.

There are a variety of factors influencing surgical decision making between breast-conserving lumpectomy and mastectomy. The goals of breast conservation can be summarized as surgical removal of all identifiable disease with good cosmesis. The tumor size and location in relation to the breast size must be taken into account. In this case, even if the mammographic calcifications were an accurate reflection of the distribution of the DCIS, complete surgical extirpation would have required removal of much of a quadrant, making a pleasing cosmetic result difficult to achieve.

CASE 8

Breast cancer presenting as architectural distortion in extremely dense breasts

A 46-year-old woman with very dense breasts was called back for bilateral magnification views of microcalcifications noted on screening mammography. These proved to be widely scattered, with morphology consistent with milk of calcium. However, right upper outer quadrant (UOQ) increased breast density was noted with architectural distortion (Figure 1), and ultrasound was performed for further evaluation. Sonography showed a 1.2-cm hypoechoic, shadowing, irregularly marginated mass in the UOQ, corresponding to the mammogram (Figure 2). Ultrasound-guided core needle biopsy confirmed infiltrating ductal carcinoma (IDC). Because of the extreme density of the patient's breast parenchyma, breast MRI was performed as an aid to presurgical staging. The known IDC was visualized as a spiculated, enhancing 1.5-cm mass in a background of diffuse fibrocystic enhancement, with innumerable scattered small foci of less intense enhancement (Figures 3, 4, 5).

After ultrasound-guided needle localization (Figure 6, specimen radiograph), a partial mastectomy was performed. The pathology showed a 1.5-cm IDC with mucinous and clear cell features, without angiolymphatic invasion, estrogen receptor and progesterone receptor positive, with margins clear for invasion and notable only for a focal close (1 mm) inferior medial margin for DCIS. Five sentinel lymph nodes were negative.

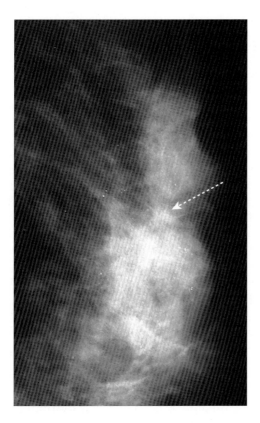

FIGURE 1. Architectural distortion (*arrow*) was suspected on the right, best seen in an exaggerated CC spot view.

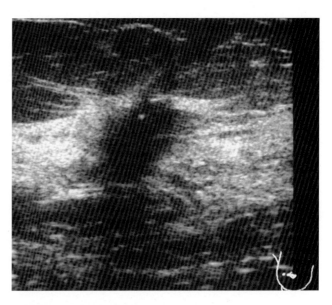

FIGURE 2. Ultrasound of the area in question shows a corresponding abnormality, with an intensely hypoechoic, taller-than-wide, irregularly marginated mass concealed within a band of hyperechoic, dense fibrous tissue. Margins show angularity and spiculations, features of malignancy. Biopsy with ultrasound guidance confirmed IDC.

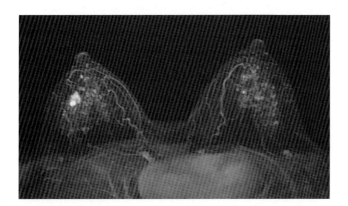

FIGURE 3. Maximum intensity projection (MIP) of an early, enhanced, fat-saturated volumetric dynamic acquisition shows a dominant enhancing mass with irregular margins in the right lateral breast, which is readily visualized despite the extensive background of diffuse fibrocystic foci of enhancement. MIP views provide an overview of a volumetric data set and can be useful as a visual "shorthand" form of communication when presenting a case in conference or discussing it with a clinician, but should never be relied on for primary interpretation.

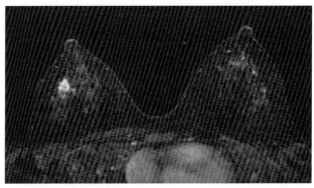

FIGURE 4. A single slice from early in the dynamic enhanced series better shows the malignant MRI features of the IDC. Margin spiculation and rim enhancement are seen.

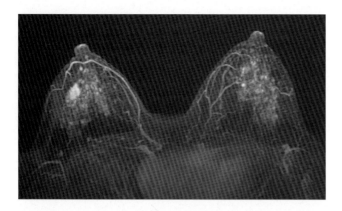

FIGURE 5. Importance of imaging early during dynamic enhanced breast MRI is well demonstrated in this patient. The lesion becomes less conspicuous with progressive enhancement of the parenchyma by 4 minutes after the contrast injection.

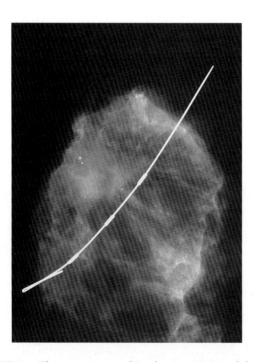

FIGURE 6. The mammographic characteristics of the IDC are best demonstrated on the specimen radiograph, which shows the spiculated mass adjacent to the localizing wire, placed under ultrasound guidance. Microcalcifications are seen throughout the specimen.

The final stage was stage I, T1N0M0 disease. The patient was treated with four cycles of doxorubicin (Adriamycin) and cyclophosphamide (Cytoxan) chemotherapy and radiation therapy, with a boost to the lumpectomy bed. Tamoxifen was started after completion of chemotherapy.

TEACHING POINTS

This case raises a variety of points for additional discussion. The patient was called back for calcifications, which were benign in morphology. Fortunately, the callback provided an opportunity for the mammographically subtle finding of architectural distortion to be suspected. In dense breasts like these, the threshold for imaging with other modalities, especially with ultrasound, of questionable areas should be low. The ultrasound is unequivocally suspicious and shows well how the position of the suspicious spiculated mass, concealed within dense fibrous tissue, enables the abnormality to be nearly occult on mammography.

The breast MRI of this patient shows a dramatic example of hormonal effects, manifested as innumerable enhancing foci, which are regularly encountered in performing breast MRI, particularly in younger and premenopausal women. Even with such expected findings, breast MRI is useful in evaluating women with dense breast tissue. The timing of performance of enhanced, subtracted dynamic imaging is particularly important in these patients. The early, intense enhancement of tumors capitalizes on angiogenesis and is best visualized in the first 1 to 2 minutes after intravenous contrast administration, when the greatest differential in enhancement between tumors with angiogenesis and normally enhancing breast tissue is encountered. With greater delays, the progressive enhancement of normal tissue will decrease the conspicuity of neoplastic lesions, as is well demonstrated here.

Another issue raised by this case is the use of specimen radiography after ultrasound-guided needle localization. Although specimens can be sonographically imaged after removal, this is less frequently used in practice. Radiography of specimens obtained after sonographic localization is used sporadically, often on a case-by-case basis, particularly if the localized abnormality, residual lesion, or clip is difficult to visualize and additional assurance is desired that the abnormality has been removed. In this case, the specimen radiograph provides the first unobstructed mammographic look at the malignant features of the lesion. Specimens should be scrutinized for the presence of localizing wires and clips as well as for the presence and position within the specimen of the abnormality. In addition to assessing the completeness of the excision, the relation of the abnormality to the margins of the specimen is assessed to determine whether to obtain additional tissue.

ILC presenting as a growing amorphous density

An asymptomatic 61-year-old woman underwent screening mammography over a 14-year period. Over the course of the patient's screening examinations, an amorphous density and focal asymmetry developed within the upper outer right breast (Figures 1, 2, 3, and 4). Although this was recalled for spot compression views, the finding was interpreted as asymmetric glandular tissue because it partially dispersed on compression and contained fat density areas (Figure 5). The area subsequently became palpable, prompting an ultrasound examination. The ultrasound demonstrated an irregular solid mass with posterior acoustic shadowing (Figure 6). Needle biopsy of the mass revealed an invasive lobular carcinoma (ILC).

TEACHING POINTS

This case illustrates several teaching points. It is important to compare screening mammograms with several prior years' mammograms. As in this case, a slowly growing cancer may not appear to change much from year to year. Comparing the current mammogram with films from several years before may reveal a developing mass.

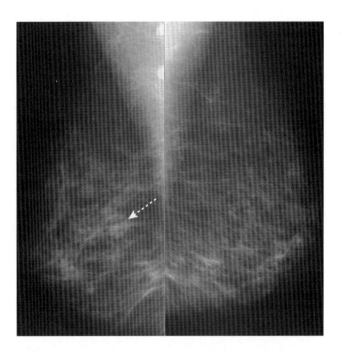

FIGURE 2. Bilateral MLO views performed in 1996. In retrospect, there is the subtle beginning of a developing asymmetry in the upper outer right breast (*arrow*).

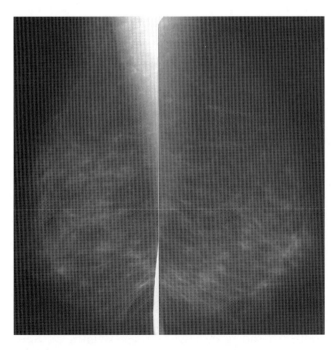

FIGURE 1. Bilateral MLO mammographic views from 1992. The breasts are mixed fat and fibroglandular density. There are no apparent abnormalities.

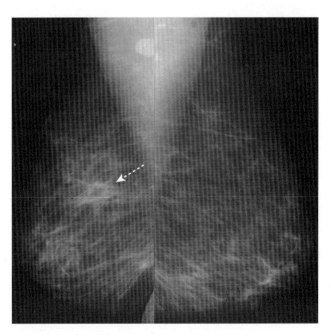

FIGURE 3. Bilateral MLO views from 2001. The asymmetry (*arrow*) in the right breast has increased in size and density since the prior examination.

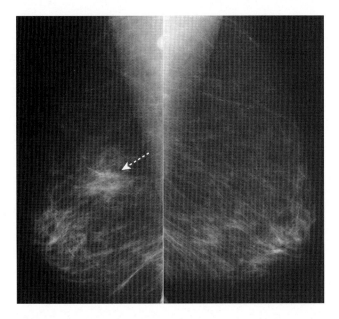

FIGURE 4. Bilateral MLO views performed in 2004. The asymmetry in the right breast continued to enlarge (*arrow*). At this point, the finding on screening mammography prompted a callback for additional evaluation.

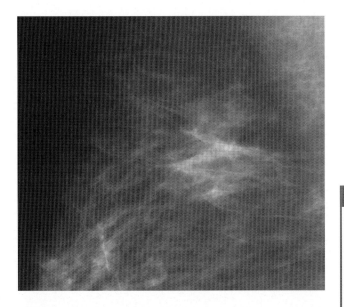

FIGURE 5. An MLO spot compression view demonstrates the asymmetry to partially disperse and to contain areas of fat. This was thought to represent asymmetrical normal glandular tissue, and the patient was returned to annual screening.

Although the mammographic finding could have been asymmetric glandular tissue, an unexplained enlarging density should prompt a biopsy. In this case, we see that invasive lobular carcinoma can mimic normal tissue, and ultrasound can

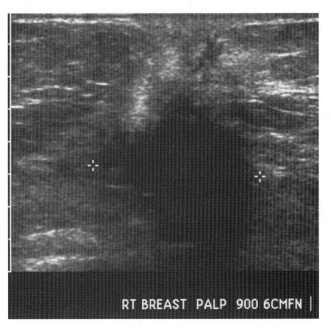

RT BREAST PALP 900 6CMFN |

FIGURE 6. In 2006, the patient presented complaining of a palpable mass in the area of mammographic asymmetry in the upper outer right breast. Ultrasound reveals a large irregular hypoechoic mass with posterior shadowing, corresponding to the palpable finding. Subsequent needle biopsy revealed an invasive lobular carcinoma.

help in differentiation. Invasive lobular carcinoma represents about 10% of invasive breast cancers.

CASE 10

Small cancer in implant patient, well seen only on implant-displaced views

An asymptomatic 51-year-old woman with bilateral silicone implants underwent annual screening mammography. The right standard views showed no definite abnormality (Figure 1). The implant-displaced MLO view demonstrated a focal asymmetry in the upper right breast (Figure 2). Spot compression MLO view confirmed a spiculated mass in the upper right breast (Figure 3). Ultrasound showed a corresponding irregular 11-mm

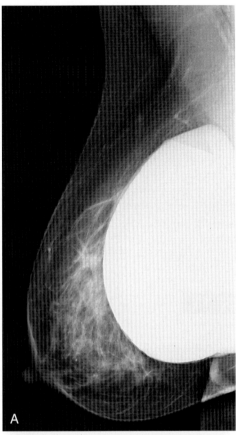

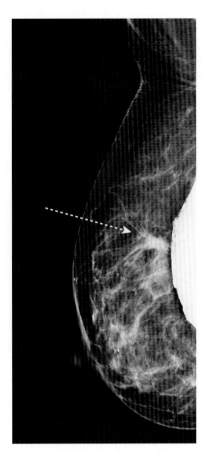

FIGURE 2. With implant displacement, a focus of increased density and architectural distortion is seen adjacent to the implant (*arrow*).

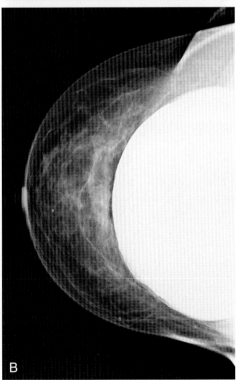

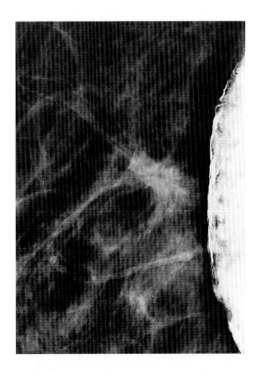

FIGURE 1. Right breast mammographic views [MLO (**A**) and CC (**B**)] show subglandular implants and moderate parenchymal density. No definite abnormality is seen.

FIGURE 3. MLO spot compression confirms a small, suspicious, spiculated mass adjacent to the implant.

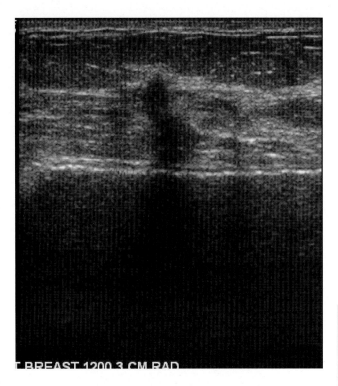

FIGURE 4. Ultrasound of the right upper breast confirms a corresponding suspicious mass that is hypoechoic, taller than wide, with irregular, angular margins.

solid mass in the 12-o'clock position (Figure 4). Subsequent biopsy confirmed an invasive ductal carcinoma.

TEACHING POINTS

This case demonstrates the need for supplemental views in patients with implants undergoing screening mammography. These include implant push-back or displacement views to better compress the breast tissue anterior to the implants. Other views may include laterally exaggerated craniocaudal views and 90-degree ML views.

CASE 11

Importance of a complete workup of new mammographic masses

A screening mammogram on an asymptomatic 49-year-old woman showed bilateral, similar-appearing upper outer quadrant breast masses (Figure 1), which were new from a prior mammo-

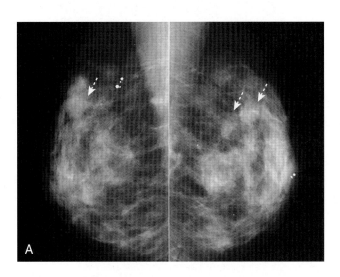

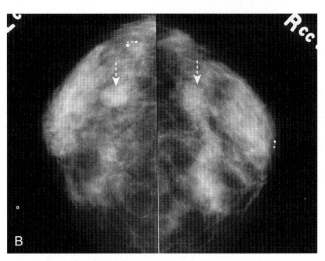

FIGURE 1. Screening mammography [MLO (**A**) and CC (**B**)] shows heterogeneous breast parenchymal density and bilateral, similar-appearing breast masses (*arrows*). Where the margins can be visualized, they appear circumscribed, suggesting cysts. Other margins are obscured by dense adjacent parenchyma. Because the masses were new compared with a mammogram taken 2 years earlier, and the patient had never been demonstrated to have cysts, sonography was recommended to characterize the masses.

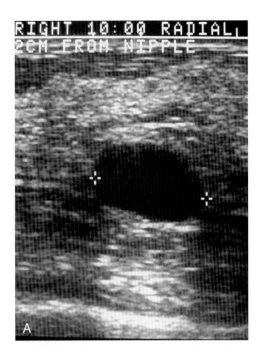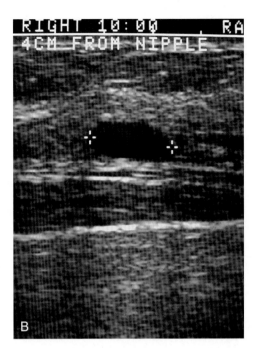

FIGURE 2. Ultrasound of the right breast (**A** and **B**) confirms two simple cysts, accounting for the right mammographic findings. These display all the hallmarks of simple cysts (sharp back wall, anechoic, and enhanced through-transmission).

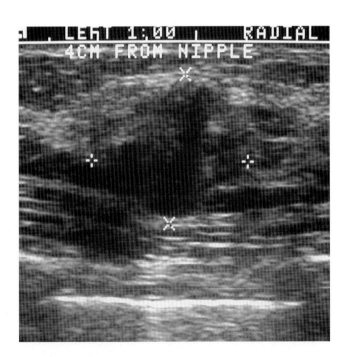

FIGURE 3. Ultrasound of the left breast shows a solid, vascular, taller-than-wide mass, without ultrasound features to suggest benignity. Although the mass shows lobular borders, it is not surrounded by the thin echogenic pseudocapsule that can often be demonstrated in benign solid masses, such as fibroadenomas. Biopsy was recommended and confirmed infiltrating ductal carcinoma.

gram taken 2 years earlier. Ultrasound was performed to further evaluate these masses (Figures 2 and 3). On the right, where mammography suggested two masses, ultrasound confirmed two simple cysts. On the left, where mammography showed a single new mass (similar in appearance to the right-sided findings), sonography identified a vascular, solid mass with indeterminate features. Biopsy was recommended. Excision of the lesion demonstrated a 1.4-cm infiltrating ductal carcinoma. In addition to lumpectomy and a negative sentinel lymph node sampling, the patient was treated with radiation therapy.

TEACHING POINTS

The case illustrates the importance of complete workups. Mammographers often refer to the "rule of multiplicity," which suggests that if there are multiple breast masses, they are all likely benign. It is difficult to correlate sonographic to mammographic masses, one for one, when the lesions are numerous. However, at least when beginning screening, it is useful to clearly establish by ultrasound that a patient with multiple masses has multiple cysts, multiple solid masses, or some combination. With this information, subsequent mammographic changes, such as waxing and waning of multiple cysts, can be more accurately assessed. However, development of a new mass or masses in a patient without such prior findings warrants a sonographic evaluation. In this case, virtually identical new bilateral mammographic findings resulted in a diagnosis of benign cysts on one side and cancer on the other.

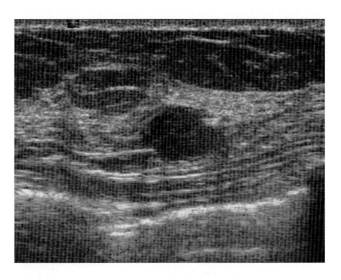

FIGURE 2. Ultrasound of the left breast identifies the correlate at 3 o'clock as an indeterminate, hypoechoic, solid mass with no well-defined capsule. Biopsy with ultrasound guidance confirmed IDC.

CASE 12

MRI high-risk screening for occult breast cancer

A 35-year-old woman who tested positive for the *BRCA1* gene mutation was followed with yearly mammograms and breast MRI after treatment 4 years earlier for right breast cancer. The tumor was a stage I, T1N0M0, node-negative 1.9-cm medullary carcinoma, treated with lumpectomy, chemotherapy, and radiation. The patient underwent hysterectomy and bilateral salpingo-oophorectomy after treatment for breast cancer.

An intensely enhancing small (5-mm) left breast nodule was noted to be new on high-risk screening MRI (Figure 1). After a 3-month delay during which a prior comparison MRI was obtained from another facility (confirming the lesion to be new), a sono-

graphic correlate was identified and biopsied, confirming infiltrating ductal carcinoma (IDC) (Figure 2). By ultrasound, the mass measured 8 × 6 mm. The patient elected to undergo bilateral mastectomies for treatment and received postoperative chemotherapy with docetaxel (Taxotere) and cyclophosphamide (Cytoxan), as well as chest wall and supraclavicular radiation therapy. The left mastectomy specimen showed a 1.6-cm, T1N1 tumor with angiolymphatic invasion and negative margins, with one of 19 lymph nodes positive. No additional tumor was found on the right.

TEACHING POINTS

This case provides a convenient launching point for a discussion of imaging surveillance of patients at high risk for breast cancer. Who is considered high risk? Patients with a genetic predisposition to breast cancer include those with genetic mutations (*BRCA1* and *BRCA2*) and those with a family history of breast cancer in one or more first- or second-degree relatives (mother, sister, daughter, maternal aunt), especially if the relative's breast cancer was premenopausal. Other patients who are considered at high risk include those with a prior personal history of breast cancer and those with prior histologic diagnoses of lobular carcinoma in situ (LCIS), atypical lobular hyperplasia (ALH), and atypical ductal hyperplasia (ADH).

The high lifetime risk for developing breast cancer faced by women with the *BRCA1* and *BRCA2*

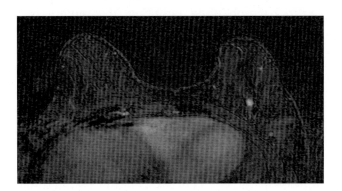

FIGURE 1. Axial, enhanced, subtracted slice from bilateral high-risk screening breast MRI shows a solitary enhancing sub-centimeter nodule with irregular margins in the left posterior breast, new from a prior year's study. Based on MRI, this was localized at 5 o'clock.

gene mutations is well recognized. Lifetime breast cancer risks of up to 85% have been predicted for *BRCA* mutation patients. As illustrated by this case, there is a substantial risk (30%) in these patients of developing a contralateral breast cancer within 5 years after diagnosis of breast cancer.

The breast cancers developing in *BRCA* mutation patients tend to occur early, in younger patients with dense breasts who are more difficult to screen with mammography. The tumors also tend to be more rapidly growing and aggressive. This is suggested in this case by noting the discrepancy between the apparent size of the new small mass on MRI (5 mm), its ultrasound correlate 3 months later (8 mm), and the 1.6-cm IDC found in the mastectomy specimen, suggesting interval growth in the 5 months that elapsed between the initial identification of the lesion and its excision.

BRCA mutation patients should undergo multipronged surveillance, with twice-yearly clinical breast examinations and yearly imaging screening, which traditionally consisted of mammography. Because of the difficulty of screening younger women with dense breast tissue with mammography, a number of investigators have reported in recent years on the use of breast MRI to supplement the imaging surveillance of these patients. These studies support the use of breast MRI as a more sensitive modality than mammography for earlier diagnosis of smaller, earlier-stage, occult breast cancers. The largest series reported to date was a prospective trial from the Netherlands by Kriege and colleagues, in which 1909 women with a cumulative lifetime breast cancer risk of 15% or greater were screened every 6 months with clinical breast examination and yearly with mammography and breast MRI. The study population included 358 patients with genetic mutations. Fifty-one cancerous lesions were identified over a median follow-up period of 2.9 years, including 44 invasive cancers, 6 cases of DCIS, 1 lymphoma, and 1 LCIS. Sensitivity for identification of invasive breast cancer with clinical breast examination (CBE) was 18%, compared with 33% for mammography and 80% for breast MRI, with specificities of 98%, 95%, and 90%, respectively. The invasive cancers identified by MRI were smaller, with a lower incidence of positive axillary nodes, than those identified by mammography.

A Canadian study of 236 *BRCA* mutation patients by Warner and associates reported similar results and included ultrasound in the comparison between modalities and CBE. In this study, CBE was performed every 6 months. Once a year, patients underwent mammography, breast ultrasound, breast MRI, and CBE on the same day. Each modality was interpreted independently, and all breast imaging reporting and data system (BI-RADS) 4 (suspicious) and 5 (highly suspicious) abnormalities detected by any modality underwent biopsy. The sensitivity and specificity of each modality were calculated, as well as the sensitivity of all four modalities together compared with mammography and CBE. Twenty-two cancers were identified, including 16 invasive cancers and 6 cases of DCIS. The sensitivity of breast MRI was 77%, compared with 36% for mammography, 33% for ultrasound, and 9% for CBE. The four screening modalities together had a sensitivity of 95%, compared with 45% for mammography and CBE together. Overall sensitivity of the combined modalities dropped to 86% with ultrasound excluded. A third of the detected cancers (7 of 22, or 32%) were demonstrated on MRI alone. Mammography and ultrasound each found two cancers not identified on other modalities.

These data suggest several approaches to the imaging surveillance of *BRCA* mutation and other high-risk patients. On the one hand, in an ideal world (with no constraints on costs), all three imaging modalities would be employed to maximize cancer detection. Because their strengths in diagnosing breast cancers derive from different approaches to imaging, it is to be expected that there will be cancers picked up on one modality that go undetected on others. An additional price to be paid with this approach would be an increase in false-positive results and additional biopsies. A more cost-effective approach might be to screen yearly with mammography and breast MRI, with ultrasound used to further evaluate abnormalities and guide biopsies when abnormalities are identified. A case can also be made for yearly performance of mammography and breast MRI, alternating every 6 months.

This case also reminds us not to be rigid about lesion localization in the breast when looking for ultrasound correlates for breast MRI abnormalities. By MRI, the new focus of enhancement was judged to be at 5 o'clock, whereas its correlate on ultrasound was found at 3 o'clock. The mobility of breast tissue and positioning differences (prone versus supine or supine oblique positioning between breast MRI and ultrasound) introduces considerable variability in apparent position of corresponding lesions. It probably is a good idea to examine with ultrasound at least a quadrant's worth of breast tissue on either side of the clock position of any concerning lesion identified on MRI.

SUGGESTED READINGS

Kriege M, Brekelmans CT, Boetes C, et al. Efficacy of MRI and mammography for breast-cancer screening in women with a familial or genetic predisposition. *N Engl J Med* 2004; 351:427–437.

Morris EA, Liberman L, Ballon DJ, et al. MRI of occult breast carcinoma in a high-risk population. *AJR Am J Roentgenol* 2003; 181:619–626.

Stoutjesdijk MJ, Boetes C, Jager GJ, et al. Magnetic resonance imaging and mammography in women with a hereditary risk of breast cancer. *J Natl Cancer Inst* 2001; 93:1095–1102.

Warner E, Plewes DB, Hill KA, et al. Surveillance of *BRCA1* and *BRCA2* mutation carriers with magnetic resonance imaging, ultrasound, mammography, and clinical breast examination. *JAMA* 2004; 292:1317–1325.

Warner E, Plewes DB, Shumak RS, et al. Comparison of breast magnetic resonance imaging, mammography, and ultrasound for surveillance of women at high risk for hereditary breast cancer. *J Clin Oncol* 2001; 19(15):3524–3531.

CASE 13

MRI high-risk screening for occult breast cancer

An asymptomatic 57-year-old high-risk woman underwent screening mammography and screening MRI. The patient was considered high risk because of breast cancer history in multiple family members. The patient had heterogeneously dense breasts, and the mammogram was unrevealing (Figure 1). Subsequent MRI showed a suspicious enhancing mass in the upper outer left breast (Figures 2 and 3). Directed ultrasound confirmed the presence of an irregular, 12-mm, hypoechoic solid mass (Figure 4). Ultrasound-guided core needle biopsy yielded a diagnosis of intermediate-grade invasive ductal carcinoma (IDC).

TEACHING POINTS

There is no established role for breast MRI in screening of the general population. However, breast MRI has gained credence in recent years for screening of higher-risk patients. Recently published American Cancer Society guidelines recommend annual screening MRI as an adjuvant to mammography in high-risk patients. High-risk

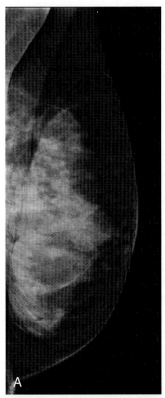

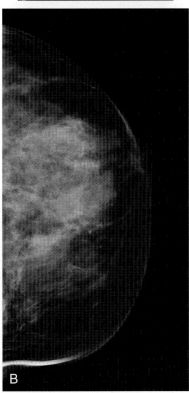

FIGURE 1. Left mammographic views [MLO (**A**) and CC (**B**)] show dense breast parenchyma, but no findings particularly suggestive of malignancy.

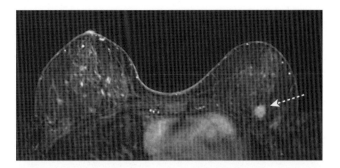

FIGURE 2. High-risk screening breast MRI shows an enhancing mass in the upper outer left breast (*arrow*).

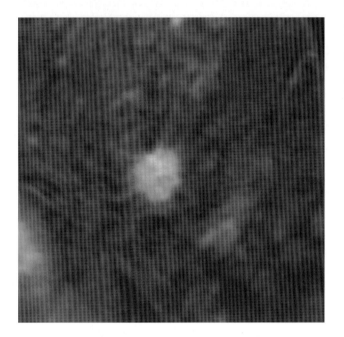

FIGURE 3. Close-up view of the MRI mass shows its irregular margins and heterogeneous enhancement.

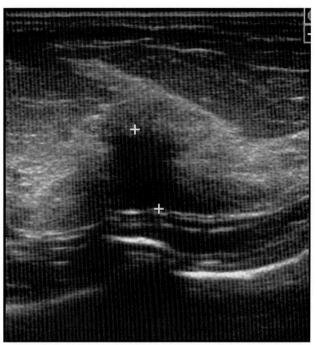

FIGURE 4. Targeted ultrasound demonstrates a suspicious, solid, very hypoechoic, irregularly marginated mass, corresponding to the MRI finding. Because it could be seen on ultrasound, ultrasound-guided core needle biopsy was performed to obtain a tissue diagnosis of IDC.

cases, MRI can identify DCIS that is mammographically occult.

SUGGESTED READING

Saslow D, Boetes C, Burke W, et al. American Cancer Society guidelines for breast screening with MRI as an adjunct to mammography. *CA Cancer J Clin* 2007; 57:75–89.

women were defined as women with an approximately 20% to 25% or greater lifetime risk for breast cancer. These patients include those with *BRCA* genetic mutations, strong family history (especially premenopausal breast cancer or breast cancer in two or more primary relatives), or prior treatment for Hodgkin's disease. Increased breast density has recently been recognized as an independent risk factor for development of breast cancer and limits the efficacy of mammographic screening, as in this case. It should be emphasized that MRI is recommended as an adjuvant rather than a replacement for mammography. Given the variable sensitivity of MRI for DCIS, mammography may find areas of DCIS not detected by MRI. Conversely, because DCIS may not be calcified in up to two thirds of

CASE 14

Breast cancer presenting as a growing small mass on screening MRI

A 57-year-old woman who was due for routine screening mammography requested breast MRI as

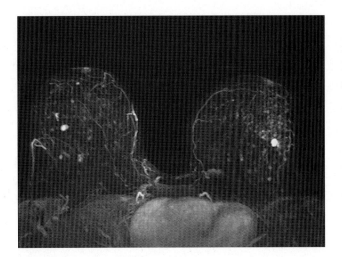

FIGURE 1. Axial maximal intensity projection (MIP) from the first minute of an enhanced, subtracted dynamic MRI series shows a background of innumerable, scattered, tiny foci of fibrocystic enhancement. Bilateral, solitary, sub-centimeter, benign-looking masses are noted in the lateral aspects of both breasts.

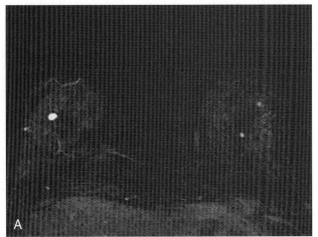

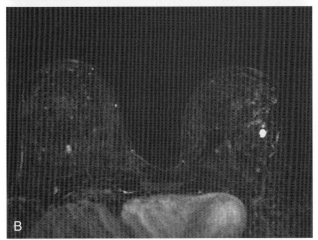

FIGURE 2. Source images from early in the dynamic series show similar-appearing, oval, benign-appearing bilateral masses, one each in the lower outer quadrants of both breasts [right (**A**) and left (**B**)]. With windowing, faint nonenhancing septa were suggested within these masses, which were bright on STIR images. These were thought to be benign, probably fibroadenomas. No correlates were found on mammography or ultrasound, and 6-month follow-up MRI was recommended.

an alternative because of concerns about radiation. She had previously had a benign right stereotactic breast biopsy for new microcalcifications, 1.5 years before.

The breast MRI showed small, scattered bilateral enhancing nodules, thought to be benign (Figure 1). The largest was 8 × 6 mm in the right lower outer quadrant (LOQ), with a similar lesion in the left LOQ (Figure 2). A workup with bilateral mammography and ultrasound showed no suspicious findings or definite corresponding lesions. A repeat breast MRI in 6 months was recommended.

The follow-up breast MRI showed interval growth of both of the lower outer quadrant small masses (Figures 3, 4, and 5). They were both sub-centimeter in size, and similar in appearance, being bright on short tau inversion recovery (STIR) imaging, with faint nonenhancing internal septa, suggesting fibroadenomas. A sonographic correlate was found on ultrasound for the larger (9 ×

9 mm) nodule in the right LOQ (Figure 6). Ultrasound-guided core needle biopsy revealed invasive ductal carcinoma (IDC). Sonographic evaluation of the left breast showed a possible correlate at 3 o'clock, a hypoechoic, round, 7-mm complex cyst

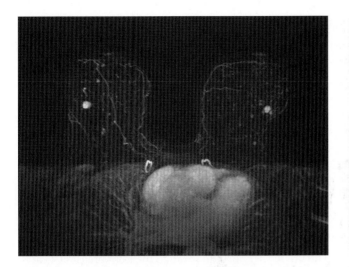

FIGURE 3. Axial MIP from enhanced, subtracted, dynamic breast MRI, 6 months later, is similar to the prior study, with a single, rounded, benign-appearing mass in each breast, seen against a background of fibrocystic enhancement.

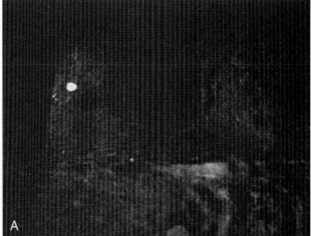

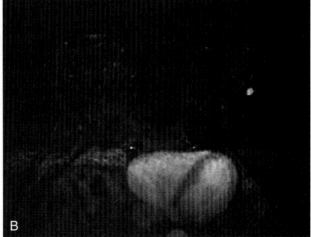

FIGURE 4. Source images from the enhanced subtracted dynamic series, from the 6-month follow-up study, showed nonenhancing septa on windowing within the oval breast masses [right (**A**) and left (**B**)]. Both of these lesions showed interval growth. The larger one, on the right, measured 9 × 9 mm, compared with 8 × 6 mm previously.

versus solid mass (Figure 7). However, it aspirated, proving it was a complex cyst and not a correlate for the enhancing (and thereby solid) nodule on MRI. No solid sonographic correlate was found for the left LOQ lesion, which by MRI was nearly identical in appearance to the contralateral proven cancer.

MRI-guided biopsy (Figure 8) of the left LOQ enhancing mass initially returned a diagnosis of cribriform atypical ductal hyperplasia and atypical lobular hyperplasia. A clip was placed to mark the site. The pathologic diagnosis was revised subsequently (after review by Dr. David Page of Vanderbilt) to atypical lobular hyperplasia.

Surgical therapy was accomplished by bilateral ultrasound-guided needle localizations of the residual mass on the right and the clip and postbiopsy hematoma site on the left (Figure 9). A sentinel lymph node procedure was performed on the right.

Pathology of the right lumpectomy specimen showed a 7-mm infiltrating ductal carcinoma, with clear margins. The single sentinel lymph node was negative for malignancy. The left excisional biopsy specimen again showed atypical lobular hyperplasia.

An Oncotype DX assay indicated a recurrence score of 19, in the low-intermediate risk group, with the rate of recurrence using the assay estimated at 12% at 10 years. The patient declined chemotherapy and was begun on anastrozole (Arimidex) for her estrogen receptor–positive disease and further treated with radiation therapy.

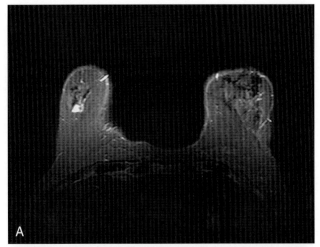

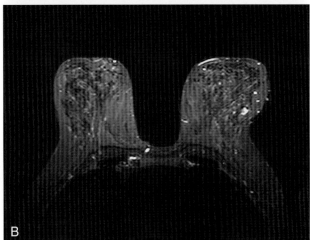

FIGURE 5. Corresponding STIR axial MRI [right (**A**) and left (**B**)] through the same levels show the small bilateral masses to be hyperintense in signal.

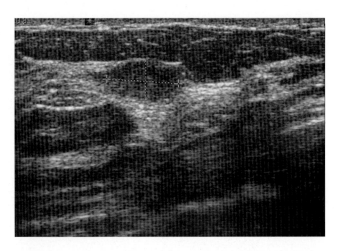

FIGURE 6. Ultrasound through the right breast LOQ at 8 o'clock shows a subtle, oval, solid, fairly benign-appearing mass (demarcated by cursors), isoechoic to subcutaneous fat, which seemed to correspond to the MRI finding. Biopsy was performed with ultrasound guidance, identifying IDC.

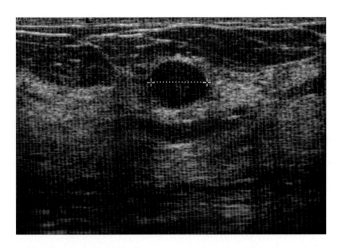

FIGURE 7. Ultrasound of the left breast at 3 o'clock shows a 7-mm, round, hypoechoic, benign-looking complex cyst versus solid mass, which readily aspirated, proving it was a complex cyst and not a correlate for the enhancing, solid nodule on MRI.

TEACHING POINTS

There are a variety of teaching and discussion points raised by this case. This patient requested MRI as an alternative to mammography because of concerns about radiation. She had had a prior benign biopsy of calcifications but had no prior pathologic diagnosis of atypical ductal hyperplasia (ADH) or other borderline histology to suggest she was a higher-risk patient. There are no data supporting the use of breast MRI for breast cancer screening in the general (non-high-risk) popula-

tion. Thus, in a perfect world (in which patients heed the advice of medical professionals), this patient would not have undergone breast MRI as an alternative to mammography, which remains the only imaging modality that excels at detecting microcalcifications as a harbinger of potential

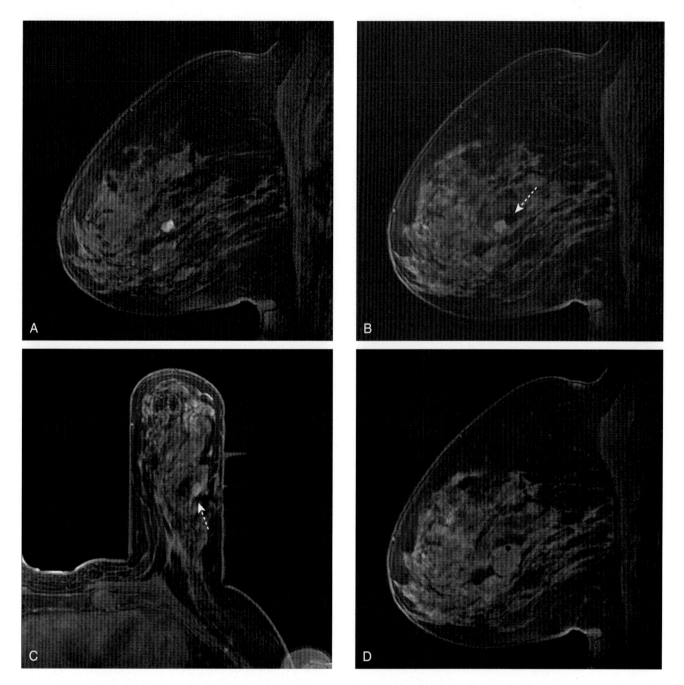

FIGURE 8. **A,** A fat-saturated, enhanced, gradient echo image from the sagittal localizer series identifies the lobular, sub-centimeter mass in question for biopsy. **B,** Repeat sagittal fat-saturated series after placement of the localizing obturator shows signal void adjacent to the enhancing nodule, at the posterosuperior margin (*arrow*). **C,** Axial fat-saturated image shows the breast in compression, with lateral skin indentations from the localizing grid. The mass is enhanced, and the signal void from the localizing obturator is immediately posterior to it (*arrow*). **D,** Repeat sagittal series after sampling with a 9-gauge Suros vacuum-assisted system shows the signal void of the obturator at the superior margin of a small postbiopsy cavity. The enhancing mass is no longer seen. Atypical lobular hyperplasia (ALH) was obtained on analysis of the specimens.

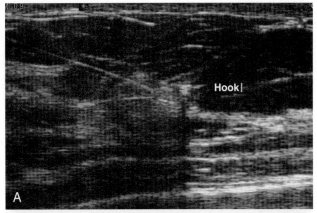

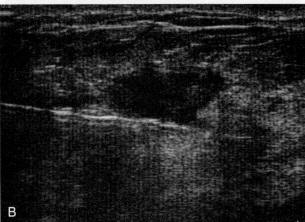

FIGURE 9. **A,** Image from the ultrasound-guided needle localization of the proven right breast IDC at 8 o'clock shows the hookwire in place (entering from the left), traversing the residual mass. **B,** Image from the ultrasound-guided needle localization of the left breast postbiopsy cavity at 3 o'clock shows the needle deep to the collection, entering from the left. The procedure was performed four days after MRI-guided vacuum-assisted biopsy. ALH was again obtained from the excision specimen.

malignancy. In cases of extreme patient anxiety (cancer phobia), a better but not completely supportable case could be made for supplementing mammographic surveillance with periodic breast MRI. That said, there likely are patients in many practices who may insist, for radiation-related or other reasons, on having an imaging alternative to mammography. If, after appropriate counseling, these patients cannot be dissuaded, we generally take the view that some imaging screening is better than none.

This patient's breast MRI showed no dominant mass or highly suspicious findings to suggest an occult invasive breast cancer. Fairly typical, faint, scattered, tiny fibrocystic-type foci of enhancement were noted diffusely. The significance of such foci, less than 5 mm in size and showing progressive enhancement, depends on the context. That is, they are not likely to be significant in a screening population because they are present in 80% of studies in healthy, premenopausal women, but such findings need to be scrutinized with a higher level of suspicion in a cancer patient.

Larger foci, such as the lesions identified in each LOQ of this patient, warrant workup, with mammographic correlation and targeted ultrasound. If corresponding targets are identified (generally on sonography), histologic sampling is recommended.

In this case, the initial workup did not identify targets for sampling, and 6-month follow-up breast MRI was recommended. The overall findings on repeat breast MRI were very similar, with the imaging features of both of the LOQ lesions again suggesting probable fibroadenomas. However, there was interval growth of both lesions, appropriately triggering repeat targeted breast ultrasounds. This time, a subtle, fairly benign-looking ultrasound correlate was found for the larger, right-sided lesion. Biopsy proved this growing mass was a sub-centimeter IDC.

Correlation on the left for the contralateral mirror-image lesion was more problematic. The initially identified correlate proved on aspiration to be a complex cyst, and so could not be the same lesion as this small enhancing (thereby solid) mass. Given the similarity in its MRI appearance and behavior (growth) to the proven IDC in the opposite breast, this prompted further preoperative investigation in the form of MRI-guided biopsy. This proved to be a proliferative lesion with foci of ADH and atypical lobular hyperplasia (ALH), illustrating the nonspecificity of MRI findings. (This histologic diagnosis was subsequently revised to ALH after review by Dr. David Page of Vanderbilt.)

It is also of interest to observe how benign in appearance small breast cancers can be, as this case illustrates. It is important to remember that apparent margins of a lesion seen on MRI are actually a map of enhancement and angiogenesis and do not correspond to actual anatomic borders of a lesion.

Finally, this case illustrates a variety of image-guided procedures used for diagnosis and in needle localization for surgery. Depending on their size, biopsy cavities can be visualized for ultrasound localization for several weeks after a biopsy and may in some cases be easier to relocate and target than clips placed after a biopsy.

CASE 15

CT identification of unknown breast cancer in an asymptomatic patient

An 83-year-old woman had an abdomen and pelvis CT for left lower quadrant (LLQ) pain. An enhancing nodule was noted in the right breast on the most superior image (Figure 1). The patient had not had a mammogram for 4 years. A diagnostic workup was performed, including mammography and ultrasound.

On mammography, extreme breast density was noted, attributable to the patient's use of conjugated estrogens (Premarin) for more than 40 years (Figure 2). The new mammogram showed a change in contour at the posterior margin of dense retroareolar tissue, suggesting a poorly visualized new mass. Ultrasound readily demonstrated a corresponding suspicious mass (Figure 3). Multiple features of malignancy were noted of the solid, vascular mass, including marked hypoechogenicity, taller-than-wide dimensions, and microlobulation of the margins. Ultrasound-guided biopsy confirmed infiltrating ductal carcinoma (IDC).

After ultrasound-guided needle localization, the IDC was treated surgically with lumpectomy, confirming a 1.1-cm IDC with negative margins and two benign sentinel lymph nodes. Radiation therapy consisted of brachytherapy, with interstitial catheters. No chemotherapy was given, and the patient declined hormonal therapy for her weakly estrogen receptor– and progesterone receptor–positive tumor.

TEACHING POINTS

CT is an uncommon modality to be the first indication of breast cancer, but it does happen on occasion. Cross-sectional imagers interpreting chest

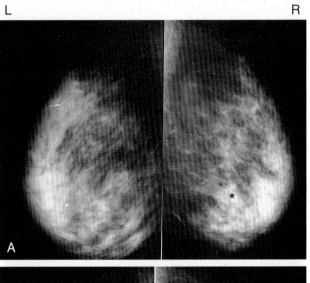

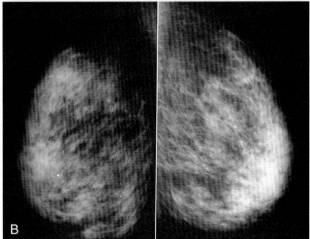

FIGURE 2. Mammograms [MLO projection (**A**)] obtained to evaluate the CT finding show marked breast density for an older patient, presumably owing to her decades of hormone therapy replacement. Only by comparing with the patient's prior mammogram (**B**), from 4 years earlier, is an abnormality suspected to correspond with the CT scan. At the posterior edge of the extremely dense retroareolar tissue on the right is seen an ill-defined mass (*asterisk*), manifested primarily as a contour change from the prior mammogram.

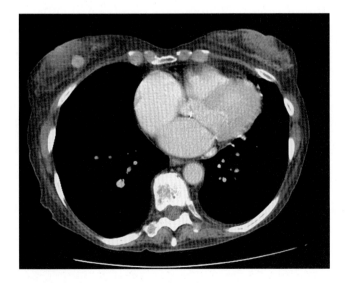

FIGURE 1. Contrast-enhanced image from an abdominal CT scan obtained for LLQ pain shows an enhancing discrete mass in the right breast.

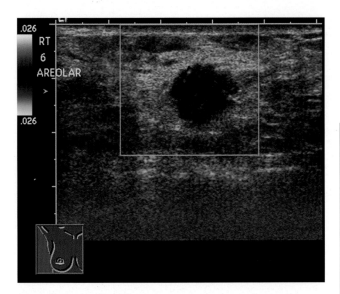

FIGURE 3. Ultrasound of the mass shows suspicious characteristics. The solid, vascular mass is markedly hypoechoic and taller than wide, and the margins show microlobulation.

and abdominal CT scans should include in their search pattern a review of the breast parenchyma for density, symmetry, and masses. Although breast cancers can often be seen on enhanced CT scans, the contrast generally achievable between an enhancing cancer and the surrounding breast tissue is not as advantageous as the contrast routinely obtained with fat-saturated or enhanced-subtracted breast MRI. For this reason, CT is not generally relied on for initial identification of breast lesions or local staging of known cancers, although it is an imaging mainstay in identifying axillary, interpectoral (Rotter's), and supraclavicular lymph nodes in initial staging of locally advanced disease, often in conjunction with positron emission tomography.

If a new or unknown mass is found in the breast on CT, it needs to be worked up in the conventional way, generally beginning with mammography and ultrasound. The CT appearance should not be relied on to predict whether a visualized mass is benign or malignant (with rare exceptions, such as a densely calcified fibroadenoma). The proven cancer in this case does not appear particularly malignant on CT (no necrosis or margin irregularity) and could have been a benign mass, such as a fibroadenoma.

SUGGESTED READING

Harish MG, Konda SD, MacMahon H, et al. Breast lesions incidentally detected with CT: What the General Radi-ologist Needs to Know *RadioGraphics*, Oct 2007; 27: S37–S51.

CASE 16

PET identification of occult breast cancer in an asymptomatic patient*

A 73-year-old woman was referred for positron emission tomography (PET) imaging for suspicion of recurrent lung cancer. Eighteen months after undergoing right lower lobe resection for lung cancer, she developed shortness of breath and a small right pleural effusion. PET scan demonstrated an unexpected hypermetabolic left breast focus (Figure 1). Subsequent evaluations confirmed breast cancer, which was excised by lumpectomy.

TEACHING POINTS

PET, typically performed as a whole-body examination, affords the occasional opportunity to identify unexpected but significant findings that are unrelated to a patient's known diagnoses. Focal, intense breast activity such as seen here mandates further evaluation and is generally readily differentiated from the lower-level, more diffuse physiologic activity that can be seen normally in breast tissue. Knowledge of the typical patterns of disease spread for any given histology must be weighed in assessing the significance of activity encountered in an unexpected location. Not infrequently, investigation of such serendipitous active foci will identify significant additional diagnoses.

A series reported by Agress and Cooper addresses the frequency and significance of such unexpected PET findings. These investigators identified 58 FDG-avid unexpected sites of uptake in 53 patients on review of 1850 whole-body PET scans. Of these, 45 were followed up with correlative imaging, and

*Case from: Kipper MS, Tartar M. Case 1: Focal breast activity due to an unsuspected breast cancer. In *Clinical Atlas of PET*. Philadelphia, WB Saunders, 2004.

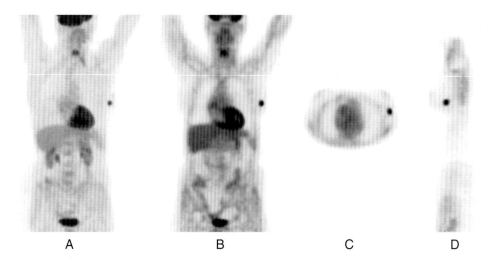

FIGURE 1.   PET imaging shows an intensely hypermetabolic, unexpected left breast focus, which was subsequently proved to be a breast cancer. Projection image (**A**) and coronal (**B**), transaxial (**C**), and sagittal (**D**) views are shown.

histopathologic confirmation was obtained in 42. Of these, 30 (71%) were malignant or premalignant; colonic adenomas (18) and colonic adenocarcinomas (3) were the most frequently encountered unexpected diagnoses. Other previously unsuspected carcinomas diagnosed as a result of unexpected PET findings in this series included two breast carcinomas, two laryngeal squamous cell carcinomas, one gallbladder carcinoma, one endometrial adenocarcinoma, one ovarian adenocarcinoma, one fallopian tube adenocarcinoma, and one papillary thyroid carcinoma. Nine benign diag-noses were also confirmed to explain unexpected PET uptake encountered in this series, including three with clinical significance (one case each of cholecystitis, knee pigmented villonodular synovitis, and Hashimoto's thyroiditis).

SUGGESTED READING

Agress H, Cooper BZ. detection of clinically unexpected malignant and premalignant tumors with whole-body FDG PET: histopathologic comparison. *Radiology* 2004; 230:417–422.

CHAPTER 2

Evaluation of the Symptomatic Patient: Diagnostic Breast Imaging

Screening mammography is used to detect breast cancer in asymptomatic women. In order to be cost-effective and efficient, screening mammography is performed by a technologist and batch-read at a later time by the radiologist. Most screening mammography findings for which patients are called back prove to be benign. The average callback rate for screening mammography is about 8% to 10%.[1] Of these callbacks, only about 15% will prove to be suspicious after diagnostic workup and require biopsy. Of the biopsies, about one third (30% to 35%) will yield a diagnosis of cancer. Screening mammography is intended for detection, not analysis, of potential abnormalities. Diagnostic evaluations involve the use of additional mammographic views, such as spot compression and magnification, and other breast evaluation techniques, such as ultrasound, physical exam, and ductography, to analyze potential abnormalities identified on screening mammography and to evaluate symptomatic patients. A diagnostic study is directed and supervised by a radiologist, and patients are given their results at the conclusion of the examination. Questions to be addressed through workup of a screening mammography finding are:

1. Is the finding real or simply superimposition of overlying normal structures?
2. How suspicious are the morphologic features of the finding?
3. What is the location of the finding within the breast?

Magnification views are utilized to evaluate morphologic features, such as the margins of masses and the shapes of microcalcifications. The Breast Imaging Reporting and Data System (BI-RADS) lexicon is a classification scheme used to help standardize the description and disposition of breast lesions seen on mammography, ultrasound, and MRI.[2] BI-RADS categories 1 and 2 are used to describe a negative study and a study in which there are benign findings, respectively. Category 3 is used to describe probably benign findings, with a less than 2% chance of malignancy, which can be followed in 6 months.[3] Patients with new or enlarging solid masses or increasing clustered microcalcifications that are not classically benign require biopsy. Category 4 is used to describe suspicious findings (greater than 2% chance of malignancy) that require biopsy. BI-RADS category 5 lesions are highly suspicious findings, having a 95% or higher likelihood of malignancy. Category 6 is used in patients with a known breast cancer who are undergoing neoadjuvant chemotherapy or additional imaging studies (Table 1).

Another primary role of diagnostic workups is to evaluate symptomatic patients. Commonly evaluated complaints include palpable lumps, an area of thickening, pain, and nipple discharge. The use of ultrasound in combination with mammography is extremely important in the symptomatic patient because some breast cancers may not be detected mammographically. Real-time evaluation by the radiologist is often necessary to detect subtle cancers. A report by the Physicians Insurers Association of America (PIAA) noted that a large percentage of suits involve women presenting with clinical symptoms and that a common reason for litigation was the claim that the physical symptoms "failed to impress" the physician.[4] The negative predictive value of a negative mammography and ultrasound is estimated to be 95% to 99%.[5–8] However, despite this high negative predictive value, a biopsy may still be warranted in the setting of a suspicious clinical finding.

MAGNETIC RESONANCE IMAGING (MRI) OF THE BREAST

Dynamic contrast-enhanced (DCE) MRI of the breast has been shown to be extremely sensitive in the detection of invasive breast cancer and is not limited by breast tissue density. Current indications include high-risk screening, evaluation for an unknown primary carcinoma, preoperative evaluation in patients with known breast cancer, evaluating response to neoadjuvant therapy, and suspected recurrence. However, the utility of DCE MRI has been limited by its variable sensitivity

Table 1   BREAST IMAGING-REPORTING AND DATA SYSTEM (BI-RADS) CATEGORIES

Category	Assessment	Description	Recommendation
1	Negative	Nothing to comment on	Routine screening
2	Benign	Benign finding noted	Routine screening
3	Probably benign	Findings with a high probability of benignity (>98%)	Six-month short-interval follow-up
4	Suspicious abnormality	Not characteristic of breast cancer, but reasonable probability of malignancy	Biopsy should be considered
5	Highly suspicious of malignancy	Lesion with a high probability of being malignant (≥95%)	Take appropriate action
6	Known, biopsy-proven malignancy	Lesion known to be malignant and being imaged before definitive treatment	Ensure treatment is completed

for ductal carcinoma in situ (DCIS). In general, the role of DCE MRI as a problem-solving tool in the evaluation of suspicious imaging or clinical findings is unclear. A negative MRI should not be used to avoid biopsy of suspicious findings on mammography or ultrasound or of a suspicious clinical finding.

NEEDLE BIOPSY PROCEDURES

Lesions categorized as suspicious following diagnostic workup require biopsy. Image-guided percutaneous needle biopsy techniques are firmly established as a valid replacement for surgical excisional biopsy, both in the evaluation of suspicious imaging findings and in diagnosing breast cancer.[9–19] Multiple studies have demonstrated the accuracy of percutaneous large-core breast biopsy for nonpalpable lesions to be comparable to that of needle localization and open surgical biopsy. Percutaneous needle biopsy is less expensive and less invasive than surgical biopsy and does not deform or significantly scar the breast. Its use has decreased the number of unnecessary surgical biopsies for benign lesions and reduces the number of surgeries required to treat patients with cancer. Instead of two surgical procedures to diagnose and treat breast cancer (excisional biopsy for diagnosis, followed later by a separate sentinel node biopsy or axillary dissection), a single surgical procedure can often be performed. The average number of surgeries performed in women with cancers diagnosed preoperatively using percutaneous needle biopsy is significantly lower than in women whose cancer was surgically diagnosed.[20–24] In addition, a preoperative tissue diagnosis allows patients to have a more informed and thorough discussion of cancer treatment options before surgery.

Ultrasound is the guidance method of choice for percutaneous interventional procedures of nonpalpable breast lesions. In addition, ultrasound guidance may be useful for selected palpable masses that are small, mobile, or vaguely palpable, in which palpation-guided biopsy may prove difficult.[25,26] Ultrasound as a guidance modality for cyst aspiration, needle localization, and biopsy procedures is preferred for several reasons. These include patient tolerance, accuracy, speed, real-time visualization, accessibility to all areas of the breast and axilla, relatively low cost, and lack of ionizing radiation. Most ultrasound-guided biopsy procedures are performed for masses. Even when seen on ultrasound, microcalcifications are usually best biopsied stereotactically, unless an associated mass is identified on ultrasound.

Cyst Aspiration

Benign (simple) cysts can be accurately characterized using high-resolution ultrasound imaging and do not require aspiration or biopsy.[27,28] Incidental complicated cysts (circumscribed round or oval masses with posterior enhancement, homogeneous low-level internal echoes, or mobile debris) can be safely followed.[29–32] Aspiration is reasonable for isolated complicated cysts that are enlarging or newly palpable. In addition, simple cysts may be aspirated in patients desiring symptomatic relief. For incidental nonpalpable lesions that cannot be reliably classified as simple or complicated cysts, and would require biopsy if solid, ultrasound-guided cyst aspiration is indicated for differentiation.

Routinely sending aspirated cyst fluid to cytology can lead to unnecessary surgical biopsies because of false-positive fluid analysis. Unless the fluid is unusually bloody, it can be discarded.[33–35] Bloody cyst fluid, although most likely benign, has been associated with intracystic papillomas. In cases in which bloody fluid is obtained upon aspiration and the cyst does not completely resolve, core needle biopsy of the residual cyst may yield a more definitive diagnosis than fluid analysis, possibly averting unnecessary surgical biopsy.

Fine-Needle Aspiration Biopsy

High-quality, fine-needle aspiration breast biopsies (FNABs) require both a skilled cytopathologist and on-site evaluation to establish adequacy of sampling. Although FNAB can provide quicker results and reduce patient anxiety because of faster processing time, accuracy should not be compromised for the sake of speed. Several studies, including the multicenter randomized trial performed by the Radiation Oncology Diagnosis Group V (RDOGV), have shown large-core needle biopsy to be superior to FNAB.[36–38] In addition, unlike core needle biopsy, FNAB cannot reliably distinguish in situ from invasive carcinoma. Patients whose cancer has been diagnosed as invasive preoperatively can undergo a lumpectomy and lymph node dissection in a single surgical procedure, as opposed to two separate surgeries when diagnosed using FNAB. Given its superior accuracy, diagnostic utility, and safety, with few significant complications, core needle biopsy is preferred over FNAB.

14-Gauge Core Needle Biopsy

Image-guided percutaneous needle biopsy is a less invasive and less expensive alternative to surgical excisional biopsy in the diagnosis of breast cancer. Fourteen-gauge needles have been found to be more accurate than smaller-diameter core biopsy needles.[39] To ensure accurate sampling, it is important to obtain an adequate number of samples and to be certain that the biopsy needle traverses the mass.

With the advent of large core needles, particularly with vacuum-assisted devices, it is not uncommon to remove most of the visible signs of a lesion during the biopsy. In these cases, a marker clip should be placed to allow localization in the event that the lesion requires subsequent surgical excision. In addition, it is recommended that a marker be placed in cancers before neoadjuvant chemotherapy to enable localization in the event the cancer is no longer visible after therapy.

Vacuum-Assisted Core Biopsy

Vacuum-assisted core biopsy devices allow the acquisition of larger amounts of tissue per core biopsy specimen. Compared to 14-gauge spring-loaded biopsies, which on average yield 18 mg of tissue per core specimen, the 11-gauge vacuum-assisted devices can obtain core samples averaging 95 mg.[40] Complication rates for 11-gauge vacuum-assisted biopsy have not been shown to be significantly different than those for 14-gauge automated core needle biopsy.[41,42]

Larger tissue volume devices have facilitated the sampling of microcalcifications during stereotactic biopsy. In addition, the frequency of histologic underestimation, imaging-histology discordance, and rebiopsy is lower for 11-gauge vacuum-assisted stereotactic biopsy than for 14-gauge core needle biopsy.[43–48] However, because these types of sampling errors occur in only a small percentage of patients who undergo 14-gauge ultrasound-guided biopsy, improvements in these rates may benefit relatively few patients. Philpotts and colleagues[42] reported no significant differences in the outcomes of sonographically guided core biopsies performed with the automated gun compared with those performed with a vacuum-assisted device, in terms of missed cancers, underestimation, or the need (immediate or delayed) for a second biopsy.

If enough samples are taken, vacuum core biopsy devices can remove a large portion of a lesion. However, they are only approved for diagnostic purposes and not for excision or removal. Although there is little data available, removal of most of a lesion through vacuum core biopsy has been suggested for possible relief of painful, symptomatic fibroadenomas. Removing all imaging evidence of a lesion does not equate to complete excision of the pathologic abnormality. Liberman and colleagues[49] reported that for cancers in which the imaging findings had been removed by vacuum-assisted biopsy, 79% had residual cancer at excision. The use of large-volume vacuum core biopsy, instead of open surgical excision, to evaluate high-risk lesions found at 14-gauge biopsy (papillomas, radial scars, atypia, or suspected phyllodes tumors) has not been extensively studied. Further investigation is needed to assess the potential benefits of completely removing the imaging findings of lesions versus sampling them.

Imaging-Histology Correlation and Follow-up

The false-negative rate for ultrasound-guided core-needle biopsy procedures is between 0% and 1.26%.[50] It is important to remember that needle biopsy of breast lesions is a sampling procedure and that undersampling can occur. Low false-negative rates and high accuracy are only attained by combining precise targeting and sufficient sampling with systematic radiologic and pathologic correlation.

In order for needle biopsy procedures to attain a level of accuracy similar to that of needle localization and surgical excisional biopsy, pathology results must be correlated with the imaging findings.[18,51–53] A discordant finding, one in which the histopathologic findings do not provide a sufficient explanation for suspicious imaging findings, warrants a repeat biopsy. This is usually in the form of a surgical biopsy, owing to the possibility of a second discordant result on repeat needle biopsy. Imaging-histologic discordance rates for 14-gauge ultrasound-guided needle biopsy have been reported as high as 7.7%. Crystal and associates[18] found that 12 of 323 cancers were missed at initial ultrasound-guided 14-gauge needle biopsy. Of these missed cancers, 7 were found immediately at rebiopsy prompted by discordant results, 2 at immediate rebiopsy because of indeterminate pathology findings, and 3 at later follow-up. Sauer and coworkers,[51] in their study of 962 lesions that underwent 14-gauge core biopsy under three-dimensional ultrasound guidance, reported a 3% discordance rate, of which 27.6% proved to be malignant on rebiopsy. Additionally, Liberman and colleagues[52] reported a 3.3% discordance rate out of 580 lesions biopsied under ultrasound guidance. At rebiopsy, 10.5% of these discordant lesions proved to be carcinoma. Therefore, careful imaging-histologic correlation will allow the detection of a significant number of false-negative results immediately after needle biopsy, thereby avoiding delays in diagnosis.

HIGH-RISK LESIONS FOUND AT CORE NEEDLE BIOPSY

Lobular Neoplasia and Atypical Ductal Hyperplasia

Underestimation of disease occurs when a lesion diagnosed as benign or atypical by core needle biopsy is upgraded to cancer upon surgical excision. Although the upgrade rate of atypical ductal hyperplasia (ADH) at needle biopsy to DCIS at surgical excision has decreased because of larger tissue volumes obtained with 11-gauge vacuum-assisted technique, upgrade rates as high as 21% have been reported.[54,55] Even when 100% of the mammographic lesion was removed at stereotactic biopsy, 8% of cases with ADH were still upgraded from ADH to DCIS at excision.[54] Therefore, a diagnosis of ADH at core needle biopsy warrants surgical excision.

The diagnosis of lobular neoplasia (lobular carcinoma in situ [LCIS] and atypical lobular hyperplasia) confers an increased risk for developing infiltrating carcinoma (ductal or lobular) in either breast. However, recommendations for surgical excision following a diagnosis of lobular neoplasia on core needle biopsy have not been standardized. Recent studies have suggested that, similar to ADH, surgical excision may be warranted when a diagnosis of lobular neoplasia is obtained at core needle biopsy.[56–58] However, as more data is accumulated, the decision to excise may be further refined based on the variety of LCIS and the relationship of the pathology to the radiographic findings that prompted biopsy.

Radial Scars and Papillary Lesions

Radial scars, also termed *complex sclerosing lesions* when larger than 1 cm, are not infrequently associated with DCIS, tubular carcinoma, ADH, and LCIS.[59–61] Therefore, surgical excision is recommended when a diagnosis of radial scar is obtained at core needle biopsy. Although further data are needed, recent studies have suggested that in selected subsets of patients, incidental radial scars found at core needle biopsy can potentially be safely followed rather than excised.[62–65]

A diagnosis of benign papilloma found at core needle biopsy of a radiographically suspicious mass should be considered discordant and calls for surgical excision. In addition, atypical papillary lesions should be excised.[66,67] For benign papillary lesions that are incidental or concordant with the imaging findings, recommendations for imaging follow-up versus excision have not been standardized. A recent study and literature review reports upgrade rates for benign papillomas diagnosed by core biopsy of 5% and 8%.[68] However, upgrade rates of benign papillomas diagnosed by large-gauge vacuum core biopsy may be lower.

Cellular Fibroadenomas and Phyllodes Tumors

Phyllodes tumors are relatively uncommon, accounting for less than 1% of all breast neoplasms.[69] Although they are most often benign, they can be locally aggressive. An actively growing cellular fibroadenoma may be difficult for the pathologist to distinguish from a phyllodes tumor when sampled by core biopsy. Therefore, surgical excision should be considered when a diagnosis of cellular fibroadenoma is obtained at core biopsy of a mass that is rapidly growing, clinically discordant, or has unusual imaging features.[70]

REFERENCES

1. Rosenberg RD, Yankaskas BC, Abraham LA, et al. Performance benchmarks for screening mammography. *Radiology* 2006; 241:55–66.

2. American College of Radiology (ACR) Breast Imaging Reporting and Data System Atlas (BI-RADS® Atlas). Reston, Va, American College of Radiology, 2003

3. Sickles EA. Periodic mammographic follow-up of probably benign lesions: results in 3,184 consecutive cases. *Radiology* 1991; 179(2):463–468.

4. Report from the Physician Insurers Association of America (PIAA), 2005.

5. Dennis MA, Parker SR, Klaus AJ, et al. Breast biopsy avoidance: the value of normal mammograms and normal sonograms in the setting of a palpable lump. *Radiology* 2001; 219:186–191.

6. Soo MS, Rosen EL, Baker JA, et al. Negative predictive value of sonography with mammography in patients with palpable breast lesions. *AJR Am J Roentgenol* 2001; 177:1167–1170.

7. Moy L, Slanetz PJ, Moore R, et al. Specificity of mammography and US in the evaluation of a palpable abnormality: retrospective review. *Radiology* 2002; 225:176–181.

8. Houssami N, Irwig L, Simpson JM, et al. Sydney breast imaging accuracy study: comparative sensitivity and specificity of mammography and sonography in young women with symptoms. *AJR Am J Roentgenol* 2003; 180:935–940.

9. Liberman L, Kaplan JB. Percutaneous core biopsy of nonpalpable breast lesions: utility and impact on cost of diagnosis. *Breast Dis* 2001; 13:49–57.

10. Mainiero MB, Gareen IF, Bird CE, et al. Preferential use of sonographically guided biopsy to minimize patient discomfort and procedure time in a percutaneous image-guided breast biopsy program. *J Ultrasound Med* 2002; 21:1221–1226.

11. Rubin E, Mennemeyer ST, Desmond RA, et al. Reducing the cost of diagnosis of breast carcinoma: impact of ultrasound and imaging-guided biopsies on a clinical breast practice. *Cancer* 2001; 91(2):324–332.

12. Parker SH, Jobe WE, Dennis MA, et al. US-guided automated large-core breast biopsy. *Radiology* 1993; 187.

13. Parker SH, Burbank F, Jackman RJ, et al. Percutaneous large-core breast biopsy: a multi-institutional study. *Radiology* 1994; 193.

14. Crowe JP Jr, Rim A, Patrick RJ, et al. Does core needle breast biopsy accurately reflect breast pathology? *Surgery* 2003; 134:526–528.

15. Meloni GB, Dessole S, Becchere MP, et al. Ultrasound-guided Mammotome vacuum biopsy for the diagnosis of impalpable breast lesions. *Ultrasound Obstet Gynecol* 2001; 18.

16. Simon JR, Kalbhen CL, Cooper RA, Flisak ME. Accuracy and complication rates of US-guided vacuum-assisted core breast biopsy: initial results. *Radiology* 2000; 215.

17. Buchberger W, Niehoff A, Obrist P, et al. Sonographically guided core needle biopsy of the breast: technique, accuracy and indications. *Radiology* 2002; 42.

18. Crystal P, Koretz M, Shcharynsky S, et al. Accuracy of sonographically guided 14-gauge core-needle biopsy: results of 715 consecutive breast biopsies with at least two-year follow-up of benign lesions. *J Clin Ultrasound* 2005; 33.

19. Smith DN, Rosenfield Darling ML, Meyer JE, et al. The utility of ultrasonographically guided large-core needle biopsy: results from 500 consecutive breast biopsies. J Ultrasound Med 2001; 20.

20. Smith DN, Christian R, Meyer JE. Large-core needle biopsy of nonpalpable breast cancers. The impact on subsequent surgical excisions. *Arch Surg* 1997; 132:260.

21. Kaufman CS, Delbecq R, Jacobson L. Excising the reexcision: stereotactic core-needle biopsy decreases need for reexcision of breast cancer. *World J Surg* 1998; 22:1028.

22. Liberman L, LaTrenta LR, Dershaw DD, et al. Impact of core biopsy on the surgical management of impalpable breast cancer. *AJR Am J Roentgenol* 1997; 168.

23. Lind DS, Minter R, Steinbach B, et al. Stereotactic core biopsy reduces the reexcision rate and the cost of mammographically detected cancer. *J Surg Res* 1998; 78(1):23–26.

24. Yim JH, Barton P, Weber B, et al. Mammographically detected breast cancer. Benefits of stereotactic core versus wire localization biopsy. *Ann Surg* 1996; 223:697–700.

25. Liberman L, Ernberg LA, Heerdt A, et al. Palpable breast masses: is there a role for percutaneous imaging-guided core biopsy? *AJR Am J Roentgenol* 2000; 175.

26. Lorenzen J, Welger J, Lisboa BW, et al. Percutaneous core-needle biopsy of palpable breast tumors. Do we need ultrasound guidance? *Rofo* 2002; 174.

27. Hilton SV, Leopold GR, Olson LK, Willson SA. Real-time breast sonography: application in 300 consecutive patients. *AJR Am J Roentgenol* 1986; 147.

28. Vargas HI, Vargas MP, Gonzalez KD, et al. Outcomes of sonography-based management of breast cysts. *Am J Surg* 2004; 188.

29. Berg WA, Campassi CI, Ioffe OB. Cystic lesions of the breast: sonographic-pathologic correlation. *Radiology* 2003; 227.

30. Buchberger W, DeKoekkoek-Doll P, Springer P, et al. Incidental findings on sonography of the breast: clinical significance and diagnostic workup. *AJR Am J Roentgenol* 1999; 173.

31. Mendelson EB, Berg WA, Merritt CR. Toward a standardized breast ultrasound lexicon, BI-RADS: ultrasound. *Semin Roentgenol* 2001; 36.

32. Venta LA, Kim JP, Pelloski CE, Morrow M. Management of complex breast cysts. *AJR Am J Roentgenol* 1999; 173.

33. Ciatto S, Cariaggi P, Bulgaresi P. The value of routine cytologic examination of breast cyst fluids. *Acta Cytol* 1987; 31.

34. Hindle WH, Arias RD, Florentine B, Whang J. Lack of utility in clinical practice of cytologic examination of nonbloody cyst fluid from palpable breast cysts. *Am J Obstet Gynecol* 2000; 182.

35. Smith DN, Kaelin CM, Korbin CD, et al. Impalpable breast cysts: utility of cytologic examination of fluid

obtained with radiologically guided aspiration. *Radiology* 1997; 204.

36. Pisano ED, Fajardo LL, Caudry DJ, et al. Fine-needle aspiration biopsy of nonpalpable breast lesions in a multicenter clinical trial: results from the radiologic diagnostic oncology group V. *Radiology* 2001; 219.

37. Symmans WF, Cangiarella JF, Gottlieb S, et al. What is the role of cytopathologists in stereotaxic needle biopsy diagnosis of nonpalpable mammographic abnormalities? *Diagn Cytopathol* 2001; 24.

38. Clarke D, Sudhakaran N, Gateley CA. Replace fine needle aspiration cytology with automated core biopsy in the triple assessment of breast cancer. *Ann R Coll Surg Engl* 2001; 83.

39. Nath ME, Robinson TM, Tobon H, et al. Automated large-core needle biopsy of surgically removed breast lesions: comparison of samples obtained with 14-, 16-, and 18-gauge needles. *Radiology* 1995; 197.

40. Berg WA, Krebs TL, Campassi C, et al. Evaluation of 14- and 11-gauge directional, vacuum-assisted biopsy probes and 14-gauge biopsy guns in a breast parenchymal model. *Radiology* 1997; 205(1):203–208.

41. Kettritz U, Rotter K, Schreer I, et al. Stereotactic vacuum-assisted breast biopsy in 2874 patients: a multicenter study. *Cancer* 2004; 100.

42. Philpotts LE, Hooley RJ, Lee CH. Comparison of automated versus vacuum-assisted biopsy methods for sonographically guided core biopsy of the breast. *AJR Am J Roentgenol* 2003; 180.

43. Kettritz U, Rotter K, Schreer I, et al. Stereotactic vacuum-assisted breast biopsy in 2874 patients: a multicenter study. *Cancer* 2004; 100.

44. Darling ML, Smith DN, Lester SC, et al. Atypical ductal hyperplasia and ductal carcinoma in situ as revealed by large-core needle breast biopsy: results of surgical excision. *AJR Am J Roentgenol* 2000; 175.

45. Jackman RJ, Burbank F, Parker SH, et al. Atypical ductal hyperplasia diagnosed at stereotactic breast biopsy: improved reliability with 14-gauge, directional, vacuum-assisted biopsy. *Radiology* 1997; 204.

46. Jackman RJ, Nowels KW, Rodriguez-Soto J, et al. Stereotactic, automated, large-core needle biopsy of nonpalpable breast lesions: false-negative and histologic underestimation rates after long-term follow-up. *Radiology* 1999; 210.

47. Philpotts LE, Lee CH, Horvath LJ, et al. Underestimation of breast cancer with 11-gauge vacuum suction biopsy. *AJR Am J Roentgenol* 2000; 175.

48. Philpotts LE, Shaheen NA, Carter D, et al. Comparison of rebiopsy rates after stereotactic core needle biopsy of the breast with 11-gauge vacuum suction probe versus 14-gauge needle and automatic gun. *AJR Am J Roentgenol* 1999; 172.

49. Liberman L, Kaplan JB, Morris EA, et al. To excise or to sample the mammographic target: what is the goal of stereotactic 11-gauge vacuum-assisted breast biopsy? *AJR Am J Roentgenol* 2002; 179.

50. Memarsadeghi M, Pfarl G, Riedl C, et al. Value of 14-gauge ultrasound-guided large-core needle biopsy of breast lesions: own results in comparison with the literature. *Rofo* 2003; 175.

51. Sauer G, Deissler H, Strunz K, et al. Ultrasound-guided large-core needle biopsies of breast lesions: analysis of 962 cases to determine the number of samples for reliable tumour classification. *Br J Cancer* 2005; 92.

52. Liberman L, Drotman M, Morris EA, et al. Imaging-histologic discordance at percutaneous breast biopsy. *Cancer* 2000; 89.

53. Lee CH, Philpotts LE, Horvath LJ, Tocino I. Follow-up of breast lesions diagnosed as benign with stereotactic core-needle biopsy: frequency of mammographic change and false-negative rate. *Radiology* 1999; 212.

54. Jackman RJ, Birdwell RL, Ikeda DM. Atypical ductal hyperplasia: can some lesions be defined as probably benign after stereotactic 11-gauge vacuum-assisted biopsy, eliminating the recommendation for surgical excision? *Radiology* 2002; 224(2):548–554.

55. Winchester DJ, Bernstein JR, Jeske JM, et al. Upstaging of atypical ductal hyperplasia after vacuum-assisted 11-gauge stereotactic core needle biopsy. *Arch Surg* 2003; 138:622–623.

56. Lechner MC, Jackman RJ, Brem RF, et al. Lobular carcinoma in situ and atypical lobular hyperplasia at percutaneous biopsy with surgical correlation: a multi-institutional study [abstract]. *Radiology* 1999; 213(P):106.

57. Arpino G, Allred DC, Mohsin SK, et al. Lobular neoplasia on core-needle biopsy: clinical significance. *Cancer* 2004; 101.

58. Foster MC, Helvie MA, Gregory NE, et al. Lobular carcinoma in situ or atypical lobular hyperplasia at core-needle biopsy: is excisional biopsy necessary? *Radiology* 2004; 231.

59. Sloane JP, Mayers MM. Carcinoma and atypical hyperplasia in radial scars and complex sclerosing lesions: importance of lesion size and patient age. *Histopathology* 1993; 23:225–231.

60. Frouge C, Tristant H, Guinebretiere J-M, et al. Mammographic lesions suggestive of radial scars: microscopic findings in 40 cases. *Radiology* 1995; 195:623–625.

61. Hassell P, Klein-Parker H, Worth A, Poon P. Radial sclerosing lesions of the breast: mammographic and pathologic correlation. *Can Assoc Radiol J* 1999; 50:370–375.

62. Philpotts LE, Shaheen NA, Jain KS, et al. Uncommon high-risk lesions of the breast diagnosed at stereotactic core-needle biopsy: clinical importance. *Radiology* 2000; 216:831–837.

63. Kirwan SE, Denton ERE, Nash RM, et al. Multiple 14G stereotactic core biopsies in the diagnosis of mammographically detected stellate lesions of the breast. *Clin Radiol* 2000; 55(10):763–766.

64. Brenner RJ, Jackman RJ, Parker SH, et al. Percutaneous core needle biopsy of radial scars of the breast:

when is excision necessary? *AJR Am J Roentgenol* 2002; 179.

65. Cawson JN, Malara F, Kavanagh A, et al. Fourteen-gauge needle core biopsy of mammographically evident radial scars. Is excision necessary? *Cancer* 2003; 97:345–351.

66. Leung J, Margolin FR, Lester SC, et al. Benign papillary breast lesions diagnosed at large-core needle biopsy: correlation with surgical pathology and clinical outcome [abstract]. *AJR Am J Roentgenol* 2002; 178:59–60.

67. Agoff SN, Lawton TJ. Papillary lesions of the breast with and without atypical ductal hyperplasia: can we accurately predict benign behavior from core needle biopsy? *Am J Clin Pathol* 2004; 122.

68. Mercado CL, Hamele-Bena D, Oken SM, et al. Papillary lesions of the breast at percutaneous core-needle biopsy. *Radiology* 2006; 238(3):801–808.

69. Liberman L, Bonaccio E, Hamele-Bena D, et al. Benign and malignant phyllodes tumors: mammographic and sonographic findings. *Radiology* 1996; 198.

70. Meyer JE, Smith DN, Lester SC, et al. Large-needle core biopsy: nonmalignant breast abnormalities evaluated with surgical excision or repeat core biopsy. *Radiology* 1998; 206.

CASE 1

Palpable axillary IDC, presenting as a growing mammographic mass simulating a lymph node

An 82-year-old woman identified a palpable right axillary tail mass. Mammography showed interval growth of a small mass (Figure 1), which had been evaluated 9 months before and was previously thought to be a lymph node (Figure 2). Ultrasound showed a corresponding 1-cm solid mass with lobular margins, with vascularity and no well-defined capsule (Figure 3). A surgical excisional biopsy revealed a 1.3-cm infiltrating ductal carci-

noma (IDC) with ductal carcinoma in situ, most of which was within the invasive component. Carcinoma was transected at the anterior margin. The patient elected to undergo simple mastectomy to clear the margins, rather than undergo re-excision and radiation. No residual tumor was identified in

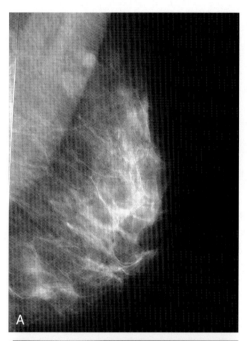

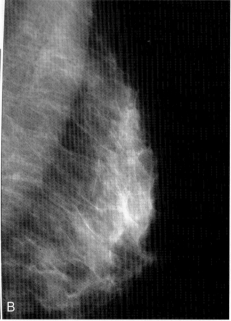

FIGURE 2. Comparison MLO mammograms from 1 (**A**) and 2 (**B**) years before show that the mass was not present 2 years before and grew from 1 year before. It had been evaluated at the time of initial appearance and was thought to be a lymph node based on a notched appearance.

FIGURE 1. MLO mammogram obtained during evaluation of a palpable axillary tail lump shows a notched mass at the level in question. The appearance is suggestive of a lymph node. However, some margins appear indistinct, and the mass is increased in density.

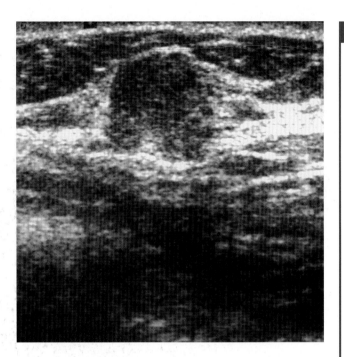

FIGURE 3. Ultrasound of the palpable lump shows indeterminate features. The mass is solid, is vascular by color Doppler (not shown), has lobular margins (simulating a lymph node notch), and has no echogenic capsule.

Palpable lump presenting as malignant microcalcifications on mammography

A 43-year-old woman presented with a palpable, painful left upper outer quadrant breast mass. Mammography showed a 3-cm region of suspicious pleomorphic microcalcifications in the corresponding location (Figures 1 and 2). Ultrasound showed no evidence of an invasive component. Stereotactic biopsy confirmed ductal carcinoma in situ (DCIS) with foci of invasion. Lumpectomy and axillary lymph node dissection were performed after needle localization with a single needle. The pathology demonstrated a stage II left breast cancer, T2N2, a 3.5-cm moderately differentiated infiltrating ductal carcinoma with high-grade DCIS, which was estrogen receptor and progesterone receptor positive, *HER-2/neu* negative, and had extensive lymphovascular invasion and multifocal

the mastectomy specimen. An axillary sentinel lymph node was negative. The final stage was stage I, T1N0, estrogen receptor positive, *HER2/neu* negative.

TEACHING POINTS

Beware the axilla! This case reinforces the need to carefully scrutinize the axilla when reviewing mammograms, especially any new "lymph nodes." Any new densities or masses that appear in the axillary tail or axilla must fulfill strict criteria to be dismissed as lymph nodes. All margins should be circumscribed and a fatty hilus clearly visualized. Differences in positioning may sometimes result in lymph nodes that seem to appear anew, but actually were never included in the imaging field. It can be worth taking an extra minute to look through additional comparison exams to see whether the lymph node might have been demonstrated before with subtle changes in positioning, thereby saving a patient unnecessary workup and anxiety.

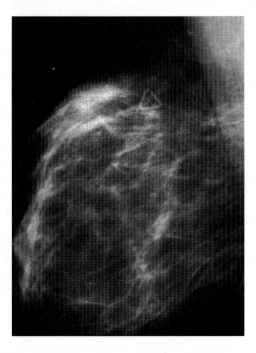

FIGURE 1. MLO mammographic view shows a radiopaque "BB" at the site of a palpable lump in the upper outer quadrant. There is increased parenchymal density at this level, containing pleomorphic suspicious microcalcifications. A triangular marker is also noted on a skin lesion in the upper inner quadrant.

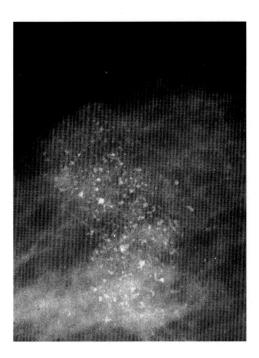

FIGURE 2. The suspicious morphology of the microcalcifications is better demonstrated on a lateral magnification view. The calcifications are extensive, irregular in shape, and variable in density. Some are elongated and linear.

margin positivity. The sentinel lymph node was positive for tumor, and subsequent axillary dissection confirmed 4 of 14 lymph nodes to be involved. A subsequent quadrantectomy was performed, with pathology showing residual intralymphatic tumor, and a lateral superficial margin was close (<0.5 mm). Chemotherapy on a study protocol and radiation were given, as well as subsequent tamoxifen therapy.

TEACHING POINTS

Evaluating microcalcification morphology is difficult and is among the more difficult assessments breast imagers make on a daily basis. It is helpful to look at classic cases of pleomorphic, highly suspicious microcalcifications and to bear in mind that microcalcification appearances are a spectrum. At the benign end are readily recognizable and classifiable morphologies, such as vascular calcification, skin calcifications, coarse fat necrosis patterns of calcification, and classic examples of milk of calcium. This case is an example of the other, classically malignant, end of the spectrum: clustered, arrayed in a ductular distribution, with

highly variable shape, size, and density of the individual calcifications, many of which are elongated and linear. Even within the middle ground between the two extremes of the microcalcification spectrum, there is a gradient of appearances. Fortunately, with the ease with which such findings can now be percutaneously sampled, today's breast imager need not agonize as much over decision making as when the only alternative available was surgical excision.

This case also reminds us that ultrasound can be useful in evaluating relatively large expanses of calcifications such as these. Although generally not particularly useful for direct evaluation of the calcifications themselves, ultrasound may on occasion demonstrate an invasive mass that is not readily apparent on mammography. If a mass is identified on ultrasound within a region of microcalcifications, a more accurate histologic diagnosis of invasive carcinoma might be obtained by using ultrasound as guidance for biopsy of the mass than by stereotactically sampling microcalcifications.

Finally, this case also illustrates the difficulty of achieving clear margins with microcalcifications. Our first line of defense is based on a clear understanding of the number and distribution of microcalcifications, achieved by motion-free, adequately penetrated and positioned magnification views during the initial workup. The initial needle localization in this case was performed with a single needle, placed in the midst of the calcifications. It could be argued that bracketing the microcalcifications with one or more additional needle placements during the localization might have helped in achieving clear margins in fewer steps.

CASE 3

Palpable ILC presenting as architectural distortion

A 47-year-old woman presented for evaluation of a growing palpable lump in the left breast, noted initially 3 to 4 months before. Architectural distortion was noted on mammography at the indicated site (Figures 1 and 2). Ultrasound showed a shadowing, ill-defined mass, with maximal dimension esti-

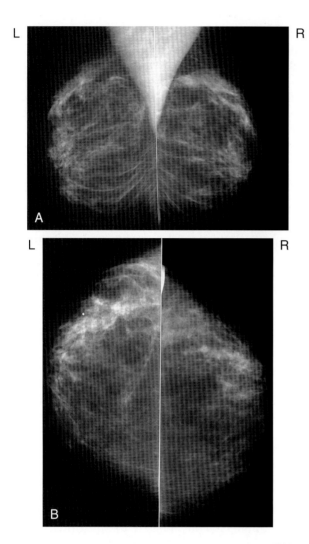

FIGURE 1. MLO (**A**) and CC (**B**) mammograms show heterogenous parenchymal density. A marker was placed at the site of a left upper outer quadrant palpable lump. Ill-defined architectural distortion is suggested at the site.

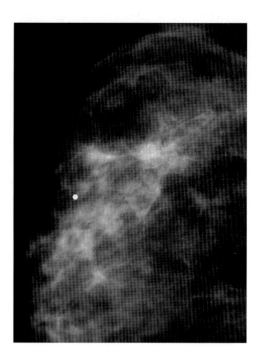

FIGURE 2. CC spot compression view confirms architectural distortion, at the level of the palpable lump, indicated by the marker.

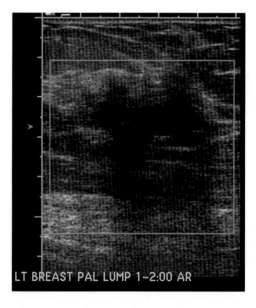

FIGURE 3. Ultrasound of the palpable lump shows a large, irregularly marginated, hypoechoic mass with shadowing.

mated of 4.6 cm (Figure 3). Palpation-guided biopsy by a breast surgeon did not confirm the suspected malignancy, and so an image-guided biopsy was performed stereotactically of the architectural distortion. Because of the ill-defined mammographic margins of the mass, a clip was placed to mark the site of the biopsy. Histology was invasive lobular carcinoma (ILC). MRI was recommended to better delineate the extent of the neoplasm and to evaluate the opposite breast. MRI showed the mass to occupy essentially the entire upper outer quadrant and to consist of irregular, strandy enhancement with architectural distortion (Figures 4, 5, 6, and 7). Strandy extension toward both the nipple and chest wall was noted.

Clinical evaluations of the patient during the course of the workup had noted the large size of the palpable mass (estimated at 3 × 4 cm when initially seen by the breast surgeon, and ranging up to 8 × 7 cm when seen by the medical oncologist, after two biopsies), and the consensus was that she was not a candidate for breast conservation. However, the patient was disinclined to undergo mastectomy and elected to undergo neoadjuvant chemother-

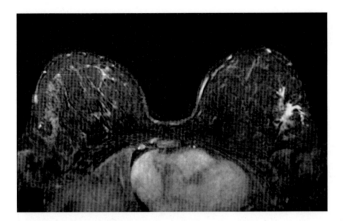

FIGURE 4. Fat-saturated axial breast MRI shows architectural distortion and strandy irregular enhancement in the left outer breast, at the level of the palpable mass.

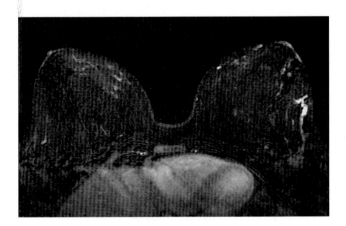

FIGURE 5. A lower slice from the same series, at the level of the nipple, shows the inferior extent of the strandy, linear enhancement.

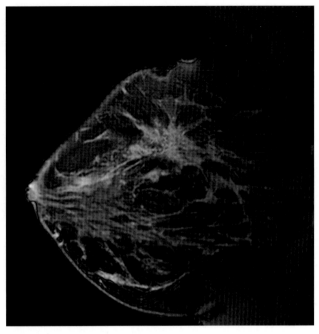

FIGURE 6. Fat-saturated, subtracted sagittal enhanced image through the left lateral breast shows the spiculated enhancing mass, with enhancing tendrils extending toward the nipple.

TEACHING POINTS

This case provides multiple interesting takeoff points for discussion. Many typical features of ILC are depicted. The mass presented as a palpable lump, which was large clinically at presentation. Its major mammographic manifestation was architectural distortion, and it was better seen on the CC projections, which generally achieve better compression. On ultrasound, it was well seen as ill-defined hypoechogenicity, with irregular margins and shadowing. However, the margins and its size were difficult to define precisely on both mammography and ultrasound. Although ultrasound guidance for performance of image-guided biopsy is preferred by many when a lesion is seen both mammographically and sonographically, there was some concern in this case about using ultrasound for biopsy guidance because of poor margin definition. Stereotactic guidance was utilized and confirmed the diagnosis of ILC. Because of the poor mammographic definition of the mass margins, a clip was placed to mark the biopsy site. With large, well-seen lesions, clip placement after biopsy is not universal. However, with increasing neoadjuvant use of preoperative chemotherapy and the attendant possibility that a mass may disappear with treatment, the universal use of clip placement after

apy. Her staging evaluation included enhanced body CT scans and positron emission tomography (PET)/CT (Figures 8 and 9). The breast mass showed only modest increased metabolic activity, and no other abnormalities were identified.

During the course of the eight rounds of neoadjuvant chemotherapy, the response of the ILC mass was periodically assessed with repeat breast MRI (Figures 10, 11, 12, 13, and 14).

After completion of neoadjuvant chemotherapy, the patient elected to undergo bilateral mastectomy. The residual ILC measured 5.2 cm, grade 6/9, estrogen receptor and progesterone receptor positive, *HER-2/neu* negative, with negative margins and two negative sentinel lymph nodes. Postoperatively, the patient was treated with left chest wall and supraclavicular fossa radiation and tamoxifen.

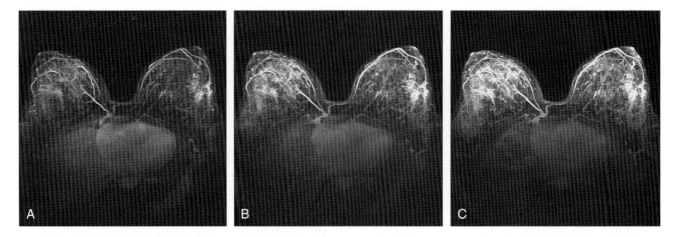

FIGURE 7. Axial maximal intensity projection (MIP) views (**A, B,** and **C**) from the dynamic enhanced axial series 1, 2, and 4 minutes after injection of contrast show the extensive irregular left lateral breast enhancement and architectural distortion against a background of fairly diffuse normal parenchymal enhancement. With increased delay after injection and progressive enhancement of the normal breast tissue, the conspicuity of the ILC diminishes.

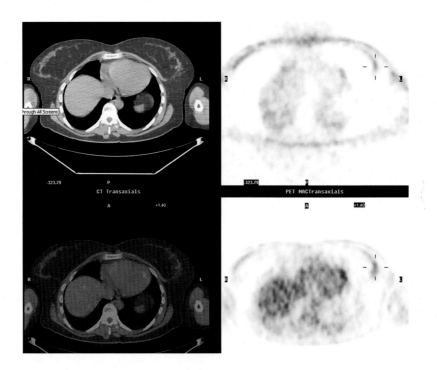

FIGURE 8. Axial images from the staging PET/CT (*upper left:* unenhanced CT; *upper right:* non-attenuation-corrected PET image; *lower left:* fused PET/CT; *lower right:* attenuation-corrected PET) show the mass to be only modestly increased in metabolic activity, being barely more active than normal breast parenchyma (*cursors* indicate the mass).

biopsy may need to be considered. Often, it is not known at the time of a diagnostic image-guided biopsy whether a patient will undergo neoadjuvant chemotherapy, but with larger lesions and a patient highly motivated for breast conservation, this possibility should be considered and a clip placed while there is access and a visible lesion. In this

case, the mass did not resolve completely and ultimately this patient elected mastectomy.

MRI was useful in this case to most precisely estimate the size of the ILC. The mass was noted clinically by all to be large, but estimates of its size increased over the course of staging evaluations. By the time the medical oncologist saw the patient,

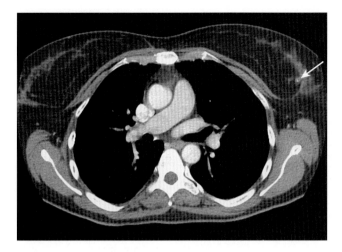

FIGURE 9. Axial image from the diagnostic contrast-enhanced chest CT performed during staging shows a clip in the left lateral breast (*arrow*). The mass is poorly delineated on CT.

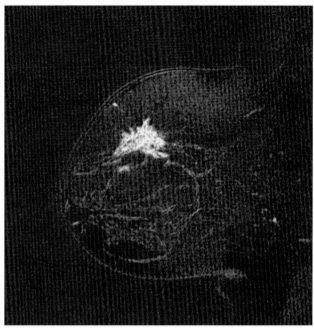

FIGURE 11. Sagittal, enhanced subtracted views of the mass, from the same postchemotherapy study, shows some contraction and shrinkage of the mass.

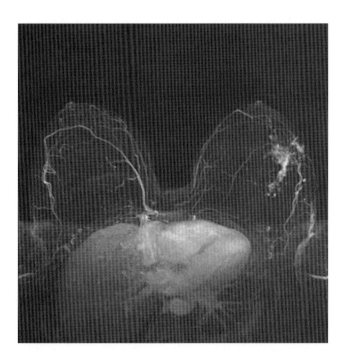

FIGURE 10. Axial MIP from early in the dynamic series from a repeat breast MRI, 2 months later, after four cycles of neoadjuvant chemotherapy. The mass is visible as strandy, spiculated, linear enhancement in the left lateral breast, now well visualized with the background breast tissue enhancement minimal.

she had undergone two percutaneous biopsies, and so it was not clear whether the mass growth was due to biopsy-related bleeding. The MRI showed that the mass was sizable, even larger than the most generous clinical estimates, and provided the best delineation of measurable disease for

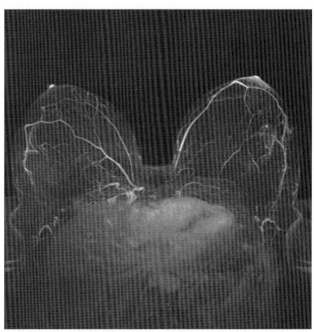

FIGURE 12. Axial MIP image from a third breast MRI, 3 additional months later, after completion of neoadjuvant chemotherapy, shows further contraction and shrinkage of the mass, with less intense enhancement.

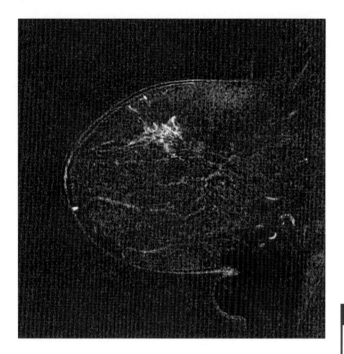

FIGURE 13. Sagittal subtracted views of the mass from the same postneoadjuvant chemotherapy study. The mass is smaller and enhances less intensely.

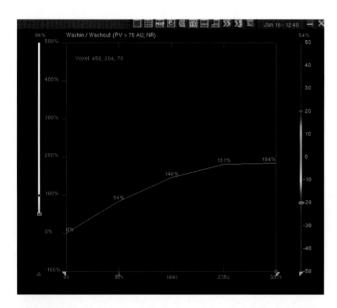

FIGURE 14. No angiogenesis could be identified within the mass. Only progressive enhancement is found, as graphically depicted.

follow-up during the course of neoadjuvant chemotherapy. MRI also is useful in such cases for evaluation of the opposite breast, given the relatively high propensity of ILC for bilaterality.

The patient's election of neoadjuvant therapy meant that her axillary nodal status would not be known. Because of this and the large size of her ILC, pretreatment staging was undertaken with PET/CT. The modesty of the metabolic activity level displayed by this sizable ILC is striking. ILC is known to be generally less metabolically active than infiltrating ductal carcinoma (IDC). ILC is three times as likely to be false negative on PET imaging as IDC. The minimal increased metabolic activity displayed by this large ILC implies lower sensitivity as well for metastases, so the reassurance provided by the otherwise negative PET/CT must be considerably tempered.

CASE 4

Palpable lump presenting as mammographic architectural distortion with microcalcifications

A 47-year-old woman with very dense breasts presented for evaluation of a newly self-noted right 12-o'clock palpable lump. Her routine screening mammogram performed 5 months before was negative (Figure 1). A diagnostic mammogram and ultrasound were performed to evaluate the palpable mass. On magnification spot compression of the mass, architectural distortion, and faint microcalcifications were appreciated, which appeared to be new (Figure 2). Ultrasound of the palpable mass showed a suspicious solid corresponding mass with angular margins and associated calcifications (Figure 3). Nearby (about 2 cm away) was a second, smaller, equally suspicious mass at 11 o'clock (Figures 4 and 5). In the axilla, a lymph node with an abnormally thickened and nodular cortical mantle was identified (Figure 6). These abnormalities were sampled with ultrasound guidance. The axillary fine-needle aspiration obtained groups of malignant cells, compatible with metastatic carcinoma of breast primary origin. The palpable mass at 12 o'clock was proved to be an infiltrating ductal carcinoma. The smaller, 11-o'clock mass was technically difficult to sample because of extreme breast density and proximity to the chest wall, and sampling yielded benign fibrotic breast tissue.

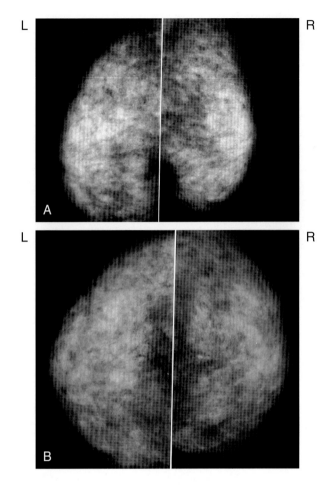

FIGURE 1. MLO (**A**) and CC (**B**) screening mammograms, performed 5 months before presentation with a palpable right breast lump, were negative. The breast tissue is extremely dense.

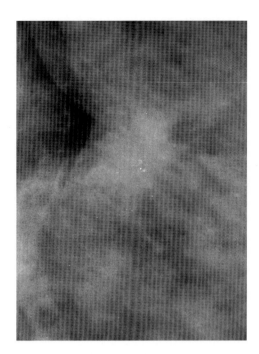

FIGURE 2. Magnification spot compression (CC projection) of the palpable right 12-o'clock breast lump shows retraction of the posterior glandular margin, with subtle architectural distortion and evidence of a mass as a double density, with associated microcalcifications. This was not seen on the screening mammogram performed 5 months earlier (see Figure 1).

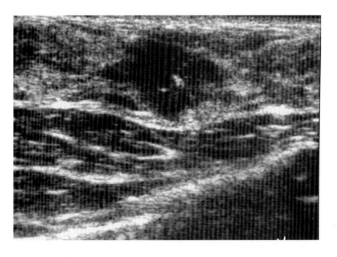

FIGURE 3. Ultrasound of the palpable lump at 12 o'clock shows findings corresponding to the mammogram. A hypoechoic, solid mass with marginal angularity and microcalcifications is highly suspicious for malignancy.

Sampling error at this level was suspected prospectively.

Because of the marked breast density, and proven node-positive disease, breast MRI was recommended preoperatively to supplement this patient's local staging. This suggested that the right breast cancer was extensive (Figure 7), with suspicious enhancement in the right upper inner and right lower inner quadrants, in addition to enhancing masses at the 11- and 12-o'clock positions. The palpable known cancer at 12 o'clock was accompanied by enhancing small suspected satellite lesions. The patient's staging was completed with performance of chest, abdomen, and pelvis enhanced CT, and positron emission tomography (PET)/CT (Figure 8), which did not suggest distant metastatic disease. Based on the MRI findings, the patient did not seem a suitable breast conservation candidate, and mastectomy and axillary dissection were performed.

The mastectomy pathology demonstrated the 12-o'clock mass to be a 1.5-cm infiltrating ductal carcinoma, and multiple foci of DCIS (ranging up to 1 cm in size) were identified, both on the periphery of the invasive cancer and in the upper inner quadrant. In addition, LCIS was found in the

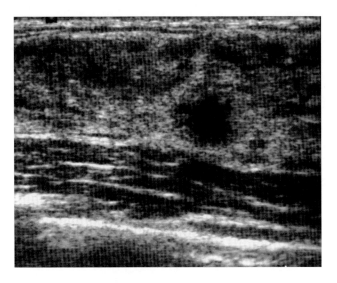

FIGURE 4.   A second suspicious smaller solid mass was noted on ultrasound in the same breast at 11 o'clock. Spiculation and angularity of the margins of this very hypoechoic solid mass indicate probable malignancy.

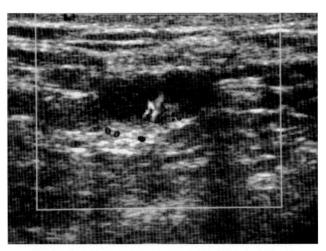

FIGURE 6.   Axillary sonography shows a suspicious lymph node for malignancy. The cortex is abnormally thickened and nodular. The hilus is seen by vascular flow but is largely effaced. Fine-needle aspiration confirmed metastatic carcinoma, enabling a sentinel node sampling procedure to be skipped. Axillary dissection was performed at the time of mastectomy.

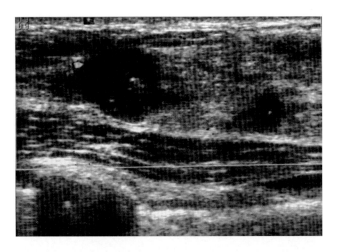

FIGURE 5.   Ultrasound shows the relationship of the two suspicious solid, hypoechoic masses.

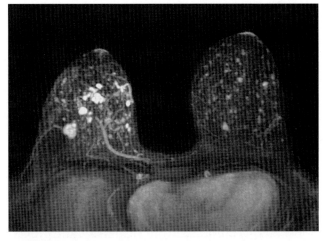

FIGURE 7.   Breast MRI axial enhanced subtracted maximal intensity projection shows multiple enhancing masses and clumped foci of enhancement in the right breast, markedly asymmetrical from the left. This study suggested the breast cancer was more extensive than known to this point.

upper inner and lower inner quadrants. One of 12 lymph nodes showed metastatic carcinoma, with a 0.8-cm tumor deposit and focal extracapsular extension. The tumor was estrogen receptor and progesterone receptor positive and *HER-2/neu* negative.

Additional therapy given included chemotherapy (four cycles of dose-dense doxorubicin [Adriamycin] and cyclophosphamide [Cytoxan], followed by four cycles of paclitaxel [Taxol]), tamoxifen, and right chest wall and supraclavicular fossa radiation.

TEACHING POINTS

This patient has extremely dense breast tissue. Ultrasound proved a valuable supplement to the mammographic evaluation, but even in combination, these two modalities underestimated the extent of disease in this patient's right breast. Breast density is not a limiting factor for breast MRI,

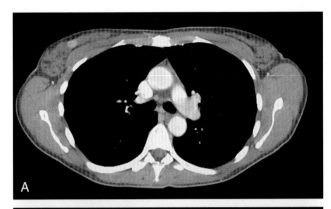

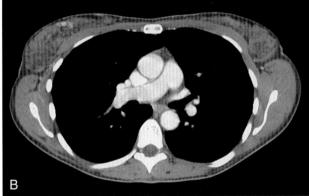

FIGURE 8. Images (**A** above **B**) from enhanced chest CT obtained for staging for node-positive disease. The breast tissue is dense. Enhancing small nodules are seen in the right breast, correlating with the known findings, but severely under-representing the extent of disease.

making it a valuable adjunct in the evaluation of such patients. Hormone-related enhancement can be limiting, making it advisable to schedule examinations when possible in the second week of the menstrual cycle (ideal is days 7 to 10). This rule is most readily enforceable when doing more elective studies, such as follow-up studies, or surveillance of high-risk patients. With new diagnoses of breast cancer in premenopausal patients, expediency in the workup will generally have to take precedence over optimal timing. This may make interpretation more challenging because there will often be many benign foci of enhancement to "read around." Use of a bilateral axial technique provides a convenient built-in control in the form of the other breast, which will be screened simultaneously. In breasts of similar mammographic density, a striking difference in the number of foci and intensity of enhancement can be significant. Such findings are seen here in the right breast, where there are multiple small, intensely enhancing masses, too large to be considered fibrocystic foci of enhancement, and accordingly suspicious.

Sonographic evaluation of the axilla at the time of breast ultrasound or to evaluate a clinically suspicious axilla may lead as in this case to identification of one or more suspicious-appearing lymph nodes. Clear preoperative establishment of axillary involvement will allow the surgeon to proceed directly to axillary node dissection without performance of sentinel node sampling. Axillary involvement may be suggested by clinically palpable nodes, abnormally enlarged or enhancing lymph nodes on preoperative staging CT or MRI, or hypermetabolism in axillary nodes on PET. Sonography is useful in identifying abnormal morphology of lymph nodes, which may not be enlarged enough to draw attention on physical examination, CT, MRI, or PET.

CASE 5

Palpable lump presenting as growing amorphous mammographic asymmetry

A 61-year-old woman was noted to have a palpable left breast mass on clinical examination by her physician. It was described as a 1-cm, irregular, firm, and mobile mass. Mammography showed amorphous parenchyma-like density at the corresponding level (Figure 1). Subsequent comparison showed that the asymmetry had been developing over the preceding years (Figures 2 and 3). The patient was seen for surgical consultation, and a palpation-guided fine-needle aspiration was performed. Atypical cells were obtained. An excisional biopsy confirmed a stage I, T1N0, 1.3-cm, well-differentiated invasive ductal carcinoma, with positive margins. Re-excision and sentinel node procedure followed, with pathology showing no residual tumor and negative sentinel nodes. External-beam radiation therapy with a boost to the lumpectomy bed was also given.

TEACHING POINTS

The mammograms showed the breasts to be largely fatty, with a small amount of retroareolar density.

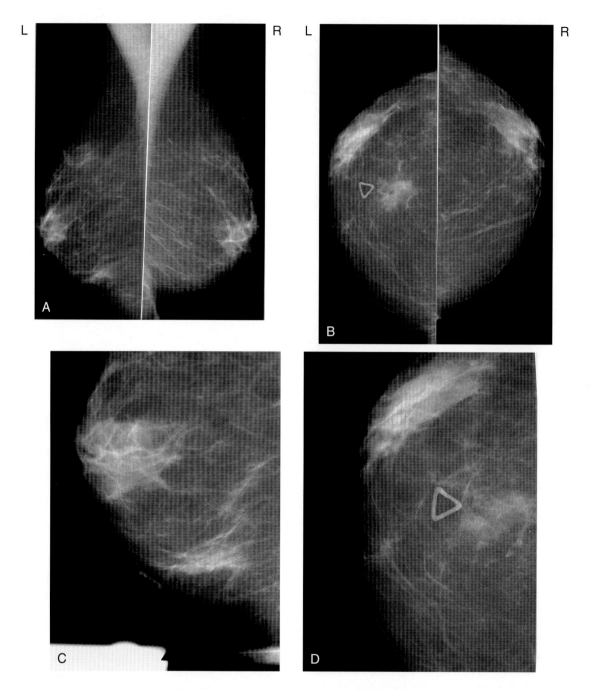

FIGURE 1. MLO (**A**) and CC (**B**) mammographic views are obtained with a triangular marker placed at the site of the palpable abnormality, at about 6 o'clock on the left. There is amorphous, tissue-like density at this level. MLO (**C**) and CC (**D**) spot compression views show the proximity of the marker to the vague density, which shows no spiculation, architectural distortion, or more specific features of malignancy.

In the inferior left breast, at the site of the lump indicated by the patient, there was amorphous, tissue-like density, with no architectural distortion or other concerning features. However, comparison showed that the asymmetry had been developing over the preceding years.

This is a recognized but less common mammographic manifestation of breast cancer. Therefore, amorphous, developing densities need to be evaluated, because occasionally they are a manifestation of a growing cancer, as in this case. Often, biopsies of similar-appearing densities return relatively nonspecific diagnoses, such as fibrosis. Short interval surveillance (typically, 6-month follow-up) is indicated if such a nonspecific diagnosis is obtained, to minimize sampling error.

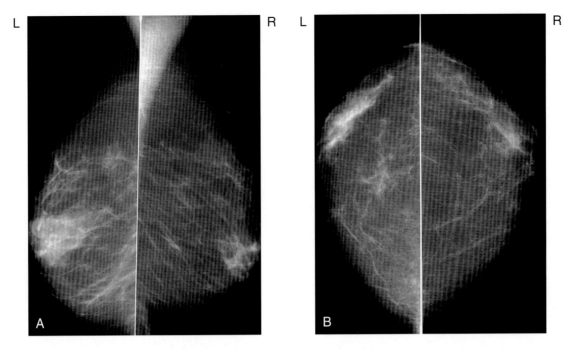

FIGURE 2.   MLO (**A**) and CC (**B**) mammograms from 2 years before.

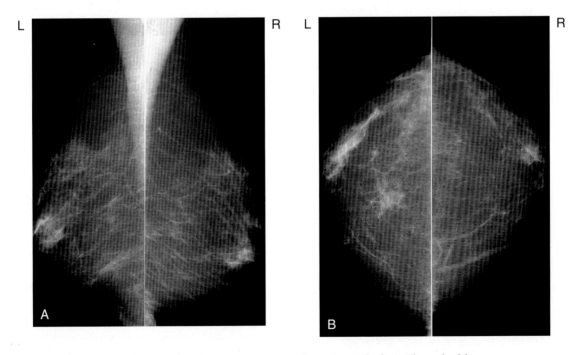

FIGURE 3.   MLO (**A**) and CC (**B**) mammograms from 1 year before. The palpable abnormality can be seen in retrospect to have been slowly developing over the preceding years. Asymmetries associated with palpable abnormalities need further evaluation.

Palpable lump presenting as developing mammographic density

A 48-year-old woman presented with a palpable mass in the lower inner left breast. Routine mammographic views demonstrated a large dense mass at the site of the palpable finding (Figures 1 and 2).

Ultrasound confirmed the presence of an irregular solid mass (Figure 3). Ultrasound-guided core needle biopsy yielded a diagnosis of low-grade invasive ductal carcinoma.

The patient was treated with lumpectomy and sentinel node biopsy. The surgical margins and sentinel node were negative. The patient went on to have radiation therapy.

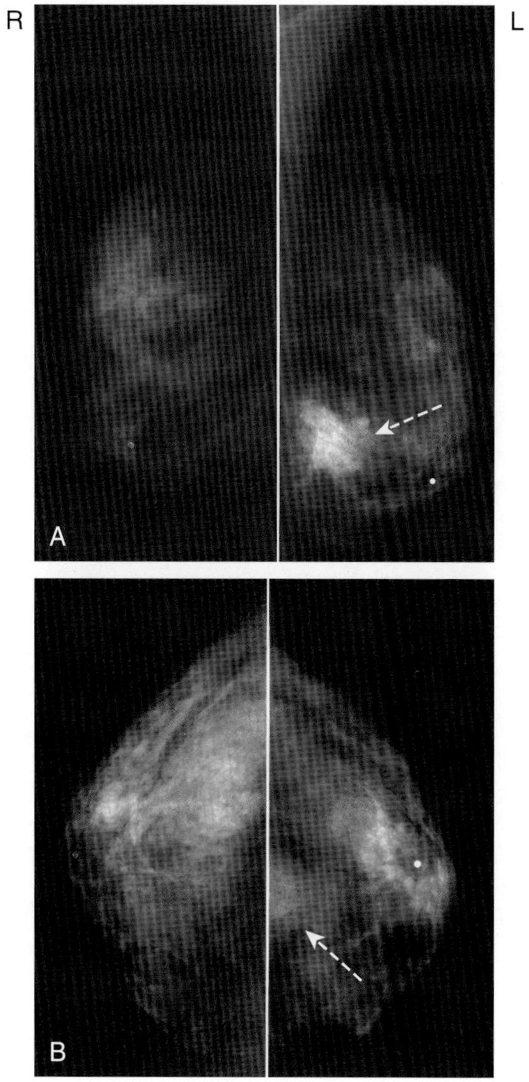

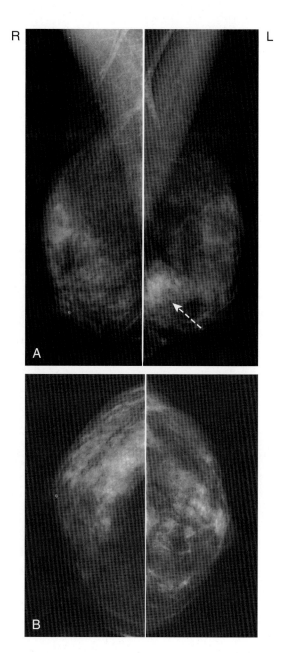

FIGURE 1. Bilateral mammographic views [MLO (**A**) and CC (**B**)] show heterogeneously dense breast tissue. A "BB" marker is noted over the lower inner left breast at the site of the patient's palpable lump. There is an underlying dense irregular mass (*arrows*).

FIGURE 2. Bilateral MLO (**A**) and CC (**B**) mammographic comparison views from the prior year's screening examination show in retrospect a focal asymmetry (seen well only on the left MLO) at the site where the patient's cancer was subsequently diagnosed.

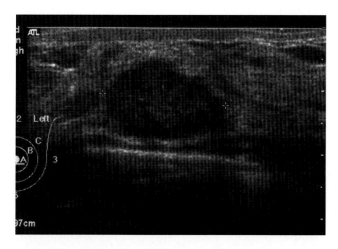

FIGURE 3. Ultrasound of the palpable lump demonstrates a hypoechoic solid mass with microlobulated, irregular margins.

TEACHING POINTS

The only mammographic sign of some breast carcinomas may be amorphous density, which may be better seen on one view than another, rather than forming a distinct three-dimensional mass. This is especially true in women with dense breasts.

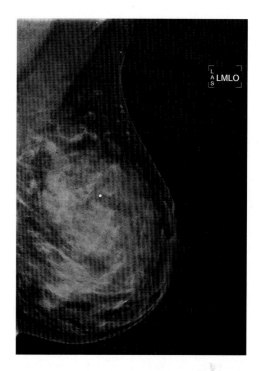

FIGURE 1. Left MLO mammographic view. A skin marker is seen at the level of the palpable mass.

CASE 7

Large, palpable, mammographically occult invasive carcinoma

A 49-year-old woman presented with a new palpable mass in the medial left breast. Mammographic evaluation showed no corresponding abnormality (Figures 1, 2, and 3). Ultrasound demonstrated a large hypoechoic solid mass, corresponding to the palpable finding, as well as a small adjacent satellite lesion (Figures 4 and 5). Subsequent ultrasound-guided core needle biopsy yielded a diagnosis of high-grade invasive ductal carcinoma. The large cancer is easily seen on a preoperative MRI examination (Figure 6).

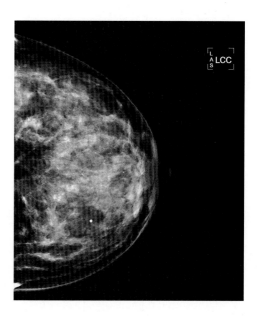

FIGURE 2. Left CC mammographic view. No mass is seen at the level of the palpable lump on either view.

TEACHING POINTS

This case illustrates that even large cancers may be occult on mammography, depending on location and the density of the patient's breast tissue. Both diagnostic mammography and targeted ultrasound

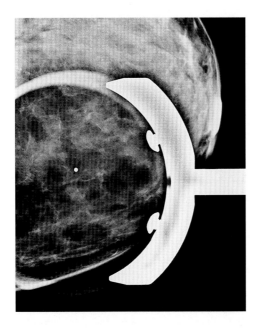

FIGURE 3. Left CC mammographic spot compression view performed of the palpable mass. The patient has dense breasts. Even with the use of spot compression to thin the dense tissue, no discrete mass is seen to account for the patient's palpable mass.

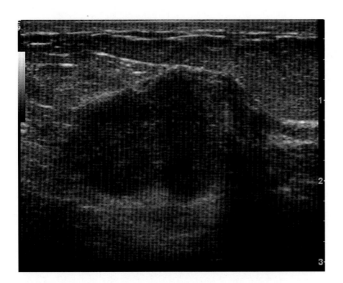

FIGURE 4. Ultrasound demonstrates a 2.5-cm hypoechoic solid mass with lobular margins and no defined capsule, corresponding to the palpable mass in the medial left breast.

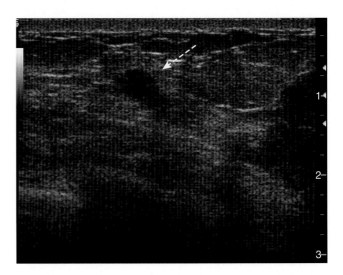

FIGURE 5. Ultrasound also showed a 5-mm satellite lesion (*arrow*) adjacent to the index lesion (*to the right*).

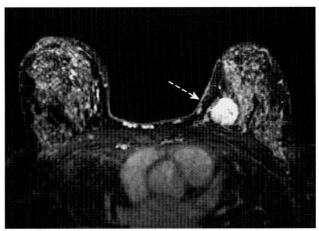

FIGURE 6. Enhanced subtracted axial MRI readily shows the dominant mass (*arrow*). A moderate amount of background parenchymal enhancement is seen, which is symmetrical.

should be used in the imaging evaluation of a palpable mass in a woman with dense breasts. Using this combined approach, mammography will permit detection of almost all cancers that display visible calcifications, as well as many noncalcified cancers. Noncalcified cancers that are obscured by dense fibroglandular tissue at mammography can usually be identified on ultrasound. In women with dense breasts and a palpable mass, the likelihood of malignancy when both mammography and ultrasound are negative is about 1% to 5%. This case also demonstrates the importance of evaluating the tissue surrounding a suspicious finding for adjacent satellite lesions. By identifying any satellite lesions, the extent of the disease can be better defined. If conservative therapy is performed, needle localization to include these satellite lesions will improve the probability of obtaining clear margins at surgery.

SUGGESTED READINGS

Dennis MA, Parker SR, Klaus AJ, et al. Breast biopsy avoidance: the value of normal mammograms and normal sonograms in the setting of a palpable lump. *Radiology* 2001; 219:186–191.

Durfee SM, Selland DG, Smith DN, et al. Sonographic evaluation of clinically palpable breast cancers invisible on mammography. *Breast J* 2000; 6:247–251.

Houssami N, Irwig L, Simpson JM, et al. Sydney breast imaging accuracy study: comparative sensitivity and specificity of mammography and sonography in young women with symptoms. *AJR Am J Roentgenol* 2003; 180:935–940.

Moy L, Slanetz PJ, Moore R, et al. Specificity of mammography and US in the evaluation of a palpable abnormality: retrospective review. *Radiology* 2002; 225:176–181.

Soo MS, Rosen EL, Baker JA, et al. Negative predictive value of sonography with mammography in patients with palpable breast lesions. *AJR Am J Roentgenol* 2001; 177:1167–1170.

Weinstein SP, Conant EF, Orel SO, et al. Retrospective review of palpable breast lesions after negative mammography and sonography. *J Womens Imaging* 2000; 2:15–18.

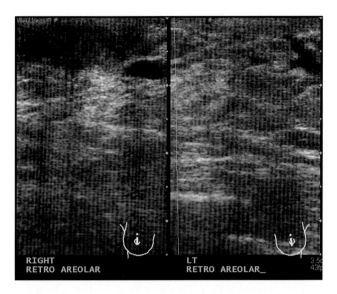

FIGURE 1. Split-screen comparison ultrasound views of the retroareolar regions bilaterally show asymmetry. There is little hypoechoic tissue on the asymptomatic left side, with a portion of a prominent duct demonstrated. On the right side, hypoechoic, asymmetrical tissue is seen, as well as a small cyst. The soft tissue asymmetry was noted but thought to be within normal variation limits.

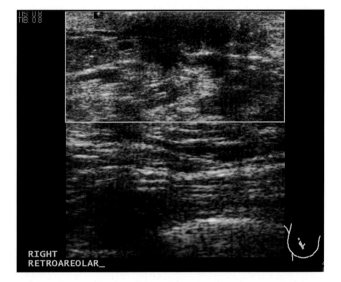

FIGURE 2. A portion of the right subareolar soft tissue could be considered mass-like, with a taller-than-wide component. A small vessel is demonstrated by color Doppler on the margin of this component.

CASE 8

Breast cancer involving the nipple-areolar complex, not identified on conventional imaging, demonstrated by MRI

A 68-year-old woman noted several months of change in the right nipple-areolar complex, with tenderness. Mammographic and sonographic evaluations were considered negative, although asymmetry was noted on ultrasound of the retroareolar area compared with the opposite side (Figures 1 and 2). It was thought to be within normal limits, and a referral for breast surgical evaluation was made. Retraction and palpable hard nodularity were noted on physical examination by the breast surgeon, who performed a palpation-guided core needle biopsy. This confirmed infiltrating ductal carcinoma (IDC).

A breast MRI readily demonstrated an intensely enhancing, irregularly shaped subareolar mass at the level in question (Figure 3).

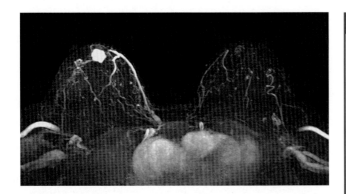

FIGURE 3.   Axial maximal intensity projection from enhanced, subtracted dynamic breast MRI shows an irregularly marginated and intensely enhancing right subareolar mass.

The patient was treated surgically with a mastectomy, which demonstrated a stage IIB, T2N1, estrogen receptor–positive, *HER-2/neu* negative IDC. Chemotherapy was interrupted after four cycles because of reactivation of chronic hepatitis B, and the patient was placed on anastrozole (Arimidex). Chest wall radiation was also performed.

TEACHING POINTS

The nipple-areolar complex can be a breast imaging blind spot. The confluence of ductular structures in the retroareolar region on mammography can make identification of coexisting abnormalities difficult. On ultrasound, the intense shadowing that the nipple-areolar complex can generate makes sonographic assessment challenging. Special maneuvers, well described by Stavros in his *Breast Ultrasound* textbook, can help in sonographically interrogating the retroareolar region. Comparison with the opposite side and evaluation with color Doppler for increased vascularity can help in the assessment. In this case, physical examination of the patient might have aided recognition that the sonographic asymmetry was a significant abnormality—namely an infiltrating carcinomatous mass.

In ambiguous cases such as this, in which the conventional breast imaging is inconclusive or discordant with clinical findings, breast MRI can be helpful to confirm that there is an abnormality and to delineate the full extent of disease.

SUGGESTED READING

Stavros AT, Rapp CL, Parker SH. *Breast Ultrasound.* 1st ed. Philadelphia, PA: Lippincott Williams & Wilkins; 2003.

Mammographically occult retroareolar breast cancer presenting as nipple retraction

A 72-year-old woman presented for evaluation of right nipple change, noted for several years, but pronounced in the last year. A mammogram performed 2 months earlier was negative (Figure 1).

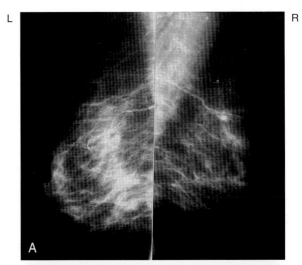

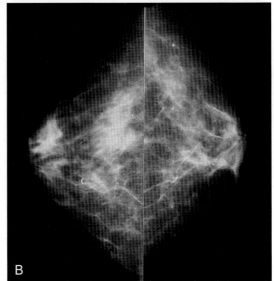

FIGURE 1.   MLO (**A**) and CC (**B**) mammograms show moderate parenchymal density and no definite abnormality.

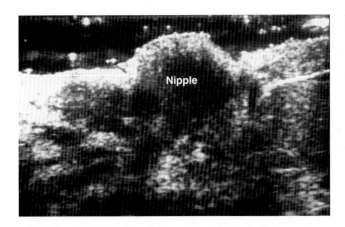

FIGURE 2. Sonography of the retroareolar region shows mass-like, hypoechoic tissue with irregular margins. No abnormality was recognized prospectively at this level. This image was obtained at the time of second-look ultrasound, after MRI was abnormal, and subsequent sonographic biopsy confirmed IDC.

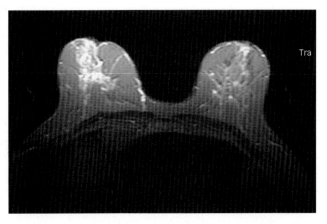

FIGURE 4. Axial short tau inversion recovery (STIR) image at the same level as Figure 3, for correlation.

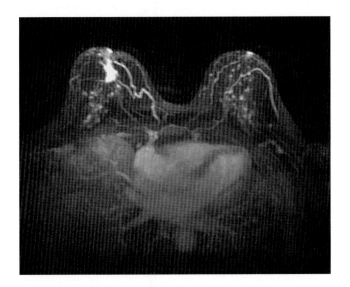

FIGURE 3. Enhanced, subtracted axial bilateral breast MRI maximal intensity projection view shows marked asymmetry, with an intensely enhancing, spiculated mass confirmed in the right retroareolar region, producing nipple retraction.

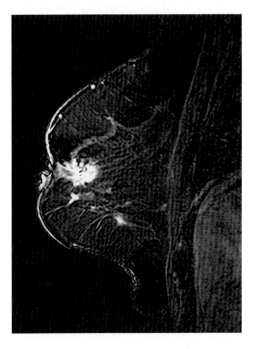

FIGURE 5. Sagittal subtracted view of the right breast demonstrates well the extension to the nipple and secondary retraction produced by the spiculated, highly suspicious mass.

Retraction of the nipple-areolar complex was confirmed on physical examination, with an area of irregular firmness on palpation at 1 o'clock. A palpation-guided core needle biopsy yielded only benign tissue and did not confirm the clinically suspected breast cancer. Sonographic examination was undertaken next and was negative (Figure 2). Breast MRI was obtained and demonstrated an irregular, intensely enhancing retroareolar mass, measuring up to 2.5 cm (Figures 3, 4, and 5). Repeat breast sonography (see Figure 2), with the MRI information, identified a 9-mm, irregularly shaped, hypoechoic retroareolar breast mass, which was successfully sampled with ultrasound guidance, confirming infiltrating ductal carcinoma (IDC).

The patient was treated with a mastectomy and sentinel lymph node sampling. The specimen showed a 2.5-cm IDC, with high-grade ductal carcinoma in situ involving 25% of the tumor, estrogen receptor positive, *HER-2/neu* negative, with clear margins and no angiolymphatic involvement. Three sentinel lymph nodes were all negative. Final stage was IIA, T2N0M0. The patient was placed on tamoxifen.

TEACHING POINTS

Similar to Case 8 in this chapter, the nipple-areolar complex proved in this case to be a breast imaging blind spot. At times, breast cancers presenting as nipple changes or retraction can be more clinically compelling than the imaging findings. The convergence of ductular structures at the nipple-areolar complex makes this region difficult to evaluate mammographically, and it can be challenging to overcome the dense shadowing that can normally emanate from the nipple-areolar complex to adequately assess this region sonographically. In such a case, with high clinical suspicion, an inconclusive biopsy and falsely reassuring imaging, the unambiguous breast MRI provides confirmation that there is a breast cancer underlying the clinical changes and serves as a roadmap for repeat ultrasound evaluation and biopsy with ultrasound guidance.

CASE 10

Importance of clear communication and accurate history; inaccurate history of biopsy "scar" leads to near-miss of a spiculated cancer

A 67-year-old woman was referred for breast imaging evaluation of a left breast palpable abnormality noted by her physician. However, the location of the area of concern was not indicated by the physician, and the patient did not seem to be aware of the clinical question. She did indicate to the technologist that she had had a previous benign biopsy. The technologist diagrammed a linear surgical scar in the left lower inner quadrant, and to physical inspection, there was a linear skin indentation at this level. Mammograms obtained with a scar marker in place showed a dense "scar" at the marked level, with architectural distortion and spiculation (Figure 1). The mammogram interpreter thought the scar was more prominent than on prior examinations and recommended ultrasound for further evaluation. The ultrasound technologist reported that she could see shadowing from the scar, but no other abnormalities (Figure 2). On physician real-time evaluation, the patient's history was reviewed, and it became apparent that the patient's prior biopsy had been stereotactic, and that she had never had breast surgery before! With this information, the presumed scar assumed increased significance as a spiculated, highly suspicious, probable breast cancer. With the room lights on, the linear scar diagrammed by both the mammographic and ultrasound technologists was revealed to be a linear pucker in the patient's skin due to retraction by the cancer.

An ultrasound-guided core needle biopsy of the suspicious shadowing mass confirmed well-differentiated invasive ductal carcinoma. Pathology from the subsequent lumpectomy showed a strongly estrogen receptor– and progesterone receptor–positive, 1.2-cm infiltrating ductal adenocarcinoma with rare small foci of intermediate-grade ductal carcinoma in situ, mostly within the invasive component, with clear margins and three negative sentinel lymph nodes. She was also treated with external-beam radiation and declined chemotherapy.

TEACHING POINTS

This case could have had a disastrous outcome because of the incomplete and misleading history. From the referral, which indicated a left breast abnormality, but not the location, to the patient's incomplete knowledge of her physician's concerns, this case was plagued by poor communication. The patient did indicate to the technologist her history of a prior benign breast biopsy. The technologist may have mistaken the linear skin retraction for a scar site, or been misled by the patient's description of her prior biopsy into diagramming a surgical scar site on her history form and marking it on her films. In any case, misinformation was conveyed to the interpreting mammographer. If the cancer was changing more slowly, this might have been passed off as the surgical scar purported by the history. The ultrasound technologist was also

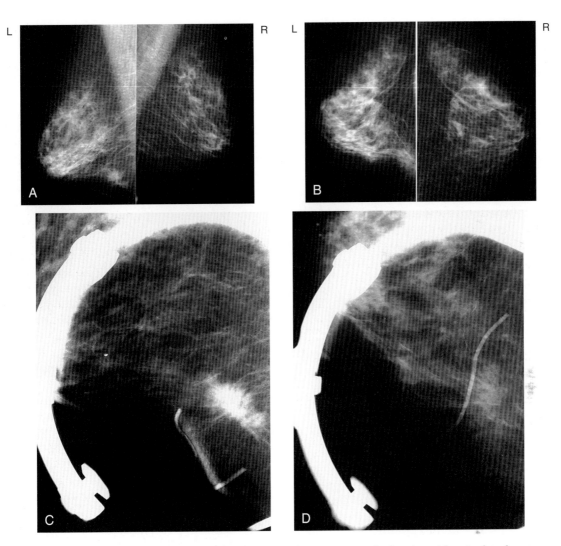

FIGURE 1.   MLO (**A**) and CC (**B**) mammograms show asymmetric density with spiculated margins at the level of a marked "scar" in the left lower inner quadrant, better seen on MLO (**C**) and CC (**D**) spot compression views where a linear scar marker can be seen.

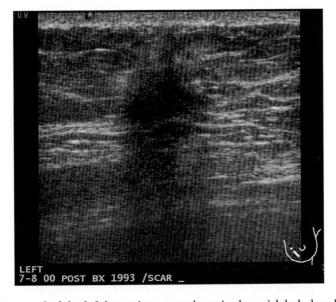

FIGURE 2.   Ultrasound of the left lower inner quadrant is also mislabeled and identifies a shadowing, intensely hypoechoic irregularly marginated mass as a "scar." The spicules do extend up to the skin, and the overlying skin showed a linear crease, presumably from retraction by the cancer.

misled by the history from the mammogram. Fortunately for the ultrasound interpreter, verifying the history by phrasing the questions differently uncovered the confusion. Although in the same quadrant, her prior biopsy had been stereotactic (reports were subsequently made available from another facility, verifying this), and she had never had breast surgery. At that point, the true significance of what had been regarded as scar became abundantly apparent.

CASE 11

Axillary nodal presentation of ILC, primary occult on conventional imaging, found by MRI

A 59-year-old woman presented to her physician with a new palpable right axillary mass. Palpation-directed fine-needle aspiration of the axillary mass revealed metastatic adenocarcinoma. Physical exam of the right breast was unremarkable except for pain noted by the patient in the lateral aspect of the right breast. Mammographic evaluation showed the enlarged right axillary node but no primary breast carcinoma (Figure 1). Ultrasound was also performed of the right breast but failed to show a breast mass (Figures 2 and 3). MRI was obtained to search for a primary breast carcinoma. The MRI demonstrated a large area of abnormal enhancement in the lateral right breast that proved on biopsy to be invasive lobular carcinoma (ILC) (Figures 4 and 5).

TEACHING POINTS

This case illustrates the use of MRI in the evaluation of patients presenting with an axillary metastasis of unknown origin. If conventional imaging by mammography and ultrasonography fails to detect a primary breast cancer, MRI can be useful. Orel and colleagues observed that MRI identified the primary breast carcinoma in 86% of 22 women

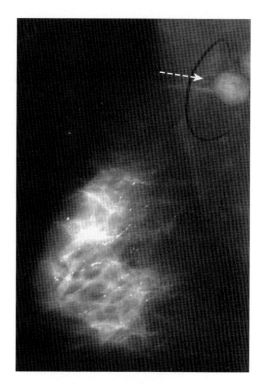

FIGURE 1. Right MLO mammographic view shows an enlarged and mammographically dense node (*arrow*) corresponding to the biopsy-proven involved node seen in the right axilla. The breast parenchyma is dense, and there are secretory calcifications, but no primary is seen.

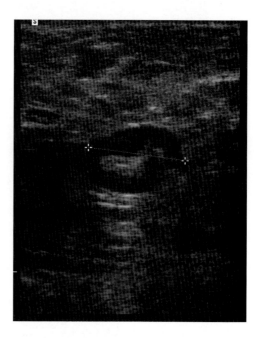

FIGURE 2. Ultrasound of the right axilla demonstrates an abnormal lymph node corresponding to the palpable metastatic lymph node. The cortex is abnormally thickened, and there is mass effect on the echogenic fatty hilus.

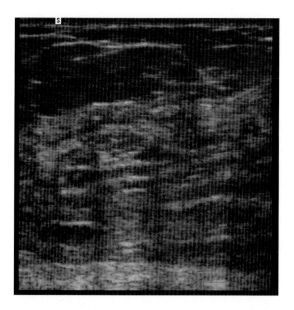

FIGURE 3. Ultrasound image of the painful lateral right breast shows no abnormality.

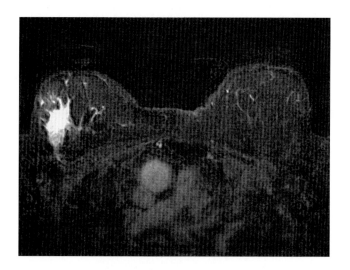

FIGURE 4. Axial contrast-enhanced, subtracted MRI image shows a large area of abnormal segmental enhancement in the lateral right breast.

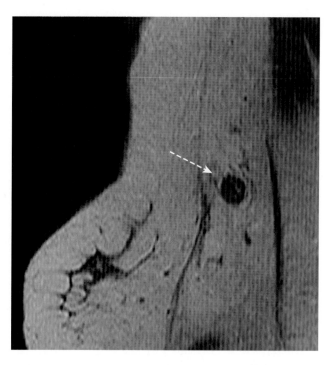

FIGURE 5. Noncontrast, T1-weighted, angled oblique sagittal MRI of the right axilla demonstrates the abnormal lymph node (*arrow*). The fatty hilus is largely effaced in this view.

ment pattern may be less characteristically malignant than in comparably sized infiltrating ductal carcinoma (IDC). Enhancement may be less intense and more progressive in pattern than in IDC. Accordingly, interpretation of breast MRI abnormalities in cases of suspected or known ILC may be based predominantly on morphology. Absence of washout or a plateauing enhancement pattern should not be regarded as reassuring if an abnormal morphologic pattern, such as this segmental enhancement, is encountered.

studied with axillary nodal presentation of breast cancer. A review of six studies suggests that MRI may have a sensitivity as high as 94% in the detection of occult breast malignancy in patients with axillary metastasis.

As demonstrated by this example, ILC can be evasive to detection by physical examination, mammography, and ultrasound. Even on breast MRI, the most sensitive modality commonly employed in the evaluation of ILC, the enhance-

SUGGESTED READINGS

Blue Cross Blue Shield (BCBSA), Technology Evaluation Center (TEC). Breast MRI for detection or diagnosis of primary or recurrent breast cancer. TEC Assessment Program, Chicago, IL: BCBSA, vol. 19(1), April 2004.

Orel SG, Weinstein SP, Schnall MD, et al. Breast MR imaging in patients with axillary node metastases and unknown primary malignancy. *Radiology* 1999; 212: 543–549.

CASE 12

Axillary nodal presentation with negative mammogram, primary found on PET*

A 39-year-old woman presented with left breast pain and axillary adenopathy. Mammography noted the enlarged lymph nodes in the axilla but did not identify a source within the breast (Figure 1). The left axilla was sampled, and metastatic carcinoma compatible with a breast primary was confirmed. She was referred for positron emission tomography (PET) to search for an unknown primary lesion.

PET imaging showed three hypermetabolic foci in the left axilla, corresponding to the known residual palpable lymph nodes (Figure 2). In addition, a separate, small, hypermetabolic focus was identified in the upper inner quadrant of the left breast (Figure 3). The mammogram was re-reviewed with this information, and a neodensity was noted in the medial breast compared with the prior year's study (Figure 4). Further mammographic and ultrasonographic workup confirmed the abnormality

(Figures 5, 6, and 7). Planned mastectomy was deferred in favor of core needle biopsy of the suspected primary lesion. Poorly differentiated invasive ductal carcinoma was confirmed. The patient's management was changed from mastectomy to lumpectomy. At pathology, a 1.5-cm poorly differentiated invasive ductal carcinoma was identified, and 3 of 12 lymph nodes from axillary dissection were positive for malignancy. The largest lymph node measured 2.1 cm. Further therapy was undertaken with adjuvant chemotherapy and radiation.

TEACHING POINTS

PET imaging was the initial study to locate this patient's breast carcinoma primary lesion. Overlooked initially on mammography, the addition of the PET information enabled the mammographic workup to be redirected and the lesion successfully localized and sampled. The PET information also changed this patient's management. Until the lesion was confirmed on mammographic and ultrasonographic workup, it was considered unable to be localized, and the patient was slated for mastectomy without consideration of breast conservation therapy. If the lesion had not been confirmed on the additional breast imaging

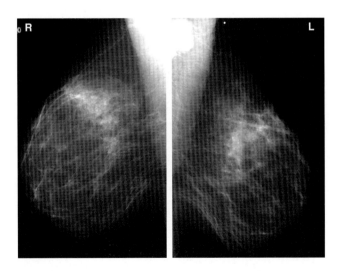

FIGURE 1. MLO mammographic views show a radiopaque marker at the level of the palpably enlarged left axillary lymph nodes. No breast parenchymal abnormality was recognized prospectively. R, right; L, left.

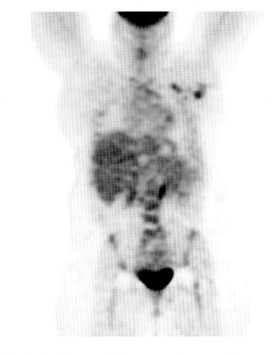

FIGURE 2. Coronal PET section shows multiple metabolically active left axillary lymph nodes.

*Case from: Kipper MS, Tartar M. Case 3. In *Clinical Atlas of PET*. Philadelphia: Saunders, 2004.

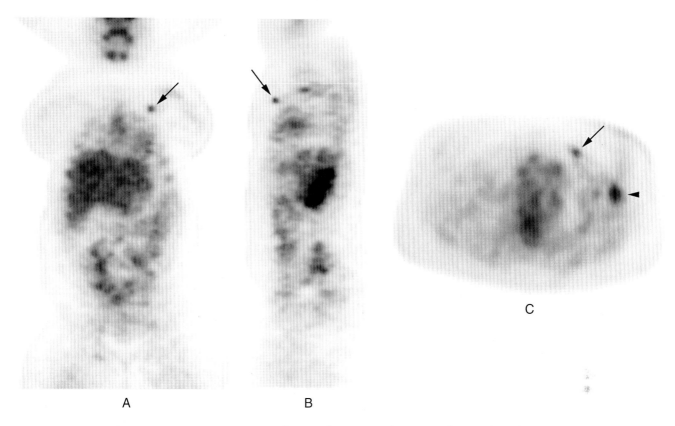

FIGURE 3.   A more anterior coronal (**A**) and corresponding sagittal (**B**) and axial (**C**) sections show a separate hypermetabolic nodule in the left breast upper inner quadrant (*arrows*). The axial slice also visualizes one of the hypermetabolic axillary lymph nodes (*arrowhead*).

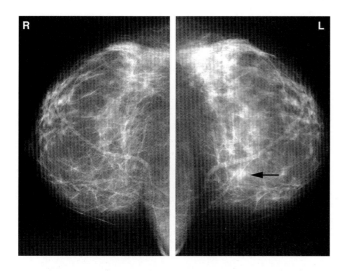

FIGURE 4.   The patient's mammogram was re-reviewed with the PET information for correlation. On the craniocaudal views, a neodensity is visualized in the medial breast, new from the prior study (*arrow*). R, right; L, left.

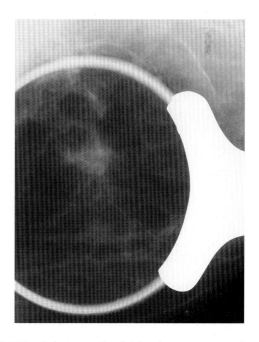

FIGURE 5.   Subsequently obtained spot compression view in craniocaudal projection shows suspicious features, with noncompressibility of the neodensity, irregular margins, and spiculation.

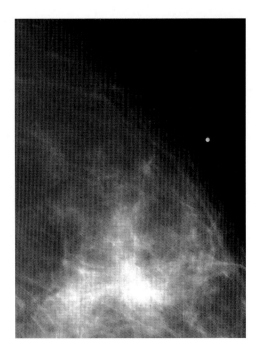

FIGURE 6.   Spot compression in the lateral projection also shows a mass with spiculation and architectural distortion.

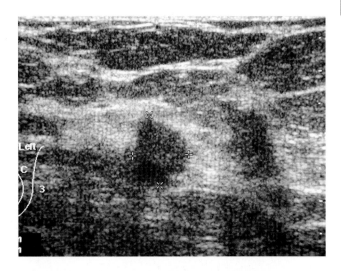

FIGURE 7.   Ultrasonography obtained before performance of ultrasound-guided core needle biopsy shows suspicious ultrasonographic characteristics. Hypoechoic 1.1-cm solid mass (*calipers*) is taller than wide, with irregular margins and no capsule.

workup, enhanced breast MRI could have been considered as an appropriate next step in the imaging pursuit of this highly persuasive PET scan abnormality.

CASE 13

Axillary nodal presentation with initially negative mammogram, medial primary found on CT

A 52-year-old woman presented to her physician with a palpable right axillary lymph node. Fine-needle aspiration of the lymph node revealed an adenocarcinoma. To search for a primary breast carcinoma as the source of the right axillary metastasis, a mammogram was performed. The mammogram showed the abnormal right axillary adenopathy, but no evidence of a primary breast carcinoma (Figures 1 and 2). The patient under-

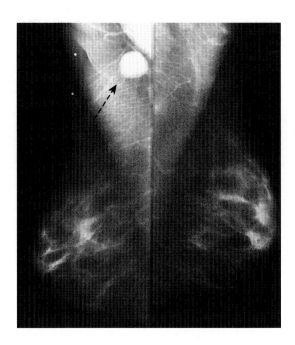

FIGURE 1.   Bilateral MLO mammographic views: The breasts are mixed fat and fibroglandular density. There is an enlarged, dense, abnormal right axillary lymph node (*arrow*).

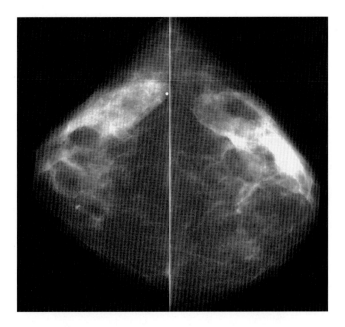

FIGURE 2.   Bilateral CC mammographic views: No obvious abnormalities are seen to suggest a source for the abnormal lymph node.

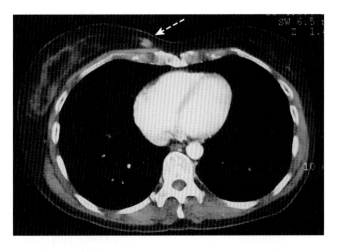

FIGURE 3.   Axial image from a contrast-enhanced CT scan of the thorax shows a small enhancing lesion in the far medial aspect of the right breast (*arrow*).

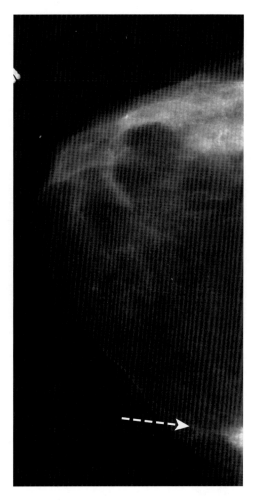

FIGURE 4.   Medial exaggerated CC mammographic view: Corresponding to the lesion seen on CT, there is an irregular, dense mass in the far posteromedial right breast.

went subsequent staging CT scan of the thorax. A small enhancing lesion was seen on the CT scan in the far medial right breast (Figure 3). Additional mammographic views were performed, including a medial exaggerated CC view (Figure 4). At the far posteromedial breast, a small irregular mass was identified, corresponding to the lesion on CT. Targeted ultrasound demonstrated a solid mass (Figure 5). Subsequent core needle biopsy confirmed an intermediate-grade invasive ductal carcinoma. The patient was treated with lumpectomy, axillary node dissection, and chemotherapy.

TEACHING POINTS

This case demonstrates the limitations of routine mammography. There can be a significant amount of breast tissue that is not routinely imaged on standard CC and MLO views. In this case, a lesion in the far medial right breast was not included on either the CC or MLO views because of its far posterior location. Ultrasound and MRI may be useful adjuvant tools when evaluating patients with an axillary metastasis of unknown origin. This primary breast carcinoma was incidentally detected on staging CT of the thorax.

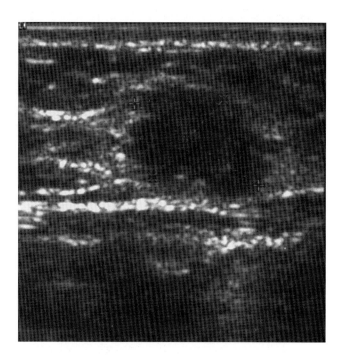

FIGURE 5. Ultrasound of the right breast: An irregular, hypoechoic solid mass is seen in the medial right breast, corresponding to the mammogram and CT.

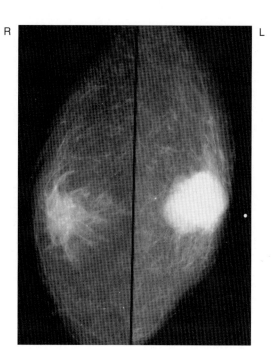

FIGURE 1. Bilateral CC mammographic views show an obvious mass in the subareolar region of the left breast. Within the subareolar right breast is a small amount of normal-appearing glandular tissue, consistent with gynecomastia.

CASE 14

Male breast cancer and gynecomastia

A 70-year-old man presented with a palpable mass in the subareolar left breast. Standard mammographic views showed a dense mass in the subareolar region, corresponding to the palpable lump (Figures 1 and 2). In the contralateral breast, gynecomastia was noted. Ultrasound confirmed the palpable finding in the left breast to be a solid, lobular mass (Figure 3). Subsequent core needle biopsy confirmed an invasive ductal carcinoma.

TEACHING POINTS

Male breast cancer is uncommon. It accounts for less than 1% of all breast cancer. Family history is a known risk factor for male breast cancer. Men with a first-degree relative with breast cancer have up to a 4 times increased risk for breast cancer.

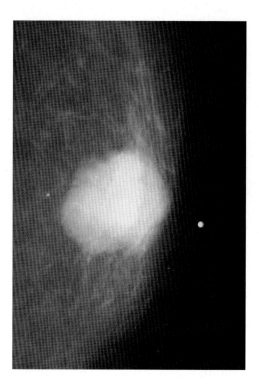

FIGURE 2. Close-up CC view of the left breast: In contrast to the gynecomastia in the opposite breast, the palpable finding in the subareolar left breast corresponds to a radiographically dense, space-occupying mass exhibiting irregular and convex margins.

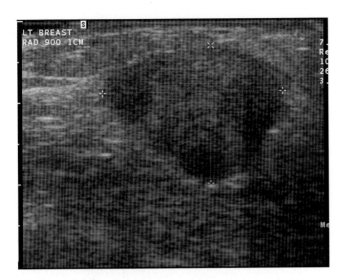

FIGURE 3. Ultrasound image of the subareolar left breast: The palpable mass corresponds to a hypoechoic solid mass with lobular margins.

Most male breast cancers are hormone sensitive, and estrogen is implicated as an etiologic agent in some cases. Known risk factors include *BRCA2* gene mutation, Klinefelter's syndrome (extra X chromosome, associated with testicular insufficiency and gynecomastia), and radiation exposure at a young age. Other risk factors include age, estrogen therapy for prostate cancer or gender reassignment, diseases associated with hyperestrogenism (e.g., liver disease), and conditions resulting in androgen deficiency (testicular dysfunction). Although a correlation between gynecomastia and male breast cancer has been suspected, with up to 40% of male breast cancer patients having gynecomastia, histologic progression from gynecomastia to cancer has never been demonstrated.

Most male breast cancer patients present with a palpable lump. Imaging of the male with symptoms of a palpable lump, breast enlargement or tenderness, or nipple discharge or bleeding begins with mammography, supplemented as necessary with ultrasound. Most male patients evaluated with mammography for breast symptoms have benign findings, most often gynecomastia, which can be accurately diagnosed with mammography. If the mammographic findings are not characteristic of gynecomastia, ultrasound can be helpful as a next step in the imaging evaluation. The potential for gynecomastia to obscure an underlying mass has been noted in the literature.

Identification of a subareolar mass at mammography or ultrasound is suspicious for malignancy, particularly if it is eccentric in relation to the nipple. Solid and complex cystic masses should undergo histologic sampling. A complex cystic lesion on ultrasound suggests the diagnosis of papillary ductal carcinoma in situ. To make the diagnosis, core needle biopsy of any solid component is more reliable than cytologic evaluation of a fluid component.

Microcalcifications are a less common manifestation of malignancy in men. When seen, they are most often in association with a mass, and their appearance may be more coarse and benign than malignant microcalcifications seen in women.

Because the axilla is involved in up to 50% of cases of male breast cancer, the axilla should be carefully scrutinized with mammography and ultrasound when suspicious imaging findings of the breast are identified in a male patient. Morakkabati-Spitz and colleagues have shown that the same techniques and interpretation criteria, although not likely to be necessary very often, can be applied to performance of breast MRI in men, in those rare cases in which there is continued clinical or imaging ambiguity after conventional imaging.

As in this case, essentially all male breast cancers are ductal. Although virtually every type of breast cancer occurring in women has been reported in men, there generally is no lobular development in men, and lobular carcinomas in men are extremely rare.

As in female breast cancer, the single most important prognostic factor is the status of the axilla. Tamoxifen is the most widely used adjuvant hormonal therapy for male breast cancer, with data available showing improved survival and improved disease-free survival compared with controls.

This case demonstrates the typical mammographic appearance of gynecomastia on one side, with a typical appearance of male breast cancer on the other. In contrast to gynecomastia, which presents as an area of subareolar fan-like or flame-edged, non-mass-like tissue density, the palpable left breast cancer in this case presents as a solid, space-occupying dense mass.

SUGGESTED READING

Jackson VP, Gilmor RL. Male breast carcinoma and gynecomastia: comparison of mammography with sonography. *Radiology* 1983; 149:533–536.

Male breast cancer with microcalcifications

A 42-year-old man presented with a palpable mass in the upper outer left breast. Mammographic views showed an area of asymmetric density with associated microcalcifications in the upper outer left breast in the area of the palpable lump (Figures 1 and 2). Ultrasound evaluation identified a solid mass corresponding to the palpable mass (Figure 3). Subsequent core needle biopsy revealed an

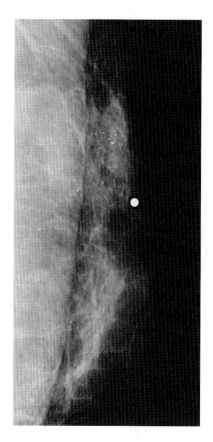

FIGURE 2. Left breast CC magnification mammographic view. On closer examination, the calcifications in the left breast are loosely grouped but display suspicious pleomorphism.

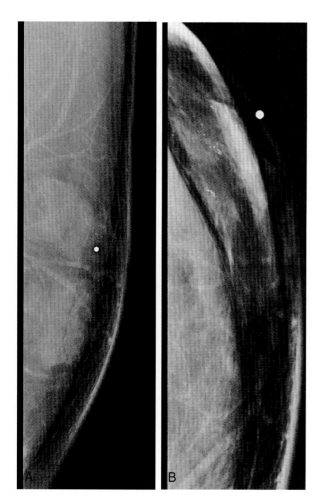

FIGURE 1. Left breast MLO (**A**) and CC (**B**) mammographic views show an area of increased tissue density with associated microcalcifications in the upper outer left breast, at the level of the palpable lump (indicated by radiopaque marker).

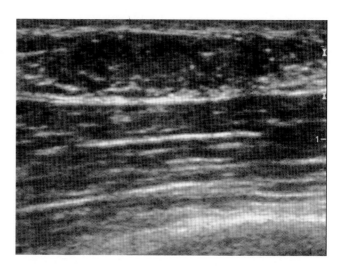

FIGURE 3. Ultrasound image of the upper outer left breast palpable lump: There is an ill-defined solid mass with associated microcalcifications.

invasive ductal carcinoma and associated ductal carcinoma in situ.

TEACHING POINTS

This case illustrates an example of male breast cancer with associated microcalcifications. Male breast cancer usually manifests as a firm, painless mass in the subareolar region that is eccentric to the nipple. Although uncommon, calcifications may be seen in male breast cancer. The calcifica-tions may be large, pleomorphic, and scattered. Seeing any microcalcifications in a symptomatic or high-risk man should heighten suspicion because malignant microcalcifications in men may be more benign in appearance and distribution than in women.

SUGGESTED READING

Langlands A, Maclean N, Kerr G. Carcinoma of the male breast: Report of a series of 88 cases. *Clin Radiol* 1976; 27:21–25.

CHAPTER 3

Local Staging: Imaging Options and Core Biopsy Strategies

Treatment planning for newly diagnosed breast cancer patients, including local and systemic therapies, is based on tumor type, extent of disease, and accurate staging. Imaging and image-directed needle biopsies play a critical role in establishing the local extent of disease and aid in staging. Surgical decision making, between breast-conserving therapy (also termed lumpectomy or segmental or partial mastectomy) and mastectomy, is primarily based on tumor size, extent and location within the breast, cosmetic implications, and patient preference. Imaging modalities, including mammography, ultrasound, MRI, and molecular imaging, are used to determine the extent of disease. However, disease extent cannot be reliably established solely by imaging. When preoperative imaging suggests more extensive disease than clinical impressions, histologic confirmation is necessary before performing a more extensive surgery.

Imaging is used to locally stage breast cancer. The TNM stage is based on the size of the tumor and whether the cancer has spread (Table 1). Identification of abnormal adenopathy (axillary, supraclavicular, or internal mammary nodes), as well as involvement of the skin, pectoralis muscle, or chest wall, affects staging and therapeutic decision making. Options for local therapies include surgery and radiation therapy, whereas systemic treatments may include chemotherapy, hormone therapy, and biologic therapy. Imaging also is used to identify distant metastases.

Selection of the appropriate imaging tests to determine tumor extent and stage are not standardized and are often based on the particulars of each case.

EXTENT OF DISEASE

Most breast cancers are evaluated by mammography, ultrasound, or both modalities. It is important to document the size, location, and distribution of the primary lesion, but also to evaluate for satellite lesions. Preoperative identification of additional lesions improves the likelihood of obtaining clear margins if breast-conserving therapy (BCT) is performed. For masses, it is important to look for associated microcalcifications, which may represent an associated noninvasive (in situ) component. The term *extensive intraductal component* (EIC) is used to refer to invasive tumors in which ductal carcinoma in situ (DCIS) makes up at least 25% of the neoplasm. Of all invasive ductal carcinomas, 15% to 30% have an EIC.[1] Tumors that are predominantly DCIS with focal invasion are also classified as EIC. The presence of EIC may have prognostic implications on the likelihood of obtaining clear margins, as well as the risk for subsequent local recurrence.[2,3]

As many as 30% to 60% of breast cancers are pathologically multifocal (more than one tumor focus, separated by normal tissue) at the time of diagnosis.[4,5] The term multicentric has been variably defined. It generally has been used to describe cancers separated by more than 4 cm or tumors located in different quadrants of the breast. BCT generally is not suitable for multicentric carcinomas because of poor cosmetic results, limitations of radiation therapy, and inability to obtain clear margins.

Synchronous contralateral breast cancer may occur in about 3% to 5% of women with breast cancer.[6,7] Identification of these lesions at the time of the contralateral index cancer diagnosis can facilitate treatment in a single surgery, thereby avoiding both delays in diagnosis, as well as the emotional stress of a later diagnosis and second surgery.

MRI is useful to identify residual disease and direct re-excision in patients with positive margins at initial lumpectomy (Figure 1).

EVALUATING ADENOPATHY

Identification of abnormal adenopathy, including axillary, supraclavicular, and internal mammary nodes, is important in staging. Metastatic adenopathy is suspected on imaging when there is cortical thickening (generally >3 mm), loss of the fatty

Table 1 AMERICAN JOINT COMMITTEE ON CANCER STAGING SYSTEM FOR PATIENTS WITH BREAST CANCER

Primary Tumor (T)

TX	Primary tumor cannot be assessed
T0	No evidence of primary tumor
Tis	Carcinoma in situ
Tis (DCIS)	Ductal carcinoma in situ
Tis (LCIS)	Lobular carcinoma in situ
Tis (Paget's)	Paget's disease of the nipple with no tumor
TI	Tumor 2 cm or less in greatest dimension
T1mic	Microinvasion 0 to 1 cm or less in greatest dimension
T1a	0.1 to 0.5 cm
T1b	>0.5 to 1 cm
T1c	>1 to 2 cm
T2	Tumor >2 to 5 cm in greatest dimension
T3	Tumor >5 cm in greatest dimension
T4	Tumor of any size with direct extension to chest wall or skin
T4a	Extension to chest wall, not including pectoral muscle
T4b	Edema (including peau-d'orange) or ulceration of the skin of the breast, or satellite skin nodules confined to the same breast
T4c	T4a and T4b
T4d	Inflammatory carcinoma

Regional Nodes (N)

NX	Regional lymph nodes cannot be assessed (e.g., previously removed)
N0	No regional lymph node metastasis
N1	Metastasis in movable ipsilateral axillary lymph nodes
N2	Metastasis in ipsilateral axillary lymph nodes fixed or matted, or in clinically apparent ipsilateral internal mammary nodes in the *absence* of clinically evident axillary lymph node metastasis.
N2a	Metastasis in ipsilateral axillary lymph nodes fixed to one another or to other structures
N2b	Metastasis only in clinically apparent ipsilateral internal mammary nodes and in the absence of clinically evident axillary lymph node metastasis
N3	Metastasis in ipsilateral infraclavicular lymph node(s) with or without axillary lymph node involvement, or in clinically apparent ipsilateral internal mammary node(s) in the presence of clinically evident axillary lymph node metastasis; or metastasis in ipsilateral supraclavicular lymph node(s) with or without axillary or internal mammary lymph node involvement
N3a	Metastasis in ipsilateral infraclavicular lymph node(s) and axillary lymph node(s)
N3b	Metastasis in ipsilateral internal mammary lymph node(s) nodes and axillary lymph node(s)
N3c	Metastasis in ipsilateral supraclavicular lymph node(s)

Distant Metastasis (M)

MX	Distant metastasis cannot be assessed
M0	No distant metastasis
M1	Distant metastasis

hilum, and enlargement, particularly with increasingly round shapes[8] (Figures 2 and 3). However, because many benign processes may cause reactive nodes with similar imaging findings, fine-needle aspiration (FNA) or core needle biopsy is necessary to confirm suspected metastatic nodal disease. Conversely, the absence of suspicious imaging findings, whether on mammography, ultrasound, MRI, or molecular imaging studies, does not exclude metastatic nodal involvement,

particularly for micrometastasis. Therefore, in addition to imaging, sampling, either with axillary dissection or sentinel lymph node biopsy, is essential in the staging of breast cancer patients.

The axillary nodes form a chain from the underarm to the collarbone (Figure 4). The axillary lymph nodes are named in relation to the pectoralis minor muscle, with level I the lowest, lateral to the pectoralis minor muscle. Level I receives the most lymphatic drainage from the breast. Level II axillary

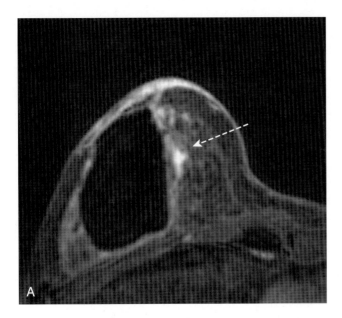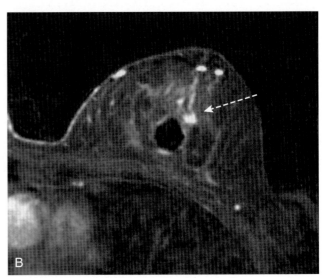

FIGURE 1. MRI evaluation can be useful in patients with close or positive surgical margins. **A**, Post-contrast, subtracted MRI of a right breast shows a focus of residual DCIS (*arrow*) along the medial aspect of a large lumpectomy cavity. **B**, Post-contrast, subtracted MRI shows residual invasive tumor (*arrow*) along the anterior lateral aspect of a small lumpectomy cavity.

nodes are beneath the pectoralis minor muscle. Level III is above and medial to the pectoralis minor muscle. A traditional axillary lymph node dissection usually removes nodes in levels I and II. Sentinel lymph node sampling involves the mapping and removal of the first lymph node or nodes (usually 1 to 3) that drain the involved area of the breast (Figures 5 and 6). Instead of removing 10 or more lymph nodes as performed in a standard dissection, the status of the axilla can be predicted by excision and close pathologic examination of the sentinel node. Sentinel lymph node biopsy has significantly reduced the number of women undergoing standard axillary dissection, avoiding dissection-associated side effects such as arm lymphedema. The identification of abnormal lymph nodes on physical exam or imaging studies favors proceeding directly to axillary dissection over sentinel node biopsy.

The use of molecular imaging studies, CT, or MRI may identify adenopathy in areas other than the axilla (Figure 7). The presence of internal mammary node adenopathy (Figure 8) affects staging and radiation therapy planning. Identification of abnormal Rotter's nodes (Figure 9), nodes between the pectoralis minor and major muscles, also has staging and therapeutic implications.

SKIN, PECTORALIS, AND CHEST WALL INVOLVEMENT

Identification of breast edema and skin thickening in patients with invasive breast cancer may represent an inflammatory component (tumor involving the dermal lymphatics). This materially affects staging and therapeutic approach. Skin punch biopsy may be necessary to confirm the diagnosis if the clinical picture is not characteristic. Identification of pectoralis muscle or chest wall involvement also affects treatment planning. Pectoralis muscle involvement should be looked for in women with posterior lesions. The diagnosis on MRI requires not just effacement or obliteration of the pectoralis fascia but also enhancement of the muscle (Figure 10). Identification of either skin or chest wall involvement classifies a tumor as a locally advanced breast carcinoma (LABC). Large (>5 cm) tumors and those with clinically matted or fixed axillary node involvement or involved supraclavicular or internal mammary nodes by imaging are also considered locally advanced. LABC is generally treated with preoperative (neoadjuvant or primary systemic) chemotherapy, which converts some patients into operative candidates. Multiple examples are presented in Chapter 5.

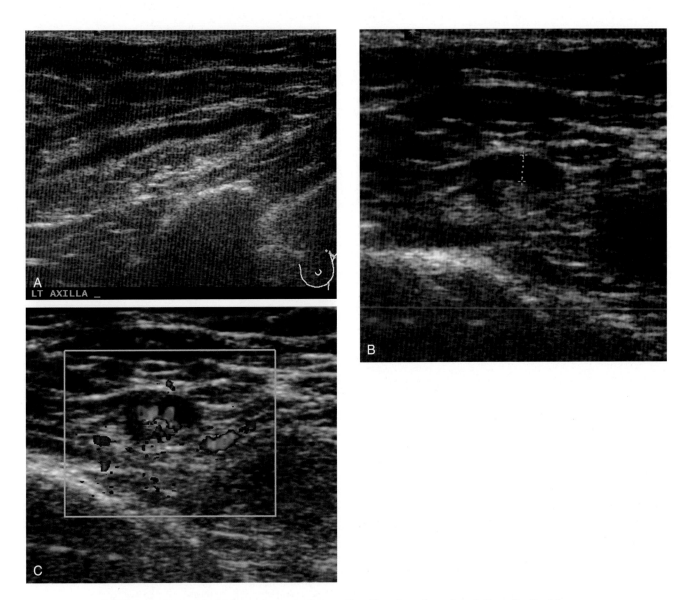

FIGURE 2.   Sonographic appearance of normal axillary lymph nodes. **A**, Longitudinal image shows uniform thickness of the hypoechoic cortex, surrounding the echogenic fatty hilus. **B**, Transverse image of the same lymph node. The cortical thickness of 2 mm is within normal limits (<3 mm). **C**, Color Doppler image shows vascularity in the hilus.

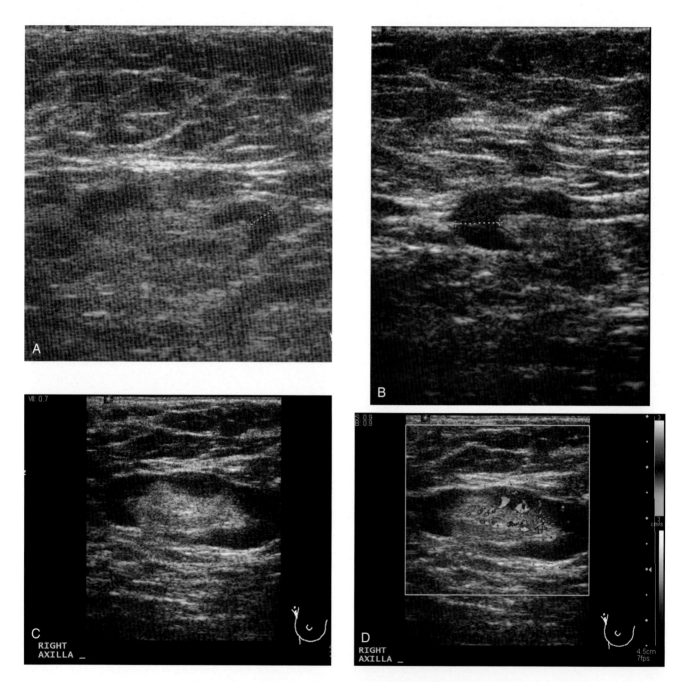

FIGURE 3.   The spectrum of abnormal axillary node sonographic findings (all FNA-proven to have breast cancer metastases). **A,** Cursors delineate borderline thickening of the hypoechoic cortex. The fatty hilus is preserved. A second, similar-appearing axillary lymph node is seen to the left. These findings are not clearly pathologic by sonographic criteria. Subtle findings on staging MRI, CT, and positron emission tomography (PET) studies (for inflammatory breast cancer) suggested axillary involvement. FNA confirmed metastatic carcinoma. **B,** Cortical thickening in this case is more eccentric and measures 5 mm. Ultrasound-guided FNA of the axillary lymph node confirmed metastatic carcinoma. **C,** Axillary node sonography of a 55-year-old woman with locally advanced breast cancer (LABC) shows highly suspicious morphology. The cortex is very hypoechoic, as well as abnormally thickened and nodular. There is a rat-bite, scalloped appearance and mass effect on the echogenic hilus. **D,** Same case as **C,** with color Doppler. Increased and abnormal vascularity is seen. Normal lymph node vascularity is seen only at the hilus.

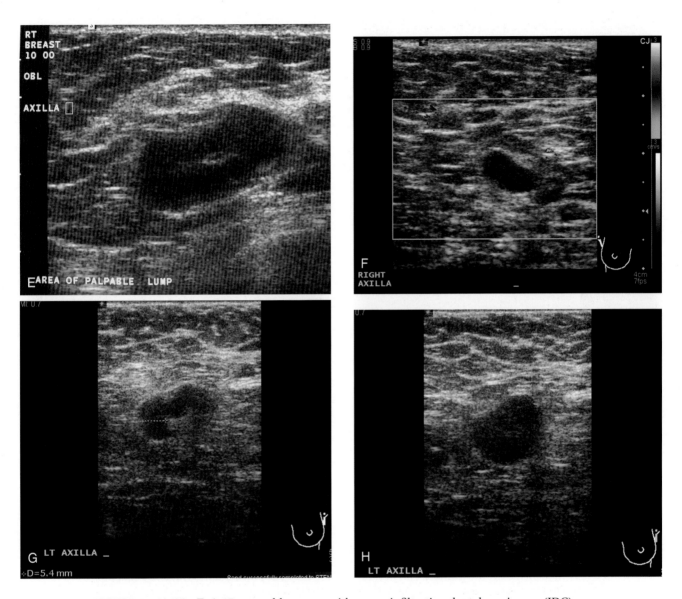

FIGURE 3, cont'd   **E,** A 45-year-old woman with a new infiltrating ductal carcinoma (IDC) diagnosis. The cortical mantle of this axillary lymph node is markedly thickened, and the echogenic hilus is nearly completely effaced. **F,** Although small, this axillary node morphology is quite abnormal. The cortex is very hypoechoic. The node is "thick-waisted," with nearly complete effacement of the fatty hilus, which is hinted at in profile. **G,** A 56-year-old woman with a neglected LABC (IDC with secondary inflammation) and multiple abnormal axillary nodes, which were FDG-avid on PET. This lymph node shows diffuse cortical thickening, without hilar effacement. **H,** Another lymph node of the same patient shows complete hilar loss and an abnormally rounded shape.

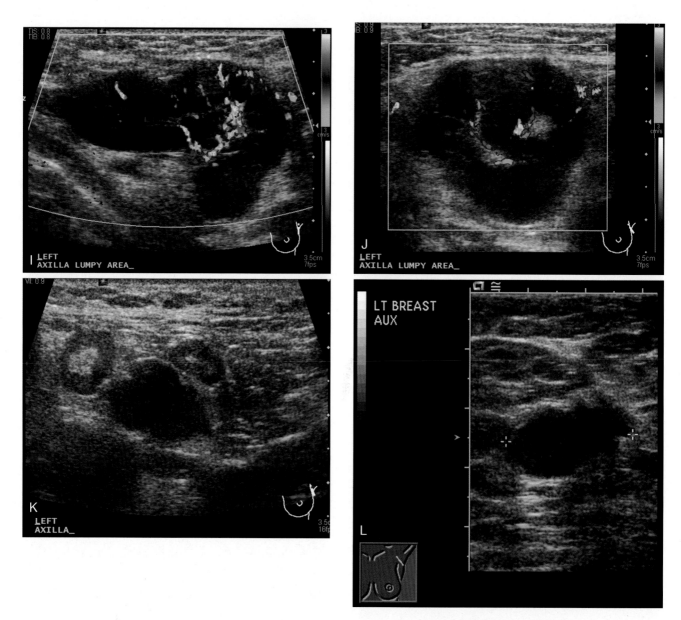

FIGURE 3, cont'd   I, A 41-year-old woman with a large postpartum pregnancy-associated breast cancer. This lymph node is massively enlarged and would be considered abnormal on any modality. Size, the primary criterion for judging normalcy on CT and MRI, is a weaker criterion by which to judge axillary nodes. Other morphologic criteria, including shape, cortical thickening and nodularity, and mass effect on or effacement of the fatty hilus, are more reliable in the assessment of the axillary lymph nodes of breast cancer patients. These more subtle findings are most easily assessed with ultrasound. This lymph node shows many of these features: marked cortical hypoechogenicity, nodularity, and thickening, with partial loss of the fatty hilus. The intracortical and peripheral vascularity is highly abnormal and also suggests malignancy. **J**, The same lymph node seen transversely shows that the hilus is incompletely effaced. Echogenic remnants are seen surrounded by the grossly thickened hypoechoic cortex. The abnormally increased vascularity, seen on the periphery of the cortex, is highly suggestive of malignancy. **K**, Even more normal-appearing adjacent lymph nodes, with visible echogenic fatty hila, have borderline thickened cortices and are notable for their ease of visualization and increased number. **L**, A 49-year-old woman with newly diagnosed, node-positive (five of eight nodes, largest 1.9 cm, with extracapsular extension), 1.8-cm left breast IDC. Her preoperative ultrasound predicted the extracapsular extension. This very hypoechoic axillary lymph node shows no echogenic hilus. The left side is rounded by a cortical nodule, and the right side has frankly angular margins.

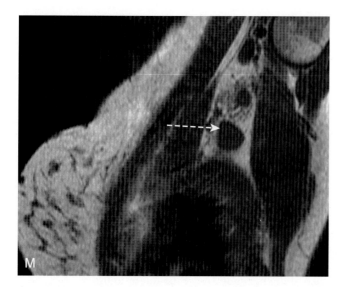

FIGURE 3, cont'd   M, Oblique, noncontrast, T1-weighted MRI of the left axilla shows an abnormal lymph node (*arrow*), notable for the loss of the fatty hilum and the rounded and expanded shape.

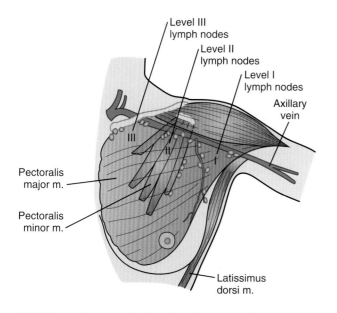

FIGURE 4. Schematic of axillary lymph node nomenclature. The axillary lymph nodes ascend from the axilla medially to the clavicle and are named in relation to the pectoralis minor muscle. Level I, the lowest, is lateral to the pectoralis minor; level II, deep to it; and level III, medial to it.

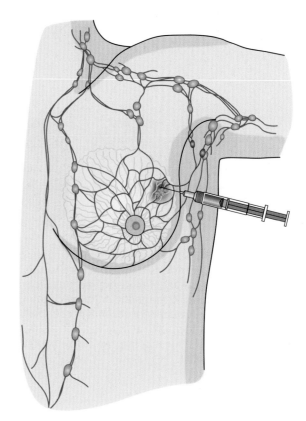

FIGURE 5. Schematic of the technique of sentinel lymph node injection. The breast lymphatics drain to the skin, and there is a rich periareolar network of lymphatics, with one or two major lymphatic channels draining to the axilla. Anatomic studies indicate 75% of the lymphatic drainage of the breast is to the axilla, with 25% to the internal mammary nodes. In this drawing, a peritumoral injection is depicted, but success has been reported for a variety of techniques (including subdermal or intradermal overlying the tumor, and periareolar), presumably owing to the rich network of the breast lymphatic plexus.

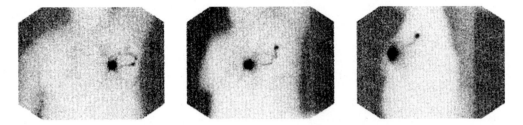

FIGURE 6.   Lymphoscintigraphy (*from left to right:* anterior, left anterior oblique, and left lateral) can be performed in conjunction with injections for sentinel lymph node identification. In this example, intense activity is seen at the injection site of the tumor in the left breast. A lymphatic drainage channel extending to the axilla is clearly delineated, as are a faint, more superior secondary channel and the axillary sentinel lymph node. If a sentinel node is identified at imaging, skin marking can save surgical dissection time. Breast cancer sentinel node mapping with lymphoscintigraphy is not universally performed, unlike in melanoma.

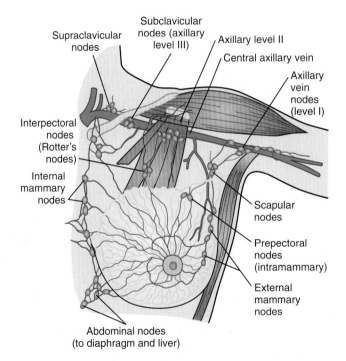

FIGURE 7.   Schematic of the lymphatic drainage pathways of the breast. By anatomic studies, 75% of the lymphatic drainage is to the axilla, with 25% to the ipsilateral internal mammary nodes. Note lymphatic communications extending across the midline of the chest to contralateral internal mammary nodes and inferiorly extending channels, which communicate with the abdomen.

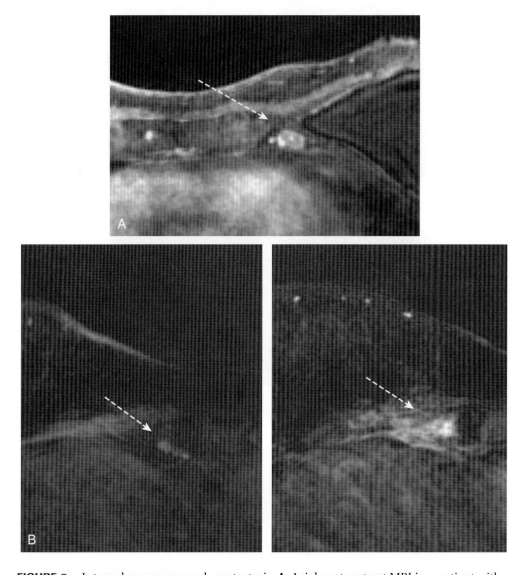

FIGURE 8. Internal mammary node metastasis. **A**, Axial postcontrast MRI in a patient with an implant with an abnormally enlarged left internal mammary node (*arrow*) adjacent to the internal mammary artery and vein, suspicious for involvement. **B**, Axial postcontrast MRI shows a small (2–3 mm) right internal mammary node (*left*). The same area, 5 years later, has a chest wall recurrence (*arrow*), presumably from metastasis to the internal mammary node (*right*).

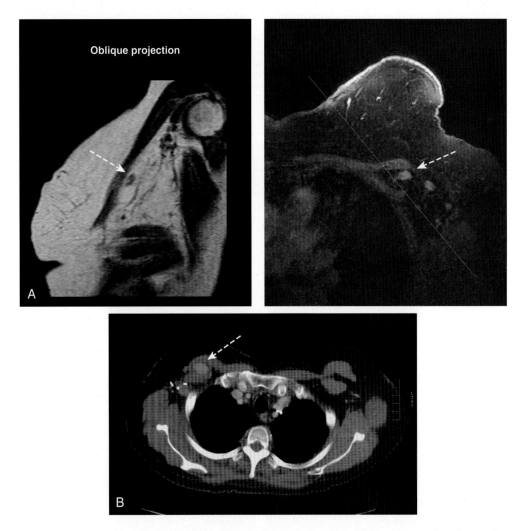

FIGURE 9.   Rotter's nodes. **A**, Oblique T1-weighted (*left*) and axial fat-saturated, enhanced T1-weighted (*right*) MRIs of the left axilla show a small Rotter's node (*arrows*) between the pectoralis major and pectoralis minor muscles. **B**, Enhanced CT scan demonstrates a metastasis to a large Rotter's node (*arrow*), as well as within the right axilla.

PREOPERATIVE MAGNETIC RESONANCE IMAGING

MRI is becoming increasingly established as a useful modality in patients with known breast cancer. However, patterns of use of preoperative MRI in women with biopsy-proven breast cancer remain highly variable in practice because of the lack of randomized control trials. It has been firmly established that preoperative MRI can detect unsuspected disease and often changes management in women with known breast cancer.[9] However, the use of preoperative MRI to alter surgical management has been criticized because of the lack of studies evaluating its effect on tumor recurrence and mortality.[10–12] Fischer and col-

leagues,[13] in a study involving more than 40 months of follow-up, reported a reduction in ipsilateral breast tumor recurrence, from 6.8% to 1.2%, in patients who underwent preoperative MRI. However, this study was a retrospective, single-institution review of only 346 patients. It has been argued that unsuspected disease detected on MRI and treated with BCT is of little clinical consequence and is controlled by radiation therapy. This argument is primarily based on the fact that 10-year local recurrence rates as low as 10% have been reported in patients with negative surgical margins.[14–16] Concerns about the use of preoperative MRI involve the potential for unnecessary biopsies, delays in treatment, and an increase in unnecessary mastectomies. Despite these arguments, there is ongoing evidence and experience

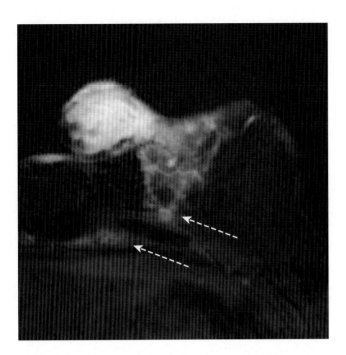

FIGURE 10. Chest wall invasion. Postcontrast axial MRI in a patient with a breast sarcoma, demonstrating enhancement of the pectoralis major muscle and intercostal muscles (*arrows*). Chest wall involvement is confirmed by identification of intercostal muscle enhancement, whereas the pectoralis muscle is considered part of the breast.

accumulating that supports its benefit in preoperative staging, as follows:

1. Although no randomized controlled trials have been performed, preoperative MRI has the potential to reduce recurrences in many patients. Recurrence rates overall are very low; however, higher recurrence rates have been reported in select patients, such as those with high-grade DCIS.[17] In addition, recurrence rates as high as 35% have been reported in younger women and in women who do not undergo radiation therapy.[18] With the increasing use of partial-breast irradiation, it will be important to monitor the recurrence rates in patients thus treated, to compare with established rates for whole-breast irradiation. Preoperative MRI may prove essential to identify patients likely to fail partial-breast irradiation because of the presence of occult disease outside of the local radiation field.

2. Preoperative MRI may help to improve surgical outcomes. The previously reported low breast cancer recurrence rates following BCT are based on patients with negative surgical margins. In the United States, the number of women requiring multiple surgeries to obtain clear margins is significant. Positive margin rates at initial lumpectomy may be as high as 40%.[19] By better defining tumor extent and providing three-dimensional information, MRI can potentially improve surgical outcomes and decrease positive margin rates.

3. In addition to better defining disease extent, preoperative MRI can improve treatment planning in other ways. By demonstrating abnormal axillary adenopathy, MRI can help to identify patients who may be better served by standard axillary dissection, rather than sentinel node biopsy. Surgical planning may also be altered in patients in whom MRI demonstrates pectoralis or chest wall involvement. MRI also has the ability to demonstrate abnormal internal mammary nodes, information that may be incorporated in radiation therapy planning.

4. Preoperative MRI has the ability to detect mammographically and clinically occult carcinoma in the contralateral breast in 3% to 5% of patients.[7,20] Failure to detect these cancers at the time of initial diagnosis exposes the patient to potential risks associated with repeat general anesthesia and surgery, as well as possible delays in diagnosis. In addition, the psychological toll of dealing with a second cancer diagnosis in the opposite breast is not insignificant.

These benefits, although individually small, together have the potential to positively affect a significant number of patients. Preoperative MRI can improve surgical clear margin rates, guide surgical and radiation therapy planning, detect occult contralateral cancers, and potentially reduce recurrences. However, the number of false-positive results and delays in treatment needs to be minimized. Other breast imaging studies, such as mammography and ultrasound, must be correlated with the MRI findings to provide the most accurate interpretation and appropriate recommendations.

FUNCTIONAL (MOLECULAR) BREAST IMAGING: BREAST-SPECIFIC GAMMA IMAGING AND POSITRON EMISSION MAMMOGRAPHY

Functional breast imaging is a growing and evolving field that is assuming a larger role in breast cancer diagnosis, providing complementary information to anatomically based breast imaging modalities. Scintimammography has matured from initial versions using standard gamma cameras, which were limited in resolution and positioning flexibility, to breast-specific gamma imaging (BSGI), which obtains higher-resolution planar images in views emulating mammography.[21–25] Similarly, positron emission mammography (PEM) is performed using a small-field-of-view, high-resolution PET scanner that resembles a mammogram unit and acquires tomographic data sets in planes analogous to mammography.[26–29] Scintimammography is performed after the intravenous administration of 25 mCi of either ^{99m}Tc-sestamibi or ^{99m}Tc-tetrofosmin, whereas PEM is performed after an hour's uptake of 10 mCi of ^{18}F-fluorodeoxyglucose (FDG) administered intravenously. The radiation dose is about the same, about 0.4 rad. Imaging time is also similar. Scintimammography planar views are acquired for 5 to 10 minutes, or at least 150,000 counts, whereas PEM tomographic data sets are acquired for 4 to 10 minutes per projection. The lower limit of BSGI detector resolution is 3 mm (although smaller lesions may be identifiable), whereas the in plane resolution of PEM is on the order of 2 mm (Table 2).

The uptake of sestamibi is dependent on regional blood flow and cellular mitochondrial density. Enhanced blood flow due to tumor-induced neo-angiogenesis results in increased delivery of radiopharmaceutical. Cancer cells have higher cytoplasmic mitochondrial density than normal breast tissue and bind more of the radiopharmaceutical than the surrounding tissue.

PEM is performed with ^{18}F-FDG, a radioactive glucose analogue in wide use as a cancer-imaging agent with whole-body PET. PEM and PET with FDG capitalize on the higher glycolytic rate of cancer cells, with FDG actively transported intracellularly through an up-regulated transmembrane GLUT-1 receptor mechanism. Once intracellular, FDG is phosphorylated by hexokinase like glucose, but because it is not metabolized further, it is trapped intracellularly in proportion to glucose utilization.

At this writing, BSGI is becoming more available, with sites with early experience finding it useful both for problem solving of ambiguous conventional breast imaging findings, and as an adjunct to local staging, looking for multifocality, multicentricity, and contralateral lesions (Figure 11). BSGI does not require a diagnosis of

Table 2 FUNCTIONAL BREAST IMAGING COMPARISON CHART

	BSGI	PEM
Radiopharmaceutical	^{99m}Tc-sestamibi (Miraluma) (^{99m}Tc-methoxyisobutylisonitrile)	^{18}F-FDG (2-[fluorine-18] fluoro-2-deoxy-D-glucose
Half-life	6 hr	110 min
Emission energy	140 keV	511 keV
Dose	25 mCi	10 mCi
Sensitivity	85%–93% (scintimammography) >90% (BSGI)	91%
Specificity	87%–89%	93%
Whole-body dosimetry	About 0.4 rad	About 0.4 rad
Acquisition	Planar	Tomographic
Binding target	Intracellular mitochondria	Intracellularly phosphorylated by hexokinase
Theoretical basis	Cancer cells have greater cytoplasmic mitochondrial density than normal breast	Higher glycolytic rate of cancer cells results in increased cellular uptake and glucose utilization
Negative predictive value (NPV)	82%–98% (scintimammography) 90%–100% (BSGI)	88%
Target population	Suspicion of breast abnormality (breast cancer diagnosis not required)	Approved for patients with known or past history of breast cancer
Mechanism of cellular transport	Passive diffusion through potassium channels	Active transport into cell
Lower limit of resolution	3-mm detector spatial resolution	2 mm

BSGI, breast-specific gamma imaging; PEM, positron emission mammography.

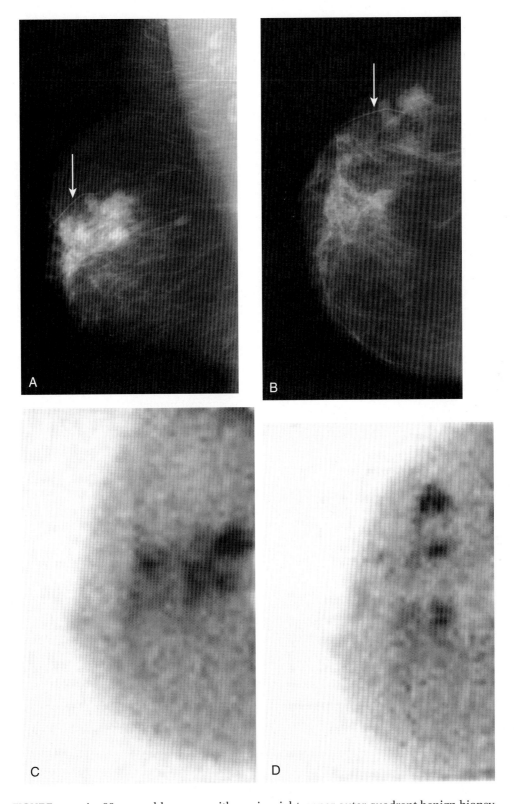

FIGURE 11.   An 89-year-old woman with a prior right upper outer quadrant benign biopsy (scar marked on mammographic views (*arrows*)—**A**, MLO; **B**, CC). Multiple lobular and circumscribed masses are seen within moderately dense breast tissue, especially in the upper outer quadrant near the scar. Ultrasound of the corresponding area suggested two cysts and one solid mass, for which biopsy was recommended. Breast-specific gamma imaging (BSGI) (**C**, MLO; **D**, CC) shows multifocal upper outer quadrant increased activity, with three discrete sites of increased uptake. At surgical pathology, a multilobed mucinous carcinoma, with ductal carcinoma in situ was confirmed. *(Case courtesy of Dilon Technologies)*

breast cancer for reimbursement, and increasingly is being performed in patients with suspicious conventional breast imaging findings as an aid to biopsy decision making (e.g., deciding how many areas need sampling). Currently, PEM is approved for patients with known or prior breast cancer diagnoses. Several cases incorporating the use of PEM have been included in this chapter. Its performance compared with MRI in preoperative local staging of apparently localized breast cancer is being assessed by a multicenter, prospective clinical trial, which at this writing is accruing patients. Early pilot studies show high sensitivity for depiction of primary breast cancers, on the order of 91%. Similarly high sensitivity for primary tumor depiction is reported for BSGI. Both modes of functional breast imaging appear to have improved specificity compared with MRI, on the order of 87% to 89% for BSGI and 93% for PEM, offering hope that increased use of functional breast imaging in the future may decrease the number of unnecessary benign biopsies now being performed.

Currently, no biopsy capability using functional imaging modalities for guidance is readily available, although feasibility studies have been done and this should be available in the near future.

DISTANT METASTASES

Routine imaging with bone scan, CT, and PET is not indicated for early-stage (stage I and II) breast cancers. Patients with limited-stage breast cancer who have symptoms, such as back or bone pain, or right upper quadrant pain; physical examination abnormalities (such as jaundice or hepatomegaly), or laboratory abnormalities can be considered for imaging to exclude distant metastatic disease. Patients with locally advanced breast cancer or evidence of axillary nodal involvement by physical examination or imaging should be considered for systemic imaging after a detailed history, physical exam, and laboratory evaluation.

REFERENCES

1. van Dongen JA, Fentiman IS, Harris JR, et al. In situ breast cancer: the EORTC consensus meeting. *Lancet* 1989; 2:25–27.
2. Schnitt SJ, Connolly JL, Recht A, et al. Breast relapse following primary radiation therapy for early breast cancer. II. Detection, pathologic features and prognostic significance. *Int J Radiat Oncol Biol Phys* 1985; 11:1277–1284.
3. Bartelink H, Borger JH, van Dongen JA, Peterse JL. The impact of tumor size and histology on local control after breast conserving treatment. *Radiother Oncol* 1988; 11:297–303.
4. Holland R, Veling SH, Mravunac M, Hendricks JH. Histologic multifocality of Tis, T1–2 breast carcinomas: implications for clinical trials of breast conserving surgery. *Cancer* 1985; 56:979–990.
5. Wilkinson LS, Given-Wilson R, Hall T, et al. Increasing the diagnosis of multifocal primary breast cancer by the use of bilateral whole-breast ultrasound. *Clin Radiol* 2005; 60:573–578.
6. Heron DE, Komarnicky LT, Hyslop T, et al. Bilateral breast carcinoma: risk factors and outcomes for patients with synchronous and metachronous disease. *Cancer* 2000; 88:2739–2750.
7. Liberman L, Morris EA, Kim CM, et al. MR imaging findings in the contralateral breast of women with recently diagnosed breast cancer. *AJR Am J Roentgenol* 2003; 180:333–341.
8. Yang WT, Chang J, Metreweli C. Patients with breast cancer: differences in color Doppler flow and gray-scale US features of benign and malignant axillary lymph nodes. *Radiology* 2000; 215:568–573.
9. Bedrosian I, Mick R, Orel SG, et al. Changes in the surgical management of patients with breast carcinoma based on preoperative magnetic resonance imaging. *Cancer* 2003; 98:468–473.
10. Morrow M. Magnetic resonance imaging in the preoperative evaluation of breast cancer: primum non nocere. *J Am Coll Surg* 2004; 198:240–241.
11. Morrow M. Magnetic resonance imaging in breast cancer: one step forward, two steps back? *JAMA* 2004; 292:2779–2780.
12. Morrow M. Magnetic resonance imaging in breast cancer: is seeing always believing? *Eur J Cancer* 2005; 41:1368–1369.
13. Fischer U, Zachariae O, Baum F, et al. The influence of preoperative MRI of the breasts on recurrence rate in patients with breast cancer. *Eur Radiol* 2004; 14:1725–1731.
14. Smitt MC, Nowels KW, Zdeblick MJ, et al. The importance of the lumpectomy surgical margin status in long-term results of breast conservation. *Cancer* 1995; 76:259–267.
15. Neuschatz AC, DiPetrillo T, Safaii H, et al. Long-term follow-up of a prospective policy of margin-directed radiation dose escalation in breast-conserving therapy. *Cancer* 2003; 97:30–39.
16. Obedian E, Haffty BG. Negative margin status improves local control in conservatively managed breast cancer patients. *Cancer J Sci Am* 2000; 6:28–33.
17. Provenzano E, Hopper JL, Giles GG, et al. Histological markers that predict clinical recurrence in ductal carcinoma in situ of the breast: an Australian population-based study. *Pathology* 2004; 36:221–229.
18. Borg MF. Breast-conserving therapy in young women with invasive carcinoma of the breast. *Australas Radiol* 2004; 48:376–382.

19. Smitt MC, MD, Horst K. Association of clinical and pathologic variables with lumpectomy surgical margin status after preoperative diagnosis or excisional biopsy of invasive breast cancer. *Ann Surg Oncol* 2007; 14(3):1040–1044.
20. Lehman CD, Gatsonis C, Kuhl CK, et al. ACRIN Trial 6667 Investigators Group. MRI evaluation of the contralateral breast in women with recently diagnosed breast cancer. *N Engl J Med* 2007; 356(13):1295–1303.
21. Schillaci O, Buscombe JR. Breast scintigraphy today: indications and limitations. *Eur J Nucl Med Mol Imaging* 2004; 31(Suppl 1):S35–45.
22. Brem RF, Schoonjans JM, Kieper DA, et al. High-resolution scintimammography: a pilot study. *J Nucl Med* 2002; 43:909–915.
23. Brem RF, Rapelyea JA, Zisman G, et al. Occult breast cancer: scintimammography with high-resolution breast-specific gamma camera in women at high risk for breast cancer. *Radiology* 2005; 237:274–280.
24. Brem RF, Fishman M, Rapelyea JA. Detection of ductal carcinoma in situ with mammography, breast specific gamma imaging, and magnetic resonance imaging: a comparative study. *Acad Radiol* 2007; 14(8):945–950.
25. Brem RF, Petrovitch I, Rapelyea JA, et al. Breast-specific gamma imaging with (99m) Tc-sestamibi and magnetic resonance imaging in the diagnosis of breast cancer: a comparative study. *Breast J* 2007; 13(5):465–469.
26. Levine EA, Freimanis RI, Perrier ND, et al. Positron emission mammography: initial clinical results. *Ann Surg Oncol* 2003; 10:86–91.
27. Rosen EL, Turkington TG, Soo MS, et al. Detection of primary breast carcinoma with a dedicated, large-field-of-view FDG pet mammography device: initial experience. *Radiology* 2005; 234:527–534.
28. Berg WA, Weinberg IN, Narayanan D, et al. High-resolution fluorodeoxyglucose positron emission tomography with compression ("positron emission mammography") is highly accurate in depicting primary breast cancer. *Breast J* 2006; 12(4):309–323.
29. Tafra L, Cheng Z, Uddo J, et al. Pilot clinical trial of 18F-fluorodeoxyglucose positron-emission mammography in the surgical management of breast cancer. *Am J Surg* 2005; 190(4):628–632.

CASE 1

Mammography: Extent of disease

A 75-year-old woman presented with a palpable left breast mass. Mammography demonstrated a dense, spiculated breast cancer, corresponding to the palpable mass (Figure 1). Closer review of the mammogram showed a second abnormality distant from the palpable mass, with suspicious linear microcalcifications in the central left breast (Figure 2). Biopsy of the mass revealed invasive ductal carcinoma and stereotactic biopsy of the calcification found intermediate-grade ductal carcinoma in situ (DCIS). Because the two areas of disease involved a large portion of the left breast, mastectomy was performed.

TEACHING POINTS

Breast imagers need to constantly guard against "satisfaction of search." By fully defining the extent of disease, the appropriate surgical therapy can be planned. The occurrence of synchronous ipsilateral or bilateral breast cancer is about 3% to 5%. For localized breast cancer, the 20-year follow-up reports of two pivotal prospective randomized trials demonstrated that survival after a lumpec-

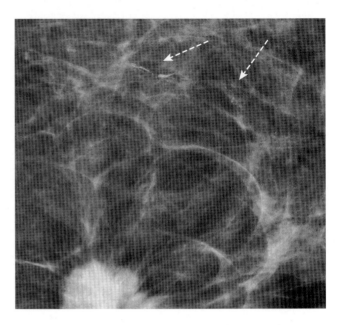

FIGURE 2. Close-up view of the CC mammographic view: An area of suspicious linear microcalcifications is seen (*arrows*) in the central breast, distant from the palpable mass. These calcifications exhibit classic linear and casting features of DCIS.

tomy with radiotherapy is equal to survival after mastectomy. However, these studies are based on patients in whom clear margins were obtained. By better defining the extent of disease preoperatively, the likelihood of obtaining clear margins at initial surgery can be improved. Pathologic margin status is the most important predictor of local recurrence after breast conservation with radiation. Even when clear margins are obtained, many patients have remaining foci of disease. The role of radiation therapy is to treat these areas of occult residual tumor. The risk for local recurrence may be diminished if the residual tumor burden after surgery is minimized. This is even more important in patients who undergo partial breast irradiation rather than whole breast irradiation.

SUGGESTED READINGS

Fisher B, Anderson S, Bryant J, et al. Twenty year follow-up of a randomized trial comparing total mastectomy, lumpectomy, and lumpectomy plus irradiation for the treatment of invasive breast cancer. *N Engl J Med* 2002; 347:1233–1241.

Holland R, Veling SH, Mravunac M, Hendriks JH. Histologic multifocality of Tis, T1–2 breast carcinomas: implications for clinical trials of breast-conserving surgery. *Cancer* 1985; 56(5):979–990.

Veronesi U, Cascinelli N, Mariani L, et al. Twenty year follow-up of a randomized study comparing breast conserving surgery with radical mastectomy for early breast cancer. *N Engl J Med* 2002; 347:1227–1232.

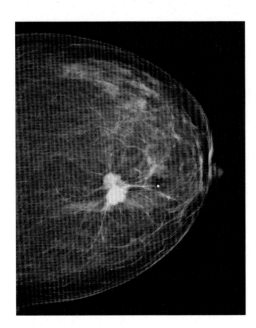

FIGURE 1. CC mammographic view of the left breast: A dense spiculated mass is seen in the medial left breast, corresponding to the palpable finding.

Wazer DE, Schmidt-Ullrich RK, Schmid CH, et al. The value of breast lumpectomy margin assessment as a predictor of residual tumor burden. *Int J Radiat Oncol Biol Phys* 1997; 38(2):291–299.

CASE 2

Use of ultrasound to find invasive disease within extensive microcalcifications; depiction of disease extent by breast MRI versus PEM versus whole-body PET

An asymptomatic 40-year-old woman had extensive new left lateral microcalcifications identified on screening mammography. These showed suspicious linear and branching pleomorphism on magnification views (Figure 1), and extensive ductal carcinoma in situ (DCIS) was suspected. Ultrasound was performed to determine whether an invasive component could be identified for biopsy. Five solid masses were identified in the left lateral breast, ranging up to 1.8 cm in size, as well as a suspicious abnormal axillary lymph node (Figure 2).

Biopsies with ultrasound guidance of the two largest upper outer quadrant masses at 2 and 3 o'clock confirmed grade 3 infiltrating ductal carcinoma, high-grade DCIS, with comedonecrosis, estrogen receptor and progesterone receptor positive, and *HER-2/neu* negative, from both sites. Axillary lymph node fine-needle aspiration confirmed metastatic carcinoma.

The patient desired breast conservation, and so extensive staging studies were performed to assess the extent of disease. These included breast MRI (Figure 3), positron emission mammography (PEM) (Figures 4 and 5), and whole-body positron emission tomography (PET) (Figure 6). These studies

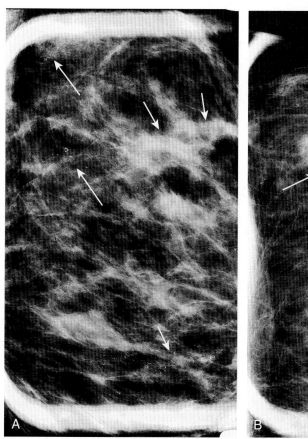 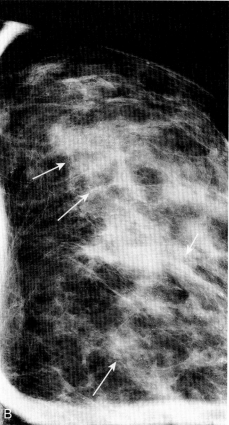

FIGURE 1. Lateral (**A**) and CC (**B**) magnification views show moderate parenchymal density. Diffuse pleomorphic microcalcifications are present throughout the left lateral breast (*arrows*).

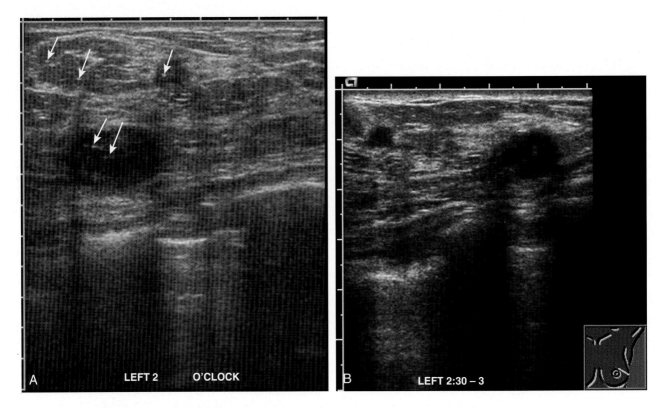

FIGURE 2.   Left lateral breast ultrasound, performed to search for invasive components within suspected extensive DCIS, identified five discrete masses, measuring up to 1.8 cm in size. (**A**) At 2 o'clock, an oval hypoechoic mass without a well-defined capsule shows tiny punctate foci of hyperechoic calcium. Similar foci within the surrounding parenchyma can also be appreciated (*arrows*). (**B**) At 2:30 to 3 o'clock, two additional, similar-appearing, solid, hypoechoic masses with ill-defined margins are seen.

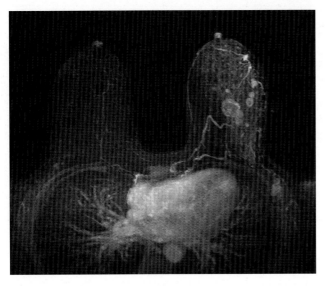

FIGURE 3.   Axial breast MRI enhanced, subtracted maximal intensity projection view shows diffuse, confluent enhancement of the left lateral breast, corresponding to the distribution of pleomorphic DCIS calcifications on mammography. Within this field can be seen a variety of intensely enhancing masses. The largest display rim enhancement and washout. Eight discrete masses could be delineated on MRI in the left upper and lower outer quadrants. An enlarged left axillary lymph node can also be seen here.

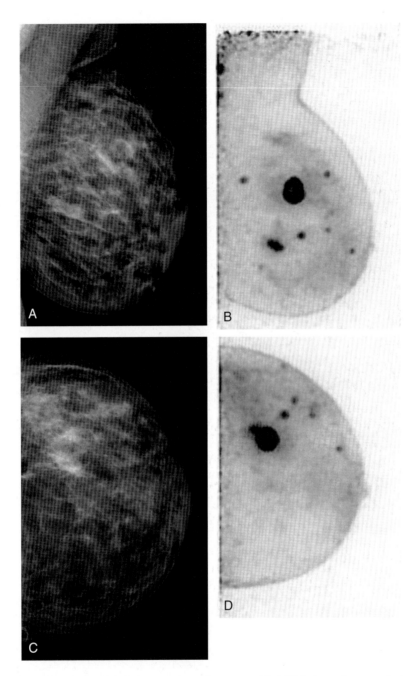

FIGURE 4. Digital mammographic views and comparable PEM views, for correlation: (**A**) MLO mammogram. (**B**) MLO "volume" PEM image. Seven discrete foci of intense increased FDG uptake are seen. (**C**) CC mammogram. (**D**) CC "volume" PEM image. The most posterior of the seven lesions seen in the MLO projection is not included in the field of view and is not seen. Lower-level uptake of FDG is seen in the upper outer breast, corresponding both to the distribution of parenchyma and the extensive microcalcifications. The mammographic parenchymal density conceals the masses which could be identified by ultrasound, MRI, and PEM.

confirmed multicentric disease with axillary nodal involvement, but showed no distant metastases. Neoadjuvant chemotherapy was given.

TEACHING POINTS

Extensive, new, suspicious microcalcifications suggested an extensive intraductal component in this case. Stereotactic biopsy of microcalcifications undoubtedly would have established a diagnosis of DCIS. However, ultrasound can be useful to search for a mass for ultrasound sampling within an area of suspicious microcalcifications, which may enable a diagnosis of invasive disease to be made.

This is a very extensive, multicentric malignancy with an extensive intraductal component. It is interesting to compare the performance of the various modalities in depicting the extent of this neoplasm. The mammogram best depicts the extensive calcified DCIS, diffusely involving the upper and lower outer quadrants, but the breast tissue density obscured the invasive components. Five masses (two proven invasive) were identified by ultrasound within the area encompassed by the microcalcifications. The microcalcifications can be recognized sonographically, but would likely not be recognized prospectively without mammographic correlation.

Both invasive and noninvasive disease components are well depicted by MRI. The DCIS mani-

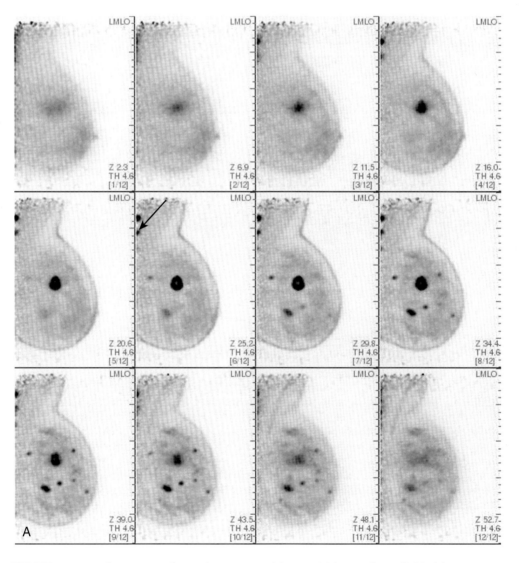

FIGURE 5. PEM data are a volumetric, tomographic acquisition and are divided into 12 slices: (**A**) MLO projection. PEM progresses from medial (*upper left*) to lateral (*lower right*). With windowing, the largest lesion, projecting above the nipple, shows a rim pattern of uptake. On the edge of the field of view (*middle row, upper left, arrow*), hypermetabolic axillary lymph nodes can be seen.

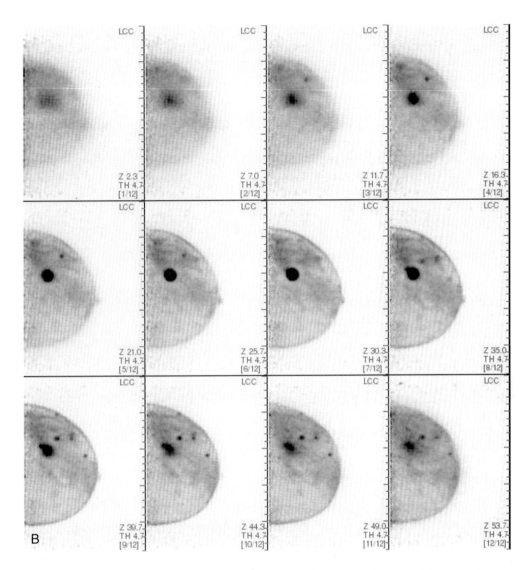

FIGURE 5, cont'd   (**B**) CC projection PEM is displayed from cranial (*upper left*) to caudal (*lower right*).

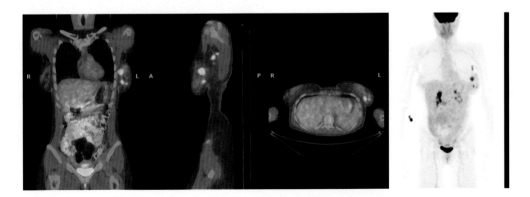

FIGURE 6.   Fused whole-body PET/CT images show three hypermetabolic foci in the left lateral breast as well as three hypermetabolic left axillary lymph nodes. No evidence of distant metastatic disease was found.

fested as confluent, segmental enhancement in the lateral breast. Eight intensely enhancing discrete masses with washout could be identified by MRI within this extensive intraductal component. PEM performed nearly as well, depicting seven discrete sites of intense increased fluorodeoxyglucose (FDG) uptake. The intraductal disease (as represented by the distribution of calcifications on mammography) would be difficult to recognize prospectively on PEM, without mammographic correlation. The lower-level segmental FDG uptake seen here in the distribution of the DCIS calcifications also corresponds to the distribution of parenchymal density and so would be difficult to differentiate from background parenchymal uptake.

PEM is essentially a small field of view, high-resolution dedicated breast PET scan. Tomographic volumetric data is acquired with gentle compression (for immobilization, not for tissue thinning) in planes analogous to mammography. Because the detectors (in compression plate-like arrays) on either side of the breast are extremely close to the radioactive source (FDG taken up by glycolytically active tumor), the resolution is considerably higher than in whole-body PET, wherein a patient's body is surrounded by a ring of detectors. State-of-the-art whole-body PET scanners have a lower limit of resolution today of about 6 mm, whereas resolution on the order of 2 mm can be expected with PEM. This is illustrated in this case. Only the three largest foci of FDG uptake could be visualized within the breast on whole-body PET, as compared with seven discrete lesions on PEM. A limitation of PEM is also illustrated here. Two hypermetabolic axillary nodes are at least partially visualized on PEM. Axillary visualization on PEM is variable, depending on patient anatomy and positioning. Whole-body PET in this patient readily demonstrated three hypermetabolic axillary nodes.

CASE 3

MRI: Extent of disease

A 54-year-old woman presented with a palpable mass in the upper outer left breast. Diagnostic mammographic and ultrasound evaluations demonstrated multiple masses in the upper outer quad-

rant of the left breast at the site of the palpable abnormality (Figures 1 and 2). Core needle biopsy confirmed invasive ductal carcinoma. Preoperative MRI suggested much more extensive involvement

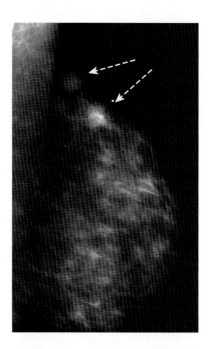

FIGURE 1.   MLO mammographic view of the left breast: Multiple masses (*arrows*) are seen in the upper outer quadrant at the site of the patient's palpable complaint.

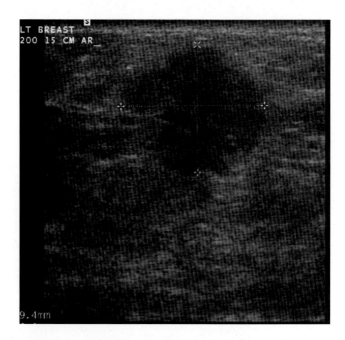

FIGURE 2.   Ultrasound evaluation of the left breast axillary tail region: A dominant mass is seen corresponding to the patient's palpable lump. The mass is highly suspicious for malignancy with its irregular shape and margin features.

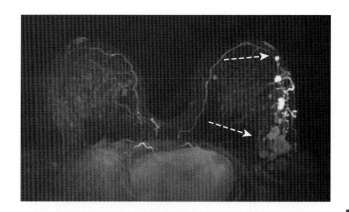

FIGURE 3. Postcontrast maximum intensity projection MRI: Multiple enhancing masses are demonstrated involving a large portion of the left breast, extending from the left axillary tail to the subareolar region (*arrows*).

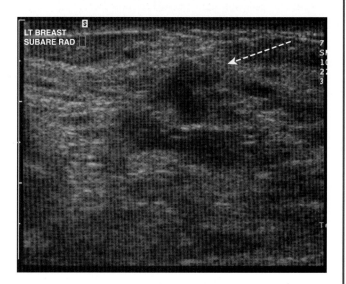

FIGURE 4. Ultrasound image of the subareolar left breast: A lobular, hypoechoic mass (*arrow*) corresponds to the MRI finding in this location.

of the left breast, with multiple enhancing masses extending from area of the known cancer toward the nipple (Figure 3). Because of the MRI findings, second-look ultrasound was performed and identified several small masses in the subareolar region (Figure 4). Core needle biopsy confirmed the extensive nature of the patient's disease, and she was treated surgically with mastectomy and axillary dissection.

TEACHING POINTS

This case illustrates the use of MRI to evaluate the extent of disease in a patient with a known carci-

noma. MRI may detect areas of additional disease unsuspected on mammography and ultrasound. In this case, MRI allowed targeting of ultrasound to identify more subtle additional lesions that could then undergo biopsy to establish the extent and aid in planning the appropriate surgical treatment.

CASE 4

Multicentric IDC and DCIS: Local staging with MRI

A 47-year-old woman was evaluated with mammography and ultrasound for a palpable lump in the right breast upper outer quadrant.

Mammography showed very dense breast tissue, with no correlate for the palpable abnormality (Figure 1). Ultrasound of the palpable lump showed a 2-cm heterogeneous, solid mass, with irregular margins and vascularity and a highly suspicious appearance (Figure 2). An ultrasound-guided core needle biopsy confirmed infiltrating ductal carcinoma (IDC), with high-grade ductal carcinoma in situ (DCIS). At initial surgical consultation, breast conservation therapy with partial mastectomy and radiation was discussed. Because of the mammographic density of the patient's breasts, the patient was referred for preoperative breast MRI to more fully evaluate her suitability for breast conservation therapy.

Bilateral enhanced subtracted breast MRI showed the known right breast carcinoma mass to be intensely enhancing, with irregular margins and spiculation. Multiple smaller, additional foci of enhancement were noted throughout the right breast, markedly asymmetric compared with the left side (Figures 3 and 4). A few of these foci were larger and more morphologically concerning, including an irregular mass at 5 o'clock (Figure 5) and clumped contiguous foci of enhancement at 9 o'clock (Figure 6). A second-look ultrasound was performed of the right breast seeking correlates for biopsy, to prove the patient's disease was multicentric and that she was not a conservation candidate.

Ultrasound identified two subtle correlates for biopsy, confirming DCIS at both sites (Figures 7

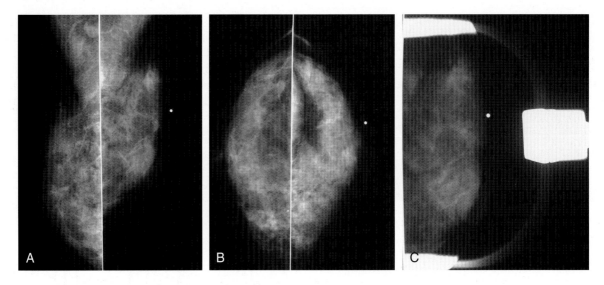

FIGURE 1. Mammography [MLO (**A**), CC (**B**), and spot compression (**C**)] shows a marker placed at the level of the palpable lump in the right upper outer quadrant. The breast tissue is very dense, and no correlate is seen.

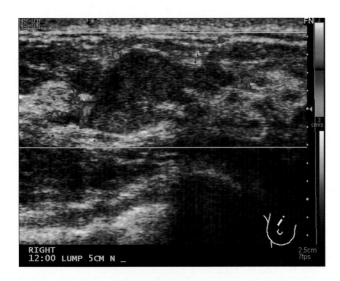

FIGURE 2. Ultrasound of the right breast palpable lump shows a mildly hypoechoic, solid mass, with lobular and irregular borders, with peripheral vascular flow on color Doppler. Several tail-like areas of suspected ductal extension are depicted.

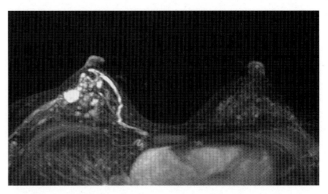

FIGURE 3. Maximal intensity projection from the enhanced, subtracted dynamic breast MRI series shows marked asymmetry between sides. The left shows no concerning finding. The right shows an irregularly marginated, dominant, intensely enhancing mass in the upper outer quadrant. Multiple smaller nodules are noted throughout the breast as well, larger than the tiny (<5 mm) foci frequently seen with physiologic and fibrocystic enhancement.

and 8). With pathologic confirmation of multicentric disease, the surgery treatment was changed to mastectomy.

Final pathology was a 2.1-cm IDC, with associated high-grade (comedo) DCIS extending into lobules. The tumor was noted to be multicentric, with 50% of the gross tumor at the index cancer site, an 8-mm residual focus at 5 o'clock, and microscopic residual at 9 o'clock. Margins were negative,

and two sentinel lymph nodes were also negative. Final stage was stage II, T2N0, and the patient was additionally treated with chemotherapy.

TEACHING POINTS

This case illustrates well how a multimodality approach can yield critical additional information

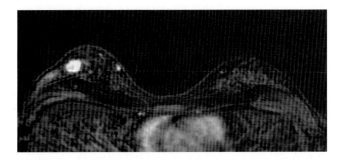

FIGURE 4. A section from the dynamic enhanced breast MRI series through the upper outer quadrants shows the known right infiltrating ductal carcinoma, with intense peripheral rim enhancement. The margins are irregular, with tiny spiculations.

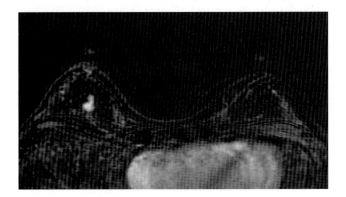

FIGURE 5. Another enhancing, irregularly bordered mass is seen just below the level of the nipple (partially visualized here). This was reported as being at 12 o'clock. However, the sonographic correlate (see Figure 7) was best seen at 5 o'clock. This discrepancy illustrates the difficulty in lesion localization between modalities, which is due both to the mobility of breast tissue and differences in positioning. This patient had very small breasts, and this is a centrally positioned lesion.

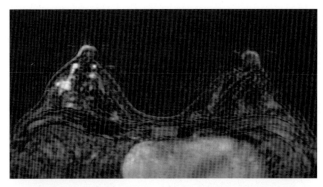

FIGURE 6. Another section from the dynamic enhanced MRI series shows additional concerning findings in the right lateral breast, at about 9 o'clock. Irregular clumped enhancement, with linear extension anteriorly toward the nipple, suggests additional disease.

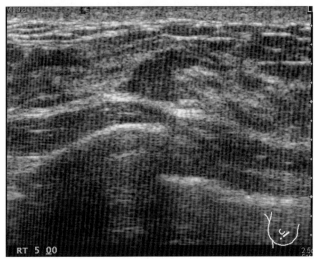

FIGURE 7. Ultrasound of the right breast at 5 o'clock: This lesion was identified using the MRI as a roadmap and was not recognized prospectively. The correlate is subtle, being minimally hypoechoic. Once located, there are some suspicious sonographic features, including being taller than wide and having marginal angularity. Core needle biopsy confirmed DCIS.

to most accurately stage a newly identified breast cancer. Mammography was not particularly useful in this patient, owing to breast density, but confirmed that there were no microcalcifications. Prospectively, ultrasound identified the index tumor and provided guidance to confirm the diagnosis of IDC. However, no additional disease sites were recognized prospectively on ultrasound to suggest multicentric disease. However, with the breast MRI as a roadmap for a directed, second-look ultrasound, more subtle correlates could be discerned and targeted for sampling, confirming two separate sites of DCIS remote from the IDC, indicating that the patient's disease should be treated surgically with mastectomy.

This case also illustrates ductal extension on ultrasound, a sonographic sign suspect for malignancy, as delineated by Stavros and colleagues. This feature is less frequently seen or recognized than other features of malignancy, such as taller-than-wide shape and shadowing.

SUGGESTED READING

Stavros AT, Thickman D, Rapp CL, et al. Solid breast nodules: use of sonography to distinguish between benign and malignant lesions. *Radiology* 1995;196: 123–134.

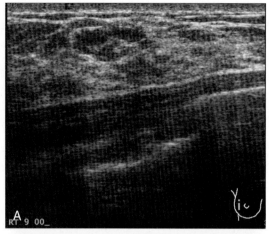

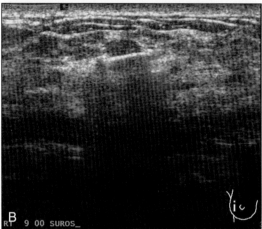

FIGURE 8. Targeted right breast second-look ultrasound at 9 o'clock showed a very subtle correlate. **A,** A lobular, minimally hypoechoic focus seemed to correlate in shape and location to the MRI findings. **B,** Because of the lack of conspicuity of this area, a larger-volume, vacuum-assisted sampling was performed, also confirming DCIS. The needle was maneuvered underneath the target. With pathology-proven multicentricity, the surgical treatment was changed to mastectomy.

CASE 5

Additional disease site identified by PEM

A 46-year-old woman was noted to have a suspicious 1-cm spiculated mass overlying the right pectoral muscle on baseline screening mammography (Figure 1). It was confirmed on spot compression views, and a suspicious sonographic correlate was found (Figure 2), as well as a second concerning ultrasound finding. Both were biopsied with ultrasound guidance, confirming infiltrating ductal carcinoma (IDC) at 12 o'clock and sclerosing adenosis at 10 o'clock.

The patient desired breast conservation and appeared by conventional imaging to be a suitable candidate. She was enrolled in a clinical trial prospectively comparing breast MRI to positron emission mammography (PEM) in preoperative staging of newly diagnosed breast cancer.

PEM identified two fluorodeoxyglucose (FDG)-avid abnormalities in the right breast. One corresponded to the known IDC. The other showed a linear and ductal pattern of uptake and was suspicious for a second site of malignancy, but did not clearly correspond to the second ultrasound abnormality in location or morphology (Figure 3).

MRI was performed subsequently. The known IDC formed a bilobed mass, but no additional abnormality was recognized prospectively (Figure 4A). When this study was then correlated with PEM, a possible correlate was recognized as localized clumped enhancement centrally, with late appearance of a 1-cm mass (see Figure 4B).

MRI-guided biopsy was recommended. At the time of biopsy, sagittal localization scans showed a clearer, branched, linear pattern of abnormal enhancement, which correlated with the morphology and location of the second PEM abnormality (see Figure 4C). Biopsy was performed with MRI guidance, confirming high-grade ductal carcinoma in situ (DCIS) as well as a complex sclerosing lesion and atypical ductal hyperplasia. This site was 8-cm away from the known IDC. Mastectomy was recommended but refused by the patient.

Double lumpectomy was performed after triple-needle localization. The 12-o'clock IDC was localized with ultrasound guidance. Ultrasound guidance was also used to place two additional needles to bracket the second abnormality. One was placed at the lateral margin of the post-MRI biopsy cavity, and the other was placed at the medial margin of this cavity, where the 10-o'clock sclerosing lesion was seen.

The 12-o'clock specimen removed a 1.2-cm IDC with DCIS. Margins were positive for DCIS inferiorly and posteriorly. The 9-o'clock specimen contained a 1.2-cm high-grade DCIS lesion as well as a complex sclerosing lesion and biopsy site changes. The medial margin was positive.

Mastectomy was again recommended, and declined. Re-excision of the positive margins was again positive for DCIS. She underwent a total of four re-excision procedures from both sites for

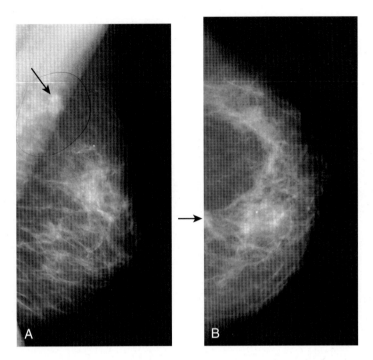

FIGURE 1. Baseline screening mammogram [MLO (**A**) and CC (**B**)] shows moderate parenchymal density. An irregularly marginated mass is seen overlying the pectoral muscle (*circled* and *arrow* on MLO view) and on the edge of the field in the CC projection (*arrow*).

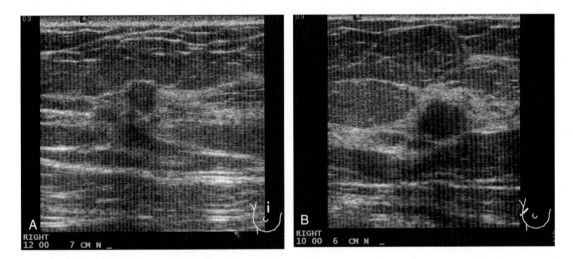

FIGURE 2. Ultrasound of the right breast identified two abnormalities. **A**, At 12 o'clock, corresponding to the mammographic abnormality, there is a taller-than-wide, hypoechoic, solid, irregularly marginated, suspicious mass. Ultrasound-guided biopsy proved IDC. **B**, At 10 o'clock, a hypoechoic mass with ill-defined margins and no capsule is indeterminate, and also a concerning finding. Ultrasound-guided biopsy identified sclerosing adenosis.

recurrently positive margins, before undergoing mastectomy.

TEACHING POINTS

PEM is an emerging modality that functionally images breast tissue. PEM is essentially a high-resolution, small-field-of-view, dedicated breast PET scan, performed after intravenous administration of FDG and an hour's uptake time. It is performed utilizing a device resembling a mammogram unit, with detector arrays in place of compression plates, which are positioned on either side of the breast. Views in projections analogous to mammographic views can be obtained, allowing

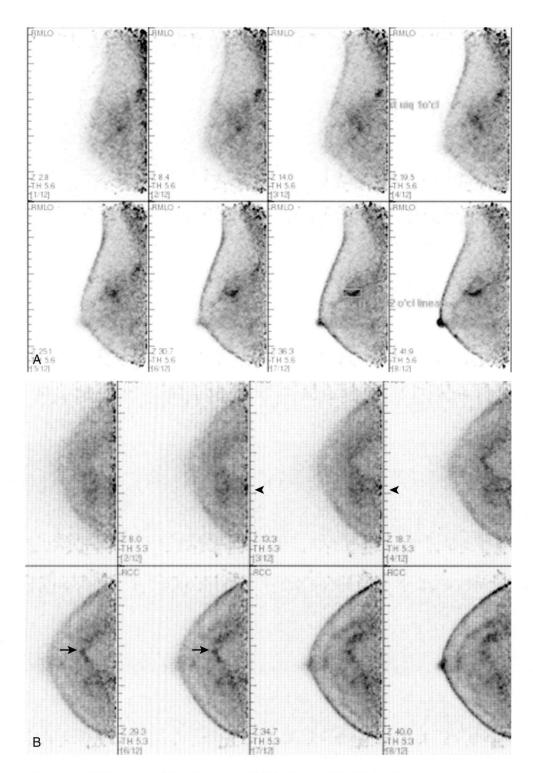

FIGURE 3. PEM images of the right breast [MLO (**A**) and CC (**B**)]. **A**, MLO views show two FDG-avid abnormalities. Regions of interest have been placed around these (*blue squares*). The scintigraphically active mass in the upper posterior breast corresponds to the known IDC. The second site, projecting above the nipple at mid-breast level, shows suspicious intensity and morphology, with a linear and ductal configuration. This did not seem to clearly correlate in either location or morphology to the sclerosing adenosis lesion known from ultrasound at 10 o'clock. **B**, Both of the abnormalities seen in the MLO projection are less clearly seen in the CC projection. The known IDC is so far posterior that it is not included in the field of view on the CC projection and can only be suspected (*arrowheads*). The arrow indicates the location suspected to correspond to the linear/ductal PEM abnormality seen in the MLO projection.

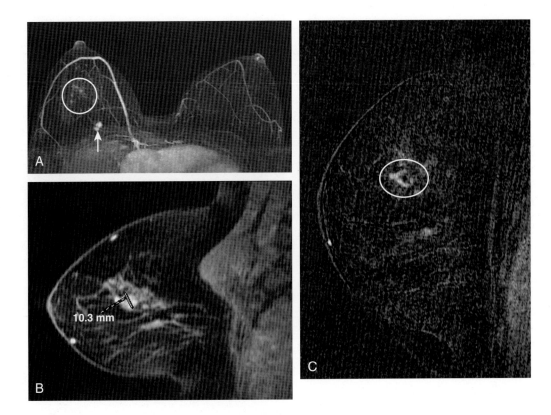

FIGURE 4. Breast MRI: **A,** Axial maximal intensity projection view shows the right posterior known IDC as a bilobed mass (*arrow*). No additional abnormality was noted prospectively. After correlation with PEM, the central region of clumped foci of enhancement (*circled*) was suspected to correspond with the second PEM abnormality. **B,** Sagittal, delayed (5 minutes after contrast), enhanced, fat-saturated image shows the clumped area of enhancement, which seemed to correlate in location with the second PEM abnormality (measured). **C,** Sagittal, enhanced, subtracted localizer image at the time of breast MRI biopsy showed a more convincing correlate for the linear-ductal PEM abnormality. A wishbone-shaped region of branched linear-ductal enhancement (*circled*) was targeted for MRI-guided vacuum-assisted sampling, confirming high-grade DCIS. This site was 8 cm away from the known IDC, indicating multicentric disease.

for ready correlation with mammograms. The breast is compressed to immobilize it, but not to the degree required to thin the tissue for optimal mammography. A volume of data is acquired tomographically. At this writing, the only U.S. Food and Drug Administration–approved device is manufactured by Naviscan PET Systems, but analogous PET and gamma camera–based devices by other manufacturers are in various stages of development. The Naviscan PEM tomographic acquisition is divided into 12 slices.

In this case, the PEM scan was the first study to indicate that this patient had multicentric disease. The MRI correlate was not recognized prospectively and was subtle to identify even with PEM correlation. PEM-guided biopsy capability is expected in the future and would provide an alter-native means of staging in a case like this, when correlation is uncertain with conventional imaging or MRI.

The multicenter prospective trial in which this patient was enrolled is accruing patients at this writing. It is hoped that the data will provide valuable information on the performance of breast MRI compared with PEM in preoperative staging of breast cancer. The precise role that PEM will play in the breast imaging armamentarium is still being defined. Pilot studies suggest sensitivity for breast cancer identification is on a par with MRI, perhaps with greater specificity, but this remains to be established. Also unclear at this point is whether PEM could function as a stand-alone modality, or whether it is best used in conjunction with conventional breast imaging correlation.

SUGGESTED READINGS

Berg WA, Weinberg IN, Narayanan D, et al. High-resolution fluorodeoxyglucose positron emission tomography with compression ("positron emission mammography") is highly accurate in depicting primary breast cancer. *Breast J* 2006; 12(4):309–323.

Tafra L. Positron emission tomography (PET) and mammography (PEM) for breast cancer: importance to surgeons. *Ann Surg Oncol* 2007; 14:3–13.

Tafra L, Cheng Z, Uddo J, et al. Pilot clinical trial of 18F-fluorodeoxyglucose positron-emission mammography in the surgical management of breast cancer. *Am J Surg* 2005; 190(4):628–632.

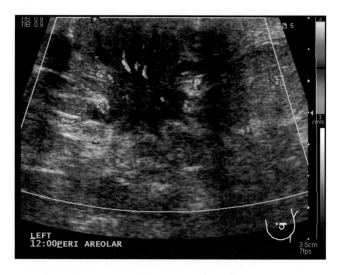

FIGURE 1. Ultrasound of the retroareolar region shows a solid, hypoechoic, highly vascular mass with irregular angular margins.

CASE 6

Subtle axillary nodal involvement

A 52-year-old woman presented with several months of left nipple change, with retraction and infra-areolar fullness. She had had tenderness and nodularity in this breast for more than a year. Her gynecologist confirmed an abnormal clinical exam and referred her to surgery, where the left side was noted to be asymmetrically enlarged, with faint peau d'orange of the periareolar area. A full, irregular, and retracted appearance of the nipple-areolar complex was noted. A large, firm, nodular mass encompassed the central breast on palpation, including the nipple-areolar complex. An axillary lymph node could be palpated. Palpation-guided core needle biopsy of the mass was performed, returning a diagnosis of infiltrating ductal carcinoma (IDC) with focal high-grade ductal carcinoma in situ (DCIS). A punch biopsy of the skin identified carcinoma in dermal lymphatics, confirming the clinical diagnosis of inflammatory breast cancer. The imaging evaluation included mammography, ultrasound, and breast MRI. Mammography showed slightly increased trabecular thickening and breast density. Sonography showed a hypoechoic, solid, irregular, highly vascular mass involving the nipple and retroareolar region (Figure 1). Multiple, sub-centimeter adjacent hypoechoic nodules were noted, and there was diffuse skin thickening. The axilla showed several lymph nodes,

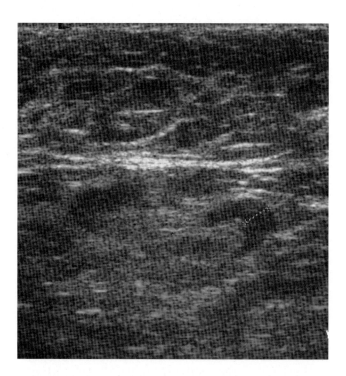

FIGURE 2. Sonography of the axilla shows two normal-sized lymph nodes. Fatty hila are readily identified, and the cortical mantles are not clearly pathologically thickened or nodular.

without clearly pathologic cortical mantle thickening or other particularly suspicious alterations in morphology prospectively (Figure 2).

The pretreatment staging of this locally advanced inflammatory breast cancer, with clinical and pathologic proof of skin involvement, was com-

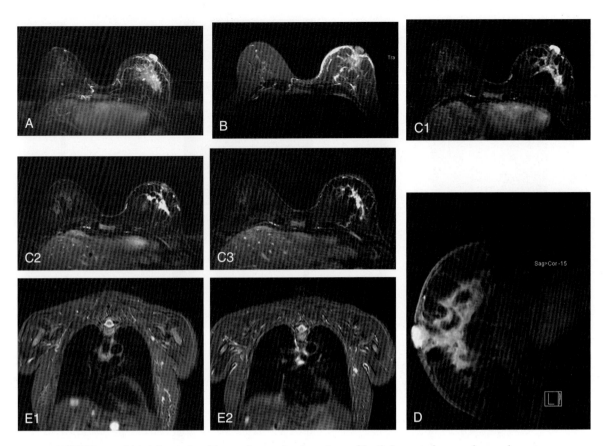

FIGURE 3. **A**, Axial maximal intensity projection view of both breasts from enhanced dynamic breast MRI series shows marked asymmetry, with intense central left breast enhancement, as well as asymmetrical nipple enhancement. An occasional, sub-centimeter, small, benign-appearing focus of enhancement is noted on the right. **B**, Axial short tau inversion recovery (STIR) image of both breasts shows marked left skin thickening and edema as well as diffuse increased edema of the entire breast. **C**, Axial, subtracted images of the breasts, from above to below (**1–3**), showing the diffusely infiltrating enhancing mass, with intense nipple enhancement and skin thickening and enhancement. **B**, Sagittal, enhanced, subtracted view (obtained about 5 minutes after contrast injection) shows diffuse infiltrative parenchymal enhancement, extending to the nipple. Enhancement of the thickened skin can be seen. **E**, Coronal STIR images through the thorax (**1** and **2**), obtained with the body coil as part of the breast MRI, show several left axillary lymph nodes. Although not clearly pathologically enlarged in size (1 cm), they are notable for the asymmetry from the opposite side. Hyperintensities in the liver are cysts.

pleted with breast MRI, body positron emission tomography (PET)/CT, and contrast-enhanced diagnostic chest, abdomen, and pelvis CT scans. Breast MRI showed a diffusely infiltrating, intensely enhancing central left breast mass, extending to and retracting the nipple (Figure 3). Breast MRI, PET/CT (Figure 4), and contrast-enhanced chest CT (Figure 5) also showed subtle but suspicious findings suggesting left axillary nodal involvement. Axillary fine-needle aspiration (FNA) of an axillary lymph node with only mild cortical mantle thickening was performed and confirmed metastatic carcinoma.

TEACHING POINTS

The imaging findings of involved axillary or regional lymph nodes can be subtle on both anatomic and functional imaging modalities. Relying on the traditional anatomic criteria of size allows us only to suggest disease when lymph nodes are clearly pathologically enlarged. Dimensions defining normalcy have been suggested previously for the axilla of less than 1 cm, or 5 mm in short axis. However, use of dimensional criteria alone will underestimate nodal involvement, which could be suspected

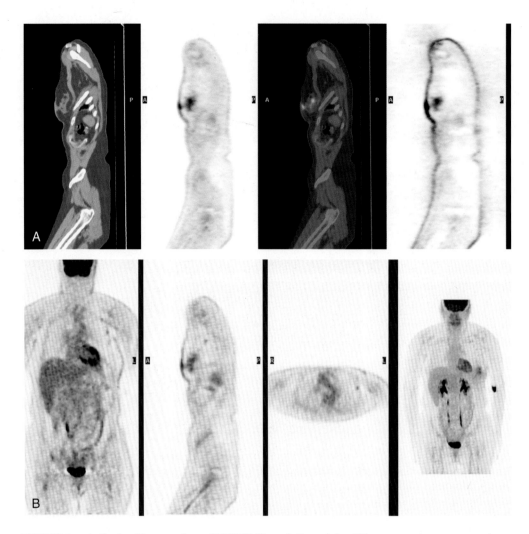

FIGURE 4. **A**, Sagittal images from PET/CT (from left to right: CT, attenuation-corrected PET, fused PET/CT, non-attenuation-corrected PET) show hypermetabolism of the central left breast mass and nipple. **B**, PET images through the axilla (from left to right: coronal, sagittal, axial, and coronal projection volume image) show a small focus of mildly increased metabolic activity at the left axillary level, suggesting nodal involvement.

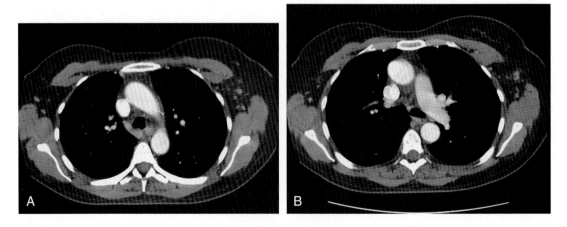

FIGURE 5. Axial contrast-enhanced chest CT images (**A** and **B**) through the axilla show an asymmetrical increased number of identifiable left axillary lymph nodes. Individual lymph nodes are not remarkably enlarged (a fatty hilus can still be seen in the largest) but are larger than the right-sided findings. In addition, there is subtle smudging of fat in the left axilla.

based on other findings, such as asymmetry from the opposite, asymptomatic side. Either an asymmetrical increase in number of lymph nodes compared with the normal side, or larger (but still "normal") size of nodes than on the opposite side, could be an imaging manifestation of nodal involvement. Extranodal extension of disease is suggested by fuzziness of nodal margins or infiltration of axillary fat. This case illustrates these more subtle findings of axillary involvement well. The PET scan also was abnormal, but not floridly so, with modest metabolic activity discernible in a normal-sized lymph node.

Preservation of the fatty hilus of a lymph node should not be regarded as complete reassurance regarding the status of that node. It is important to realize that mass effect and scalloping of the hilus, and ultimately replacement and complete effacement of the fatty hilus, are late manifestations of extensive lymph node involvement. Before these signs develop, cortical thickening, with or without nodularity, may signify a potentially abnormal lymph node and serve as a target for sampling with fine-needle aspiration.

CASE 7

Breast MRI problem solving: Deciding among sites for additional sampling

A 63-year-old woman was noted to have new right upper outer quadrant (UOQ) nodularity and increasing microcalcifications on screening mammography. Previously, she had undergone two benign stereotactic left breast biopsies for microcalcifications. Magnification spot compression confirmed the edge of a partially visualized mass as well as architectural distortion. Multiple clusters of microcalcifications were noted. At least three of these seemed to be progressive compared with prior studies, two in the right UOQ and one in the upper inner quadrant. Ultrasound of the right UOQ showed a highly suspicious, vascular, solid, hypoechoic mass at 10 o'clock (Figure 1), which correlated with the partially visualized mammographic mass.

Core needle biopsy of the right UOQ mass with ultrasound guidance confirmed invasive ductal

carcinoma (IDC), with associated calcifications. Because of the multiplicity of microcalcification clusters and prior history of two benign contralateral biopsies for microcalcifications, breast MRI was recommended after biopsy confirmation of UOQ malignancy to see where additional sampling should be undertaken, if breast conservation was considered.

Breast MRI demonstrated the known right UOQ carcinoma at 10 o'clock, with persistent enhancement (Figures 2, 3, and 4). A separate site of clumped

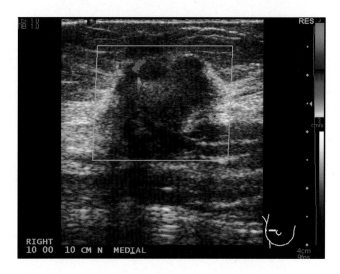

FIGURE 1. Ultrasound of the right UOQ shows a highly suspicious, vascular, solid, hypoechoic mass with ill-defined margins at 10 o'clock. Ultrasound-guided biopsy confirmed IDC.

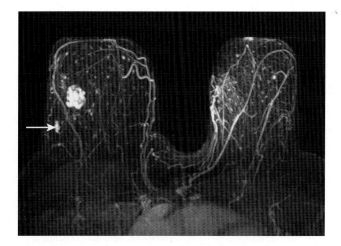

FIGURE 2. Axial maximal intensity projection view from dynamic, contrast-enhanced MRI shows a dominant, heterogeneously enhancing mass in the right lateral breast, corresponding to the known IDC in Figure 1. An oblong focus of irregular enhancement is seen in the posterior lateral right breast (*arrow*), against a background of bilateral diffuse scattered enhancing foci.

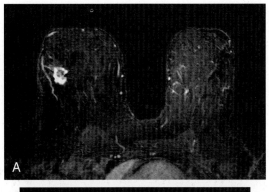

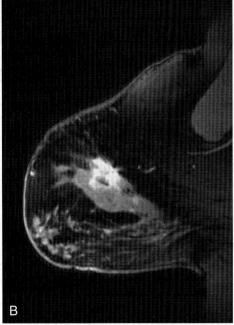

FIGURE 3. Enhanced views [axial (**A**) and sagittal (**B**)] of the right UOQ known IDC. Margins are irregular and spiculated, and there is rim enhancement, MRI features of malignancy.

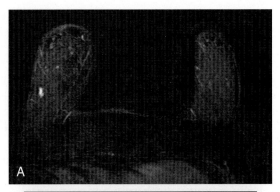

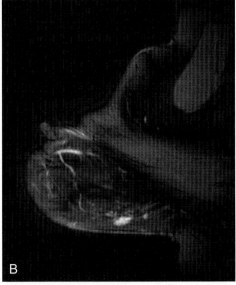

FIGURE 4. A second oblong small mass is seen in the lateral posterior LOQ right breast [axial (**A**) and sagittal (**B**)]. Biopsy was performed with MRI guidance, confirming DCIS.

enhancement was seen in the lower outer quadrant, 6 cm inferior to the known IDC, which subsequently underwent biopsy with MRI guidance (Figure 5). This proved to be ductal carcinoma in situ (DCIS), intermediate to high grade. This site did not correspond in location to the indeterminate microcalcifications.

With pathologic proof of multicentric disease established, right mastectomy was recommended. The patient ultimately opted to undergo prophylactic left mastectomy at the same time.

The pathology showed a right 2.1-cm UOQ IDC, estrogen receptor and progesterone receptor positive, with DCIS associated with the invasive cancer and in a separate 6-mm lower outer quadrant (LOQ) focus. The margins were negative, and three sentinel lymph nodes and one intramammary lymph node were negative. The left mastectomy specimen showed atypical ductal hyperplasia and one negative sentinel lymph node.

There was no indication for radiation therapy, and the patient elected not to have chemotherapy. She had an Oncotype DX score of 20, indicating intermediate to low risk (13% risk for recurrence in 10 years). She was started on anastrozole (Arimidex) but switched to tamoxifen 8 months later due to joint pain.

TEACHING POINTS

When this patient's UOQ IDC was identified, she was also seen to have at least three progressive clusters of microcalcification. In considering breast conservation, it would have been necessary to sample one or more of these microcalcification

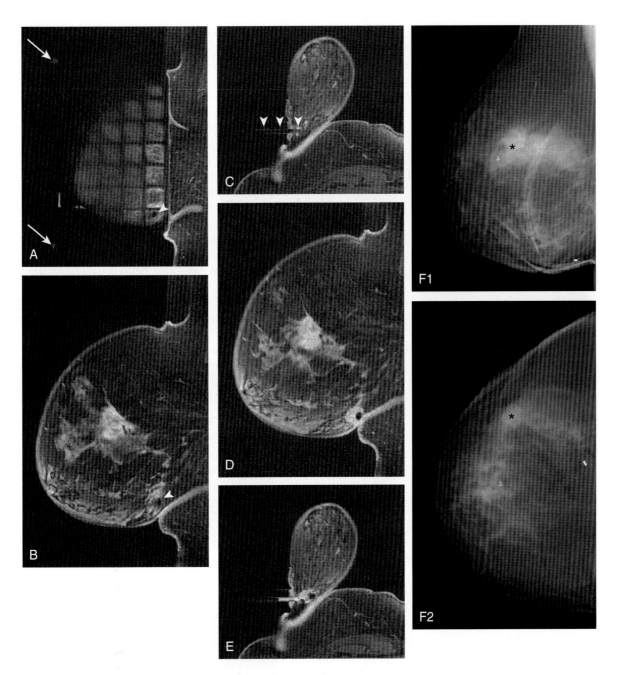

FIGURE 5.   Images from the MRI-guided biopsy of the right LOQ mass seen in Figure 4. **A**, A lateral localizing grid has been incorporated into the dedicated breast coil. Two fiducials are seen (*arrows*), as well as the hypointense obturator (seen on end, *arrowhead*) placed to the prescribed depth of the LOQ abnormality. Note how posterior the lesion is; if it had been any further posterior, it might not have been possible to access with this technique. **B**, Fat-saturated sagittal enhanced imaging after placement of the obturator shows it (*arrowhead*) in the LOQ. The known UOQ spiculated IDC is also seen on this slice. **C**, Fat-saturated axial enhanced imaging after placement of the obturator shows it in position (*arrowheads*). **D**, Repeat sagittal imaging, after the biopsy, shows a small fluid collection (postbiopsy hematoma) at the site. **E**, Repeat axial imaging, after the biopsy and clip deployment, shows a new hypointensity within the postbiopsy hematoma, representing the clip. **F**, Post-MRI-guided biopsy digital mammogram [90-degree lateral (**1**) and CC (**2**)] shows dense breast parenchyma and the MRI-placed clip in the posterior LOQ, 6 cm away from the UOQ IDC (*asterisks*), which is best seen as density and spiculation in the upper breast on the lateral view.

clusters to assess their significance. Breast MRI was obtained to see if it might help in selecting a second site for biopsy, which might avoid the need for performance of a double or triple stereotactic biopsy of the similar-appearing microcalcifications. The breast MRI did identify a LOQ suspicious abnormality, unrelated to the microcalcifications, which were all in upper quadrants. This LOQ oblong mass proved to be DCIS, indicating that the patient was best treated with mastectomy, and avoiding the need to perform a battery of stereotactic biopsies for diagnosis of the microcalcifications.

CASE 8

Breast MRI problem solving: Assessing depth of involvement of posterior breast cancer

A 47-year-old premenopausal woman noted a palpable, growing left breast mass, which was confirmed mammographically as a deep central mass. Stereotactic biopsy at another facility made the diagnosis of infiltrating ductal carcinoma (IDC). By clinical exam, the mass was on the order of 4 cm in size, occupying much of the upper outer quadrant, and seemed to be affixed to the chest wall. By ultrasound, the mass appeared to involve pectoral muscle (Figure 1).

Breast MRI was requested to assess the relationship of the mass to the chest wall. It confirmed extension of the mass into the pectoral muscle, without chest wall involvement (Figures 2 and 3). The mass enhanced intensely, had lobular margins, and displayed washout on kinetic analysis.

Neoadjuvant chemotherapy was administered with Adriamycin and Cytoxan (AC) and paclitaxel (Taxol), with shrinkage of the tumor.

Left mastectomy, with excision of some muscle, and sentinel node sampling were performed. The residual tumor was a 1-cm, well-differentiated IDC, estrogen receptor and progesterone receptor positive, *HER-2/neu* negative, with positive deep margin and perineural involvement, and two negative axillary lymph nodes.

Additional therapy given was chest wall radiation and tamoxifen.

TEACHING POINTS

It can be difficult to evaluate the extent of muscle involvement of posterior breast masses based on mammography, ultrasound, and clinical exam. This is an important determination, with implications for surgical decision making and prognostic significance. The pectoral muscle is considered part of the breast, and adequate surgical therapy of posterior breast masses superficially involving the pectoral muscle will need to include some muscle in the excision. A radical mastectomy can be considered for more extensive pectoral muscle involvement. If the chest wall (ribs, intercostal muscles, and serratus anterior muscle) is involved, the lesion is considered T4, and the patient's stage IIIB.

Breast MRI is the most accurate imaging modality currently in use for assessment of the extent of

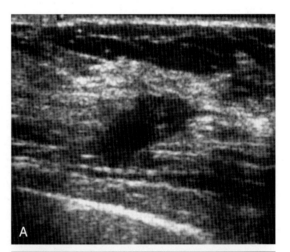

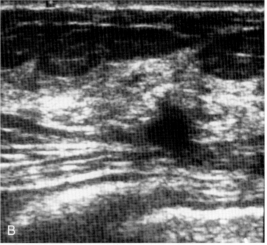

FIGURE 1.   Ultrasound [radial (**A**) and antiradial (**B**)] shows a hypoechoic, solid, irregularly marginated mass, which extends into horizontally oriented fibers of the pectoralis muscle posteriorly.

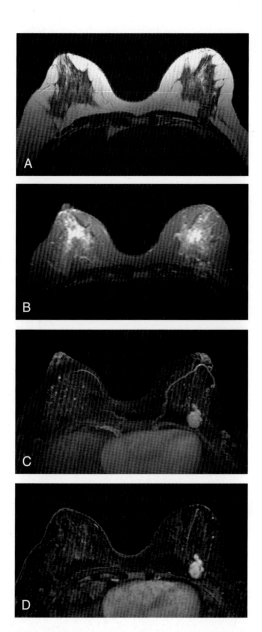

FIGURE 2. Axial breast MRI shows an intensely enhancing, posterior lateral left breast mass, which clearly involves the pectoralis muscle. No chest wall involvement was seen. **A**, Axial T2. **B**, Axial STIR. **C**, Axial maximal intensity projection from enhanced dynamic series (minute 1). **D**, Enhanced subtracted single slice from dynamic series.

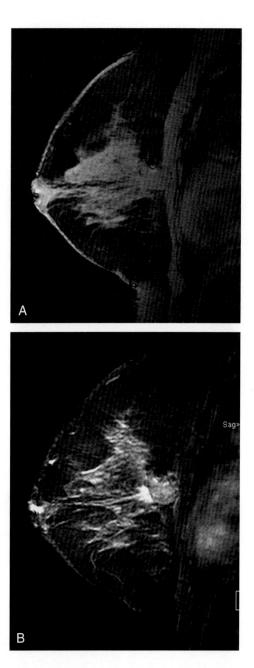

FIGURE 3. Sagittal views better show the depth of posterior muscular involvement. **A**, Fat-saturated, unenhanced, T1-weighted gradient echo. **B**, Subtracted, enhanced view shows the enhancing mass, extending into the pectoral muscle, but not into the chest wall. Susceptibility artifact associated with a clip placed at stereotactic biopsy (upper edge of the mass) is better seen on the unsubtracted view.

muscle involvement by posterior breast cancers. Morris and associates have shown that abutment or effacement of the fat plane is not sufficient imaging evidence to suggest muscle invasion. Actual enhancement in the muscle is necessary to diagnose muscle invasion. In this case, pectoral muscle involvement can be suspected from ultrasound, but the delineation of the extent of muscle invasion is more precise with MRI.

SUGGESTED READING

Morris EA, Schwartz LH, Drotman MB, et al. Evaluation of pectoralis major muscle in patients with posterior breast tumors on breast MR images: early experience. *Radiology* 2000; 214:67–72.

CASE 9

Breast MRI problem solving: Chest wall invasion

A 45-year-old woman presented with a palpable mass in the upper inner right breast. Mammography showed a partially obscured mass with associated suspicious calcifications, corresponding to the palpable mass (Figures 1 and 2). Ultrasound demonstrated the mass to be an irregularly marginated solid mass (Figure 3). Ultrasound-guided core needle biopsy identified high-grade invasive ductal carcinoma. Preoperative MRI demonstrated the known tumor to invade the pectoralis and chest wall (intercostal) muscles (Figure 4). The patient was treated with neoadjuvant chemotherapy, followed by surgery and radiation therapy.

TEACHING POINTS

This case of locally advanced breast cancer illustrates the use of preoperative MRI to aid in tumor staging. Pectoralis and chest wall involvement should be considered in patients with posterior tumors. Effacement of the intervening fat or abut-

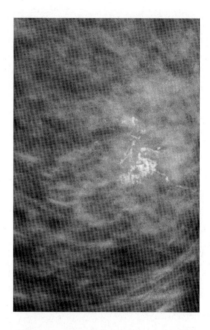

FIGURE 2. Close-up view, right CC projection: Suspicious coarse and ductal calcifications are seen within the mass.

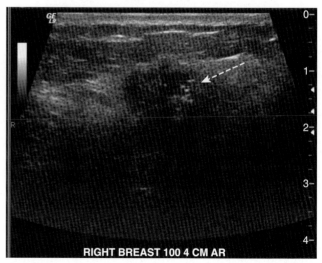

FIGURE 3. Ultrasound of the upper inner right breast demonstrates the mammographic and palpable mass to correspond to an irregular solid mass with posterior acoustic shadowing. Small echogenic foci with the mass (*arrow*) represent calcifications within the tumor.

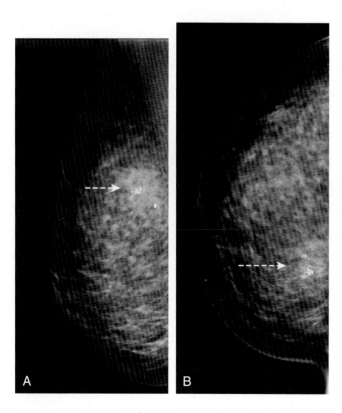

FIGURE 1. ML (**A**) and CC (**B**) mammographic views of the right breast show an ill-defined mass with associated calcifications in the upper inner right breast (*arrows*).

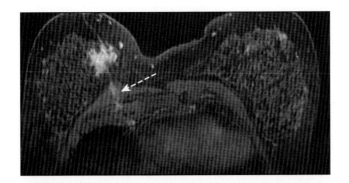

FIGURE 4. Delayed post–contrast MRI axial image: MRI demonstrates the mass in the upper inner right breast. In addition, there is linear enhancement extending into the adjacent pectoralis muscle as well as the underlying intercostal muscles. This indicates pectoralis and chest wall invasion.

ment of the pectoralis fascia does not correlate well with muscle involvement. However, enhancement of the muscle itself on MRI is highly suggestive of muscle invasion. Although pectoralis involvement alone does not change staging, chest wall (intercostal muscle) invasion would represent stage IIIB. In addition, involvement of the pectoralis or chest wall may affect surgical management as well as radiation therapy planning.

SUGGESTED READING

Morris EA, Schwartz LH, Drotman MB, et al. Evaluation of pectoralis major muscle in patients with posterior breast tumors on breast MR images: early experience. *Radiology* 2000; 214(1):67–72.

CASE 10

Breast MRI problem solving: MRI guidance for tailored lumpectomy

A 41-year-old woman underwent routine screening mammography. A nodular right upper outer quadrant (UOQ) density was questioned. Spot compression suggested persistent architectural distortion. Ultrasound of the right lateral breast at 9 o'clock

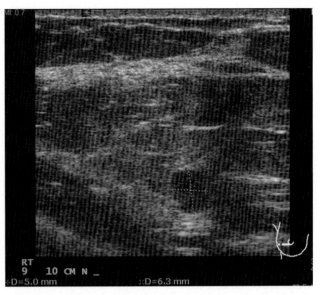

FIGURE 1. Ultrasound of the right lateral breast shows an oval, taller-than-wide, deep, hypoechoic indeterminate breast mass (*cursors*). Ultrasound-guided core needle biopsy identified IDC.

showed a subtle, hypoechoic nodule (Figure 1). The axilla was more convincingly abnormal, with a lymph node with effaced hilus and abnormal vascularity (Figures 2 and 3). Ultrasound-guided core needle biopsy of the small breast mass identified infiltrating ductal carcinoma (IDC), estrogen receptor negative, progesterone receptor positive, *HER-2/neu* negative. Malignancy was also confirmed in the axillary lymph node by fine-needle aspiration (FNA) (Figure 4).

Staging evaluations showed normal tumor markers and no evidence of distant metastatic disease by positron emission tomography, CT, and bone scans (Figure 5). Breast MRI was requested by the breast surgeon because of increased mammographic breast density. MRI showed the disease process to be larger than previously suspected. In the region identified by ultrasound, MRI showed a multinodular, clumped area of enhancement with washout (Figures 6 and 7). Individual small mass components measured on the order of 1 cm each, with the overall process measuring about 3 cm in dimension. Given the discrepancy between the volume of disease displayed by ultrasound compared with MRI, there was concern that localization for breast conservation with ultrasound guidance would lead to positive margins.

Under MRI guidance, clips were placed to bracket the MRI abnormality (Figure 8). One was placed anterolaterally and the other posteromedially. Post-MRI procedure mammograms confirmed success-

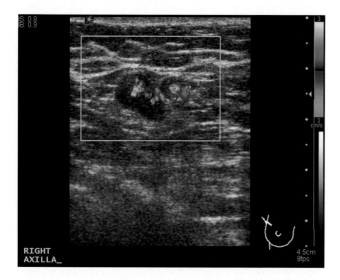

FIGURE 2. Axillary ultrasound shows two adjacent lymph nodes. The one on the left is very vascular and has complete effacement of the fatty hilus.

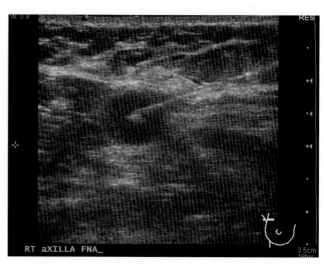

FIGURE 4. Image from an ultrasound-guided axillary lymph node FNA. The skinny needle (25 gauge) is entering from the right and can be seen within the hypoechoic node.

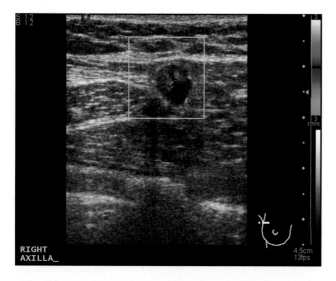

FIGURE 3. Transverse ultrasound view of the vascular lymph node in Figure 2: Note abnormal vascularity on the periphery of the node. Identification of vascularity anywhere but in the hilus is abnormal.

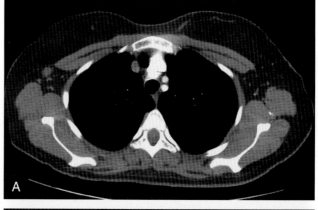

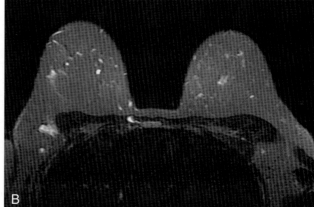

FIGURE 5. Assessment of axillary lymph nodes by size criteria, used with CT and MRI, can underestimate axillary involvement. **A,** Enhanced chest CT shows an outsized right axillary lymph node, corresponding to ultrasound. Margins appear fuzzy here, but this could be post-FNA change. **B,** Axial STIR MRI of the corresponding axillary findings.

ful clip deployment. The clips were localized with ultrasound guidance on the day of surgery.

The partial mastectomy specimen showed a 2.4-cm IDC, with ductal carcinoma in situ and angio-lymphatic invasion. The anterior and inferior margins were close (<2 mm), with others clear. Three of nine sampled lymph nodes were involved, and the largest was 1.1 cm. Re-excision was performed of the close margins, with no IDC and only biopsy site changes noted.

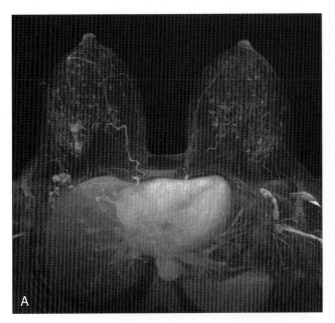

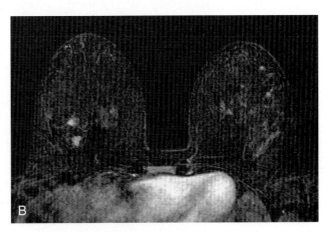

FIGURE 6. Axial enhanced subtracted T1-weighted breast MRI. **A,** Maximal intensity projection view shows a localized, multinodular abnormality in the posterior right lateral breast, seen against a background of scattered fibrocystic foci of enhancement. **B,** Single axial subtracted view of two of the larger, small, irregularly marginated masses constituting this abnormality.

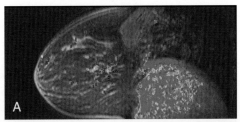

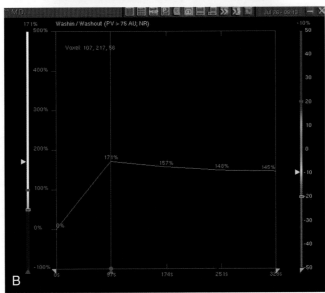

FIGURE 7. Assessment of kinetic data is made easier with color mapping. These examples use DynaCAD software. **A,** Foci of washout are colored lighter (yellow and red). **B,** Representative kinetic curve from this lesion shows rapid upstroke of enhancement and washout.

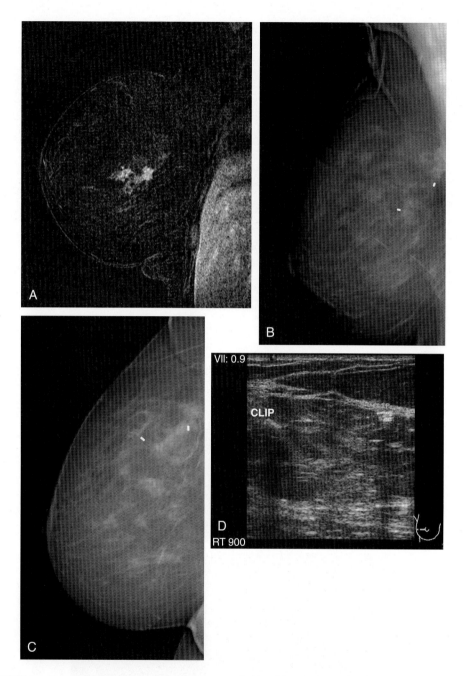

FIGURE 8. Images from MRI-guided biopsy and clip placement and subsequent ultrasound-guided needle localization. **A,** Sagittal subtracted view obtained in a coil with a lateral localizing grid in place to reidentify the target lesions. Targets anterolateral and posteromedial to the enhancement were selected for clip placement. **B,** Post-MRI-guided clip placement lateral digital mammogram confirms both clips to be successfully deployed, in the posterior upper outer quadrant, at 9 to 10 o'clock. **C,** Exaggerated craniocaudal mammogram shows both clips. **D,** On the day of surgery, ultrasound was used to identify the MRI-placed clips. The clips are hyperechoic, and annotated here. They can be difficult to visualize with ultrasound if not placed against a hypoechoic tissue background.

The final stage was stage II, T2N1. Chemotherapy was begun on a study protocol.

TEACHING POINTS

The intent of the MRI-guided clip placement was to maximize the likelihood of achieving clear margins at partial mastectomy. Similar in principle to bracketing of microcalcifications seen on mammography, the larger extent of disease seen by MRI suggested positive margins would be a likely outcome if localized any other way. In this case, clear but close margins were actually achieved on the first attempt, although that was not known with certainty until re-excision was performed subsequently.

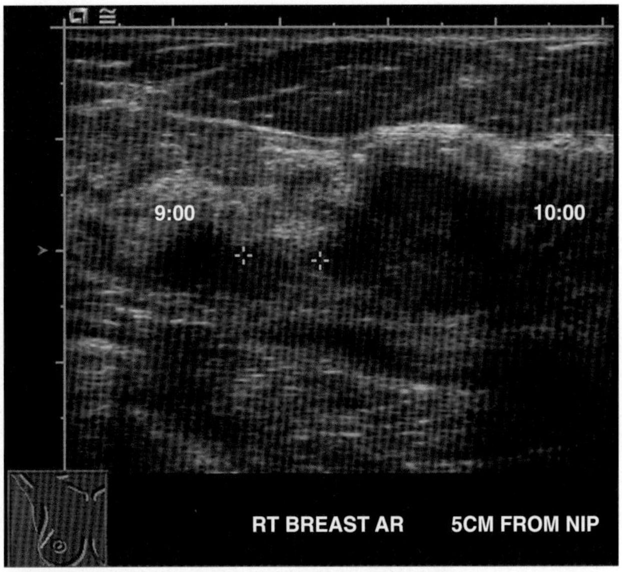

FIGURE 1. Antiradial ultrasound of the right lateral breast shows adjacent hypoechoic, highly suspicious masses with irregular margins at 9 and 10 o'clock. Subsequent core biopsy with ultrasound guidance confirmed IDC from both masses.

CASE 11

Breast MRI problem solving: Assessment of completeness of breast cancer excision

A 48-year-old woman noted a palpable right breast lump, which on her physician's physical exam was assessed to be 1 cm in the upper outer quadrant (UOQ) and possibly a cyst. Mammography showed dense breast tissue only. Ultrasound at the site of the palpable lump was negative. However, a sonographically suspicious 1.5-cm mass was found nearby, localizing to 10 o'clock, with a second nearby 7-mm nodule at 9 o'clock (Figure 1). Both were sampled with ultrasound-guided core biopsy, confirming infiltrating ductal carcinoma (IDC) at both sites.

MRI was ordered to assess the extent of tumor because the known IDC was mammographically and clinically occult. MRI suggested multifocal tumor, with three UOQ intensely enhancing tumor nodules, two of which were immediately adjacent to each other and could have been components of a bilobed mass (Figure 2).

The largest mass measured 1.8 cm, with the adjacent mass or component 1.2 cm in maximal dimension. Another smaller mass was identified 2.5 cm superolaterally. Second-look ultrasound was then undertaken and showed an additional 5 mm nodule at 10 o'clock, 2 cm away from the largest index lesion (Figure 3).

Because the patient desired breast conservation, triple-needle localization with ultrasound guidance was performed. The initial pathologic interpretation was confusing and reported as IDC and ductal carcinoma in situ (DCIS), larger than 2 cm and smaller than 5 cm, with no mention of multiple components. After discussion at breast conference, this was clarified, with pathology ultimately reporting a 2.8-cm IDC, consisting of a continuous region of admixed IDC and DCIS (only one of the localized regions was abnormal by gross). DCIS was present less than 1 mm from the final lateral margin. Angiolymphatic invasion was noted. One sentinel lymph node was negative.

Re-excision was performed 2 weeks later. The new superior and lateral margins were negative, with no residual IDC.

The patient was started on chemotherapy with Adriamycin and Cytoxan (AC) because of the angiolymphatic invasion and her intermediate-range Oncotype DX recurrence score of 21.

Because of the confusion resulting from the apparent multifocality of the tumor on imaging compared with the single tumor mass on pathology, breast MRI was obtained to assess the completeness of the resection before beginning

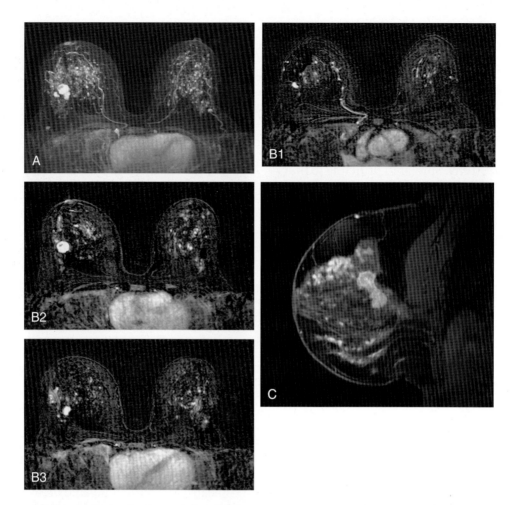

FIGURE 2. Enhanced, subtracted, axial T1-weighted gradient echo MRI shows apparent multifocal tumors in the right UOQ with a background of diffuse, stippled, fibrocystic foci of enhancement. Three discrete (versus one bilobed and a separate smaller focus) tumor masses were suspected based on this study. **A**, Axial maximal intensity projection (MIP) view. **B**, Axial enhanced subtracted views, from above to below (**1–3**), show rim enhancement of the largest enhancing mass. The most inferior mass was immediately below this, and the most superior, smaller mass was 2.5 cm superolateral. **C**, Sagittal subtracted enhanced view, obtained about 5 to 6 minutes after contrast administration, shows the two larger masses. Although they appeared separate by earlier axial imaging, enhancing bridging joining the two masses is now seen.

radiation therapy. By this time, two cycles of AC had been given.

The breast MRI showed a 7-mm enhancing nodule medial to the postoperative seroma, suspicious for a residual tumor focus (Figure 4). Biopsy with MRI guidance confirmed IDC (Figure 5). A clip was placed, which was subsequently localized with two bracketing wires. The specimen showed a 0.6-cm residual IDC, and the margins were clear.

A total of four cycles of AC were completed while the patient was undergoing these procedures. Radiation therapy was completed subsequently,

and the patient was started on tamoxifen. Final stage was stage IIA, T2N0M0, estrogen receptor and progesterone receptor positive, and *HER-2/neu* negative.

TEACHING POINTS

Although it took three surgical excisions, this patient ultimately was successfully treated with breast conservation. Breast MRI was instrumental in enabling this patient to be thus treated. Breast

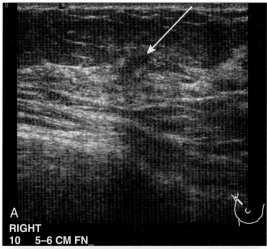

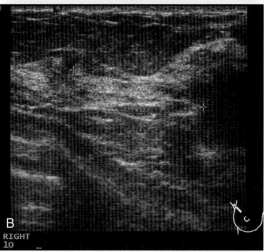

FIGURE 3. Second-look ultrasound. **A**, Ultrasound shows a subtle correlate for the separate, superolateral small mass seen on MRI as a vague, 5-mm hypoechoic focus within dense fibrous tissue, which by ultrasound was 2 cm from the index lesion (*arrow*). **B**, Additional ultrasound image shows the relationship between the new additional tumor nodule and the index lesion (*cursors*).

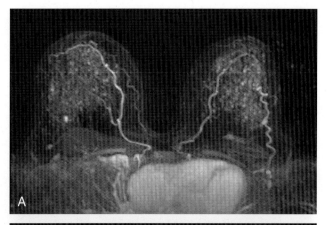

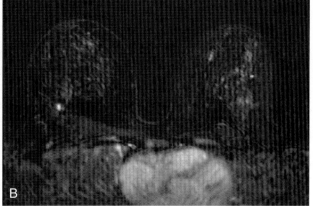

FIGURE 4. Repeat breast MRI, after two surgical excisions, the second with clear margins, after beginning chemotherapy and before radiation therapy, showed a small solitary intensely enhancing nodule in the postoperative bed, medial to a postoperative seroma (not shown). The nodule is larger and more intensely enhancing than the diffuse background lower level enhancement, and was subsequently proved to be a residual IDC by MRI-guided biopsy. **A**, Axial enhanced subtracted MIP image. **B**, Axial enhanced subtracted slice.

MRI provided the most accurate map of the extent of disease, guiding the second-look ultrasound to a third focus of disease. Ultrasound-guided triple-needle localization removed the bulk of the disease. A close margin prompted re-excision, with the new margins negative.

The apparent discrepancy between the breast MRI, which suggested multifocal tumor nodules, and pathology, which reported only a single tumor mass, caused the pathology to be re-reviewed and a tighter correlation to be made. The tumor was admixed IDC and DCIS. A possible explanation could be that the enhancing components seen on MRI represented invasive components, with the DCIS poorly delineated. The ensuing discussion of this case led to the consensus that a repeat breast MRI study should be obtained to assess the completeness of the resection.

With subsequent confirmation of residual disease, and the patient still desirous of breast conservation, localization and excision of the confirmed residual were undertaken. Whether such small-volume residual disease as this, which undoubtedly would have gone undetected in the pre–breast MRI

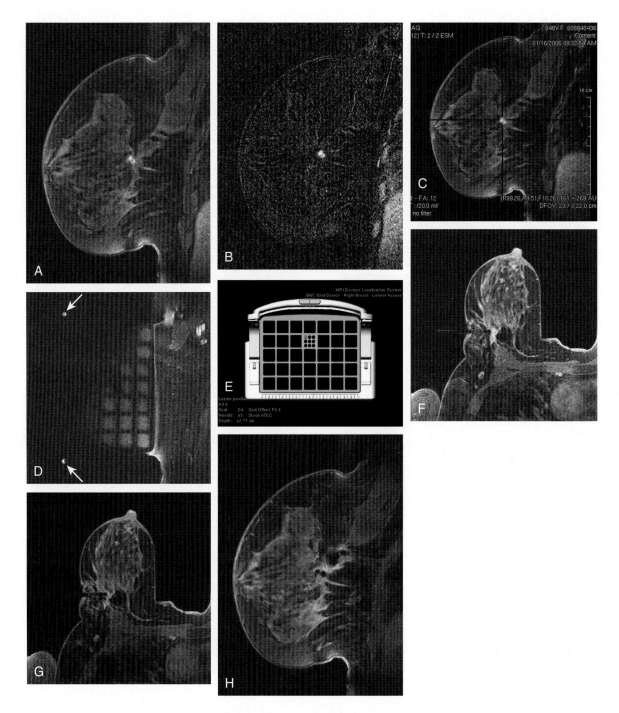

FIGURE 5. Images from MRI-guided vacuum-assisted core needle biopsy, which confirmed residual IDC, despite negative margins at prior excision. **A**, Enhanced, fat-saturated sagittal localizer shows the enhancing target. **B**, The target is initially easier to confirm and visualize with subtraction. **C**, The lesion is targeted for sampling with the aid of a software program (DynaCAD). **D**, The software calculates the depth from the lateral localizing grid, which contains two fiducials (*arrows*). **E**, The appropriate skin entry site and depth are determined. **F**, After placement of the localizing obturator, axial images are obtained to verify its position. The hypointense linear obturator is seen in the lateral breast, with the end at the level of the enhancement. This marks the center of the sampling notch. **G**, Repeat axial imaging after sampling. The enhancement is no longer seen. **H**, Repeat sagittal imaging after sampling and clip placement shows two adjacent hypointense foci at the level of the sampled target (compare with **A**). One represents the obturator and the other the deployed clip.

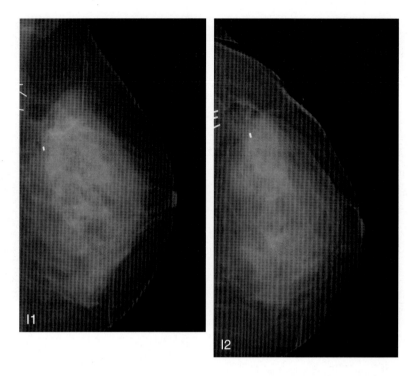

FIGURE 5, cont'd   I, Verification of successful clip deployment with a postbiopsy mammogram is advisable. Digital lateral (**I1**) and CC (**I2**) mammograms show three adjacent surgical clips in the posterior UOQ, on the edge of the field in both views. These were from the prior excisions. Anterior to the surgical clips is the MRI-placed clip, projecting at the inferomedial margin of the postoperative seroma.

era, would have been adequately treated with radiation and chemotherapy or would have predisposed this patient to local recurrence in subsequent years, we can only speculate. The rationale of breast conservation is predicated on the surgical removal of all identifiable disease, a task that has become increasingly complex now that we are better able to identify disease. There is support in the literature that indicates that patients treated with breast conservation using preoperative breast MRI have fewer local recurrences. To date, no studies evaluating the effect of the use of preoperative breast MRI on overall survival have been reported.

SUGGESTED READING

Fischer U, Zachariae O, Baum F, et al. The influence of preoperative MRI of the breasts on recurrence rate in patients with breast cancer. *Eur Radiol* 2004; 14(10):1725–1731.

CASE 12

Contralateral breast carcinoma found on MRI; not seen on second-look ultrasound

A 48-year-old woman with mammographically detected ductal carcinoma in situ in the right breast underwent preoperative MRI. The MRI revealed a suspicious enhancing mass in the contralateral left breast (Figure 1). Subsequent targeted ultrasound was performed of the lateral left breast in the area of the MRI lesion (Figures 2 and 3). Because no discrete lesion was seen on ultrasound, MRI-guided biopsy was performed of the left breast mass (Figure 4). Core needle biopsy revealed an 8-mm intermediate-grade invasive ductal carcinoma.

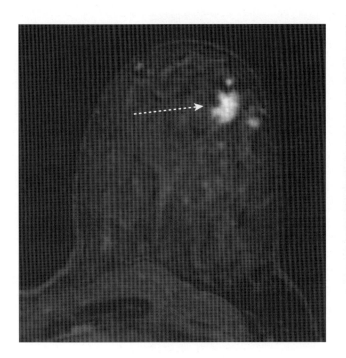

FIGURE 1.   Detail view of the subtracted postcontrast MRI. There is an irregularly shaped enhancing mass in the lateral left breast (*arrow*).

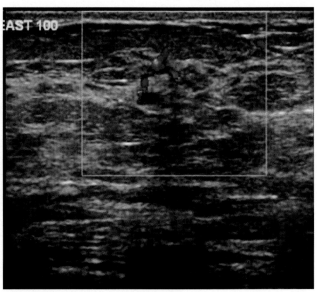

FIGURE 3.   Color Doppler ultrasound image of the lateral left breast. Increased vascularity is seen in the area of the MRI finding.

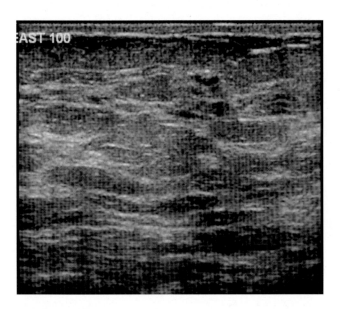

FIGURE 2.   Ultrasound image of the lateral left breast. No discrete lesion is seen to account for the MRI finding.

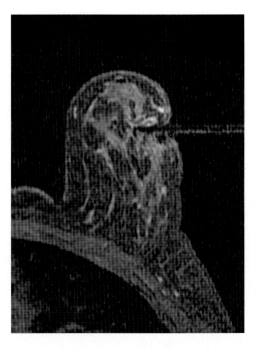

FIGURE 4.   Axial image from an MRI-guided core biopsy of the lateral left breast. The biopsy needle is seen entering the lateral left breast with its tip at the level of the targeted mass.

TEACHING POINTS

This case illustrates the limitations of ultrasound in detecting correlates for suspicious MRI lesions. Although this patient had not had a prior ultrasound of the left breast, the term *second-look* *ultrasound* is used when targeted ultrasound is performed to find an ultrasound correlate to a finding on MRI. In this case, although some vascularity was detected on Doppler ultrasound in the corresponding area in the lateral left breast, this finding is not enough to allow confident correlation with the lesion seen on MRI. In general, ultrasound-guided needle biopsy is preferred over MRI-guided biopsy because of patient comfort, time, and cost. However, depending on the size of the lesion seen on MRI and the quality of the ultrasound evaluation, second-look ultrasound may fail to identify a sonographic correlate in as many as 77% of MRI-detected lesions referred for biopsy. Therefore, a suspicious lesion seen on MRI requires biopsy despite a negative ultrasound. For programs performing breast MRI, it is essential that there also be MRI-guided biopsy capability to assess sonographically occult lesions.

SUGGESTED READINGS

Dhamanaskar KP, Muradall D. MRI directed ultrasound: a cost effective method for diagnosis and intervention in breast imaging [abstract]. *Radiology* 2002; 225:653.

LaTrenta LR, Menell JH, Morris EA, et al. Breast lesions detected with MR imaging: utility and histopathologic importance of identification with US. *Radiology* 2003; 227:856–861.

Panizza P, De Gaspari A. Accuracy of post MR imaging second-look sonography in previously undetected breast lesions [abstract]. *Radiology* 1997; 205:489.

CASE 13

Evaluation of the other breast with MRI

A 43-year-old woman with 10-year-old breast implants noted left axillary lumpiness. Similar complaints had been evaluated 5 years before. When the resurgent axillary complaints failed to improve after antibiotic therapy, the patient was referred for breast imaging evaluation.

Mammography showed asymmetrical density and nodularity at the levels indicated by the patient. Ultrasound showed multiple abnormal axillary lymph nodes as well as round lymph nodes at the lateral margins of the implant (Figure 1). Two vascular, dominant, highly suspicious breast masses were identified in the upper outer quadrant (UOQ) at 1 and 2 o'clock (Figure 2). At least three additional discrete, 4- to 5-mm, hypoechoic nodules

were noted in the same quadrant, interposed between and adjacent to the dominant masses. The two dominant breast masses were sampled with ultrasound-guided core needle biopsy, confirming infiltrating ductal carcinoma (IDC) from both sites. Two axillary lymph nodes were also sampled with fine-needle aspiration technique, confirming metastatic poorly differentiated carcinoma (consistent with breast primary) from both sampled sites (Figure 3).

Based on these evaluations, the patient's best surgical treatment option appeared to be a mastectomy, with removal of the implant. A breast MRI was obtained to assess the proximity of the disease to the implant and to look for additional disease sites.

Breast MRI showed extensive left UOQ and axillary disease and correlated well with the sonogram (Figures 4, 5, 6, 7, 8, and 9). The two known foci of IDC manifested as intensely rim-enhancing, spiculated masses with washout kinetics. They were accompanied by an entire quadrant filled with enhancing smaller masses and clumped enhancement, extending down to the level of the nipple. Multiple, intensely enhancing lymph nodes were identified, also correlating with the ultrasound, both along the lateral margin of the implant and extending up into the axilla.

A suspicious, as yet unsuspected, contralateral abnormality was identified in the right breast on MRI, manifesting as a 2 × 2.6-cm region of clumped progressive enhancement, within which was a 6-mm nodule with washout (see Figures 7, 8C, and 9G and 9H). Targeted sonography identified tiny hypoechoic nodules in the expected region. The most suspicious measured 5 mm in maximal dimension and showed irregular, angular margins (Figure 10). Core needle biopsy under ultrasound guidance identified focal (1.5 mm) invasive ductal carcinoma (in one of six cores) and intermediate-grade ductal carcinoma in situ (DCIS) in all the cores.

Additional preoperative staging was obtained, including bone scan, enhanced chest, abdomen and pelvis CT scans, and positron emission tomography (PET)/CT (Figures 11, 12, 13, 14, 15, and 16). The PET scan showed the two known left UOQ IDCs to be hypermetabolic, as were multiple level I and II left axillary lymph nodes. No evidence of systemic breast cancer was seen. Hypermetabolism identified of the uterine lining was followed up with ultrasound, which was unremarkable, and the activity was presumed to be physiologic variation.

With the new contralateral breast information, the patient elected to undergo bilateral

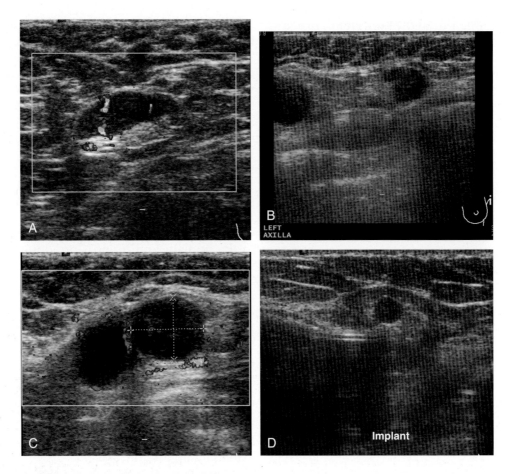

FIGURE 1. A variety of abnormal ultrasound manifestations of axillary metastases were demonstrated in this case. **A**, Color Doppler of an enlarged axillary lymph node shows abnormal thickening of the cortical mantle (up to 8 mm in this case). The fatty hilus can still be visualized. Color Doppler features of this vascularity further confirm the suspicious nature of this lymph node. Instead of vascular flow confined to the hilus, flow can be readily identified at the periphery of the thickened cortex. **B**, Additional left axillary nodal findings suggest (as subsequently proved pathologically) that multiple lymph nodes are involved. This section shows two very hypoechoic, rounded lymph nodes, with the one on the right retaining only a hint of a reniform shape and hilar notch in profile. **C**, Two additional, abnormal, enlarged, adjacent rounded left axillary lymph nodes show peripheral vascularity and complete loss of the fatty hilus. **D**, Even small, completely round lymph nodes like this, adjacent to the implant margin, should be regarded as suspicious in the appropriate setting.

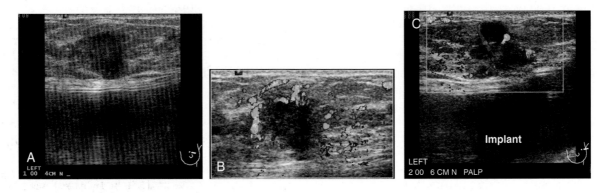

FIGURE 2. Sonographic images of the left UOQ show two dominant, vascular, highly suspicious masses at 1 (**A** and **B**) and 2 o'clock (**C**). Both are solid, hypoechoic, taller than wide, irregularly marginated, and highly vascular and both were confirmed to be IDC. The relationship of the masses to the underlying sonolucent implant can be appreciated in **A** and **C**.

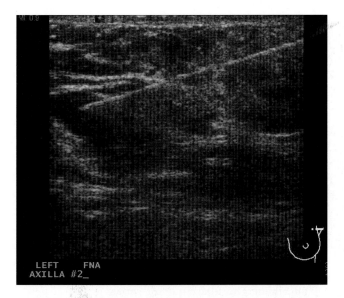

FIGURE 3. Image obtained from ultrasound-guided fine-needle aspiration of one of the abnormal axillary lymph nodes shows the skinny needle within the hypoechoic, rounded lymph node.

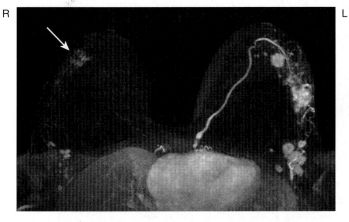

FIGURE 4. Enhanced subtracted axial maximal intensity projection view of both breasts shows large implants with extensive left lateral disease, with multiple enlarged axillary lymph nodes. A large draining vein extends to the internal mammary level. On the right, a localized, segmental region of enhancement is seen in the anterior lateral breast on the surface of the implant (*arrow*).

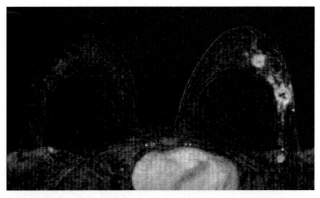

FIGURE 5. Axial subtracted image shows the two known rim-enhancing left UOQ IDC lesions, one near the midline and the other lateral to it. The entire region shows clumped enhancement in addition, suggesting an extensive intraductal component.

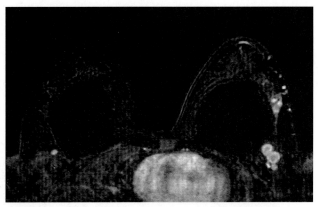

FIGURE 6. An additional slice from the same series shows two adjacent, rim-enhancing, round lymph nodes at the lateral margin of the implant, corresponding to the ultrasound findings depicted in Figure 1C. Anterior to these, in the lateral breast tissue adjacent to the implant, is a cluster of three tiny enhancing masses.

FIGURE 7. An additional section, obtained 3 minutes after contrast injection, shows tiny foci of clumped enhancement throughout the left breast, lateral to the nipple. A similar localized region of clumped enhancement is seen in the right breast, lateral to the nipple (*arrow*). Targeted ultrasound was recommended to evaluate the concerning right-sided findings.

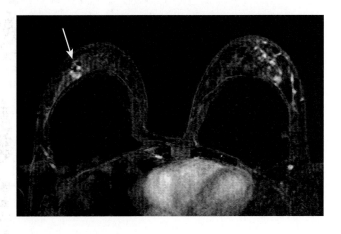

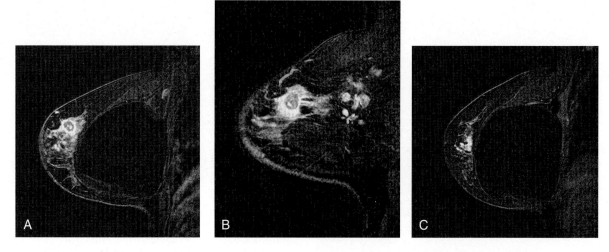

FIGURE 8. Sagittal enhanced subtracted images of these findings. **A,** Slice through the left 1-o'clock IDC mass, which is seen here with rim enhancement. The adjacent tissue shows confluent, clumped enhancement as well. **B,** A more lateral section of the left breast, through the 2-o'clock IDC mass, also displays rim enhancement of the mass. Enhancing spicules project posteriorly from it, and there is lower-level confluent enhancement throughout the quadrant, both anterior and posterior to the IDC mass. Multiple adjacent enhancing nodules and lymph nodes are noted posteriorly. **C,** Sagittal view of the clumped localized enhancement in the right lateral breast.

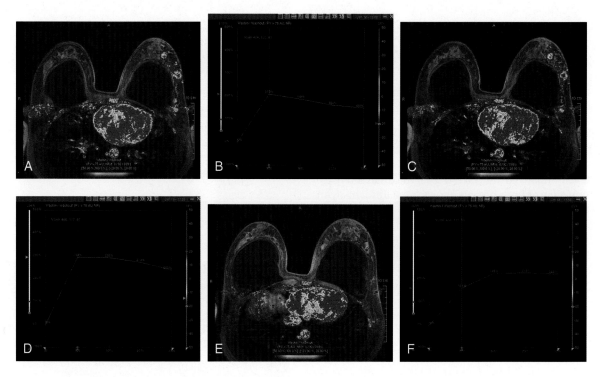

FIGURE 9. Kinetic information is consistent with the known multifocal nature of the left-sided malignancy and heightens suspicion about the more indeterminate right breast MRI findings. Color map (**A**) and signal intensity–time curve (**B**) of the left UOQ mass at 1 o'clock show early, intense enhancement and washout, evidence of angiogenesis. **C** and **D,** The left UOQ mass at 2 o'clock shows similar kinetics. **E** and **F,** The lower-level, more confluent UOQ clumped enhancement shows a plateauing pattern of enhancement.

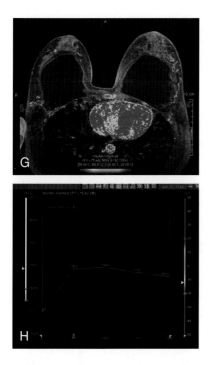

FIGURE 9, cont'd **G** and **H**, Within the clumped localized right-sided enhancement is a small region of washout.

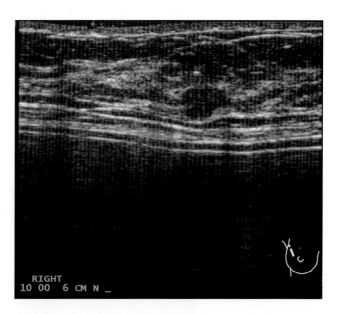

FIGURE 10. Ultrasound of the right UOQ identified tiny hypoechoic nodules. This one had the most concerning appearance, with irregular margins and ductal extension suggested medially. This was cored with ultrasound guidance and a 1.5-mm IDC focus, and DCIS was confirmed.

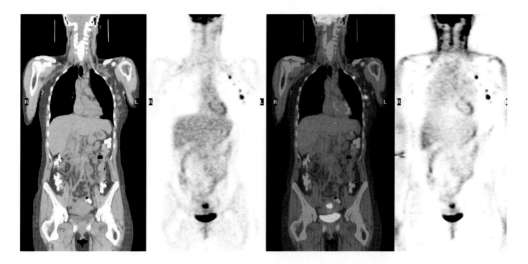

FIGURE 11. Coronal PET/CT images (left to right: CT, PET, fused PET/CT, and NAC-PET) show multiple hypermetabolic left axillary lymph nodes. A midline focus of increased activity in the pelvis above the bladder localized to the uterine lining, a physiologic normal variant.

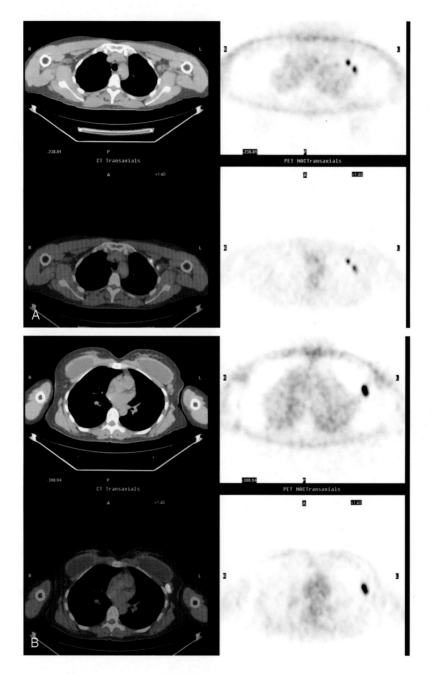

FIGURE 12. Axial PET/CT images better depict the location of the axillary disease. **A**, Hypermetabolic level I (lateral to the pectoralis minor [PM] muscle) and level II (beneath the PM muscle) left axillary lymph nodes are depicted. **B**, More inferior axillary level I hypermetabolic nodes are lateral to the implant.

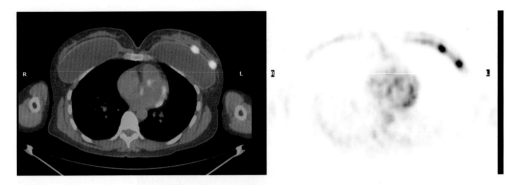

FIGURE 13.   Axial PET/CT images through the two sites of known IDC in the left breast show corresponding hypermetabolism.

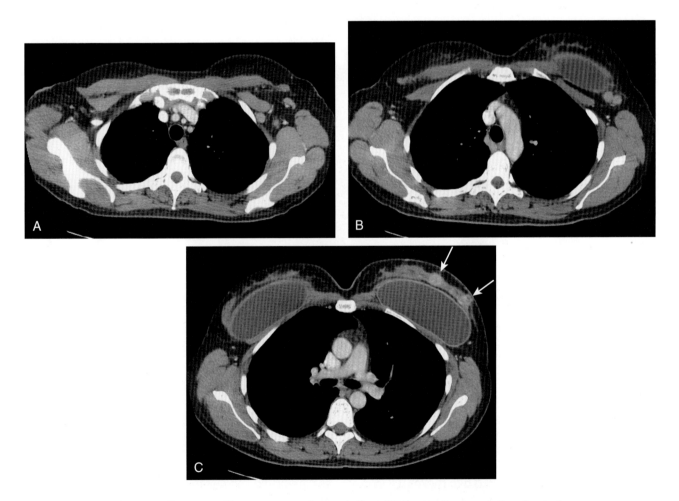

FIGURE 14.   Corresponding contrast-enhanced chest CT images for correlation, from above to below. **A**, Enlarged left axillary level I and II lymph nodes are strikingly asymmetrical compared with the right side. Several show fuzzy margins. **B**, At the upper margin of the implant, adjacent lymph nodes with fuzzy margins correspond with findings depicted on ultrasound (see Figure 1C) and MRI (see Figure 6). **C**, The two IDC masses can be seen on CT owing to differential enhancement from the rest of the parenchyma, but not to the same advantage as on breast MRI (*arrows*).

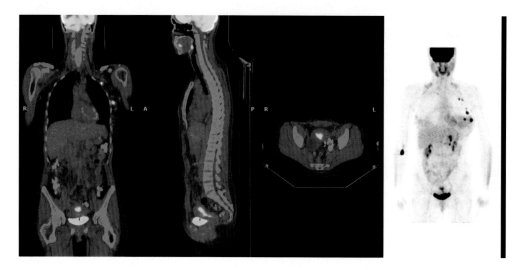

FIGURE 15. Three-plane fused PET/CT images show increased metabolic activity in the pelvis, localizing to the uterine lining (*cursors*). The axial projection shows a right adnexal corpus luteum cyst, which is not hypermetabolic in this case.

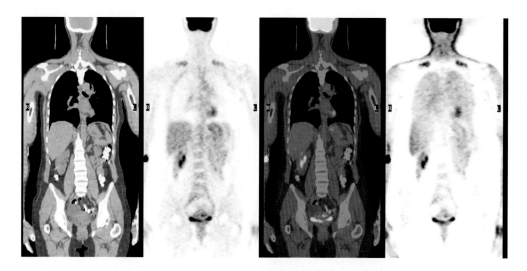

FIGURE 16. Coronal PET/CT images show symmetric mildly increased activity of "brown fat" in the supraclavicular regions bilaterally, localizing to fat on the corresponding CT.

mastectomy and implant removal. The simple mastectomy pathology on the right showed a 2-cm high-grade DCIS lesion extending into lobules, and two sentinel lymph nodes were negative. The left mastectomy specimen showed two foci of IDC, one described as in the lower outer quadrant (LOQ) measuring 1.5 × 1.4 × 1.4 cm. A second IDC was 2 cm medial and superior to the first focus (in the mid-breast posterior to nipple) and measured 2.1 × 2.0 × 1.5 cm. There was extensive angiolymphatic invasion. DCIS (solid, with foci of comedo necrosis) was associated with the invasive tumors

and extended into lobules. Nine of 18 lymph nodes showed metastatic tumor, with the largest 1.4 cm with extranodal extension. Margins were negative, by at least 5 mm. The tumors were estrogen receptor negative, progesterone receptor positive, and *HER-2/neu* negative.

After surgery, the patient was treated with chemotherapy (six cycles of Taxotere, Adriamycin, Cytoxan (TAC)), after which left chest wall and peripheral lymphatic radiation therapy to the supraclavicular and posterior axillary regions was performed. Additionally, the patient was placed on tamoxifen.

TEACHING POINTS

Implants in patients with newly diagnosed breast cancer introduce additional complexity into the therapeutic option decision making. In addition to the usual determinates of whether the patient is a lumpectomy candidate or not, the relationship of the disease to the implant and the impact of the implant on the ultimate cosmesis must be considered. If the patient is a candidate for breast conservation based on clinical and imaging assessments of the disease extent, the effect of radiation on a conserved breast with an implant must be taken into account. Breast radiation with an implant in place can be performed but may lead to contracture and an undesirable cosmetic result. In this case, the patient's reconstruction options were further limited by a prior "tummy tuck" procedure.

In this case, ultrasound accurately suggested the extensive involvement of the left breast. Prospective ultrasound of the right breast (not performed) might have successfully identified the right-sided disease, but clearly, it is easier to find a target with a map in hand (namely, breast MRI). The localized nature of the clumped enhancement in the right breast by itself would have been concerning, given how "quiet" the rest of the breast was. Coupled with the small focus of angiogenesis, our suspicion level is appropriately heightened, and any reasonably concordant sonographic correlate should be sampled. If no ultrasound correlate had been identified, it might have been technically possible to undertake MRI-guided biopsy in this region, given its anterior location. MRI-guided clip placement for subsequent localization would have been another consideration.

The correlation of the ultrasound and MRI findings with the final pathologic results is quite good in this case. The right-sided MRI findings of clumped enhancement suggested DCIS as the primary diagnosis of concern, and the small focus of invasion found at pathology correlates with the small nodule with angiogenesis on MRI kinetics and the small but suspicious ultrasound mass. Similarly, the two known IDC lesions on the left were accompanied by an entire quadrant of additional nodules and lower-level, clumped, plateauing enhancement, suggested a significant component of DCIS as well as invasion, as was subsequently confirmed.

One apparent discrepancy, of the locations of the left-sided IDC masses compared with the final pathology, is probably artifactual because of the presence in vivo of the implant. The lesion identified by pathology as in the LOQ apparently corresponds with the lesion identified as the UOQ 2 o'clock IDC, whereas the other lesion, described by pathology as 2 cm medial and superior to the LOQ IDC and in the mid-breast posterior to the nipple, correlates with the 1-o'clock IDC. In this case, the pathologist contacted radiology and reviewed the MRI to resolve the apparent discrepancy.

Systemic staging studies obtained in this patient included PET/CT and enhanced body CT scans. This case shows one source of normal variant PET increased activity, which can be seen in the pelvis of premenopausal patients. Physiologic endometrial activity can be seen, as well as activity in uterine fibroids (see Chapter 4, Case 7) and in corpus luteum cysts (see Case 17 in this chapter). In this case, PET/CT allows us to localize the uterine activity to the endometrium. Subsequent pelvic sonogram showed a normal appearance of the endometrium, and the patient was asymptomatic, so this is presumed to be normal variant activity. This has been documented to occur most commonly during menstruation and ovulation (weeks 1 and 3 of the menstrual cycle). Right adnexal findings compatible with a corpus luteum cyst were seen in this patient, but no associated hypermetabolism was apparent. Another commonly seen source of normal variant activity, brown fat, is also demonstrated in this patient.

SUGGESTED READING

Lerman H, Metser U, Grisaru D, et al. Normal and abnormal 18F-FDG endometrial and ovarian uptake in pre- and postmenopausal patients: assessment by PET/CT. *J Nucl Med* 2004; 45:266–271.

CASE 14

Use of body coil STIR imaging for local staging of new diagnoses of breast cancer

A 51-year-old woman noted a palpable lump in her right breast for 2 to 3 months, which was confirmed by her physician as a palpable 1-cm mass above the nipple at 11 to 12 o'clock. Mammography of the area showed increased density and possible architectural distortion in a region of mammographically stable microcalcifications (Figures 1, 2, and 3). Sonography confirmed a suspicious, dominant, solid, vascular, irregularly marginated, palpable mass, measuring up to 2.3 cm (Figures 4 and 5). Because it was palpable, the patient was referred to surgery for a palpation-guided biopsy, which diagnosed infiltrating ductal carcinoma (IDC).

Because of the marked breast density, completion of the evaluation was undertaken with breast MRI. This showed the known IDC to be a dominant, spiculated, intensely enhancing mass. The disease appeared to be unifocal (Figures 6 and 7). However, 1-cm bilateral supraclavicular lymph nodes (one on each side) were suggested on a coronal STIR sequence of the thorax (Figure 8). Positron emission tomography (PET)/CT was obtained for further evaluation and showed hypermetabolism only at the site of the known IDC (Figure 9).

The patient was treated surgically with lumpectomy and axillary node dissection, finding an estrogen receptor– and progesterone receptor–positive, *HER-2/neu*-negative, 2.1-cm IDC, with 1 of 12 lymph nodes positive. Final stage was IIB, T2N1M0.

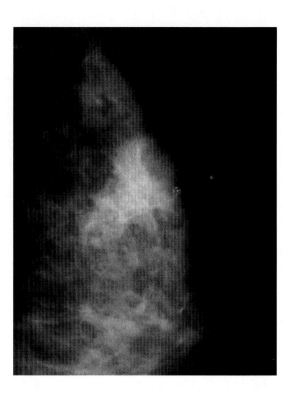

FIGURE 2. Lateral spot compression view of the palpable lump shows a marker. Underlying it, there is locally increased breast density and a suggestion of architectural distortion.

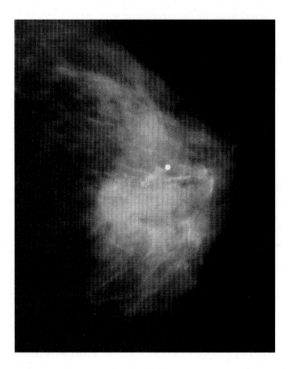

FIGURE 1. Mammogram in the CC position with a marker at a palpable lump identified by the patient shows marked increased breast tissue density. Increased density and microcalcifications are noted at the marked level. The microcalcifications had been mammographically stable for 10 years.

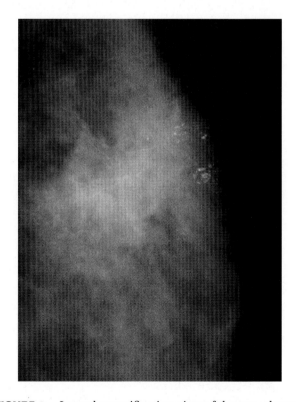

FIGURE 3. Lateral magnification view of the area shows increased density, possible architectural distortion, and microcalcifications. Some represent milk of calcium. The calcifications were mammographically stable for 10 years.

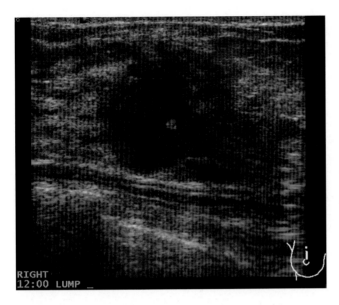

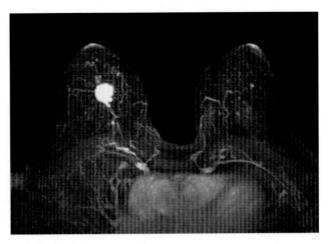

FIGURE 6. Axial maximal intensity projection from dynamic enhanced breast MRI shows a dominant, intensely enhancing mass with irregular margins.

FIGURE 4. Ultrasound of the palpable mass shows it to be highly suspicious—solid, very hypoechoic, and irregularly marginated.

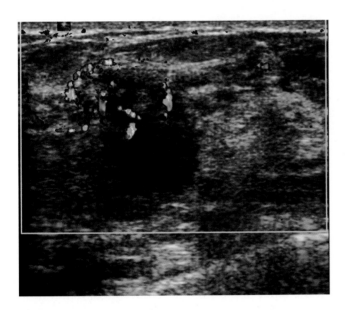

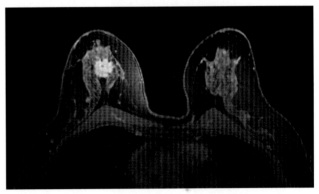

FIGURE 7. Fat-saturated, enhanced, high-resolution MRI of the mass better shows the marginal spiculation.

TEACHING POINTS

A variety of protocols are used for performance of breast MRI, with little standardization across institutions. That said, most protocols have certain critical elements in common. In general, breast MRI should be performed on a high-field magnet (at least 1.0 Tesla) in a dedicated breast coil. At a minimum, the protocol must include at least a fluid-sensitive sequence (T2 or STIR), and fat-saturated or subtracted enhanced T1-weighted sequences. Acquisition can be sagittal or axial, unilateral or bilateral. We have a strong preference for axial imaging performed bilaterally to allow for ease of comparison with the opposite side. Choices for fluid-sensitive sequences include T2-weighted, fat-saturated T2 weighted, and STIR sequences. These sequences permit identification of fluid,

FIGURE 5. Color Doppler evaluation shows the suspicious mass to be highly vascular.

Two cycles of Cytoxan, methotrexate, 5-fluorouracil (CMF) chemotherapy were administered. The patient's therapy was changed to hormonal ablation with sulindac (Zoladex) and tamoxifen because of her desire to discontinue chemotherapy.

External-beam radiation therapy, with a boost to the lumpectomy bed, was also performed in this case.

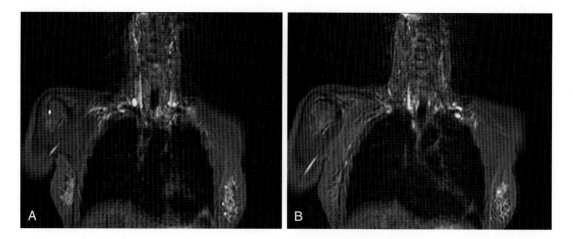

FIGURE 8. Coronal STIR images of the thorax (**A** anterior to **B**), obtained with the body coil with breast MRI, show oval hyperintense foci bilaterally, suggesting supraclavicular nodes.

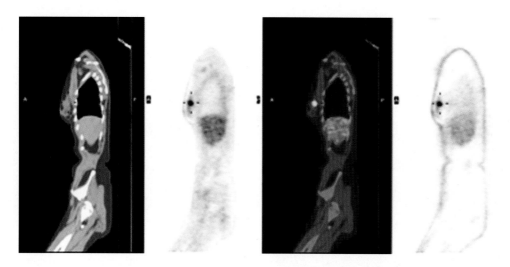

FIGURE 9. The known right IDC is hypermetabolic and well seen on sagittal PET/CT (left to right: CT, AC-PET, fused PET/CT, NAC-PET). No other abnormality was seen.

such as in cysts or in postoperative collections. Bright signal intensity on STIR of common encountered enhancing benign entities, such as fibroadenomas and lymph nodes, aids in characterization.

All protocols evaluating the breast parenchyma rely on early differential enhancement between suspicious lesions and the normal breast parenchyma, which enhances more slowly. For this reason, imaging must commence soon after the intravenous administration of Gd-chelate contrast agents, with the peak enhancement of most cancers occurring 1 to 2 minutes after injection. Dynamic, repetitive imaging before and at multiple time points after injection of the contrast enables the before and after series to be subtracted from each other, increasing the visual conspicuity of any enhancement. Three-dimensional, T1-weighted gradient echo sequences can image both breasts in the axial plane in 60 to 90 seconds, depending on acquisition parameters. This type of sequence is commonly used for performance of dynamic imaging, with the sequence built to run once before the contrast injection is triggered, and then again 3 to 5 times after the contrast is given. The sequence can be performed with or without fat saturation. However, if the patient moves during the dynamic series, subtractions will be unsuccessful, and the interpretation will have to be made from the source images, for which reason fat saturation is preferred.

As an example of how different breast MRI protocols can be, here are the current protocols in use at our institutions:

University of California, San Diego

Angled T1-weighted parasagittal oblique through each axilla (using the body coil)

Unilateral T1-weighted axial series through each breast

Unilateral fat-saturated T2-weighted series through each breast

Dynamic, fat-saturated, enhanced, bilateral axial T1-weighted gradient recalled series, run 6 times, once before and 5 times after contrast given (each series 60 seconds)

High-resolution, fat-saturated, three-dimensional axial series

25 minutes total of imaging

Scripps Clinic

Bilateral axial STIR series (5 minutes, 34 seconds)

Bilateral sagittal, T1-weighted series (precontrast) (4 minutes, 58 seconds)

Dynamic, fat-saturated, enhanced bilateral axial T1-weighted gradient recalled series, run 5 times, once before and 4 times after contrast given (each series 1 minute, 12 seconds)

Repeat bilateral sagittal, T1-weighted series (postcontrast) (4 minutes, 58 seconds)

20 minutes of total imaging

OPTIONAL (bail-out sequence for the patient suspected of having moved during the dynamic series, or if fat saturation fails): high-resolution, fat-saturated, three-dimensional axial series (3 minutes, 6 seconds)

Another choice that can be considered in creation of breast MRI protocols is concurrent performance of a limited chest MRI, in the form of a coronal STIR series through the thorax, encompassing the sternum and internal mammary vessels anteriorly and the thoracic spine posteriorly. This approach is advocated by Dr. Bruce A. Porter of First Hill Diagnostic Imaging in Seattle, who has had considerable success in identifying unsuspected stage IV disease (e.g., bone metastases in the sternum or thoracic spine) and in assessment of regional lymph nodes. At the time of this case, we included this sequence in our protocol, but overall did not find it to be as helpful in our patient population as in Dr. Porter's experience. As in this case, which suggested supraclavicular nodal involvement, we found that it not infrequently raised questions that required other imaging studies (in this case, a PET and CT) to answer them, without increasing the yield in terms of identifying more extensive disease than previously suspected. Another approach, which could have been considered in this case, would be to search sonographically for supraclavicular nodes, which could then undergo fine-needle aspiration.

CASE 15

MRI depiction of axillary and internal mammary node involvement

Annual screening mammography of a 72-year-old woman demonstrated suspicious masses in the medial left breast (Figure 1). Ultrasound confirmed these to be solid and demonstrated an abnormal left axillary node (Figures 2 and 3). An MRI confirmed the left breast masses and the abnormal axillary node (Figure 4). The constellation of findings was suspicious for multifocal carcinoma with axillary metastasis. In addition, MRI showed an abnormal-appearing left internal mammary lymph node (Figures 5 and 6). Ultrasound-guided core needle biopsy of the left breast confirmed multifocal invasive ductal carcinoma. The patient was treated with left mastectomy and radiation therapy.

TEACHING POINTS

This case illustrates the ability of MRI to demonstrate both axillary and internal mammary node (IMN) metastasis. Because normal-appearing nodes may harbor metastasis, MRI cannot be used to rule out nodal involvement. However, abnormal-appearing nodes may suggest metastasis. Internal mammary chain nodes may be seen incidentally in normal patients. Internal mammary nodes larger than 5 mm should be considered suspicious. In general, IMN metastases are located in the first or second intercostal spaces. More than 90% of women with metastases to the internal mammary nodes also have axillary node metastasis. Of the 5% to 10% of women who have isolated IMN involvement, most have tumors involving the medial aspect of the breast. Involvement of IMN nodes may indicate a worse prognosis and may benefit from radiation therapy.

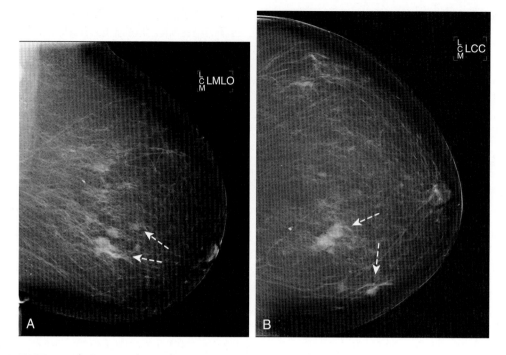

FIGURE 1.   MLO (**A**) and CC (**B**) mammographic views of the left breast show multiple irregular masses in the medial left breast (*arrows*).

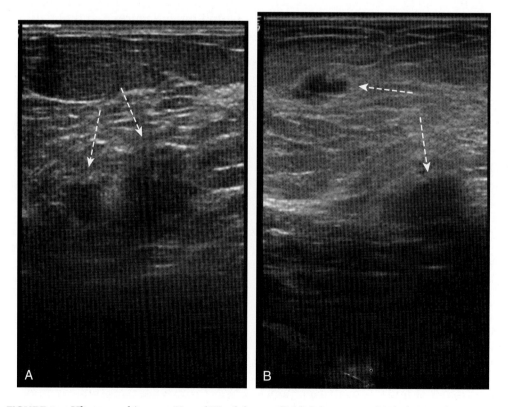

FIGURE 2.   Ultrasound images (**A** and **B**) of the medial left breast: multiple hypoechoic solid masses correspond to the mammographic masses (*arrows*). The findings are highly suspicious for multifocal carcinoma.

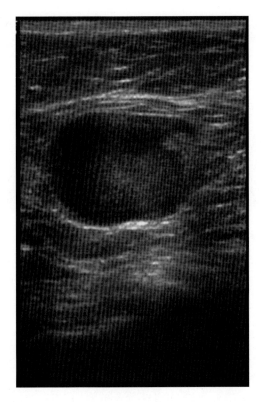

FIGURE 3. Ultrasound of the left axilla demonstrates an enlarged, abnormal lymph node with suspicious morphology for metastatic involvement. The lymph node is rounded, with effacement of the hilus.

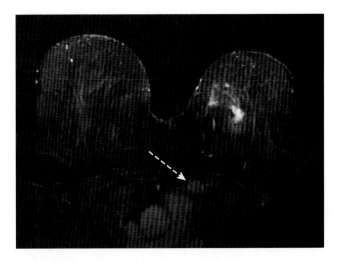

FIGURE 5. Postcontrast subtracted axial MRI. An enlarged left internal mammary node is demonstrated (*arrow*).

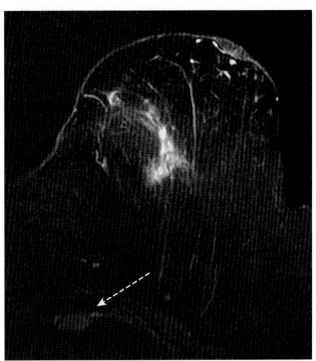

FIGURE 6. Fat-saturated, T2-weighted axial MRI of the left breast. The abnormal internal mammary node shows slight increased T2 signal intensity (*arrow*).

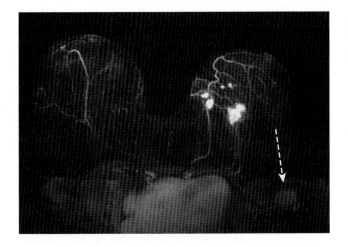

FIGURE 4. Postcontrast subtracted, maximal intensity projection MRI. Multiple intensely enhancing masses are seen in the medial left breast. In addition, an abnormal-appearing lymph node (*arrow*) is seen in the left axilla.

SUGGESTED READINGS

Bundred NJ, Morgan DAL, Dixon JM. ABC of breast diseases: management of regional nodes in breast cancer. *BMJ* 1994; 309:1222–1225.

Jatoi I. Internal mammary sentinel nodes in primary breast cancer. *Curr Med Res Opin* 2003; 19(6):567–569. © 2003 Librapharm Limited.

CASE 16

Cautionary notes on the use of breast MRI

A 53-year-old woman was diagnosed with left breast infiltrating lobular carcinoma (ILC) and lobular carcinoma in situ (LCIS) by stereotactic biopsy of left upper outer quadrant (UOQ) microcalcifications. The pathology specimen identified atypical ductal hyperplasia (ADH) associated with microcalcifications, with the ILC and LCIS noncalcified. The patient underwent a lumpectomy, with no residual tumor in the specimen. One sentinel lymph node was negative. She was treated with radiation therapy in addition.

While undergoing radiation therapy, breast MRI was performed to assess the opposite side. This showed a segmental region of clumped enhancement in the right medial breast, where the breast was largely fatty (Figures 1, 2, 3, and 4). An MRI-guided biopsy was performed when no ultrasound correlate could be found, and pathology showed ductal carcinoma in situ (DCIS).

Because of the extent of the abnormal segmental enhancement, over a 6-cm expanse, the patient was not thought to be a breast conservation candidate by multiple surgeons. Concurrently, microcalcifications in the right UOQ were noted to have progressed from prior studies. Two separate sites were sampled stereotactically, about 3 cm apart. One site returned a diagnosis of ADH and the other showed ADH and atypical lobular hyperplasia (ALH).

Despite multiple second opinions advising her to undergo mastectomy, the patient was quite reluctant to do so. Eventually, 16 months after her MRI-guided breast biopsy establishing the diagnosis of DCIS, she did undergo a simple mastectomy and placement of a tissue expander.

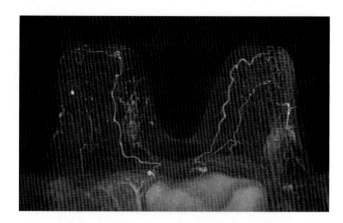

FIGURE 1. Axial enhanced subtracted maximum intensity view of both breasts shows low-level enhancement on the left posterolaterally, corresponding to the patient's recent surgery site. In the right medial breast, there is a segmental region of enhancement.

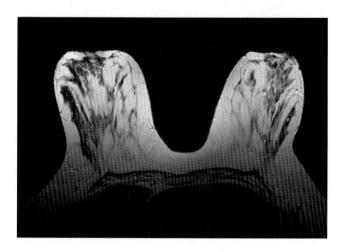

FIGURE 2. Axial T2-weighted image shows the right medial breast to be largely fatty.

The mastectomy pathology showed ADH and ALH, but no evidence of carcinoma in situ or invasive carcinoma. Two sentinel lymph nodes were negative.

TEACHING POINTS

This is an unusual outcome. Generally, when a malignant diagnosis is established by a large-volume core needle biopsy, we expect the same or worse to be obtained when the area is excised. However, the opposite is quite possible, as this case and Case 6 in Chapter 6 demonstrate. It is certainly possible in image-guided biopsies to sample a small malignant component, only to find no residual tumor in the excision. In fact, that had

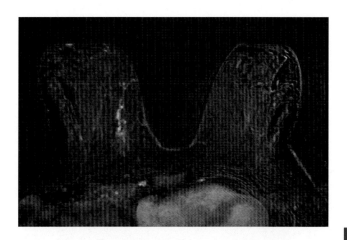

FIGURE 3. Representative enhanced subtracted image from the dynamic series shows an elongated region of clumped enhancement in the posteromedial right breast.

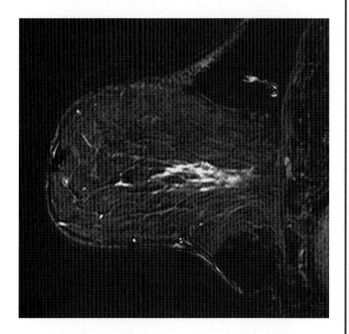

FIGURE 4. Sagittal subtracted view, obtained about 5 minutes after contrast injection, shows the right medial segmental enhancement.

the assumption that the entire process is probably all the same. Could mastectomy have been avoided in this case? A good cosmetic result would probably have been difficult to achieve, given that the patient would have required two large-volume excisions just to remove all of her known sites of disease (the right UOQ ADH and the long expanse in the right medial breast).

CASE 17

Whole-body PET as an adjunct to initial staging of node-positive breast cancer: Benign PET pelvic uptake in a corpus luteum cyst

A 41-year-old premenopausal woman presented with a few weeks' history of a palpable left upper outer quadrant breast lump. Mammography identified a dominant 2 cm mass, with irregular and spiculated margins (Figures 1 and 2). Ultrasound confirmed a 1.7-cm highly suspicious corresponding mass, as well as a small but abnormal looking axillary lymph node (Figures 3, 4, 5, and 6). Ultrasound-guided biopsy of the breast mass confirmed invasive lobular carcinoma (ILC), and fine-needle aspiration of the axillary lymph node showed metastatic adenocarcinoma.

Breast MRI was obtained because of the ILC histology. The known tumor mass showed intense rim enhancement and washout (Figures 7, 8, and 9). Tissue anterior to the known tumor showed an asymmetrical, less intense, plateauing pattern of more indeterminate enhancement (see Figure 7; Figure 10). MRI-guided biopsy was recommended.

Positron emission tomography (PET)/CT was ordered because of the known axillary involvement. The known breast cancer mass was quite hypermetabolic and readily identified. No additional breast abnormality was seen. A small punctate left axillary focus of activity was also seen, corresponding to the known involved lymph node (Figures 11 and 12). An additional focus of hypermetabolism in the pelvis appeared to corre-

happened in this patient in her original left breast diagnosis of ILC and LCIS. The targeted microcalcifications corresponded to ADH at pathology, whereas the ILC and LCIS were noncalcified but present in the stereotactic specimen. No residual tumor was found at pathologic examination of her lumpectomy specimen.

Presumably, the most intensely enhancing component visualized on breast MRI on the day of biopsy was targeted and proved to be DCIS. Because it would be difficult to sample multiple areas within such a large target area, we frequently must make

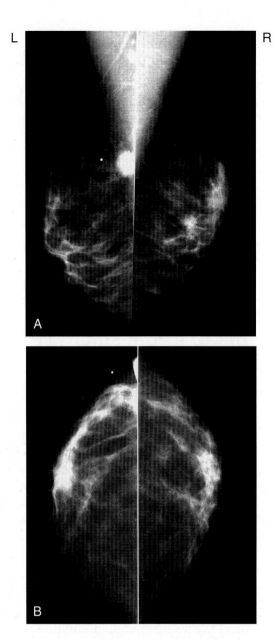

FIGURE 1.   MLO (**A**) and CC (**B**) mammograms show moderate breast parenchymal density. A dominant mass with spiculated margins is seen posteriorly overlying the left pectoral muscle on the MLO view but is largely excluded from the field of view on the CC view. This corresponds in location to the palpable lump, marked with a radiopaque BB.

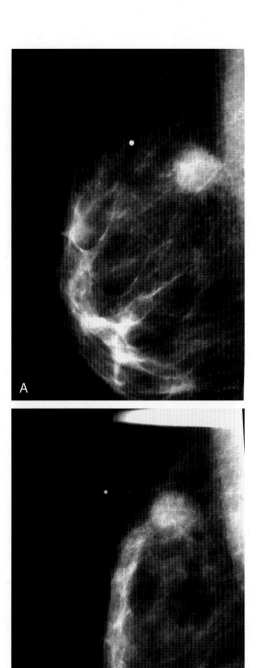

FIGURE 2.   Additional mammographic views include a 90-degree lateral view (**A**) and an exaggerated CC spot view (**B**). The margins can be better seen. Although some are obscured by adjacent parenchyma, where they can be seen, they range from indistinct to spiculated.

spond to a right ovarian cyst (Figures 13 and 14). This was presumed to be a corpus luteum cyst, a known cause of normal variant benign PET activity.

A second-look left breast ultrasound showed no additional anterior abnormality. It was elected to sample more anterior tissue at the time of lumpectomy and axillary dissection. The pathology showed a 2-cm infiltrating ductal carcinoma (IDC) with angiolymphatic invasion and high histologic grade (8 of 9) with close (<2 mm) deep margin and other margins clear by more than 1.5 cm. The invasive tumor was noted to extend close to the deep margin at two levels, both of which contained skeletal

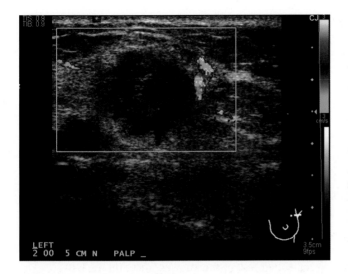

FIGURE 3. Ultrasound of the left upper outer quadrant palpable lump shows a highly suspicious appearance. The mass is solid, vascular, and very hypoechoic and has irregular, angular margins.

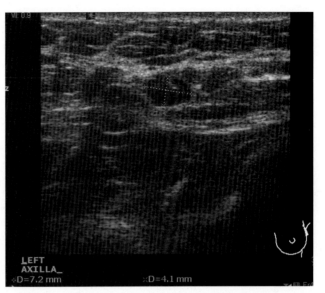

FIGURE 4. Axillary ultrasound shows a hypoechoic lymph node (*cursors*). Although not very large by size criteria (7 × 4 mm), its morphologic features are concerning. There is partial effacement of the fatty hilus.

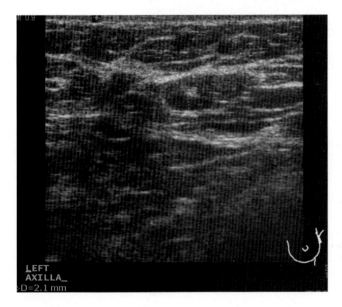

FIGURE 5. Another ultrasound view shows a cortical thickness of 2 mm, also not clearly pathologic. In other regions, it measured up to 3 mm.

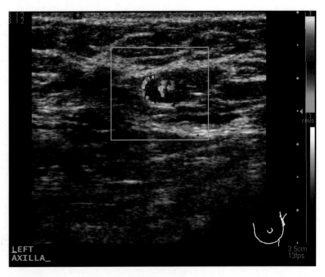

FIGURE 6. Color Doppler shows abnormal vascularity of this lymph node. In addition to expected hilar flow, there is peripheral, cortical flow. Ultrasound-guided fine-needle aspiration confirmed metastatic involvement.

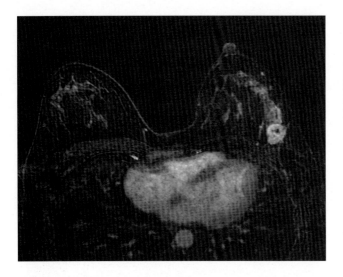

FIGURE 7. Enhanced subtracted axial breast MRI shows central necrosis (rim enhancement) of the left posterior lateral dominant mass. A concerning swath of lower-level enhancement is seen extending anteriorly toward the nipple from the known tumor.

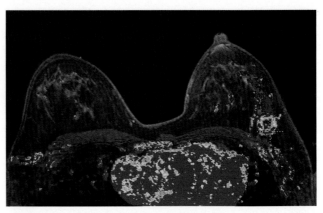

FIGURE 8. Color map of the enhancement (DynaCAD software) shows intense rim enhancement with washout (color-coded *red*) of the known cancer on the left posterolaterally. Less intense asymmetrical enhancement is seen anterior to the dominant mass (color-coded *blue*).

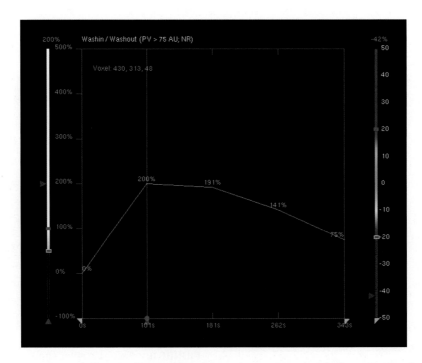

FIGURE 9. Corresponding signal intensity change versus time graph from the dominant mass shows a washout pattern of angiogenesis, with rapid upstroke (here to 200% of baseline) and subsequent decline (washout).

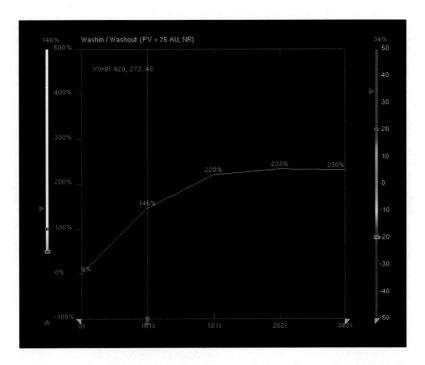

FIGURE 10.   Signal intensity change versus time graph from the less intensely enhancing tissue anterior to the known cancer shows a plateauing pattern of enhancement. MRI-guided biopsy was recommended.

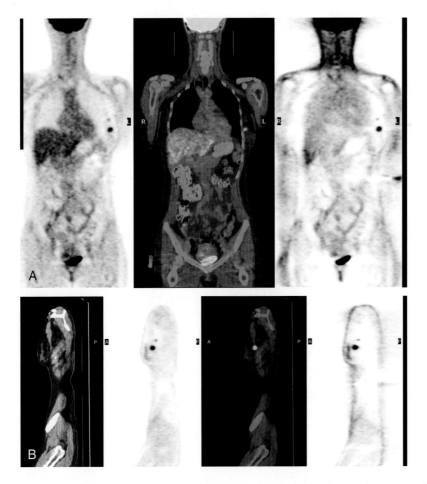

FIGURE 11.   Coronal (**A**) and sagittal (**B**) PET/CT images show the intense hypermetabolism of the known left breast cancer as well as the small, involved axillary lymph node.

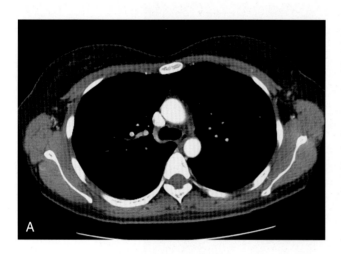
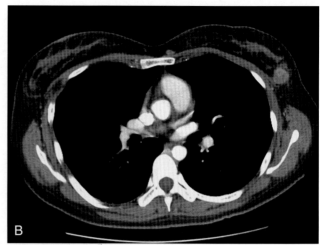

FIGURE 12. Corresponding enhanced chest CT images (**A** through axilla, and **B** through left breast mass) show the counterpart CT findings.

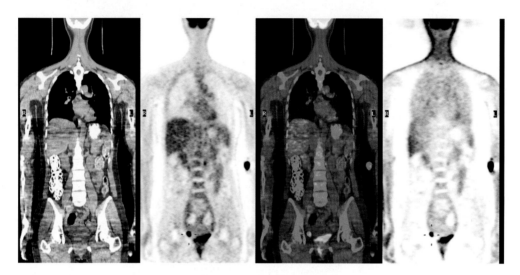

FIGURE 13. Coronal PET/CT images show an intense focus of hypermetabolism in the right hemipelvis, separate from the bladder (*cursors*).

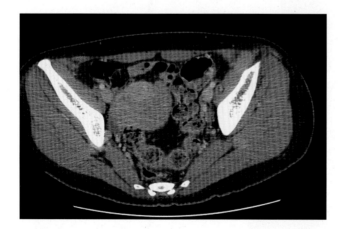

FIGURE 14. Corresponding enhanced pelvic CT image shows a right ovarian cyst at the same level. Corpus luteum cysts can be hypermetabolic on PET and are a known source of benign PET scan activity in the pelvis.

muscle at the deep surface. Fibrocystic changes and fibroadenomatoid changes were also noted in the specimen. Metastatic carcinoma was found in 1 of 17 lymph nodes.

The patient was additionally treated with chemotherapy (four cycles of dose-dense Adriamycin and Cytoxan (AC)) and radiation to the left breast and supraclavicular fossa. The final cycle was poorly tolerated by the patient. Planned additional chemotherapy with a taxane was declined, and the patient instead began tamoxifen.

TEACHING POINTS

This case provides many takeoff points for discussion. The characteristics of the index lesion in this case are entirely typical for malignancy with all modalities. The MRI did raise a question of more extensive disease extending anteriorly from the index lesion. The negative second-look ultrasound did not identify a correlate. This does not entirely resolve the question because correlates for MRI abnormalities which prove to be cancer are found in as few as 23% of cases. Rather than delay this patient's planned surgery with an MRI-guided biopsy, the surgeon used the MRI information to extend the excised area, which showed fibrocystic and fibroadenomatoid changes on histology.

Preoperative identification of axillary node involvement is desirable because patients who are known to have axillary metastases can proceed directly to axillary dissection and not undergo a sentinel node sampling. As this case illustrates, malignancy in lymph nodes can be suspected and confirmed histologically even in relatively small lymph nodes. Lymph nodes should be assessed for morphologic characteristics, which may suggest malignancy. Size itself can be misleading, but thickening or formation of nodules of the cortex, mass effect, effacement or loss of the fatty hilus, and abnormal vascularity (anywhere but at the hilus) are all features that may indicate involvement. Identification of such features should lead one to consider histologic sampling preoperatively.

The pathology of this malignancy was revised from ILC at ultrasound-guided core biopsy to IDC at partial mastectomy. The particular histology should not influence one unduly in interpretation of breast MRI. In the setting of a known IDC, the segmental regional enhancement noted here anterior to the index lesion could be due to DCIS, whereas the propensity of ILC to infiltrate regionally is well known.

This case also illustrates a fairly commonly encountered source of benign PET scan activity, with the right ovarian corpus luteum cyst showing hypermetabolism. Other sources of benign PET scan activity that may be seen in the pelvis of women being imaged systemically for breast cancer include physiologic activity of the endometrium, which will be most intense during the first (menstrual) and third (ovulatory) weeks of a premenopausal patient's cycle, and activity in uterine fibroids. Endometrial activity is a more concerning finding in a postmenopausal patient, in whom it may reflect endometrial cancer, and should prompt further evaluation. Similarly, PET hypermetabolism in an ovary is a concerning finding in a postmenopausal patient and should prompt further evaluation for possible neoplasia.

SUGGESTED READING

LaTrenta LR, Menell JH, Morris EA, et al. Breast lesions detected with MR imaging: utility and histopathologic importance of identification with US. *Radiology* 2003; 227:856–861.

CASE 18

Whole-body PET as an adjunct to initial staging of node-positive breast cancer: Rotter's node involvement

A 37-year-old woman found a right UOQ palpable breast lump. Mammography showed a dominant lobular breast mass, with some margins obscured by dense adjacent parenchyma (Figure 1). Sonography demonstrated highly suspicious features, including taller-than-wide shape, and angular and irregular margins (Figure 2). In addition, an axillary lymph node with a thickened (7-mm) cortical mantle was found (Figure 3). Ultrasound-guided core needle biopsy of the dominant mass proved infiltrating ductal carcinoma (IDC), and ultrasound guided fine-needle aspiration of the axillary lymph node confirmed malignant cells, consistent with metastatic breast carcinoma.

Because of the size of the patient's cancer relative to her breast size, mastectomy was favored for surgical therapy over lumpectomy. Breast MRI confirmed unifocal disease (Figures 4, 5, 6, 7, and 8). Staging workup showed elevated tumor markers (CEA and CA27.29). A positron emission tomography (PET)/CT scan and enhanced diagnostic chest, abdomen, and pelvic CT scans showed intense hypermetabolism in the known breast cancer (Figures 9, 10, 15) and abnormal right axillary lymph node (Figures 8, 11, and 12). Increased metabolic activity was also seen in a 5-mm right interpectoral (Rotter's) lymph node (Figures 13 and 14). A commonly seen normal variant source of PET activity was also seen, with symmetrical supraclavicular brown fat uptake (Figure 16).

The mastectomy specimen demonstrated a 3-cm infiltrating ductal adenocarcinoma, with clear margins. Because the patient was known

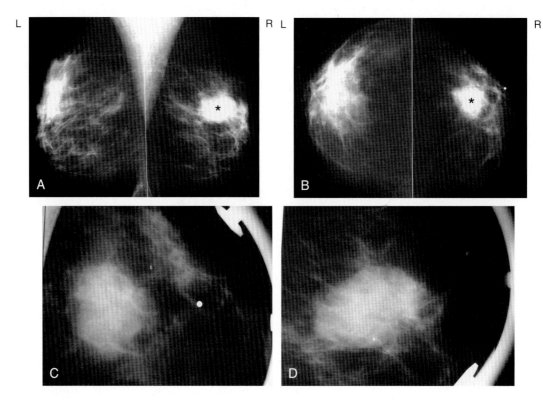

FIGURE 1. MLO (**A**) and CC (**B**) mammograms show dense anterior breast parenchyma. A dominant mass is seen in the right upper outer quadrant (*asterisk*), at the level of a marker identifying a palpable lump. Some margins appear lobular, but many are obscured. MLO (**C**) and CC (**D**) spot views of the palpable lump better show the margins, which are variably circumscribed, indistinct, and obscured by adjacent parenchyma.

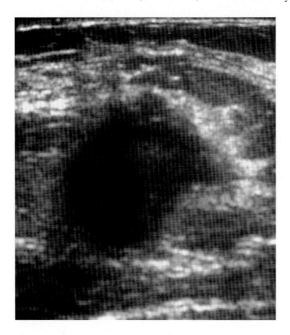

FIGURE 2. Ultrasound shows the mass to have highly suspicious features. It is taller than wide and hypoechoic, and the margins are angular and ill-defined, with no surrounding capsule. Ultrasound-guided biopsy confirmed IDC.

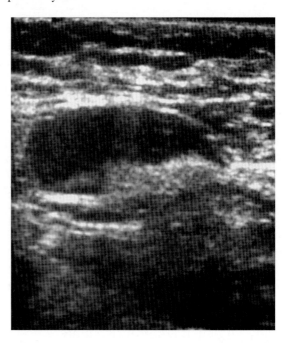

FIGURE 3. Sonography of the ipsilateral axilla shows an abnormal lymph node. Although the fatty hilus is not effaced, the cortical mantle is abnormally thick (7 mm; normal <3 mm). Well-seen, abnormal lymph nodes like this are amenable to sampling with fine-needle (20–25 gauge) aspiration (FNA). FNA of this lymph node revealed malignant cells, consistent with metastatic breast carcinoma.

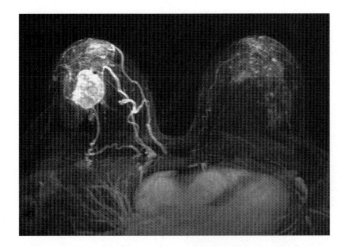

FIGURE 4. Maximal intensity projection from the enhanced, subtracted dynamic portion of a staging breast MRI shows a large, dominant, rim-enhancing right breast cancer mass. Note the marked asymmetry in vascularity of the right breast. Small scattered foci of enhancement are noted bilaterally. The pattern and low level of enhancement of these tiny foci are typical of fibrocystic enhancement.

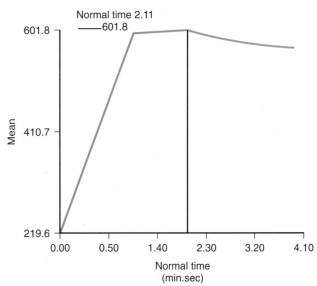

FIGURE 6. A signal intensity change versus time curve graphically confirms washout of the index tumor, another MRI feature of malignancy.

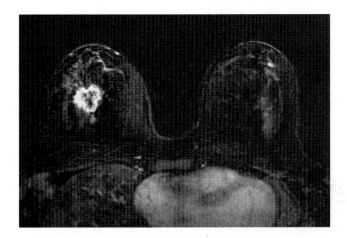

FIGURE 5. A slice from the dynamic series (T1-weighted, fat-saturated, three-dimensional gradient echo sequence) through the right IDC shows the margin irregularity and rim enhancement of this lesion well.

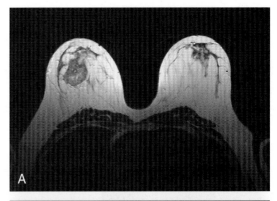

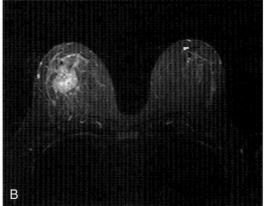

FIGURE 7. Axial T2-weighted turbo spin echo (TSE) (**A**) and STIR (**B**) images show the dominant right breast mass to be predominantly isointense to breast parenchyma. Central hyperintensity suggests necrosis.

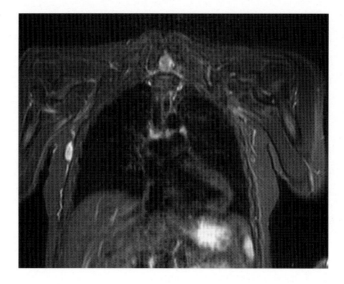

FIGURE 8.   A coronal STIR image (limited chest MRI performed in conjunction with the breast MRI, using the body coil) shows an enlarged right axillary lymph node.

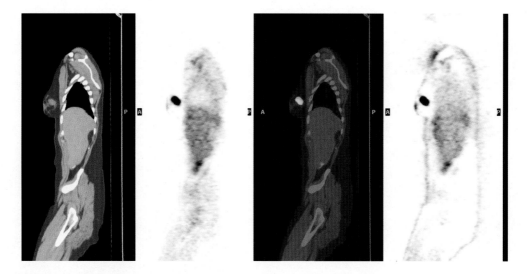

FIGURE 9.   Sagittal images from PET/CT (from left to right: noncontrast CT, PET, fused PET/CT; non-attenuation-corrected PET) show intense hypermetabolism of the right breast infiltrating ductal carcinoma. Activity at the inferior tip of the liver is physiologic, in bowel.

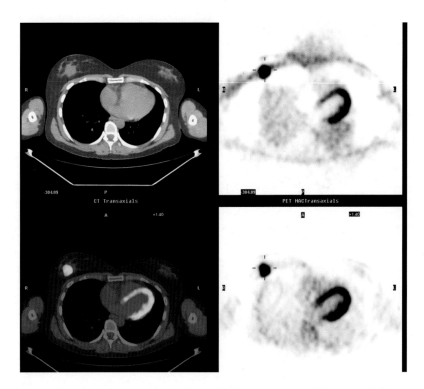

FIGURE 10.   Axial images from PET/CT (upper left: noncontrast CT; upper right: non-attenuation-corrected (NAC) PET; lower left: fused PET/CT; lower right: PET) show the dominant right IDC to be intensely metabolically active. Physiologic myocardial activity is noted on these PET views.

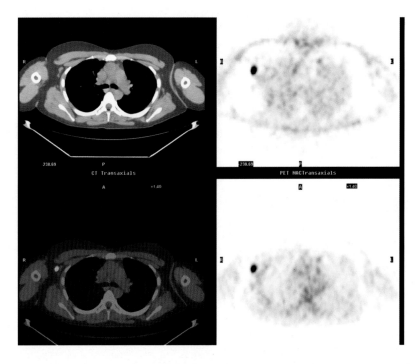

FIGURE 11.   Axial PET/CT slices through the axilla (upper left: noncontrast CT; upper right: NAC PET; lower left: fused PET/CT; lower right: attenuation-corrected PET) show marked hypermetabolism of a right level I axillary lymph node.

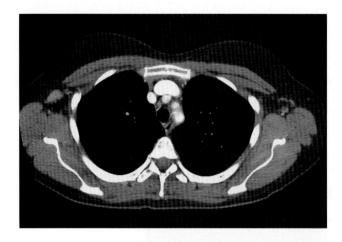

FIGURE 12. Diagnostic chest CT with intravenous contrast enhancement better shows the right axillary lymph node, corresponding to PET. It is enlarged, with no discernible fatty hilus, and corresponds to the abnormal lymph node seen on ultrasound, which was malignant on FNA.

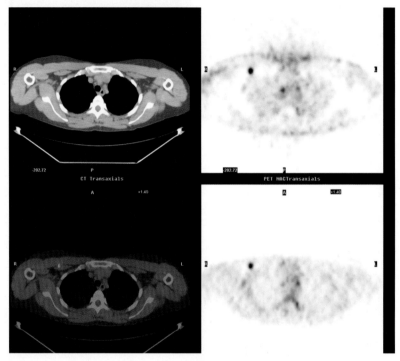

FIGURE 13. Another axial slice from PET/CT (upper left: noncontrast CT; upper right: NAC PET; lower left: fused PET/CT; lower right: attenuation-corrected PET) shows a separate small focus of Rotter's node hypermetabolism, interposed between the right pectoralis major and minor muscles.

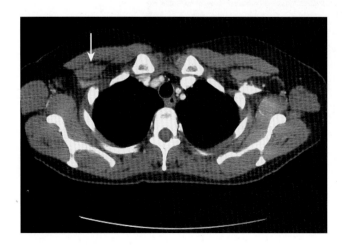

FIGURE 14. Corresponding section from enhanced chest CT shows the right interpectoral (Rotter's) lymph node (*arrow*) to be on the order of 5 mm in size.

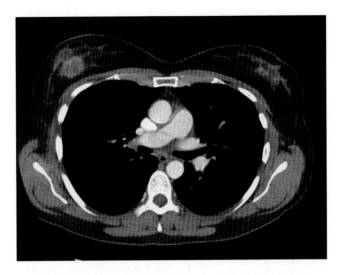

FIGURE 15. Another slice from the enhanced chest CT shows the right IDC, with central hypodensity. Although breast cancers can often be seen on CT, the soft tissue contrast is generally insufficient to rely on CT for primary identification and local staging of breast cancers.

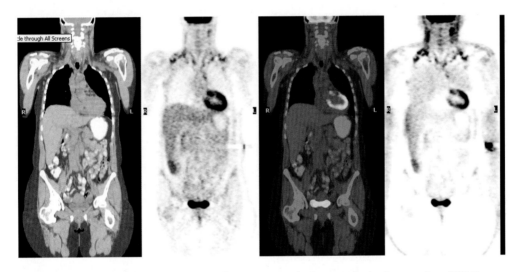

FIGURE 16. Coronal PET/CT images show symmetrical supraclavicular uptake of FDG, localizing on CT to fat. The appearance and distribution are typical of brown fat, which is a commonly observed normal variant source of benign activity on PET. Although it can be seen in any PET patient, younger female patients who are cold appear to be more prone to such uptake. Note also the left mediastinal brown fat uptake.

preoperatively to have axillary involvement, axillary dissection was performed at the same time. Three of 22 lymph nodes showed metastatic adenocarcinoma. The largest involved lymph node measured 1.5 cm.

The patient was treated postoperatively with aggressive chemotherapy (four cycles of Adriamycin and Cytoxan [AC] chemotherapy and four cycles of paclitaxel [Taxol]), followed by right chest wall, supraclavicular fossa, and posterior axillary boost radiation.

Subsequently, the patient underwent genetic testing and proved to have a *BRCA1* gene muta-

tion. Her family history consisted of premenopausal breast cancer in a maternal aunt. Ten months after finishing radiation therapy, she underwent prophylactic left mastectomy, bilateral transverse rectus abdominis myocutaneous (TRAM) flap reconstruction, hysterectomy, and oophorectomy. Her postoperative course was complicated by development of abdominal wall infection, twice requiring operative débridement of infected, necrotic tissue and intravenous antibiotic therapy (see Case 3 in Chapter 6 for imaging features of the TRAM flap donor site complications). She also developed pulmonary embolism.

Nearly concurrent with these events, the patient developed right upper arm and shoulder pain, and she noted development of an infraclavicular lump. Recurrence was subsequently confirmed in right infraclavicular and mediastinal nodal regions. See Case 7 in Chapter 10 for the recurrent disease imaging findings.

TEACHING POINTS

At initial diagnosis, the patient was considered to have stage IIB disease, T2N1M0. The increased tumor markers and evidence of axillary involvement at initial diagnosis of this breast cancer led to a comprehensive initial staging evaluation with enhanced chest, abdomen and pelvic CT scans, and PET/CT.

Historically, comprehensive imaging staging of a newly diagnosed locally advanced breast cancer (LABC) would have included a chest x-ray, bone scan, and either ultrasound or CT of the liver. Today, arguments can be made for comprehensive initial staging with PET, enhanced body CT, and bone scan. Body CT with enhancement will allow simultaneous optimal evaluation of the lung parenchyma and solid viscera (especially the liver), and the bone windows provide tomographic radiographic evaluation of axial skeletal bone. PET imaging allows for the assessment of the metabolic (glycolytic) activity of any lesions encountered on CT.

Why not do PET alone? One argument is that PET scans have a lower limit of resolution, on the order of 1 cm, depending on location in the body and a tumor's intrinsic metabolic activity. Current state-of-the-art body PET scan units have a lower limit of resolution of 6 mm, but other limitations may prevent malignant lesions of this size from being reliably visualized. One example is in the liver, which has a moderate level of intrinsic metabolic activity. Another is in the lung bases, where there is considerable respiratory excursion.

What about PET/CT? Can it substitute for PET and enhanced body CT? One limitation of PET/CT alone is in lung parenchymal evaluation. PET/CT is acquired over multiple respiratory cycles, at tidal lung volumes, rather than at full lung expansion and suspended respiration, as in diagnostic chest CT scanning.

Because PET scans are tomographic and can image the entire body, why do bone scanning? PET scans are sensitive for identification of bone marrow involvement and lytic bone metastases, areas where

bone scans frequently underestimate disease. However, blastic bone metastases that are readily demonstrated on bone scans may not show increased activity on PET.

Without the hypermetabolism displayed by the PET scan, it is doubtful that this interpectoral (Rotter's) node would have been seen. An interpectoral (Rotter's) lymph node is considered a level II axillary node. The PET scan activity is powerful presumptive evidence of involvement of a lymph node in a difficult position to sample.

CASE 19

Bracketing needle localization of microcalcifications

A 62-year-old woman was referred to an orthopedic surgeon for evaluation of right shoulder pain. The surgeon noted asymmetry of the left breast and nipple inversion and referred the patient for a mammogram. Mammography demonstrated extensive microcalcifications, with an associated mass, in the left upper outer quadrant (UOQ) (Figures 1 and 2). Palpation-guided biopsy by a breast surgeon of UOQ firmness did not confirm a malignancy, and the patient had an excisional surgical biopsy after needle localization (Figures 3 and 4). The pathology showed an estrogen receptor–positive, *HER-2/neu*-positive, 1.5-cm infiltrating ductal carcinoma (IDC), associated with solid and comedo ductal carcinoma in situ (DCIS), which extended to the margin of resection. An intramammary lymph node removed in the specimen was involved with tumor. Mastectomy was performed subsequently, showing extensive residual comedo DCIS in the specimen and negative margins. Three of 15 lymph nodes proved to be positive. Tumor stage was IIA, T1N1. The patient was further treated with chemotherapy and 5 years of tamoxifen therapy. Subsequent aromatase inhibitor therapy with letrozole was discontinued because of side effects.

TEACHING POINTS

What a difference a few years makes! This patient was treated in 1998. Palpable firmness in the same

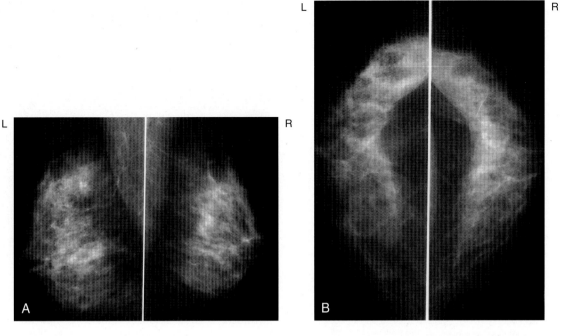

FIGURE 1. Mammograms [MLO (**A**) and CC (**B**)] show dense breast tissue, with extensive microcalcifications and a suggestion of an underlying mass in the left upper outer quadrant (UOQ), better seen in detail (Figure 2).

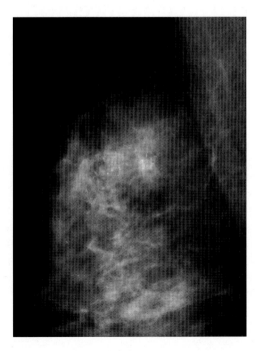

FIGURE 2. Detail of the left upper breast, MLO projection, shows an ill-defined mass with pleomorphic microcalcifications.

quadrant as the highly suspicious mammographic findings led appropriately to palpation-guided biopsy, but the suspected malignancy was not confirmed. Today, this scenario would be cause for referral for an image-guided biopsy. Ultrasound would be an important component of the workup, to identify any associated mass. When no mass is seen on mammography within a large area of suspicious microcalcifications, there is utility in evaluating the area with ultrasound to determine whether a mass can be identified to target for biopsy. If there is a mass seen on ultrasound, sampling it with ultrasound guidance may increase the likelihood of obtaining a diagnosis of invasive cancer than sampling microcalcifications stereotactically.

In this case, the patient had a diagnostic surgical excision biopsy. The abnormality is extensive. An attempt to encompass its full extent was made by bracketing the abnormality with more than one localization needle. From the specimen x-ray, we can predict the margins will be involved.

With a smaller abnormality, the bracketing needle localization illustrated here may be more successful, helping guide the surgeon's excision and, in some cases, achieving clear margins in fewer steps.

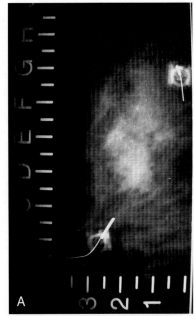

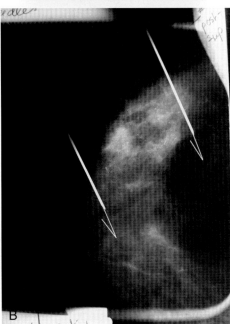

FIGURE 3. Images [lateral (**A**) and CC (**B**)] from the needle localization. An attempt was made to encompass the entire area with bracketing localization wires, placed at opposite ends of the abnormality.

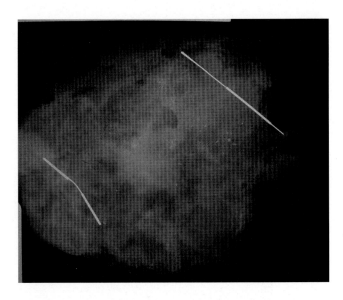

FIGURE 4. Specimen x-ray shows a large mass within the specimen, with many pleomorphic calcifications, with the localizing wires at opposite ends of the specimen.

CASE 20

Medial breast cancer with internal mammary drainage on lymphoscintigraphy*

A new, suspicious mass was identified in the lower inner quadrant of the right breast in an 83-year-old woman on screening mammogram (Figures 1 and 2). Biopsy was performed under ultrasound guidance, confirming mucinous carcinoma. A clip placed at the time of biopsy was subsequently used to guide needle localization for excision. Lympho-scintigraphy was performed at the time, through peritumoral and subdermal injections. Imaging was carried out to 4 hours and showed evidence of drainage to a right lower internal mammary lymph node (Figure 3).

TEACHING POINTS

There is little consensus in the literature on the optimal technique for breast cancer sentinel lymph

*Case courtesy of Dr. Eva Lean, Tri City Medical Center, Oceanside, CA.

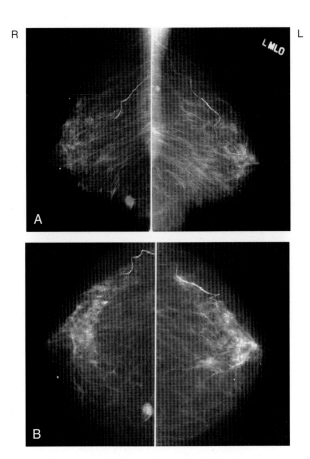

FIGURE 1. MLO (**A**) and CC (**B**) mammograms show a dense mass in the posterior lower inner quadrant of the right breast, which is readily visualized in this fatty portion of the breast.

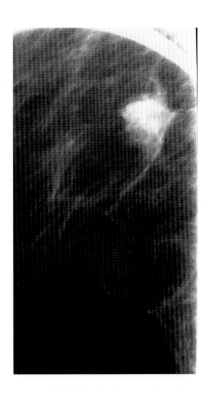

FIGURE 2. The margins are seen to be indistinct on spot compression.

node identification, other than that utilization of both radiopharmaceutical and intraoperative blue dye injection identifies more sentinel lymph nodes than protocols using either approach solely. A variety of radiopharmaceutical injection techniques, including peritumoral, subareolar, and intradermal injections, solely or in combination, have been advocated. The good news is that it seems that all these methods can work. Povoski and colleagues report a single-institution, prospective trial of 400 patients randomized to undergo either intradermal, intraparenchymal, or subareolar injection of ^{99m}Tc-sulfur colloid administration for sentinel lymph node mapping and biopsy in breast cancer. In this series, intradermal injection demonstrated significantly greater frequency of localization, decreased time to first localization on preoperative lymphoscintigraphy, and decreased time to harvest the first sentinel node.

Performance of lymphoscintigraphy is not universal. In this example, peritumoral and subdermal injections were performed, and imaging was carried

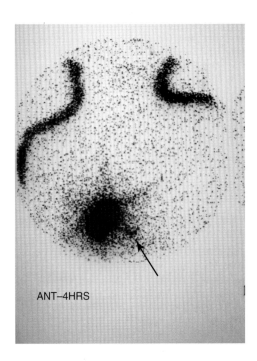

FIGURE 3. Lymphoscintigraphy shows intense activity at the peritumoral injection site. A small focus of separate activity is inferomedial to the tumor site (*arrow*), suggesting drainage of this medial tumor to an internal mammary lymph node.

out to 4 hours. At Scripps Clinic, our practice is to perform a single intradermal injection of 500 µCi of filtered ^{99m}Tc-sulfur colloid in the smallest volume possible, administered at the areolar edge of the breast cancer–involved quadrant.

In this case, lymphoscintigraphy suggests internal mammary node drainage, not a surprising result given the lower inner quadrant location of this breast cancer. Because no clear advantage has been demonstrated from surgical series of extended internal mammary dissections, what to do with this information remains controversial. Even without lymphoscintigraphic evidence of internal mammary sentinel node drainage, many radiation oncologists would plan for inclusion of internal mammary basins in designing treatment ports for such far medial lesions. This case also illustrates one of the possible limitations of lymphoscintigraphic imaging: if the draining lymph node is close to the primary and peritumoral injection has been performed, the primary site injection activity may obscure uptake in a draining lymph node. In such a case, imaging with the primary site shielded may aid in recognition of sentinel nodes.

SUGGESTED READING

Povoski SP, Olsen JO, Young DC, et al. Prospective randomized clinical trial comparing intradermal, intraparenchymal, and subareolar injection routes for sentinel lymph node mapping and biopsy in breast cancer. *Ann Surg Oncol* 2006; 13(11):1412–1421.

CASE 21

Biopsy quality control: Mammographic lesion, wrong ultrasound correlate biopsied; rationale for post–ultrasound biopsy clip placement and mammogram

An asymptomatic 71-year-old woman underwent yearly screening mammography, which showed a small mass in the posterior lateral right breast (Figure 1). Ultrasound showed a small irregular

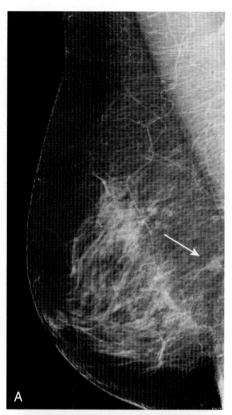

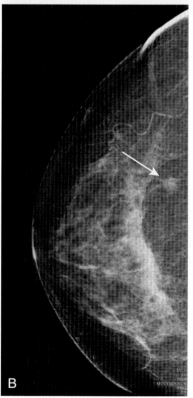

FIGURE 1. Right MLO (**A**) and exaggerated CC (**B**) mammographic views show a small mass (*arrow*) in the posterior lateral breast.

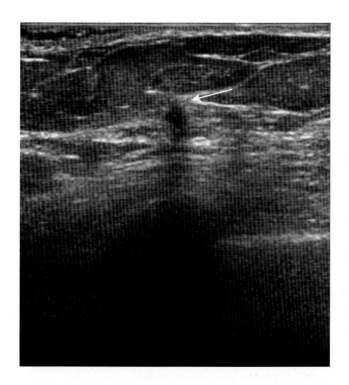

FIGURE 2. Ultrasound image of the right breast at 9 o'clock demonstrates a small 5- to 6-mm mass with irregular margins and posterior acoustic shadowing (*arrow*). This was thought to correspond to the mammographic finding.

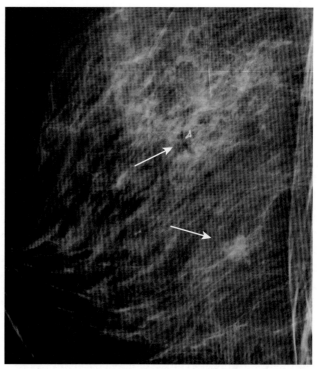

FIGURE 3. Post-biopsy right breast 90-degree lateral mammographic view demonstrates that the biopsy marker clip location does not correlate with the mammographic lesion (*arrows*).

mass in the 9-o'clock position, thought to correspond to the mammographic finding (Figure 2). An ultrasound-guided 14-gauge core needle biopsy was performed. Because of the lesion's small size, a marker clip was placed. A postbiopsy mammogram showed that the marker clip location did not correspond to the lesion seen on mammography (Figure 3). Subsequently, additional ultrasound imaging demonstrated a second lesion at 8 o'clock (Figure 4). A second core biopsy and clip placement was performed. On the postbiopsy mammogram, this clip conformed to the site of the original mammographic lesion (Figure 5). Pathology reported atypical ductal hyperplasia for the 9-o'clock lesion and invasive ductal carcinoma for the 8-o'clock lesion. The patient went on to have a preoperative MRI (Figures 6 and 7). This showed a small contralateral left breast lesion. A correlate was found on second-look ultrasound (Figure 8). On core biopsy, invasive ductal carcinoma was

confirmed. The patient decided to undergo bilateral mastectomies.

TEACHING POINT

This case illustrates the importance of careful correlation of findings seen on ultrasound with suspicious mammographic findings. In this example, the use of postbiopsy marker clips allowed the location of ultrasound findings to be correlated with the original mammographic abnormality. This is particularly important with small or subtle mammographic findings. It is also important to remember that a significant number of breast cancers are multifocal or multicentric at presentation. In this case, the patient also had a mammographically occult contralateral carcinoma.

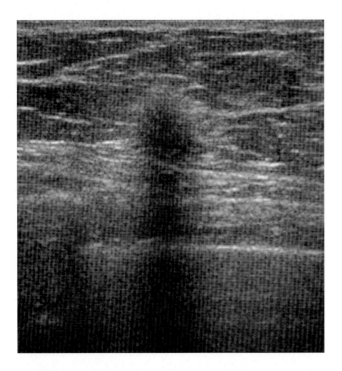

FIGURE 4. Ultrasound image of the right breast. Upon further evaluation, a second suspicious lesion was seen on ultrasound, in the 8-o'clock position.

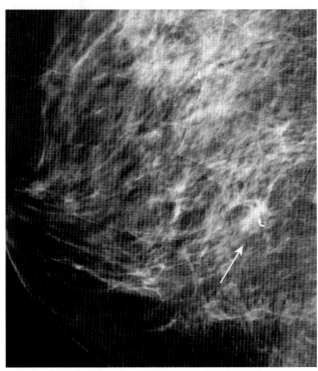

FIGURE 5. Postbiopsy mammogram following the second core biopsy demonstrates that the lesion in the 8-o'clock position on ultrasound corresponds to the original mammographic lesion (*arrow*).

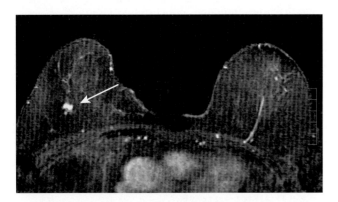

FIGURE 6. Subtracted axial postcontrast MRI demonstrates a lobular enhancing mass at 8 o'clock in the right breast (*arrow*), corresponding to the known carcinoma.

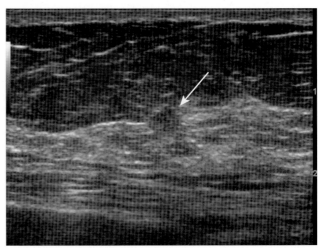

FIGURE 8. Second-look ultrasound image of the medial left breast. A small hypoechoic solid mass in seen at 9 o'clock, corresponding to the MRI finding. Subsequent core biopsy showed invasive ductal carcinoma.

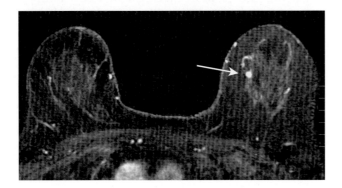

FIGURE 7. Subtracted postcontrast MRI image also showed a small enhancing round 5-mm mass in the medial left breast (*arrow*).

CASE 22

Biopsy quality control: DCIS presenting as disappearing microcalcifications and subsequent development of a mass

An 82-year-old woman presented with clustered suspicious microcalcifications in the lateral left breast on routine screening mammography. After magnification, stereotactic biopsy was recommended (Figures 1 and 2). The biopsy was technically difficult because the patient had trouble tolerating the biopsy position. Multiple sets of core samples were obtained; however, no microcalcifications were identified in the samples (Figures 3 and 4). Pathology results indicated benign breast tissue with no calcifications. Given the patient's age, 6-month follow-up was recommended over surgical excisional biopsy. At follow-up, the calcifications were seen to decrease in number, and there was interval development of an associated irregular solid mass (Figure 5). Subsequent ultrasound-guided core needle biopsy revealed an intermediate-grade invasive ductal carcinoma and DCIS (Figure 6). The patient was treated surgically with sentinel node biopsy and lumpectomy.

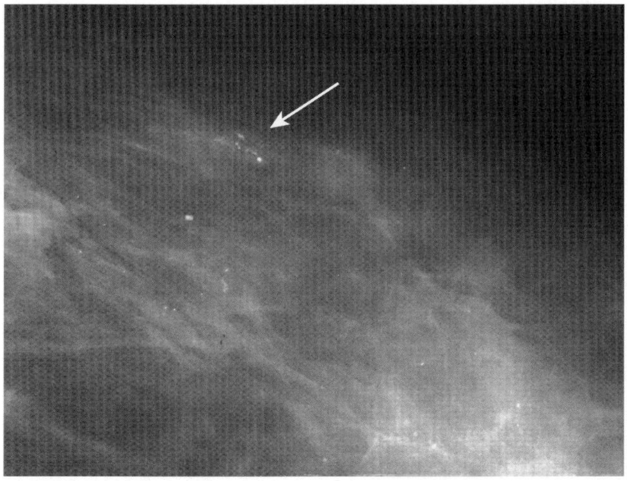

TEACHING POINTS

About 40% to 50% of mammographically detected nonpalpable breast cancer manifests as microcalcifications. If there is an associated mass, soft tissue density, or dense overlying tissue, the use of ultrasound should be considered. By identifying a mass associated with suspicious calcifications, the diag-

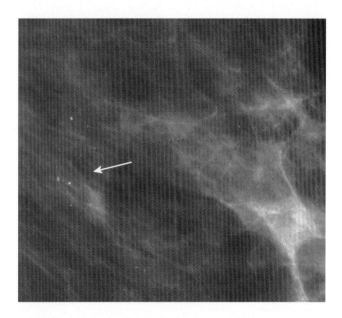

FIGURE 2. On the left 90-degree mammographic magnification view, the calcifications appear loosely grouped (*arrow*).

FIGURE 1. Left CC mammographic magnification view shows clustered suspicious pleomorphic microcalcifications (*arrow*).

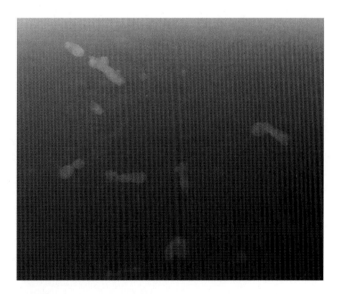

FIGURE 3. Specimen x-ray of the core samples obtained by stereotactic needle biopsy shows no obvious calcifications in the specimens.

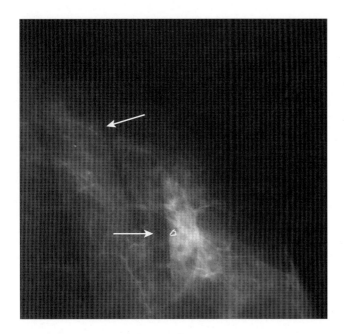

FIGURE 4. Postbiopsy left CC mammographic view. The biopsy marker is seen medial to the targeted microcalcifications (*arrows*). This immediate postbiopsy image confirmed that the biopsy missed the targeted calcifications.

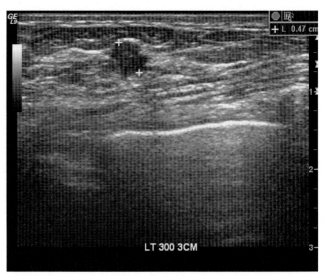

FIGURE 6. Ultrasound imaging confirms a suspicious solid mass in the lateral left breast near the prior biopsy site. The mass demonstrates irregular, angular margins, and is taller than wide.

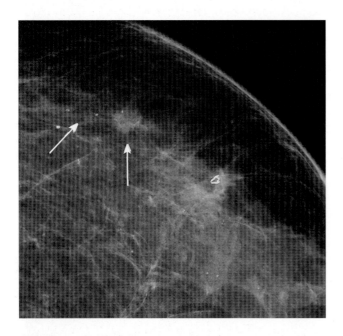

FIGURE 5. Six-month follow-up left CC mammographic view demonstrates the previously targeted calcifications to have decreased in number and interval development of an associated irregular mass (*arrows*). In retrospect, on the original mammographic CC magnification view, there is a suggestion of a partially visualized associated density.

nosis of an invasive component within an area of DCIS may be possible through the use of ultrasound-guided core needle biopsy. Preoperative diagnosis of a carcinoma as invasive alters surgical management. A single-step surgery is possible, in which lumpectomy and sentinel node biopsy are performed. Had only the in situ component been known preoperatively, the invasive component might only be diagnosed after surgical excision, requiring a second surgery for lymph node staging.

This case reminds us of the limitations of core needle biopsy. Undersampling may occur. Additional biopsy is warranted when needle biopsy of a suspicious lesion yields discordant pathology results. Specimen radiography and postbiopsy mammograms are important quality control measures that aid in recognition of a discordant biopsy.

SUGGESTED READING

Kaplan C, Matallana R, Wallack MK. The use of state-of-the-art mammography in the detection of nonpalpable breast carcinoma. *Am Surg* 1990; 56(1): 40–42.

CHAPTER 4

Unusual and Problematic Types of Breast Cancers: DCIS, Intracystic Papillary Carcinoma, Benign-appearing Breast Cancers, ILC, Inflammatory Breast Cancer, and Breast Cancer in Implant Patients

Certain subtypes of breast cancer can be particularly challenging to detect on routine mammography. This can have implications for staging and surgical outcomes.[1] Although the use of supplemental imaging tools, such as ultrasound and MRI, help to improve cancer detection and delineation of the extent of disease,[2] cancers such as invasive lobular carcinoma (ILC) and ductal carcinoma in situ (DCIS) continue to be problematic. Other generally readily detected carcinomas, such as medullary, papillary, and mucinous (colloid), may be difficult to recognize as malignant because of their propensity for relatively benign-appearing morphologic features.

Although ILC represents only about 10% of all breast tumors,[3] it is known to be one of the most common reasons for a false-negative mammogram.[4] The infiltrating growth pattern of single-file strands of malignant cells, often with minimal fibrotic reaction, is one of the reasons that ILC can be difficult to detect (Figure 1). In addition, if an ILC does produce a mammographically detectable finding, it may not form a mass and may be of relatively low or equal density to normal fibroglandular tissue.[3] Even large lesions may still be occult on mammography.[5] Mammographic sensitivity for ILC ranges between 57% and 89%.[4–8] In addition, ILC has a higher propensity for multifocal and bilateral involvement. Its extent is often underestimated by mammography.[9,10] Understaging can significantly affect surgical outcomes and patient treatment. MRI has been shown to be useful in better defining the extent of disease in patients with ILC.[10,11]

The increasing use of screening mammography has led to an increase in the detection of DCIS, usually presenting as clustered microcalcifications. However, establishing the extent of disease can be problematic because DCIS is commonly multifocal and is often noncalcified. A recent study suggested that MRI may be more useful in detecting DCIS than previously thought.[12]

Mucinous carcinoma, also termed *colloid carcinoma*, is relatively uncommon.[13] Because it often presents as a circumscribed mass, it may potentially be misinterpreted as a benign lesion, such as a fibroadenoma. However, close inspection usually reveals features that should distinguish mucinous carcinoma from benign entities, such as marginal irregularity or heterogeneous echotexture on ultrasound. In a similar manner, medullary carcinoma can present as a well-circumscribed mass. Medullary carcinomas account for about 3% to 5% of breast cancers and have a prognosis that is generally better than more common types of invasive breast cancer.

Another problematic breast cancer is papillary carcinoma, which can also present as a well-circumscribed mass on mammography. Ultrasound usually reveals an intraductal or intracystic mass. However, because papillary carcinoma cannot generally be differentiated on the basis of imaging from the more common benign papilloma, biopsy is required for all complex breast masses.

Some carcinomas may have features on ultrasound that could be confused with benign entities. Purely hyperechoic lesions on ultrasound, such as a lipoma, are invariably benign. However, some invasive carcinomas may have a hyperechoic halo that may simulate a benign lesion. On close inspection, a hypoechoic "nidus" or central region is generally present to distinguish carcinomas from

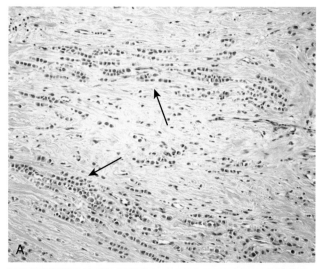

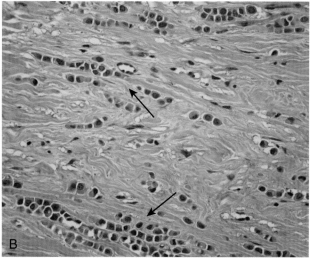

FIGURE 1. **A** and **B** (*close up*): H&E stains of an invasive lobular carcinoma demonstrating the classic single-file pattern of malignant cells extending into normal parenchyma (*arrows*).

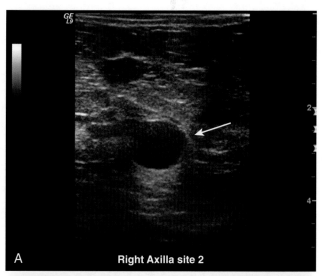

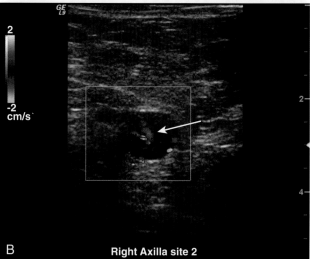

FIGURE 2. **A,** Ultrasound of an extremely hypoechoic right breast axillary tail lesion (*arrow*). **B,** Color Doppler evaluation demonstrates internal vascularity within the lesion, indicating it is solid and thereby excluding a cyst (*arrow*). Biopsy proved this to be a metastatic lymph node.

completely hyperechoic benign lesions. Some carcinomas, particularly high-grade cancers and metastatic lymph nodes, may be extremely hypoechoic on ultrasound and could be mistaken for anechoic cysts. In addition to proper gain settings and margin analysis, color Doppler helps in distinguishing solid masses from cysts (Figure 2).

Coexisting medical conditions, such as infection, trauma, and lactational changes, may hinder the detection and diagnosis of breast cancer. In addition, inflammatory breast cancer can be difficult to distinguish from benign infection process (mastitis). Careful correlation of the clinical history and physical examination findings should be made with the imaging findings. In some cases, distin-guishing between benign and malignant may not be possible solely based on imaging features.

REFERENCES

1. Veltman J, Boetes C, van Die L, et al. Mammographic detection and staging of invasive lobular carcinoma. *Clin Imaging* 2006; 30(2):94–98.
2. Berg WA, Gutierrez L, NessAiver MS, et al. Diagnostic accuracy of mammography, clinical examination, US, and MR imaging in preoperative assessment of breast cancer. *Radiology* 2004; 233(3):830–849.
3. Newstead GM, Baute PB, Toth HK. Invasive lobular and ductal carcinoma: mammographic findings and stage at diagnosis. *Radiology* 1992; 184(3):623–627.

4. Krecke KN, Gisvold JJ. Invasive lobular carcinoma of the breast: mammographic findings and extent of disease at diagnosis in 184 patients. *AJR Am J Roentgenol* 1993; 161(5):957–960.

5. Holland R, Hendriks JH, Mravunac M. Mammographically occult breast cancer: a pathologic and radiologic study. *Cancer* 1983; 52(10):1810–1819.

6. Hilleren DJ, Andersson IT, Lindholm K, Linnell FS. Invasive lobular carcinoma: mammographic findings in a 10-year experience. *Radiology* 1991; 178(1):149–154.

7. Paramagul CP, Helvie MA, Adler DD. Invasive lobular carcinoma: sonographic appearance and role of sonography in improving diagnostic sensitivity. *Radiology* 1995; 195(1):231–234.

8. Le Gal M, Ollivier L, Asselain B, et al. Mammographic features of 455 invasive lobular carcinomas. *Radiology* 1992; 185(3):705–708.

9. Lee JSY, Grant CS, Donohue JH, et al. Arguments against routine contralateral mastectomy or undirected biopsy for invasive lobular breast cancer. *Surgery* 1995; 118:640–648.

10. Boetes C, Veltman J, van Die L, et al. The role of MRI in invasive lobular carcinoma. *Breast Cancer Res Treat* 2004; 86(1):31–37.

11. Mann RM, Veltman J, Barentsz JO, et al. The value of MRI compared to mammography in the assessment of tumour extent in invasive lobular carcinoma of the breast. *Eur J Surg Oncol* 2008; 34(2):135–142 Epub 2007 Jun 15.

12. Kuhl CK, Schrading S, Bieling HB, et al. MRI for diagnosis of pure ductal carcinoma in situ: a prospective observational study. *Lancet* 2007; 370(9586):485–492.

13. Dhillon R, Depree P, Metcalf C, Wylie E. Screen-detected mucinous breast carcinoma: potential for delayed diagnosis. *Clin Radiol* 2006; 61(5):423–430.

DCIS, calcified and noncalcified

A 50-year-old woman was found on screening mammography to have suspicious pleomorphic microcalcifications in the 12-o'clock position of the right breast (Figure 1). Biopsy was performed with stereotactic technique, confirming intermediate-

grade ductal carcinoma in situ (DCIS) (Figure 2). There was a family history of breast cancer, most notably in a sister at age 31.

Breast MRI was obtained to evaluate for occult invasive components and extent of disease. Ultrasound had not shown an associated mass. The breast MRI showed clumped, small masses of intense enhancement with washout at the expected level of the residual known DCIS (Figures 3 and 4). There was a second, separate site of concerning, clumped enhancement in the same breast, with plateauing enhancement, thought suspicious for possible additional, noncalcified DCIS. MRI-guided biopsy was performed, and pathology showed two tiny foci of high-grade DCIS, the largest 1 mm in size. A clip was placed to mark the MRI-guided biopsy site, and postbiopsy mammography confirmed it to be removed in location from the remaining microcalcifications (Figure 5).

These evaluations showed the patient had proven multicentric DCIS, including noncalcified DCIS. She was recommended to have a mastectomy but was strongly desirous of breast conservation. Accordingly, lumpectomies were performed after a triple-needle localization, in which the remaining microcalcifications at 12 o'clock were bracketed with two needles (Figure 6), and the clip at 9 to 10 o'clock from the MRI-guided biopsy was separately localized (Figure 7). The specimen at 12 o'clock contained both of the bracketing localization wires and the remaining pleomorphic microcalcifications. These were noted to approach a

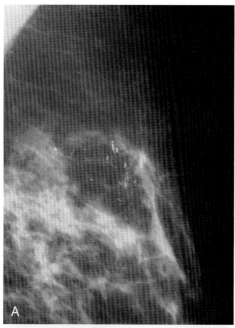

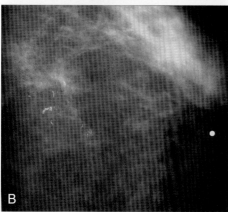

FIGURE 1. Mediolateral (**A**) and cranial-caudal (CC) (**B**) magnification views of the 12-o'clock position of the right breast show highly suspicious, clustered, pleomorphic microcalcifications. Many of the calcifications are linear, casting forms.

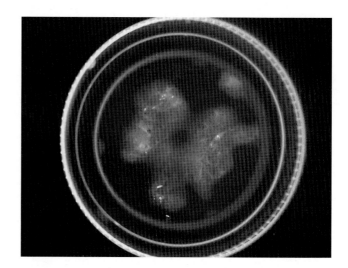

FIGURE 2. Specimen radiograph from the stereotactic biopsy confirms that the calcifications were successfully sampled and provides an unobstructed second look at the morphology of the microcalcifications. They vary in size and shape, and several of the linear forms vary in density.

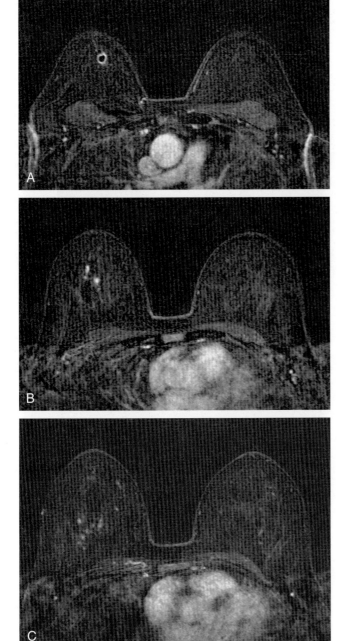

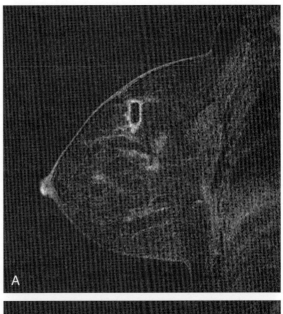

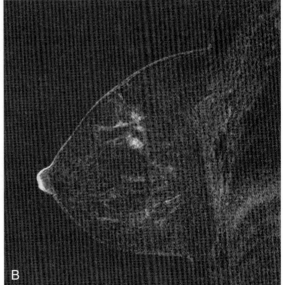

FIGURE 3. Axial enhanced, subtracted images from above to below. **A,** Rim enhancement outlines the clip placed during stereotactic biopsy. Presumably, the large-gauge (8-gauge) biopsy incited a reaction, which surrounds the collagen plug type clip. **B,** Just below the level of the clip, adjacent small enhancing masses are seen, which appear to correspond to the location of the residual microcalcifications. **C,** At a lower level, there is a regional grouping of small foci of enhancement that enhance more than other regions of the breast.

FIGURE 4. Sagittal, enhanced, subtracted breast MR images, from medial to lateral. **A,** An oblong void in the 12-o'clock position is outlined by a thin enhancing rim and corresponds to the clip placed at stereotactic biopsy. Enhancement at the inferior aspect of the clip corresponds in location to the known residual DCIS (microcalcifications remaining in the breast after stereotactic biopsy). **B,** An adjacent section, lateral to the clip, shows clumped additional enhancement and corresponds to the known residual DCIS.

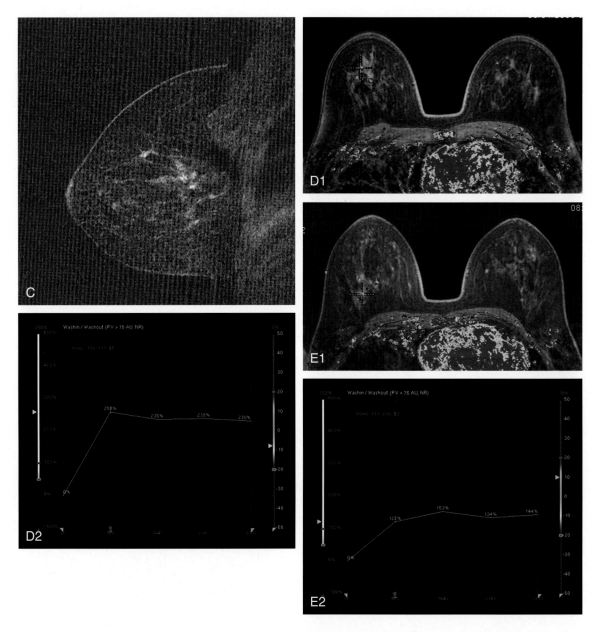

FIGURE 4, cont'd **C,** A more lateral section shows more posterior clumped enhancement, not directly contiguous with the known, calcified DCIS. **D,** Analysis [region of interest (**1**) and kinetic curve (**2**)] of the enhancement curve of the known residual DCIS shows washout, indicating angiogenesis. **E,** A plateauing pattern of less intense enhancement is seen at the level of the suspected noncalcified DCIS [region of interest (**1**) and kinetic curve (**2**)].

margin, from which additional tissue was obtained. The initial specimen from the 9- to 10-o'clock localization showed the hook wire, but not the MRI-placed clip. The surgeon was advised of this, additional tissue was obtained and radiographed, and the clip was found in the second specimen (Figure 8).

The pathology of the 12-o'clock specimen showed a 2.7-cm region of high-grade DCIS, with extension into lobules and with close lateral, infe-

rior, and deep margins. The specimen from 9 o'clock showed atypical ductal hyperplasia (ADH), with no residual DCIS and biopsy site changes.

Mastectomy was again recommended for this patient, who desired re-excision and breast conservation. The 12-o'clock lumpectomy site was re-excised. The re-excised lateral margin showed three microscopic foci of high-grade DCIS (largest, 0.5 cm), two of which were closer than 2 mm to the new lateral margin. The new inferior margin was

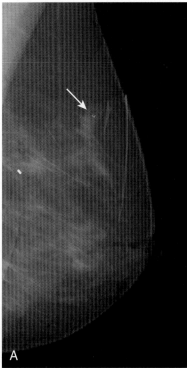

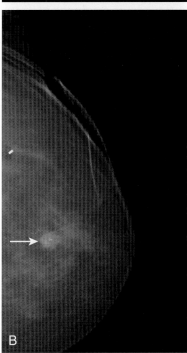

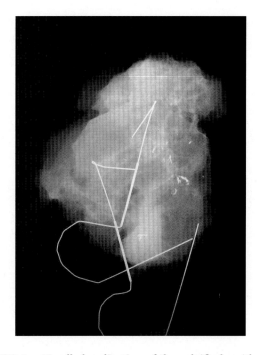

FIGURE 6. Needle localization of the calcified residual DCIS at 12 o'clock was accomplished by placement of two bracketing wires. The specimen radiograph shows the two hook wires, as well as the remaining microcalcifications, which approach a margin. The beaded appearance of an irregular linear casting calcification is well demonstrated here. The clip (collagen plug–type) is seen on one edge of the specimen as well.

FIGURE 5. Lateral (**A**) and CC (**B**) digital mammograms obtained after MRI-guided biopsy of the suspected noncalcified DCIS show the clip to be in the posterior upper outer quadrant. The clip placed at the time of stereotactic biopsy is more anterior, at 12 o'clock (*arrows*), and projects at least 4 cm away.

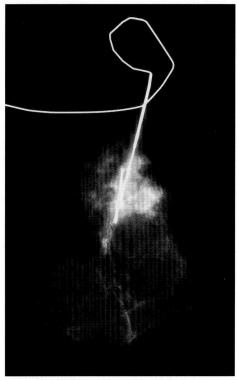

FIGURE 7. The initial specimen from the localization of the MRI-placed clip showed the hook wire, but not the clip.

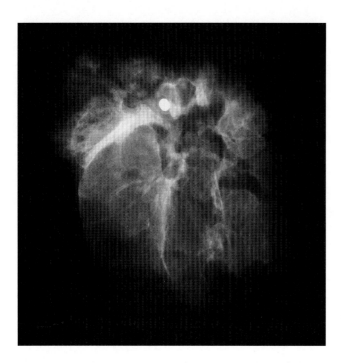

FIGURE 8. An additional specimen obtained after the surgeon was informed of the above shows the MRI-placed clip.

clear, and this specimen showed a single microscopic focus of DCIS. The additional deep margin excision showed three foci of invasive ductal carcinoma (IDC) (largest, 0.4 cm), with multifocal high-grade DCIS involving greater than 50% of the lesion (extensive intraductal component), DCIS focally at the new deep margin, and multiple foci of DCIS and IDC closer than 2 mm to the new deep margin.

Mastectomy was again recommended for this patient, who strongly desired re-excision and breast conservation. Re-excision of the lateral, inferior, and deep margins was performed. The specimens showed a single duct with high-grade DCIS and an additional focus of ADH in the lateral margin specimen, but the new margins were clear.

TEACHING POINTS

The use of MRI to evaluate DCIS has been controversial. The diagnosis of DCIS always carries with it the possibility of associated invasive disease, whether recognized or not. Invasive foci may or may not be found at pathology, depending on how extensive the sampling is. This is presumed to underlie the small percentage of DCIS patients who have axillary nodal involvement.

In this case, use of breast MRI led to a more complete preoperative understanding of the extent of this patient's disease. Before breast MRI, the patient's DCIS was delineated mammographically as a localized region of highly suspicious, pleomorphic, casting microcalcifications. The separate area of additional disease suggested by MRI led to biopsy and confirmation of a second region of localized DCIS and ADH. This area of abnormal enhancement did not correspond to calcifications on mammography.

Most DCIS discovered by mammography (90%) is heralded by microcalcifications. However, DCIS is frequently noncalcified, as indicated by pathology studies showing that only about one third of DCIS is associated with microcalcifications. Recent studies using high-resolution breast MRI indicate there may be more of a role for MRI in evaluating the extent of DCIS than suggested by earlier studies. Menell and associates evaluated the performance of mammography compared with breast MRI in identifying 39 sites of pure DCIS in 33 breasts. In this study, MRI was significantly more sensitive than mammography, detecting DCIS in 29 of 33 breasts (88%), compared with 9 of 33 breasts using mammography (27%; $P < .00001$).

In this case, the foci of microinvasion showed washout, whereas the noncalcified DCIS showed plateauing enhancement. Most DCIS shows the most benign pattern of enhancement, the persistent or progressive pattern. Accordingly, most DCIS on MRI will be recognized by an abnormal pattern of enhancement, typically linear, ductal, or clumped enhancement in a segmental distribution.

SUGGESTED READINGS

Harms SE, Harms SS. MRI evaluation and surgical planning. *Semin Breast Dis* 2004; 7:159–171.

Menell JH, Morris EA, Dershaw DD, et al. Determination of the presence and extent of pure ductal carcinoma in situ by mammography and magnetic resonance imaging. *Breast J* 2005; 11(6):382–390.

CASE 2

Extensive intraductal carcinoma presenting as a palpable, tumor-filled ductal system

A 74-year-old woman was evaluated for right upper inner quadrant (UIQ) palpable firmness. Mammography showed a segmental region of tubular nodularity with suspicious microcalcifications, spanning 5 cm, extending from the retroareolar region to the UIQ (Figures 1 and 2). On ultrasound,

dilated retroareolar soft tissue containing ducts extended into the UIQ (Figure 3). Ultrasound-guided biopsy obtained intermediate-grade intraductal carcinoma with papillary and cribriform features. The patient was a part-time resident of the area and had multiple medical problems, including severe atherosclerotic disease with prior

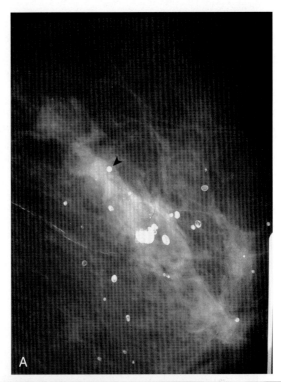

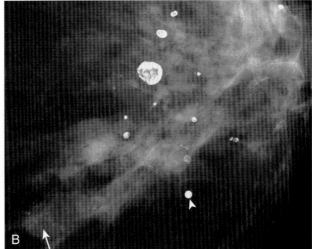

FIGURE 1. Mediolateral oblique (MLO) (**A**) and CC (**B**) mammograms show heterogeneous parenchymal density. A variety of coarse, scattered, benign calcifications are seen. A segmental zone of increased density is seen in the right UIQ. Note the marked asymmetry of the medial breasts in the CC projection. The left breast is largely fatty medially.

FIGURE 2. Magnification views of the right UIQ [lateral (**A**) and CC (**B**)] show a marker (*arrowheads*) delineating the location of the palpable abnormality. Thickened tubular structures suggesting abnormally distended ducts are particularly well depicted in the CC projection. Clusters of indeterminate microcalcifications project within these abnormal ducts (largest indicated by *arrow*).

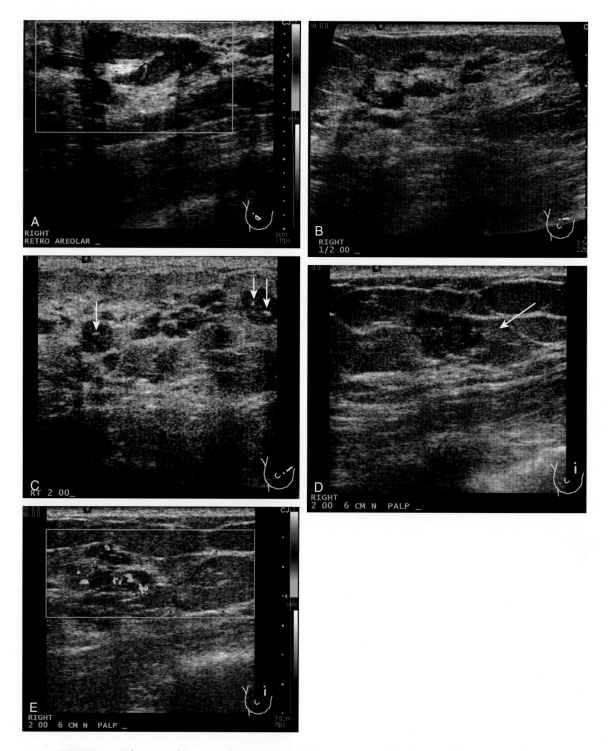

FIGURE 3.   Ultrasound images show the correlating sonographic abnormality. **A,** Branching distended retroareolar ducts are filled with soft tissue. Blood flow within the echogenic ductular contents delineates it from complex fluid. **B,** Ectatic tubular structures containing hypoechoic tumor extend into the UIQ. **C,** Punctate echogenic foci (calcification) can be seen within the hypoechoic solid tumor distending these ectatic ducts (*arrows*). **D,** A hypoechoic mass, with microlobular borders and echogenic punctate microcalcifications, is the largest discrete abnormality at the level of the palpable firmness (*arrow*). **E,** Vascular flow is readily demonstrated within the distended ducts in the UIQ as well as at the retroareolar level.

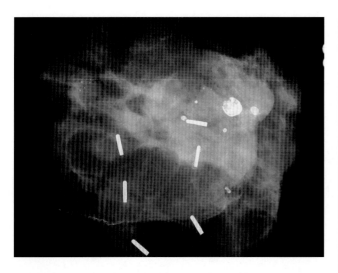

FIGURE 4. Specimen radiograph contains most of the mammographic abnormality. A conventional localization procedure was not performed because the lesion was palpable as a cord-like abnormality.

coronary artery bypass graft, stents, and abdominal aortic aneurysm repair. She elected treatment with partial mastectomy and interstitial brachytherapy (Figure 4).

The pathology showed two negative sentinel lymph nodes. A 0.9-cm mucinous (colloid) carcinoma was found, with extensive (6 cm) intermediate-grade DCIS extending into lobules, estrogen receptor and progesterone receptor positive, *HER-2/neu* negative. The margins were focally positive for DCIS posteriorly, and multiple margins were close (<1 mm) for DCIS.

TEACHING POINTS

This imaging manifestation of extensive DCIS is not commonly seen. The involved ductal system could easily be visualized because of its expansion and filling by intraductal tumor. Microcalcifications were a feature of this abnormality, but not as impressive a component as the mammographically dense and cord-like distended ductular system. The sonographic findings of vascular, tumor-filled branching ducts are well within the spectrum of described possible imaging manifestations of intraductal tumor, but such clear depiction is uncommon. The utility of color Doppler to reveal vascularity, allowing differentiation of hypoechoic solid tissue from complex fluid, is well demonstrated here.

CASE 3

BRCA1 patient, abnormal whole-body PET leading to diagnosis of DCIS

A 53-year-old woman with a past medical history of right breast cancer 15 years before and ovarian cancer 5 years previous, underwent positron emission tomography (PET)/CT for surveillance of ovarian cancer. Her prior breast cancer was infiltrating ductal carcinoma (IDC), which had been treated with lumpectomy and radiation. Whole-body PET/CT showed asymmetrical, relatively focal, mildly increased uptake in the left lateral breast (Figure 1). Correlation with a recent mammogram showed no corresponding abnormality. Left breast ultrasound was also negative.

Breast MRI was obtained 6 months later. Segmental, clumped, plateauing enhancement was found in the left lateral breast (Figures 2, 3, and 4). A positron emission mammography (PEM) scan with fluorodeoxyglucose (FDG) was obtained as well (Figures 5 and 6).

MRI-guided biopsy was performed (Figure 7). Pathology showed high-grade ductal carcinoma in situ (DCIS), with comedonecrosis and cribriform types, and lobular cancerization and multiple foci suspicious for microinvasion. The tumor was estrogen receptor and progesterone receptor negative.

Subsequently, the patient underwent *BRCA* gene testing and was confirmed to have a *BRCA1* genetic mutation. Her mother and sister had previously had breast cancer.

Breast conservation was attempted, with initial lumpectomy and subsequent margin re-excision both showing DCIS at the margins.

TEACHING POINTS

During these evaluations, the patient was not known to be a *BRCA1* mutation carrier. Her personal history of both breast and ovarian cancer and strong family history of breast cancer in both her mother and sister certainly suggested genetic predisposition. Interestingly, the initial results of *BRCA* testing of this patient were negative, but retesting proved her to be *BRCA1* positive.

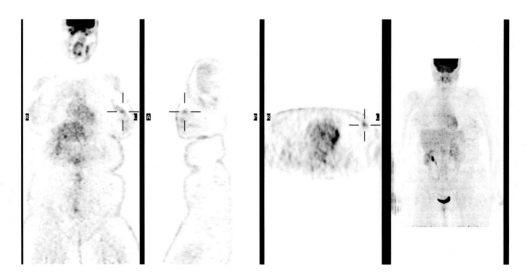

FIGURE 1. Whole-body PET images show focal, asymmetrical, mildly increased, left lateral breast uptake of FDG (*cursors*).

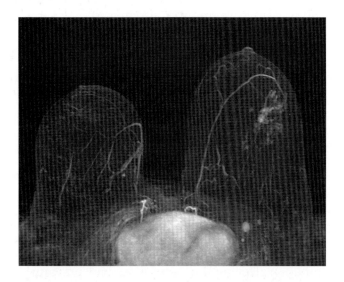

FIGURE 2. Axial maximal intensity projection breast MRI view from early in the enhanced, dynamic series shows localized, segmental, clumped left lateral breast enhancement. The right breast is smaller than the left from prior lumpectomy for IDC.

The patient's high-grade DCIS was picked up as an unsuspected finding on whole-body PET scan, obtained for surveillance for ovarian cancer. Initial workup with mammography and sonography showed no correlate. Breast MRI is the appropriate next breast imaging step in the evaluation, given the patient's high risk profile and the unexplained PET scan finding.

The MRI pattern of segmental, clumped enhancement along a ductal ray is highly suspicious.

Because there was no mammographic or sonographic correlate, MRI-guided biopsy is the appropriate next step.

A PEM scan was also obtained in this patient, before the MRI-guided biopsy. The patient was a volunteer test subject during applications for a newly installed device. It is interesting to compare the information available from the whole-body PET study to the higher-resolution PET data obtained with PEM scanning. On whole-body PET, the breast abnormality is heralded primarily by asymmetry and focality of activity in the left breast. It is somewhat difficult to precisely localize the activity because of the supine and dependent positioning of the breasts and lack of compression. Little fine detail is available from the whole-body study, but it does alert the observer to the area requiring additional evaluation.

The PEM study is obtained in gentle compression, applied only to immobilize the breasts. Because the modality is tomographic, there is no need to thin the breast tissue as much as in mammography. The resolution of PEM is on the order of 2 mm in plane, compared with 6 mm in a state-of-the-art whole-body PET scanner. The detectors are closer to the imaged tissue than in the ring array of a whole-body scanner, being located in "compression plates" of detector arrays on either side of the breast. Projections analogous to mammographic views can be obtained.

As of this writing, PEM devices have only recently become available and are limited in distribution. There is little collective experience with the capabilities and limitations of PEM scanning. A

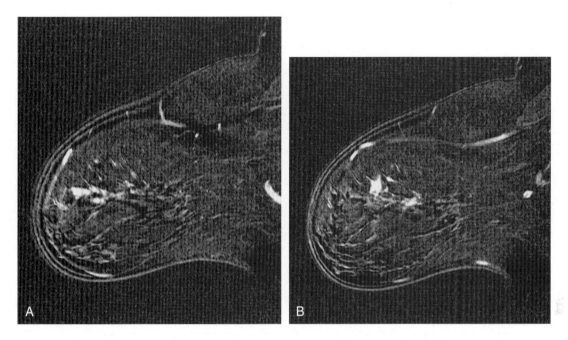

FIGURE 3. Sagittal, subtracted, enhanced images (**A** lateral to **B**) show a suspicious pattern of enhancement, with clumped, linear, ductal distribution.

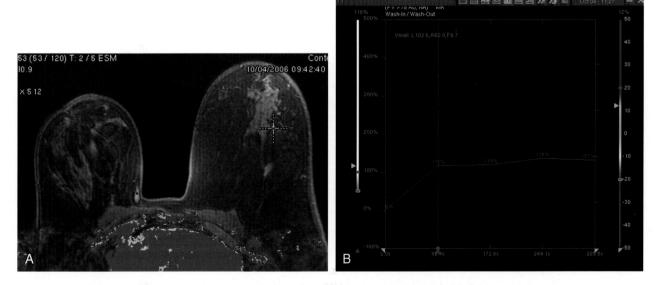

FIGURE 4. Enhancement pattern is graphically represented by color overlay (**A**) and signal intensity change–time curve (**B**), showing plateauing enhancement.

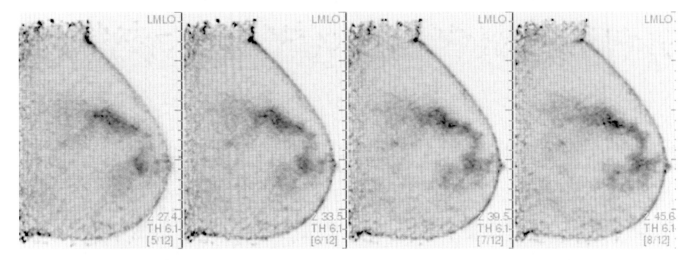

FIGURE 5. Representative PEM images of the left breast, MLO projection. In the upper breast, mild, segmental increased metabolic activity is seen.

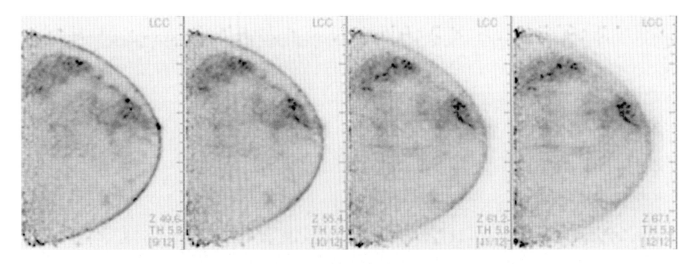

FIGURE 6. PEM images of the left breast, CC projection. The LCC marker indicates the lateral side. Segmental uptake of FDG corresponding to the MRI abnormality is seen laterally.

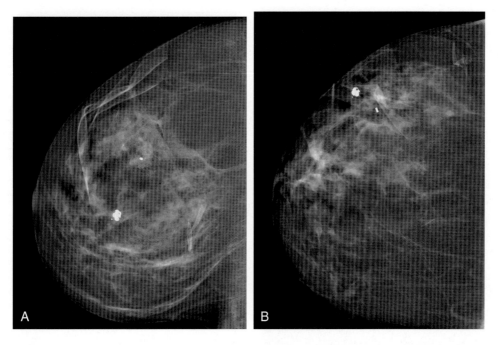

FIGURE 7. Digital mammographic images [90-degree lateral (**A**) and CC (**B**)], obtained after performance of MRI-guided biopsy, show the clip projecting in the upper outer quadrant. A large coarse benign calcification associated with a fibroadenoma also projects in the lateral breast. No mammographic abnormality is identifiable in the area of the MRI and PET abnormality.

multicenter prospective trial comparing the performance of PEM to breast MRI in preoperative staging of newly diagnosed breast cancers is accruing patients, and data from this trial will hopefully help in delineating the appropriate role of PEM in the breast imaging armamentarium.

CASE 4

Intracystic papillary carcinoma

A 51-year-old woman underwent breast imaging evaluation for a clear right nipple discharge. Two years before, she was diagnosed with right breast intracystic papillary neoplasm, estrogen receptor positive (Figure 1), and treated with lumpectomy only. On physical examination, a serous fluid dis-

charge could be readily elicited by palpation of the right lateral breast, in the region of her surgical scar. No clear imaging correlate could be identified on diagnostic mammography or breast ultrasound, with scarring noted on ultrasound at the lumpectomy site (Figure 2). Breast MRI was obtained and showed an unusual focus of branched, linear right retroareolar enhancement, with washout (Figures 3 and 4). A second focus of abnormal mass enhancement measuring 8 mm was identified, at the 9-o'clock right breast posterolateral level, with washout (Figure 5). MRI-guided biopsy was performed of the retroareolar branched enhancement, identifying intracystic papillary carcinoma, considered in situ, with no invasion identified. The second site was too posterior to reach with a grid MRI-localizing device. A second breast ultrasound was performed to find a correlate for the posterior MRI abnormality (Figure 6). A 6-mm hypoechoic nodule was identified on ultrasound at 10 o'clock, thought to be the probable correlate for the MRI finding. This had not been noted on a prior right breast ultrasound, obtained before the MRI. Ultrasound-guided core needle biopsy identified low-grade, cribriform ductal carcinoma in situ (DCIS), similar in histology to the patient's prior specimens.

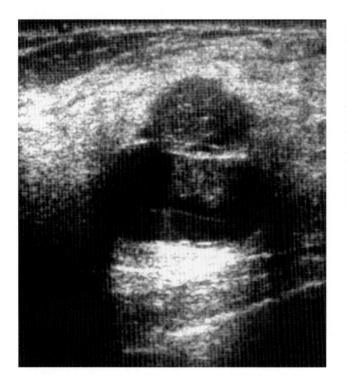

FIGURE 1. Ultrasound of the patient's original lesion, in the right breast at 9 o'clock, shows a complex, solid, and partially cystic mass. The cystic component yielded bloody fluid and contains a mural nodule. Vacuum-assisted core biopsy of the solid component identified intracystic papillary carcinoma (IPC), considered in situ and not invasive.

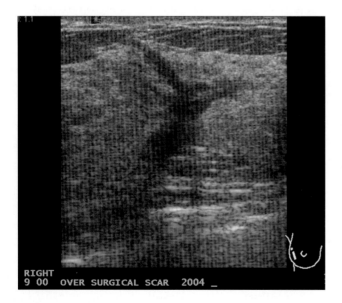

FIGURE 2. Ultrasound of the right lumpectomy site shows a complex branching linear scar, extending close to the skin surface.

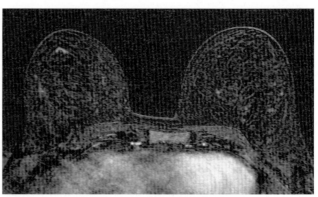

FIGURE 3. A V-shaped branched linear focus of enhancement, which could be ductular, is seen in the retroareolar right breast on enhanced, subtracted axial MRI. Biopsy with MRI guidance obtained IPC.

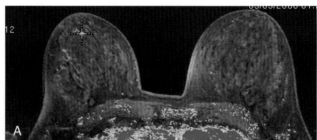

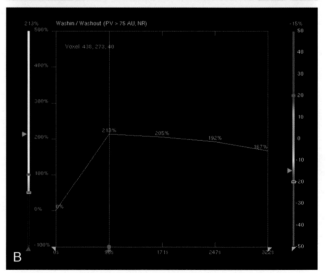

FIGURE 4. Analysis of the kinetic data with the aid of DynaCAD software. **A,** Kinetic information is color coded and overlain on breast MRI. A region of interest has been placed in the focus of branched enhancement. **B,** Graph of the enhancement (change in signal intensity versus time) shows a washout pattern: rapid early upstroke and subsequent decline.

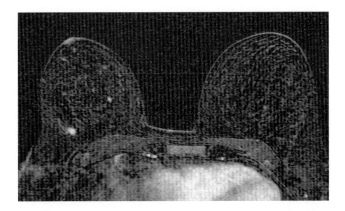

FIGURE 5. Enhanced, subtracted axial breast MRI shows a second indeterminate finding in the right lateral breast at 9 o'clock: an 8-mm mass with washout. A lymph node was considered in the differential. It could not be reached for performance of MRI-guided biopsy in the same procedure.

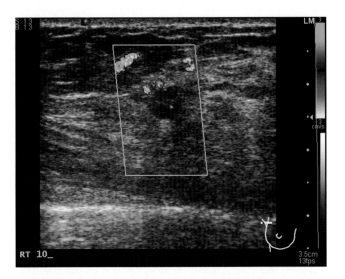

FIGURE 6. Targeted, second-look ultrasound of the right lateral breast identifies a 6-mm indeterminate, solid-appearing nodule with adjacent vascularity. Biopsy identified low-grade, cribriform DCIS, similar in histology to the patient's prior specimens.

With two proven sites of right breast intracystic papillary carcinoma (IPC)/DCIS, the patient was treated with modified radical mastectomy. She elected to undergo prophylactic mastectomy on the left at the same time, with immediate reconstruction with tissue expanders. On the right, one sentinel and one additional lymph node were negative. The right mastectomy specimen showed focal residual intracystic papillary carcinoma and focal low-grade micropapillary DCIS at the subareolar level. The left prophylactic mastectomy specimen was negative.

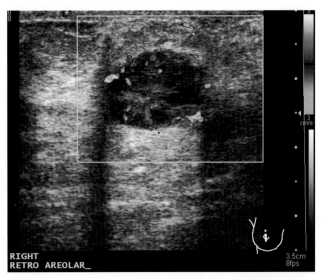

FIGURE 7. Another case of low-grade IPC, without invasion, in an 83-year-old woman who developed a new retroareolar mass, initially noted on mammography. Ultrasound of the mass shows it to be solid and vascular, with small cyst-like spaces within it and microlobulated borders. There is enhanced through-transmission.

An additional example of this less common histology is illustrated in Figure 7.

TEACHING POINTS

This patient's original IPC shows typical imaging features of these rare lesions, with a complex cyst with septations and solid components. These lesions can vary in appearance from predominantly cystic (often complex, with septations and mural nodules, as here) to predominantly solid (another example, different patient, Figure 7).

MRI can occasionally be useful to assess nipple discharge if a conventional workup does not identify a source. The MR finding in this patient is distinctly unusual in morphology but probably represents a form of ductular enhancement.

IPC can be found in isolation or in combination with DCIS or invasive disease. It can be noninvasive or invasive. Noninvasive (in situ) disease can be intraductal or intracystic. It presents most commonly with a palpable mass, as this patient did initially. Nipple discharge is also a known feature of this disease and may be bloody. Most patients are postmenopausal.

Associated DCIS or invasive cancer is found 40% of the time, and there is potential for axillary nodal involvement. These tumors are often estrogen receptor positive. The prognosis for IPC without

DCIS or infiltrating ductal carcinoma is excellent. No influence on recurrence or survival using radiation therapy has been demonstrated.

SUGGESTED READING

Soo MS, Williford ME, Walsh R, et al. Papillary carcinoma of the breast: imaging findings *AJR Am J Roentgenol* 1995; 164:321–326.

CASE 5

Colloid cancer, two cases

A 46-year-old woman, with a known left breast sarcoma history, underwent preoperative bilateral MRI. The MRI demonstrated a previously unknown mass in the contralateral breast (Figures 1, 2, 3, and 4). Ultrasound identified a solid corresponding mass in the lower outer right breast (Figure 5). Ultrasound-guided core needle biopsy diagnosed an invasive mucinous carcinoma. The patient was treated with bilateral lumpectomies and radiation therapy.

TEACHING POINTS

This case is an example of a mucinous carcinoma, also termed *colloid carcinoma*, which consists of

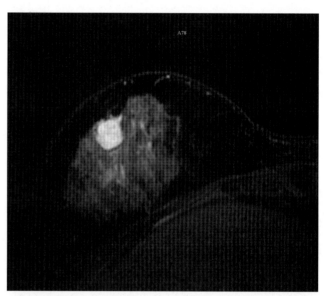

FIGURE 2.   Fat-saturated T2-weighted spin-echo image of the right breast. The mass in the lower outer right breast demonstrates high T2 signal.

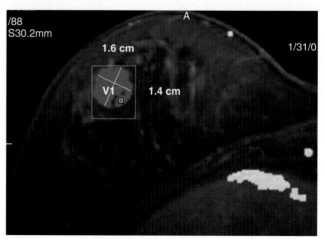

FIGURE 3.   MRI with CAD kinetic color overlay. The mass in the lower outer right breast is seen to have a uniform kinetic pattern as demonstrated by the *blue* color overlay. The blue color indicates a type I (progressive) or benign enhancement pattern.

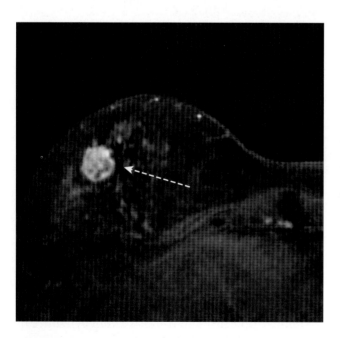

FIGURE 1.   Five-minute postcontrast subtracted axial MRI demonstrates an enhancing 1.6-cm mass in the lower outer right breast (*arrow*). The mass has partially circumscribed and partially irregular margins. In addition, the internal enhancement pattern is heterogeneous, with rim enhancement.

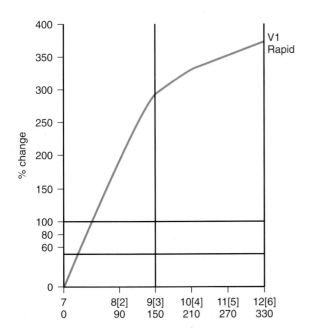

FIGURE 4. Quantitative analysis demonstrates the enhancement kinetics of the mass. There is rapid uptake and progressive enhancement pattern.

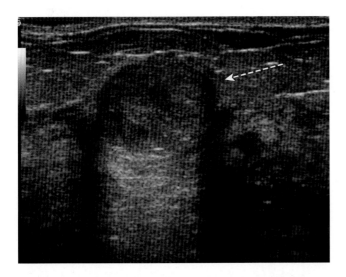

FIGURE 5. Ultrasound image of the lower outer right breast demonstrates a hypoechoic solid mass (*arrow*) corresponding to the mass seen on MRI. The mass has a mildly heterogeneous internal echotexture and microlobularity of anterior margins. There is increased acoustic through-transmission.

tumor cells floating within pools of mucin. On imaging, mucinous carcinomas potentially can be misinterpreted as benign. Features suggestive of benignity illustrated by this lesion include relatively well circumscribed margins, high T2

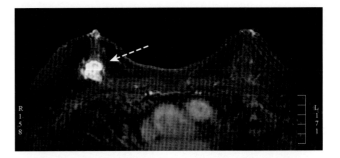

FIGURE 6. Five-minute postcontrast subtracted axial MRI demonstrates a rim-enhancing, 1.7-cm mass in the central right breast (*arrow*). The mass demonstrates irregular margins.

signal on MRI, and posterior acoustic through-transmission on ultrasound. However, detailed examination helps to prevent confusing this lesion for a fibroadenoma. Close inspection of both the MRI and the ultrasound shows that the margins of the mass are not as well circumscribed as expected for a fibroadenoma. In addition, unlike classic fibroadenomas, the internal architecture of this mucinous carcinoma is heterogeneous on both the MRI and ultrasound. Mammographically, mucinous carcinomas often present as well-circumscribed, relatively low-density masses, which may delay their diagnosis. Pure mucinous carcinoma is an uncommon form of breast malignancy, accounting for 1% to 2% of all breast cancers. They tend to occur in older patients. In contrast to mixed mucinous carcinomas, pure mucinous carcinomas have a favorable prognosis, are often low-grade tumors, and rarely metastasize.

Not every colloid carcinoma is as innocent in appearance as this example. Another case of an invasive mucinous carcinoma, in a 72-year-old woman with a palpable right breast mass, also shows bright signal on T2-weighted MRI, but other features of malignancy are notable (Figures 6, 7, 8, and 9).

TEACHING POINTS

This case demonstrates a less benign imaging appearance of a mucinous carcinoma than the preceding case. The bright signal on T2-weighted sequences might lead one to consider a fibroadenoma in the imaging differential diagnosis. However, the heterogeneity of the enhancement, with rim and internal septation enhancement, and

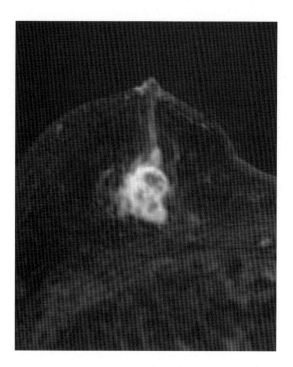

FIGURE 7. Delayed postcontrast image. The mass in the central right breast displays heterogeneous rim enhancement and enhancing septa, with areas of contrast washout.

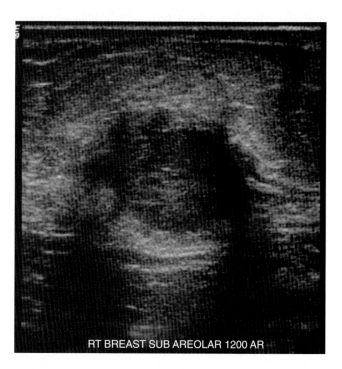

RT BREAST SUB AREOLAR 1200 AR

FIGURE 9. Ultrasound image of the central right breast demonstrates a hypoechoic solid mass corresponding to the mass seen on MRI. The mass has irregular and angular margins.

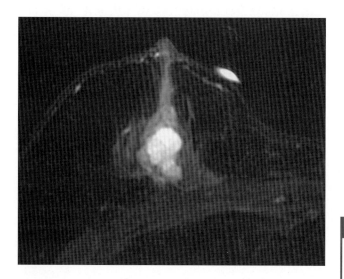

FIGURE 8. MR T2-weighted spin-echo image of the right breast. The mass demonstrates high T2 signal intensity.

the marginal irregularity, are features highly suggestive of malignancy. As always in breast imaging, a lesion should be judged by the most sinister feature it displays, and one should not be reassured by other, more typically benign characteristics.

SUGGESTED READINGS

Dhillon R, Depree P, Metcalf C, Wylie E. Screen-detected mucinous breast carcinoma: potential for delayed diagnosis. *Clin Radiol* 2006; 61(5):423–430.

Kawashima M, Tamaki Y, Nonaka T, et al. MR imaging of mucinous carcinoma of the breast. *AJR Am J Roentgenol* 2002; 179:179–183.

CASE 6

Medullary cancer, question of liver metastases on breast MRI; FDG uptake on PET in a fibroid

A 48-year-old premenopausal female noted a palpable left breast lump she had never identified before. Mammography and ultrasound confirmed

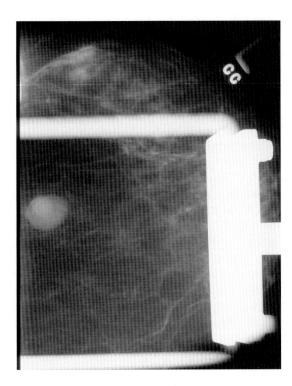

FIGURE 1. CC spot compression view of the palpable lump shows it to have lobular, relatively circumscribed margins.

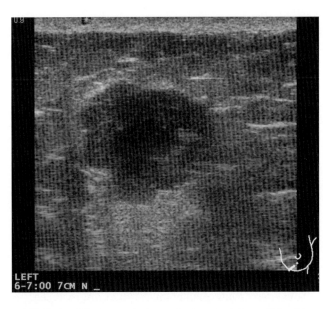

FIGURE 2. Ultrasound shows the mass to be solid, with indeterminate characteristics. The lobulations are too numerous (>3) and not gentle enough to be considered probably benign, and there is no defined thin echogenic capsule. Ultrasound-guided core needle biopsy confirmed a poorly differentiated malignant neoplasm.

a left inferior breast mass, measuring 2.5 cm on ultrasound (Figures 1 and 2). Ultrasound-guided core needle biopsy confirmed poorly differentiated malignant neoplasm, estrogen receptor negative, progesterone receptor weakly positive, *HER-2/neu* negative.

Breast MRI was requested because of the patient's age, premenopausal status, and moderate breast density (Figures 3, 4, and 5). In addition to the index cancer, a separate concerning focus of clumped enhancement was noted in the lateral breast. This was subsequently targeted for biopsy with MRI guidance, obtaining fibrocystic changes (Figure 6). Two liver lesions were also questioned on breast MRI (Figure 7). Positron emission tomography (PET)/CT and enhanced body CT scans were obtained to further evaluate the liver. No liver abnormality was confirmed on either modality. The liver findings questioned on breast MRI appeared to be relatively prominent vessels. On PET, an unexpected focus of hypermetabolism was noted in the pelvis, localizing to the uterus and corresponding with a uterine fibroid (Figures 8 and 9). The known left breast cancer was intensely hypermetabolic, but no PET evidence of nodal or metastatic disease was seen (Figures 10 and 11).

Palpation-guided lumpectomy and sentinel lymph node sampling were performed. The speci-

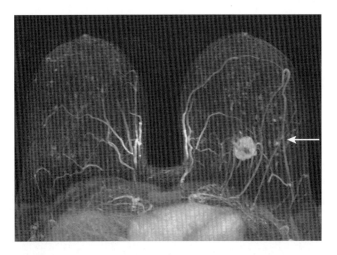

FIGURE 3. Axial enhanced breast MRI maximal intensity projection view of both breasts shows the posterior, intensely enhancing left dominant mass at 6 o'clock. A separate region of concerning clumped enhancement was noted anterolateral to the index tumor (*arrow*), better seen in Figure 4.

men contained a 2.5-cm medullary carcinoma, grade 9/9, with negative margins. One sentinel and two additional axillary lymph nodes were negative for malignancy. The final stage was stage II, T2N0M0. Additional therapy was given in the form of four cycles of doxorubicin (Adriamycin) plus

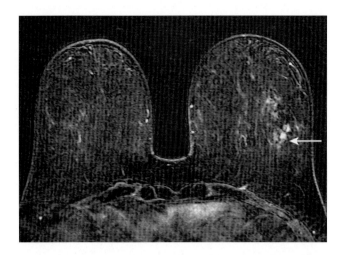

FIGURE 4. Above and anterolateral to the level of the index left breast cancer, a localized region of clumped enhancement, with small nodules (up to 7 mm), is seen in the lateral left breast (*arrow*). Biopsy was performed with MRI guidance, obtaining fibrocystic change.

cyclophosphamide (Cytoxan) (AC) chemotherapy, radiation, and tamoxifen.

TEACHING POINTS

This case illustrates many of the typical features of medullary carcinomas. Medullary carcinomas are a variant of ductal carcinoma and account for less than 10% of breast cancers overall. They are more common in younger women (11% of all breast cancers in women younger than 35 years) and are rare in elderly women. They typically present as a well circumscribed mass and may mimic a fibroadenoma, both clinically and by imaging. These features have given rise to the term *circumscribed carcinoma*. Mammographically, this medullary carcinoma displays the typical innocuous appearance. Even by ultrasound, typical features of malignancy are not seen. This lesion did not adhere to

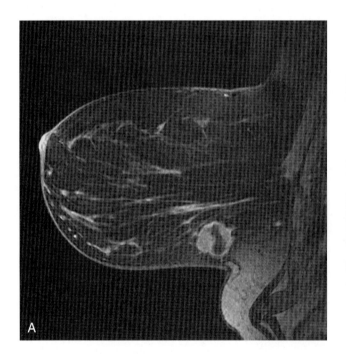

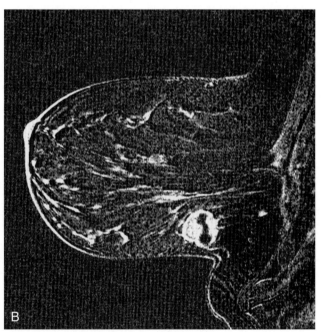

FIGURE 5. Sagittal, delayed, enhanced, fat-saturated, T1-weighted gradient echo views of the left breast. **A,** Unsubtracted. **B,** Subtracted. Rim enhancement is seen of the inferior breast cancer as well as spiculation of posterior margins. The subtraction is suboptimal, presumably because of a slight change in the patient's position between the precontrast and postcontrast imaging (about 5 minutes elapsed, during which an axial dynamic series was obtained). The imperfect subtraction can be recognized by the prominence of the inferior skin surface and alternating light and dark bands at fibroglandular interfaces. Contrast this appearance with Figure 4 from the axial dynamic series, which shows near-perfect registration and no corresponding subtraction artifacts.

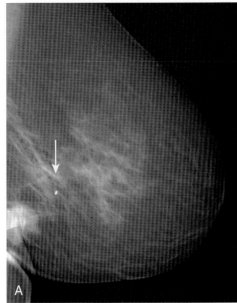

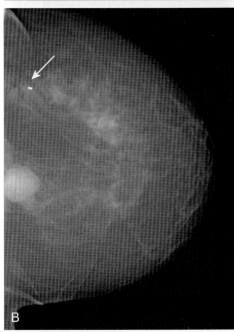

FIGURE 6. Post-MRI-guided biopsy digital mammogram films [90-degree lateral (**A**) and CC (**B**)] show the clip placed at MRI biopsy to be successfully deployed, projecting superior, anterior, and lateral to the separate known breast cancer (*arrow*).

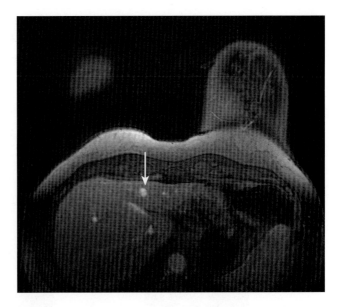

FIGURE 7. Image from the axial dynamic enhanced series (unsubtracted) shows one of the questioned liver lesions (*arrow*). No corresponding abnormality was found in the liver on subsequent enhanced abdominal CT scan or PET/CT scan.

Stavros' probably benign criteria and was considered indeterminate sonographically, leading to biopsy. As in this case, the diagnosis may not be firmly made on core biopsy.

Medullary carcinomas tend to be estrogen receptor negative and *HER-2/neu* negative. They are locally aggressive, but pure medullary carcino-

mas have a better prognosis than not otherwise specified infiltrating ductal carcinomas.

The breast MRI raised several additional questions needing resolution before the patient could be definitively treated. In the breast itself, a separate concerning site of enhancement was seen, consisting of an aggregation of small nodules, up to 7 mm in size. Targeted ultrasound did not show a correlate, which emphasizes the need to have MRI-guided biopsy capability to evaluate such additional findings. MRI-guided biopsy proved fibrocystic changes at the level in question. This was done with a large-gauge (9-gauge) vacuum-assisted device, which requires less precise targeting than other types of MRI-compatible core biopsy needles and ensures a generous sampling of questionable areas. It also enables a marker clip to be left for subsequent localization by either mammography or ultrasound, should the histology require it.

Depending on the breast MRI coil design and coverage and the patient's anatomy, a variable portion of the liver will be visualized on breast MRI. This portion may be partially obscured by phase artifact from the heart, which generally is directed right to left, rather than anterior to posterior, to minimize obscuring the breasts. The breast imager needs to carefully scrutinize the liver for lesions that could possibly represent metastases. In this case, the questioned liver lesions were seen only on

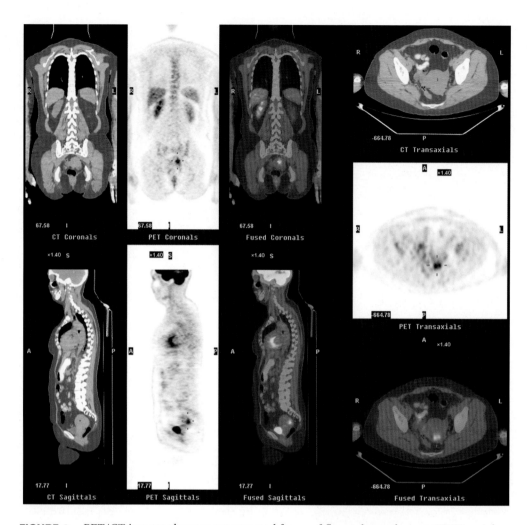

FIGURE 8. PET/CT images show an unexpected focus of fluorodeoxyglucose (FDG) uptake within the pelvis, seen posterior to the bladder on the sagittal images and localizing to the uterus (*cursors*).

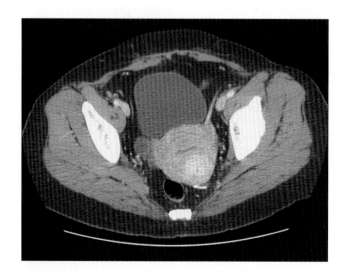

FIGURE 9. Correlation with enhanced pelvic CT shows an enhancing posterior uterine intramural fibroid. A right ovarian cyst is seen, which displayed no associated hypermetabolism on PET.

enhanced series and were not confirmed on corresponding short tau inversion recovery (STIR) images. They likely represented hepatic veins, which appeared larger and rounder in the liver periphery than expected.

This case also illustrates the image quality degradation resulting from even slight patient movement and imperfect subtraction. In this protocol, precontrast and postcontrast sagittal sequences were run before and after a dynamic series of 1-minute axial sequences, which were obtained once before and 4 times after contrast administration. Thus, the precontrast and postcontrast sagittal series were separated in time by 5 to 6 minutes, introducing more opportunity for slight patient movement. Recognition of subtraction artifacts is important, and when necessary, interpretation may need to be based on unsubtracted, fat-saturated sequences. In this case, this was not necessary, because the axial dynamic series was well registered.

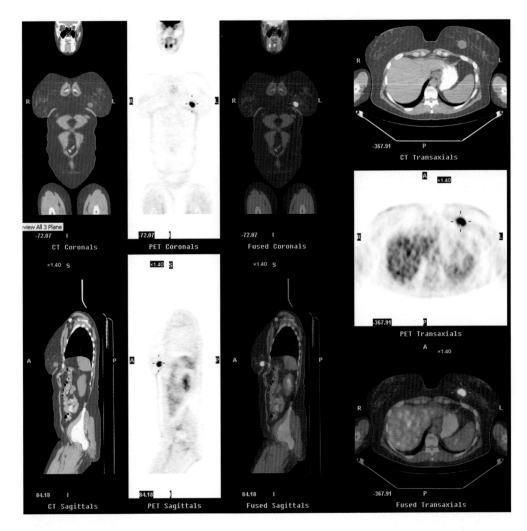

FIGURE 10.   PET/CT images show the left breast cancer to be intensely hypermetabolic (*cursors*).

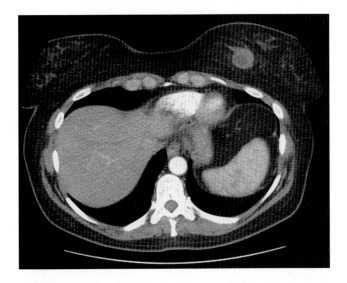

FIGURE 11.   Corresponding enhanced CT image shows the rim enhancement of the left breast cancer.

Finally, this case illustrates a source of benign pelvic activity seen occasionally on PET, which should not be mistaken for pathology. Fibroids can unpredictably show hypermetabolism on PET. PET/CT generally permits confident localization of such activity to the myometrium, allowing differentiation from other sources of uterine activity, such as the normal variant endometrial activity that can be seen in premenopausal women during menstrual and ovulatory phases of the cycle (weeks 1 and 3).

SUGGESTED READING

Subhas N, Patel PV, Pannu HK, et al. Imaging of pelvic malignancies with in-line FDG PET–CT: case examples and common pitfalls of FDG PET. *RadioGraphics* 2005; 25:1031–1043.

CASE 7

Invasive lobular carcinoma

A 68-year-old woman presented with left breast nipple retraction and palpable fullness. Mammographic views demonstrated increased density in the medial subareolar left breast and mildly prominent left axillary nodes (Figures 1, 2, 3, and 4). Ultrasound of the left breast demonstrated scattered areas of acoustic shadowing and small solid masses (Figures 5 and 6). MRI revealed diffuse abnormal enhancement of the central left breast as well as enlarged left axillary nodes (Figures 7 and 8). Subsequent ultrasound-guided core needle biopsy of multiple areas of the left breast confirmed multicentric invasive lobular carcinoma. The patient was treated surgically with mastectomy and lymph node dissection.

TEACHING POINTS

Invasive lobular carcinoma represents about 10% of all invasive breast cancers. However, because

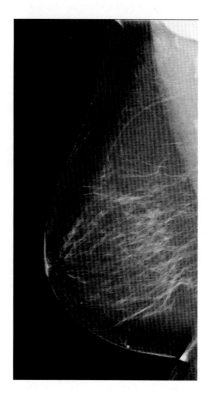

FIGURE 1. Right MLO mammographic view shows scattered glandular tissue, with no abnormality.

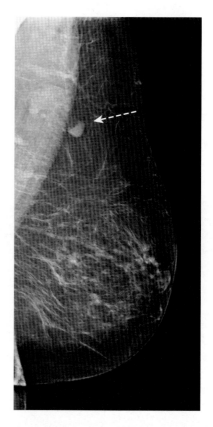

FIGURE 2. Left MLO mammographic view. Left axillary lymph nodes appear mildly prominent. The nodes are somewhat dense for size and demonstrate mild cortical thickening (*arrow*). Asymmetrical reticular subareolar density is noted.

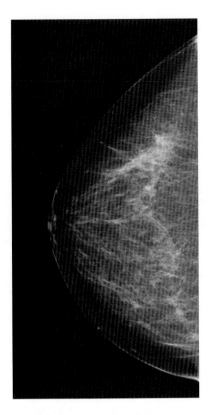

FIGURE 3. Right CC mammographic view shows no abnormality.

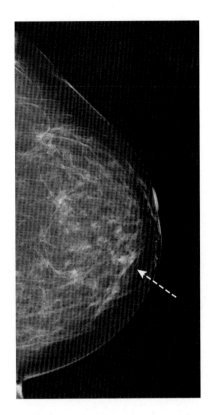

FIGURE 4. Left CC mammographic view. There is increased density in the medial subareolar left breast (*arrow*). There is also a slight generalized increase in breast tissue density compared with the right.

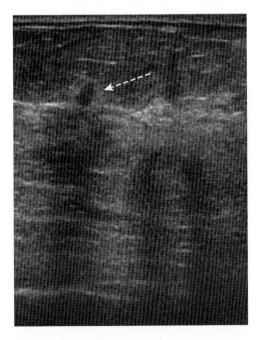

FIGURE 5. Ultrasound of the medial subareolar left breast. There is a 4-mm, ill-defined, taller-than-wide, solid mass, with a hyperechoic rim (*arrow*) as well as areas of mild acoustic shadowing.

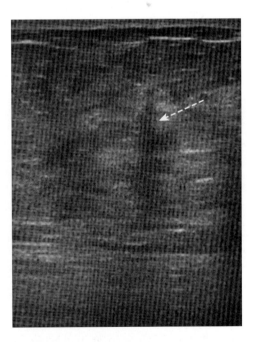

FIGURE 6. Ultrasound image of the central left breast. Multiple areas of acoustic shadowing are seen (*arrow*). A discrete mass is not seen.

they are frequently diffusely infiltrating and may not present as a discrete mass, they can be difficult to detect. In addition, invasive lobular carcinoma has a higher rate of multicentricity and bilaterality than ductal carcinoma. This example of invasive lobular carcinoma illustrates the limitations of mammography and ultrasound to accurately delineate the extent of breast involvement in some cases.

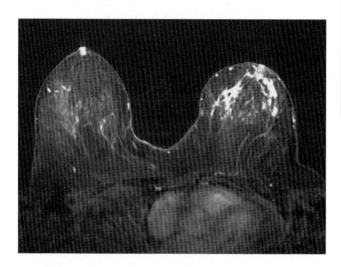

FIGURE 7. Postcontrast, subtracted, axial MRI of the breasts. MRI reveals diffuse nonmass enhancement of the central left breast.

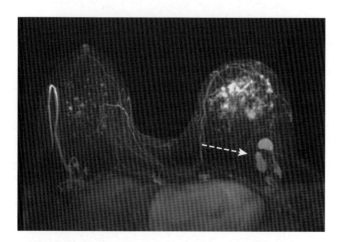

FIGURE 8. Maximal intensity projection subtracted MRI view of both breasts shows extensive abnormal left breast enhancement, along with abnormally enlarged and enhancing left axillary lymph nodes (*arrow*).

CASE 8

ILC presenting with orbital metastasis, bilateral shrinking breasts

A 72-year-old woman presented to her physician for evaluation of right eye pain. Prior routine screening mammograms had been reported as normal. Ophthalmic evaluation and orbital imaging showed a right intraconal mass, accounting for the patient's symptoms (Figures 1 and 2). The mass was biopsied and revealed adenocarcinoma, suspicious for a breast cancer metastasis. Review of the patient's mammograms was performed (Figure 3), as well as ultrasound and MRI. Bilateral, nonmass

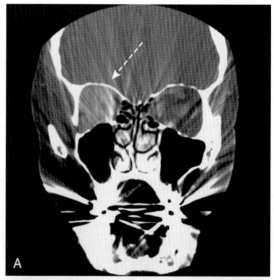

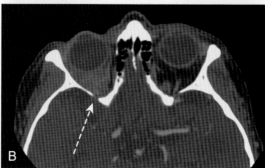

FIGURE 1. Coronal (**A**) and axial (**B**) contrast-enhanced CT images of the orbits. A right intraconal mass is seen (*arrows*), which obliterates fat planes.

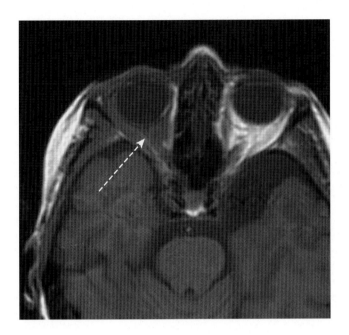

FIGURE 2. Axial T1-weighted MRI of the orbits. The right intraconal mass replaces bright signal fat in the orbit (*arrow*).

areas of enhancement on MRI (Figure 4) corresponded to dense shadowing areas in the subareolar regions on ultrasound (Figure 5). Subsequent core needle biopsies confirmed bilateral invasive lobular carcinoma (ILC).

TEACHING POINTS

This case illustrates the insidious nature of invasive lobular carcinoma. Because ILC often invades the breast as sheets of single cells rather than forming a distinct mass, it may be difficult to detect and tends to be larger at diagnosis when compared with invasive ductal carcinomas. Fortunately, ILC accounts for only 6% to 9% of breast cancers, and their stage at diagnosis is similar to that of invasive ductal carcinomas. Mammography commonly underestimates the size of ILCs. As sheets of tumor cells infiltrate the breast, they may make the breast less compressible and appear smaller on mammography than the unaffected breast. This has been termed the "shrinking breast" sign on mammography. Diffuse involvement of the breast by ILC is usually obvious clinically, with the patient describing a hardening, lump, or thickening of the breast. This example is unusual in that the patient had involvement of both breasts simultaneously. Because of the gradual and symmetrical nature of the clinical changes, the patient did not seek

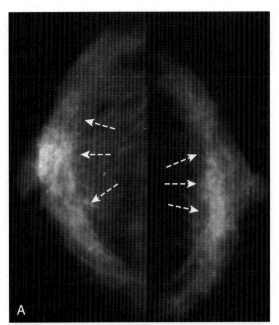

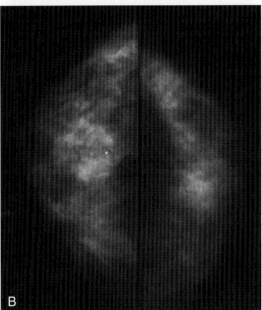

FIGURE 3. Bilateral CC views from the patient's concurrent screening mammogram (**A**). No abnormality was recognized prospectively. Subtle, symmetrical, central increased density and contraction (*arrows*) can be recognized only in comparison to a prior mammogram (**B**). No discrete mass is seen.

medical attention. It was only when she began experiencing right eye pain that she consulted her physician. Metastatic disease accounts for about 2.5% to 13% of all orbital tumors. Breast carcinoma is the most common primary source of orbital metastasis. This case highlights the importance of an awareness of breast cancer as a source for orbital

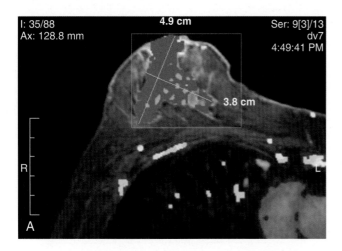
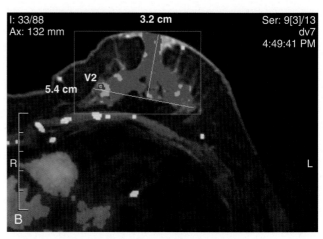

FIGURE 4. Bilateral postcontrast MRIs demonstrate non-mass-like areas of enhancement in the subareolar regions bilaterally [right (**A**) and left (**B**)], which display a mostly benign (progressive) enhancement pattern as designated by the *blue* kinetic color overlay.

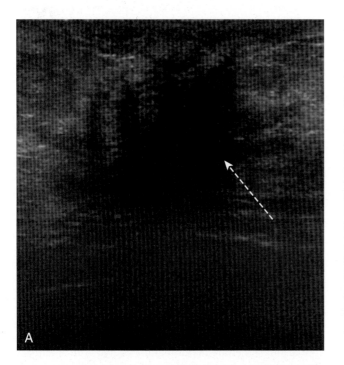
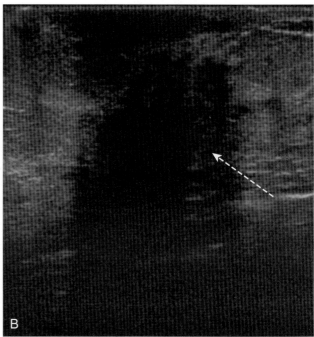

FIGURE 5. Bilateral ultrasound images of the subareolar regions [right (**A**) and left (**B**)]. There are dense areas of acoustic shadowing (*arrows*) in the subareolar regions bilaterally.

metastasis, not only in patients with a prior history of breast cancer, but also in patients with no prior history. This case is also unusual in that most patients with orbital metastasis have concomitant nonorbital metastasis. The patient in this example had no known metastasis elsewhere in the body at the time of presentation.

SUGGESTED READINGS

Harvey JA. Unusual breast cancers: useful clues to expanding the differential diagnosis [review]. *Radiology* 2007; 242(3):683–694.

Saitoh A, Amemiya T, Tsuda N. Metastasis of breast carcinoma to eyelid and orbit of a postmenopausal woman: good response to tamoxifen therapy. *Ophthalmologica* 1997; 211:362–366.

Talwar V, Vaid AK, Doval DC, et al. Isolated intraorbital metastasis in breast carcinoma: case report. JAPI 2007; 55.

Toller KK, Gigantelli JW, Spalding MJ. Bilateral orbital metastases from breast carcinoma: a case of false pseudotumor. *Ophthalmology* 1998; 105:1897–1901.

Because of the ILC histology, breast MRI was obtained preoperatively to screen the opposite breast and evaluate the extent of the known ILC (Figures 2, 3, and 4). The known left lateral ILC manifested as an 11-mm irregularly marginated mass with plateauing enhancement. Anteromedial to the index tumor was an additional enhancing 5-mm nodular focus, also with plateauing enhancement.

At the time of presentation for ultrasound-guided needle localization, a second-look ultrasound showed a 3-mm indeterminate sonographic

CASE 9

ILC presenting as a mass; postoperative changes on CT and PET

A 51-year-old asymptomatic woman underwent routine mammographic screening, which suggested a possible 1-cm mass overlying the pectoral muscle on the left MLO view. Additional mammographic spot compression and ultrasound confirmed a suspicious abnormality (Figure 1). Biopsy with ultrasound guidance confirmed infiltrating lobular carcinoma (ILC).

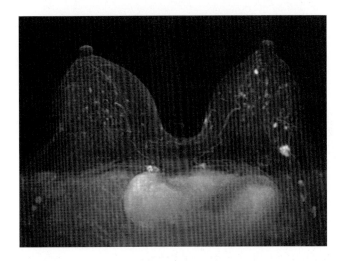

FIGURE 2. Axial enhanced, subtracted, maximal intensity projection MRI of both breasts shows the index ILC in the posterior left lateral breast. There is a background pattern of scattered, stippled fibrocystic enhancement. On the left, a few of the scattered foci of activity are more prominent, including a 5-mm focus anterior to the index ILC.

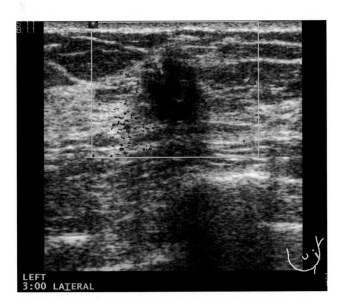

FIGURE 1. Ultrasound of the left lateral breast at 3 o'clock shows a highly suspicious 9-mm mass. Malignant features displayed by this tumor include marked hypoechogenicity, angular and irregular margins, taller-than-wide shape, faint shadowing, and vascularity.

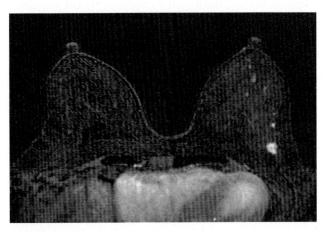

FIGURE 3. Enhanced, subtracted section through the left lateral index ILC, which is irregularly marginated. Anterior to it is a 5-mm nodular focus of enhancement.

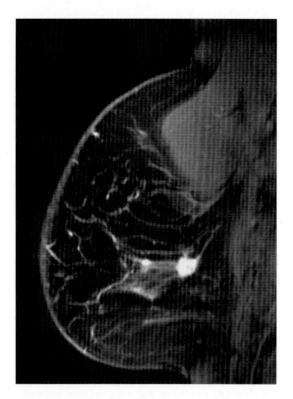

FIGURE 4. Sagittal, enhanced, fat-saturated section through the left lateral breast shows the relation of the index ILC posteriorly and the 5-mm additional focus anterior to it. On this delayed series (5 minutes after contrast injection), there appears to be a localized region of low-level parenchymal enhancement in the immediate vicinity, connecting the two lesions.

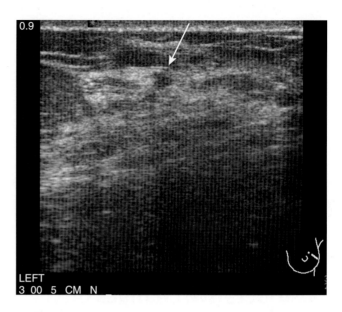

FIGURE 5. Second-look ultrasound of the left breast, on the day of needle localization, shows a 3-mm nodular focus with irregular margins in a corresponding location (*arrow*).

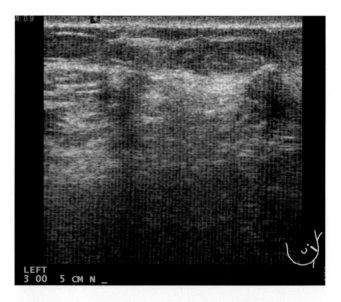

FIGURE 6. Additional left ultrasound image from the same study shows the relationship of the new finding to the known ILC. Both were needle localized with ultrasound guidance.

finding near the index lesion (Figures 5 and 6). This seemed to correlate with MRI and was needle-localized at the same time.

Pathology of the lumpectomy specimen showed a 2.7-cm ILC. Note was made by pathology that this dimension was obtained by measuring off the glass slides of the embedded specimen and was larger than the gross tumor, which measured 11 mm. The tumor was estrogen receptor and progesterone receptor positive and *HER-2/neu* negative. Margins were negative. Sentinel lymph node sampling showed two of six lymph nodes to have metastases, the largest 5 mm.

Axillary dissection performed 2 weeks later obtained 14 additional lymph nodes, all negative for tumor, for a total of 2 of 20 lymph nodes involved.

Because of the nodal involvement, systemic staging studies were obtained, including bone scan and PET/CT. PET/CT showed changes compatible with a 1-week-old axillary dissection, as well as 3-week-old postlumpectomy changes (Figures 7, 8, and 9).

TEACHING POINTS

How do we account for the apparent size discrepancy between the tumor seen on mammography, sonography, and MRI, which measured 1.1 cm, and the tumor at final pathology, which measured

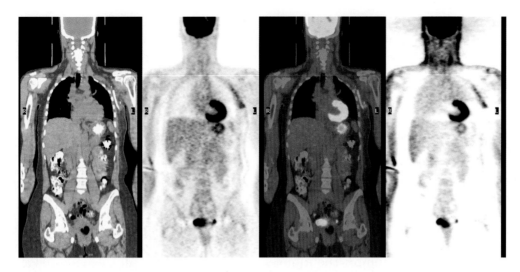

FIGURE 7. Coronal PET/CT images, obtained 1 week after left axillary dissection, show linear hypermetabolism at the operative level.

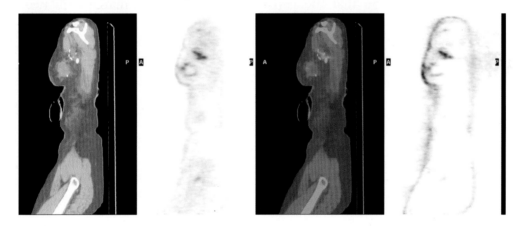

FIGURE 8. Sagittal PET/CT images through the left lateral breast and axilla show photopenia with a faint metabolically active rim in the left breast at the site of a 3-week-old postoperative seroma. More intense linear hypermetabolism is seen at the level of the 1-week-old left axillary dissection site.

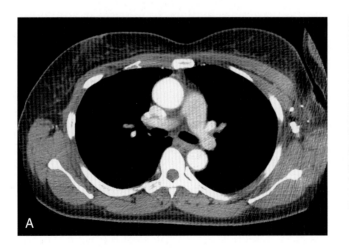
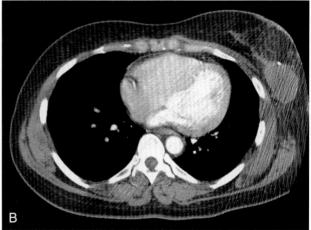

FIGURE 9. Corresponding contrast-enhanced chest CT images through the axilla (**A**) and the breasts (**B**). **A,** Surgical clips are seen in the left axilla, with ill-defined soft tissue density at the site. Axillary dissection was 1 week prior. **B,** Postoperative seroma in the left lateral breast is seen from surgery 3 weeks before. Scatter from the arm at the patient's side is noted.

2.7 cm? In this case, the gross tumor mass corresponded well to the size predicted by imaging evaluations.

If we measure the tumor size (from the sagittal MRI, Figure 4), and include both the 11-mm known ILC and the 5-mm "satellite" lesion anterior to it, and encompass the tissue between, we obtain a dimension of 2.7 cm. We know ILC can be variable in enhancement intensity on MRI. Presumably, some of this ILC did not enhance much. Conferring with the pathologist helps to suggest a resolution to questions of this nature. In this case, the gross specimen was sectioned, divided by the number of sections taken, with the tumor size estimate resulting from the number of sections taken multiplied by the number with tumor. The tumor had areas of infiltrating lines of tumor cells into fat and surrounding normal breast ducts. We can hypothesize with this information that the two tumor nodules seen on imaging represent foci within continuous tumor from the pathologic standpoint.

Review of this case suggests that the good outcome of negative margins on the first lumpectomy attempt had an element of luck involved. If there had not been an ultrasound correlate visualized for the satellite lesion suggested on MRI, which was localized at the same time as the index lesion, the desired outcome of negative margins might not have been so readily achieved.

Typical postoperative changes are demonstrated in this patient on both CT and PET. The inflammatory and reparative cellular response to surgery is visualized on FDG PET because white blood cells, typically activated monocytes, utilize glucose for fuel. The intensity of the activity at these operative sites of differing age seems proportionate, with less intense activity at the 3-week-old breast surgical site than at the 1-week-old axillary dissection level.

CASE 10

ILC presenting as architectural distortion

A 78-year-old female with two prior benign right breast biopsies had increased architectural distortion noted at the right 6-o'clock level on screening mammography (Figure 1). This was near a 20-year-old excisional biopsy site. Increased density and architectural distortion was confirmed on spot compression (Figure 2), and sonography demonstrated a corresponding shadowing mass (Figure 3). Ultrasound-guided core needle biopsy confirmed infiltrating lobular carcinoma (ILC). Because of the ILC histology, preoperative breast MRI was performed and showed the opposite breast to be clear. The known ILC manifested as a spiculated region of progressive intense enhancement, with no other sites of disease (Figure 4).

The patient elected to undergo mastectomy because the right breast was already smaller than the left (from the two prior benign biopsies) and a good cosmetic result seemed unlikely. The specimen contained a 2.5-cm ILC, estrogen receptor and progesterone receptor positive, *HER-2/neu* negative, with clear margins and two negative sentinel lymph nodes. Final stage was stage II, T2N0M0, and the patient was started on anastrozole (Arimidex).

TEACHING POINTS

Surgical scars can be tricky to evaluate. The correlation among location, appearance, and expected behavior needs to be fairly precise. Unexpected behavior (increase in prominence, density, or conspicuity on mammography) should be investigated. Ultrasound should be carefully correlated as well. This focus of shadowing did not extend to the skin surface, as most scars can be shown to do, and the increased vascularity is a tip-off that this needs further investigation. A normal old scar should not be this vascular. If there is persistent ambiguity after mammographic and sonographic evaluations, breast MRI can be very helpful in further assessment.

In this case, the diagnosis of ILC was established by ultrasound-guided core needle biopsy, and MRI was obtained to assess the extent of the known ILC and to evaluate the opposite breast. ILC has a known propensity for bilaterality, up to 30%, and is a clear indication for breast MRI. The morphology of the ILC enhancement is abnormal, with irregular, spiculated margins, and correlates well with the mammographic and sonographic manifestations of this tumor. The enhancement pattern was progressive, which is more typical of ILC than IDC. As many authors have previously noted, morphology should trump kinetic information. Kinetic data are most helpful when it is abnormal and may increase one's suspicion level regarding morphologically

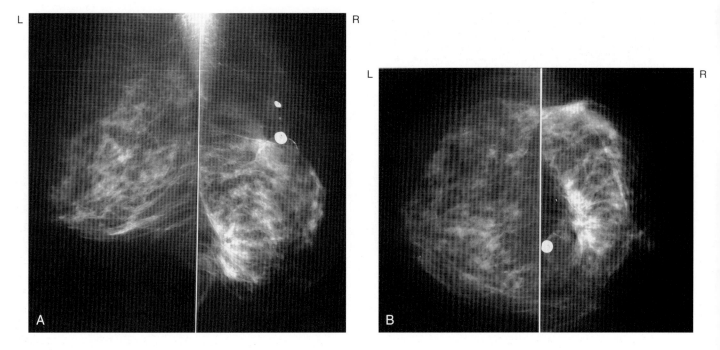

FIGURE 1.   MLO (**A**) and CC (**B**) mammograms show heterogeneously dense parenchyma. The right (R) breast is smaller than the left (L) from prior benign surgical biopsies. An oil cyst from prior surgery in seen in the upper inner quadrant. Architectural distortion is seen inferiorly on the right, at the 6-o'clock level.

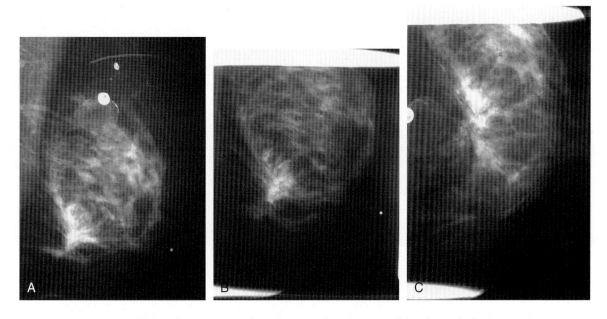

FIGURE 2.   Additional mammographic views confirm increased density, spiculation, and architectural distortion at the 6-o'clock level. **A,** 90-degree lateral view of the right breast. A scar marker had been placed in the upper breast, at the site of an excisional biopsy from 4 years before. Subjacent fat necrosis is seen (coarse benign calcification and oil cyst). **B,** 90-degree lateral spot view. **C,** CC spot view.

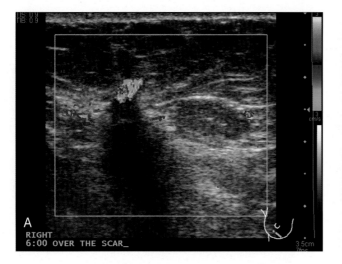
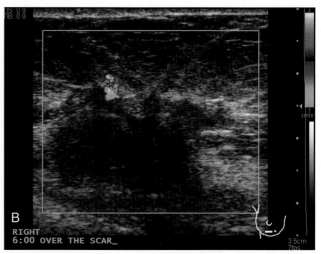

FIGURE 3. Ultrasound of the lower central breast (two views, **A** and **B**) showed a vascular, irregularly marginated, shadowing, hypoechoic mass corresponding to the region of architectural distortion on mammography. This was near the level of an old benign surgical excisional biopsy scar. No extension to the skin was seen.

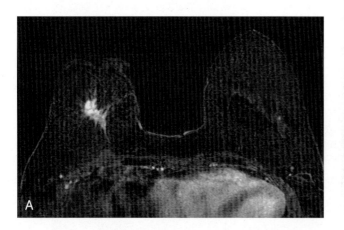
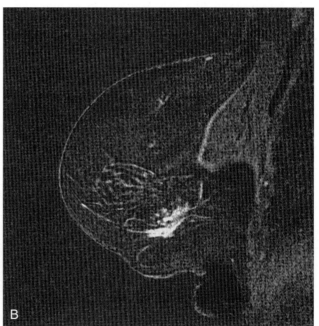

FIGURE 4. Axial (**A**) and sagittal (**B**), enhanced, subtracted breast MRIs of the right breast show the intensely enhancing, spiculated mass to be solitary and unifocal.

bland-appearing findings. Conversely, kinetic data that suggest benignity (progressive enhancement) should not reassure one about a morphologically concerning finding.

In this patient, breast MRI suggested she was a lumpectomy candidate based on extent of disease (unifocal). However, given the size of the lesion relative to the breast size, her preexisting asymmetry from prior surgeries, and its location in the inferior breast, a bad cosmetic result with partial mastectomy and radiation can be anticipated, and the patient opted for mastectomy.

ILC presenting as a palpable, predominantly hyperechoic ultrasound mass

A 55-year-old woman was referred for evaluation of firmness palpated in the right medial breast. Mammography showed heterogeneous increased breast parenchymal density, but suggested a probable mass at the level in question (Figures 1, 2, and 3). Ultrasound confirmed a discrete mass with an unusual sonographic appearance, being predominantly hyperechoic (Figure 4). The diagnosis of invasive lobular carcinoma (ILC) was made by palpation-guided core biopsy. Because of the breast parenchymal density and histology of ILC, the patient was further evaluated for breast conservation therapy with MRI. Breast MRI showed the known right ILC to have malignant features, including rim enhancement and washout (Figure 5). No indication of additional malignancy was seen in the right breast, with only scattered, fibrocystic-type tiny foci of enhancement noted. The left breast showed two small, sub-centimeter enhancing masses adjacent to each other in the anterior medial retroareolar breast (Figure 6). Ultrasound showed possible correlates of round hypoechoic masses (complex cysts versus solid masses by ultrasound) (Figure 7), which were subsequently needle-localized for excision at the time of contralateral mastectomy, and proven benign. The left breast pathology showed fibrocystic change and sclerosing adenosis. The right mastectomy specimen showed a 1.3-cm ILC, estrogen receptor and progesterone receptor positive, *HER2/neu* negative, with one negative sentinel node. Because of a close surgical margin, the patient was also treated with chest wall radiation with a boost to the surgical bed.

TEACHING POINTS

ILC represents up to 15% of all breast cancers and frequently is more difficult to diagnose than infiltrating ductal carcinoma. Clinically, it can be occult. Conversely, when it does present as a palpable mass, the clinical findings can at times be more impressive than the imaging findings, which can be relatively subtle. For this reason, clinically impressive palpable masses should be considered for palpation-guided biopsy, if the imaging evaluation is negative. Classically, ILC on histology grows as

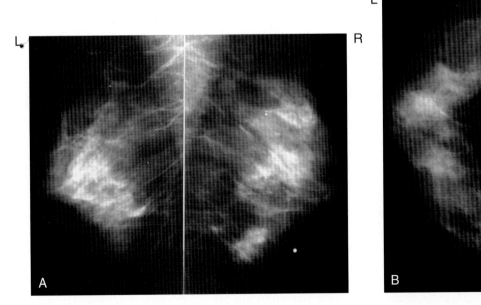

FIGURE 1.   MLO (**A**) and CC (**B**) mammograms show heterogeneous increased breast density. A radiopaque marker has been placed to identify the site of a palpable right lower inner quadrant lump. A corresponding mass is suggested, but blends into the dense adjacent parenchyma. A double density at the site is suggested on the CC view.

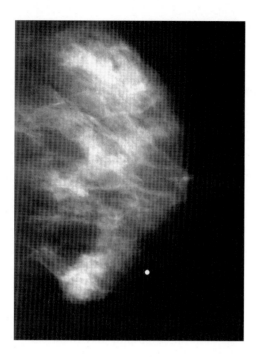

FIGURE 2. A 90-degree lateral view more convincingly shows an inferior mass of increased density at the level of the marker. Although the inferior margin appears circumscribed, the posterior and superior margins are obscured by adjacent parenchyma, into which the mass blends.

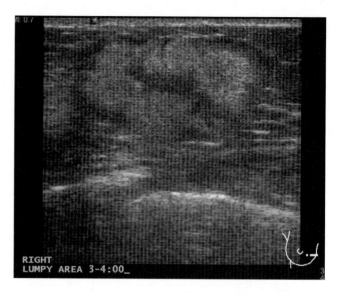

FIGURE 4. Ultrasound of the palpable mass shows an unusual appearance. The mass is lobular in shape, but with ill-defined margins and no definable capsule. The mass is predominantly hyperechoic, but shows hypoechogenicity centrally and peripherally.

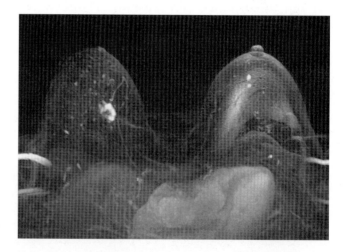

FIGURE 5. Axial maximal intensity projection of an early run from the enhanced dynamic breast MRI series shows the known ILC in the right medial breast. Rim enhancement, a morphologic feature of malignancy, is well demonstrated. Two small, adjacent, benign-appearing, enhancing masses are seen in the anterior medial left breast, behind the nipple.

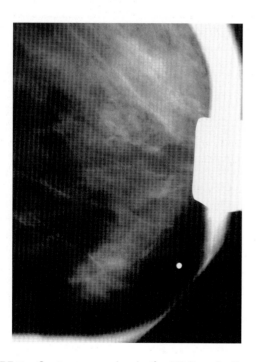

FIGURE 3. Spot compression in the MLO projection shows that the mass fails to compress or change shape.

lines of tumor cells, extending tendrils through the parenchyma in single-file manner. This growth pattern underlies the difficulty that can be encountered in diagnosing ILC on imaging. Because there may not be a concentrated mass of confluent tumor cells, 15% of ILC may manifest on mammography

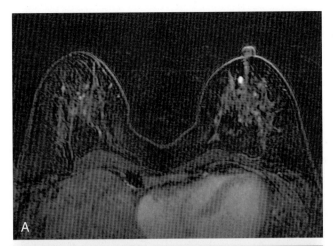

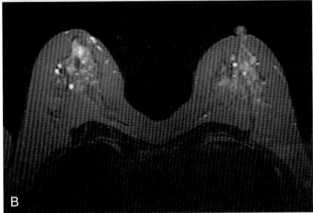

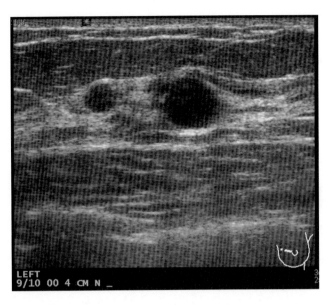

FIGURE 7. Ultrasound of the region in question on MRI on the left shows two adjacent round hypoechoic complex cysts vs. small solid nodules. These were needle-localized at the time of surgery for the contralateral ILC, and histology was benign, showing fibrocystic change and sclerosing adenosis.

FIGURE 6. Enhanced subtracted axial image (**A**) shows one of the two sub-centimeter, indeterminate masses in the left medial retroareolar breast. Corresponding axial STIR image (**B**) shows scattered, small bilateral cysts. The enhancing small nodule is of the same signal intensity as the breast parenchyma, but not nearly so bright as the adjacent cyst. The other lesion showed very similar signal intensity.

as architectural distortion alone (sometimes best seen on a CC projection), without a true mass at the center. On ultrasound, ILC producing architectural distortion may manifest as an area of ill-defined shadowing, where margins of a mass are difficult to define. On MRI, enhancement of an ILC growing in this manner may be subdued and segmental compared with ILC- and IDC-forming masses. This growth pattern may also contribute to the positron emission tomography tendency of ILC to be less hypermetabolic than IDC.

That said, at least 40% of ILCs do form a mass, and in this presentation, the imaging findings parallel those of IDC. This is such a case. The mass is suspected based on mammography, but poorly delineated from the dense parenchyma. The ultrasound appearance is interesting, being predomi-

nantly hyperechoic. It fails Stavros' criteria for benignity by virtue of being heterogeneous, with hypoechogenicity centrally and peripherally. As Stavros noted, hyperechoic masses usually are benign, but they must be uniformly hyperechoic to be characterized as benign. This appearance is not specific, and a very similar-appearing echogenic IDC is presented as a companion case in this chapter (Case 12).

The MRI features are malignant, with rim enhancement and washout. The MRI performed axially provides an opportunity for simultaneous evaluation of the opposite breast. Given both the propensity of ILC to be bilateral (up to 28% of the time) and the conventional breast imaging limitations in delineating the full extent of ILC, MRI is advocated for routine preoperative local staging of a new diagnosis of ILC, while simultaneously screening the other high-risk breast. Of course, not every focus of enhancement that turns up on breast MRI is cancer, and the use of breast MRI in such imaging evaluations will require follow-through and further workup of additional findings of concern on MRI. In this case, two small, adjacent, subcentimeter, benign-appearing but indeterminate nodules were seen on the opposite side. Ultrasound found suggestive correlates, which could have been sampled preoperatively with ultrasound guidance, but which in this case were needle-localized at the time of the contralateral lumpectomy, and proved benign. The significance of small enhancing masses like these on MRI should not be underestimated. See Case 14 in Chapter 1 for similar-appearing findings that proved to be malignant.

CASE 12

Echogenic breast cancer

A 78-year-old woman presented with a palpable left breast mass. Mammography confirmed a round mass in the lateral left breast. Ultrasound demonstrated an ill-defined, mixed echogenicity lesion, corresponding to the palpable mass (Figures 1 and 2). Core needle biopsy was performed and confirmed a low-grade invasive ductal carcinoma. The patient was treated surgically with lumpectomy.

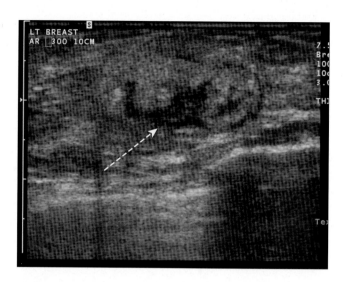

FIGURE 2. Ultrasound antiradial image of the left breast mass demonstrates that there is a central hypoechoic region within the lesion (*arrow*).

TEACHING POINTS

This case illustrates an example of invasive carcinoma with features that could potentially be misinterpreted as benign. When sonography demonstrates a purely hyperechoic lesion as the cause for a mammographic or palpable finding, it is almost certainly benign. However, one should perform close inspection for a hypoechoic component within the lesion because some small low-grade cancers may have an outer hyperechoic halo. In this example, the mass is clearly not purely hyperechoic and should not be confused with benign entities such as a lipoma.

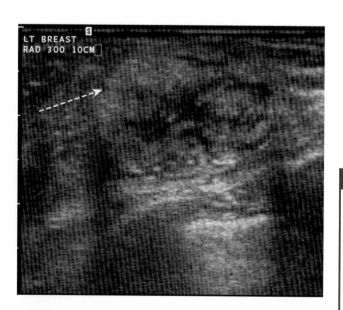

FIGURE 1. Ultrasound radial image of the 3-o'clock left breast palpable mass demonstrates a mixed echogenicity, solid mass. The lesion demonstrates a hyperechoic halo or rim (*arrow*). The mass has indistinct margins and some posterior acoustic through-transmission.

CASE 13

ILC treated with neoadjuvant chemotherapy

An asymptomatic 40-year-old woman with dense breasts underwent a routine screening mammogram (Figure 1). This raised a question of an abnormality on the left. Spot compression and ultrasound confirmed a 1.4-cm suspicious mass in the left

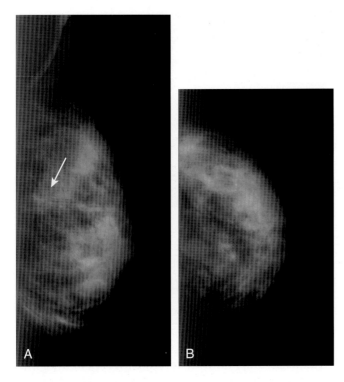

FIGURE 1. Screening mammograms [MLO (**A**) and CC (**B**)] show dense breast parenchyma. A possible mass was identified (*arrow*) in the posterior upper breast on the MLO view.

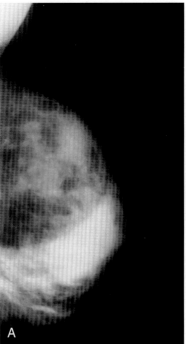

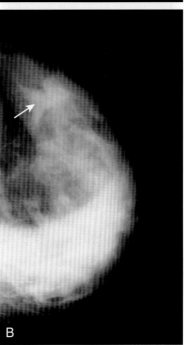

FIGURE 2. Spot compression mammographic views [MLO (**A**) and exaggerated CC (**B**)] confirm an incompressible area of increased density and architectural distortion in the posterior upper outer quadrant, best seen on the exaggerated CC spot view (*arrow*).

lateral breast at 3 o'clock (Figures 2 and 3). Ultrasound-guided biopsy proved infiltrating lobular carcinoma (ILC), estrogen receptor and progesterone receptor positive, *HER-2/neu* negative.

Because of the ILC histology and the breast density, breast MRI was performed to evaluate the full extent of disease in the involved breast and to screen the contralateral side (Figures 4, 5, and 6). Breast MRI showed the known index tumor in the posterior lateral left breast as an irregularly marginated, intensely rim-enhancing mass, with washout. Anterior to the known ILC was an additional 1-cm enhancing mass, as well as linear and clumped enhancement in a segmental distribution, extending anteriorly toward the nipple over an expanse of 6 cm.

The breast MRI results strongly suggested extensive, multifocal disease throughout the left lateral breast, indicating the patient was likely unsuitable for breast conservation therapy. To confirm multifocal disease, a second-look ultrasound was performed to determine whether a correlate for the additional disease suggested by MRI could be found. A subtle corresponding nodular focus was found anterior to the index lesion, and biopsy was performed with ultrasound guidance, also con-

firming ILC (see Figure 3). A clip was placed to mark the site.

The patient was strongly desirous of breast conservation and elected to undergo neoadjuvant chemotherapy. She was first staged with positron

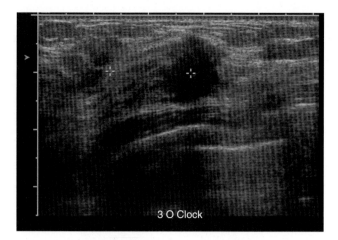

FIGURE 3.

FIGURE 3. Ultrasound of the posterior lateral left breast at 3 o'clock shows a very hypoechoic, solid, taller-than-wide mass with angular and irregular margins and no capsule, corresponding to the mammogram (*right cursor*). A few centimeters away (*left cursor*), there is a more subtle abnormality, with a vague, hypoechoic, nodular, smaller mass, which disrupts the normal breast tissue architecture. The smaller focus was not appreciated prospectively but was identified on second look after breast MRI was performed. Biopsy with ultrasound guidance of this second area also showed ILC, and was marked with a clip.

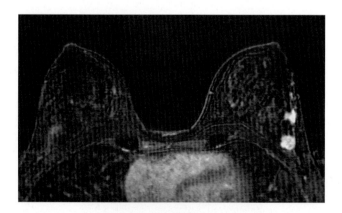

FIGURE 4. Axial enhanced, subtracted breast MRI shows two left lateral intensely enhancing masses, which are 2.5 cm apart. The more posterior mass (the index ILC) shows rim enhancement, and the smaller, more anterior mass is irregularly marginated. In addition, there is segmental linear enhancement between the two masses and extending anteriorly, toward the nipple.

emission tomography (PET)/CT and contrast enhanced chest, abdomen, and pelvis CT, which showed only faint increased metabolic activity of the known left breast ILC (Figures 7 and 8). Four cycles of doxorubicin (Adriamycin) and cyclophosphamide (Cytoxan), and four cycles of docetaxel

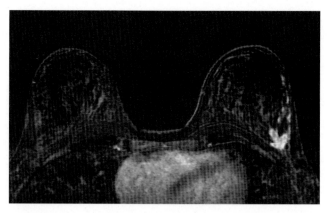

FIGURE 5. A more inferior axial, enhanced, subtracted breast MRI shows the angular and irregular margins of the known ILC mass in the posterior left lateral breast. Linear, duct-type enhancement extending anteriorly toward the nipple is well depicted on this slice.

(Taxotere) were administered, with repeat imaging assessment obtained at the midpoint and completion of chemotherapy (Figures 9, 10, 11, and 12). A partial response to chemotherapy was observed. The index lesion declined in size on ultrasound, although there was a persistent sonographically visible and vascular mass at final assessment. Serial breast MRI showed improvement as well, with progressive reduction in the size of the measurable masses, decline in enhancement intensity, and change in enhancement curve shape. There appeared to be considerable residual disease at final imaging assessment. Breast conservation was successfully achieved. Her lumpectomy specimen showed a 5-cm ILC, with no lymphovascular invasion and negative margins. Lymph node sampling showed five negative nodes. Additional treatment in the form of radiation and tamoxifen was begun subsequently.

TEACHING POINTS

This case provides many opportunities for discussion of some of the issues raised by an ILC diagnosis. This is a mammography screening success story, with mammography successfully raising alarm bells that this was a patient who needed additional imaging. Although it did not delineate the full extent of the disease, owing in part to the breast density, it succeeded in its screening role to identify the tip of a neoplastic iceberg. Prospective ultrasound, as is frequently the case, successfully found the index lesion and served to guide a biopsy

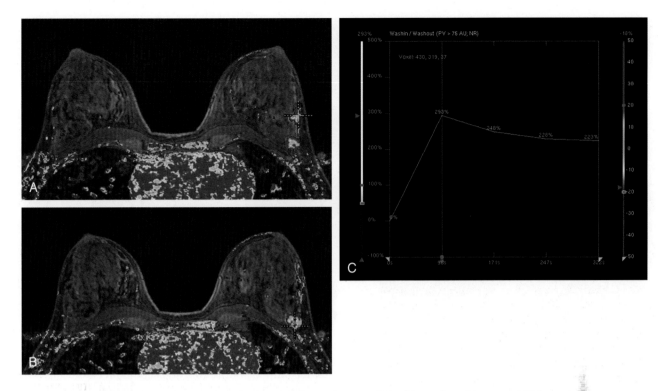

FIGURE 6. Angiogenesis color map of these abnormalities [**A,** region of interest (ROI) on the anterior mass; **B,** ROI on the posterior known ILC mass; **C,** representative signal intensity change–time enhancement graph] shows intense, early enhancement of these masses, with *red* indicating washout, as graphically depicted in **C.**

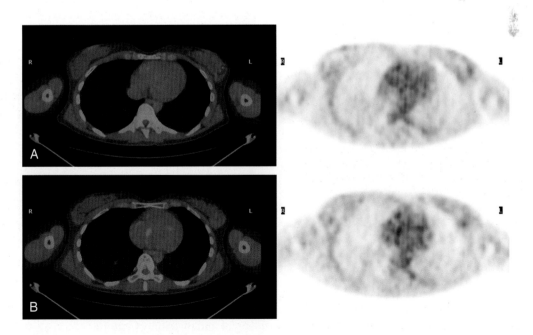

FIGURE 7. Axial PET/CT images (**A** and **B**) (*left,* fused PET/CT; *right,* attenuation corrected PET) show faint increased activity (only minimally increased over normal breast parenchymal background) in the left lateral breast at the site of the known multifocal ILC.

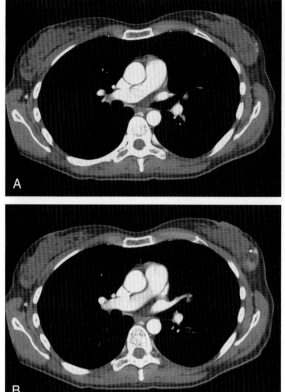
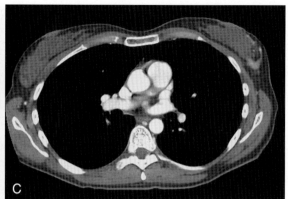

FIGURE 8. Contrast-enhanced chest CT images (**A** to **C,** from above to below, adjacent slices) show faint enhancement in the left lateral breast at the site of the known multifocal ILC. Slice **A** shows adjacent dots of enhancement, whereas **B** shows a clip placed at second-look ultrasound adjacent to an enhancing 1-cm mass, confirmed by biopsy to be a second focus of ILC. Slice **C,** just below **A** and **B,** shows the larger, faintly enhancing index ILC in the posterior left lateral breast.

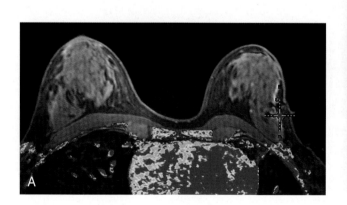
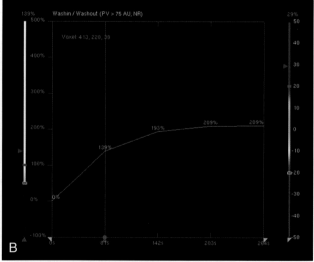

FIGURE 9. Repeat breast MRI, 4 months later, after four cycles of chemotherapy, shows evidence of a partial response to chemotherapy. Smaller masses show less intense enhancement, with enhancement curves now demonstrating a plateauing pattern and no washout. **A,** DynaCAD color map of the smaller anterior mass. **B,** Corresponding signal intensity–time curve shows blunted early enhancement and plateauing pattern.

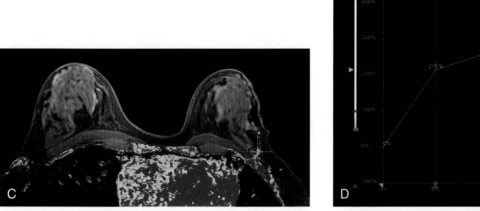

FIGURE 9, cont'd **C,** DynaCAD color map of the index posterior left lateral ILC mass. **D,** Corresponding signal intensity–time curve shows plateauing enhancement.

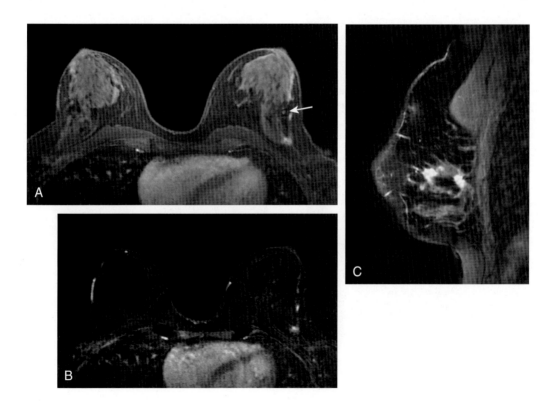

FIGURE 10. Third breast MRI, 2 additional months later, near the end of completion of chemotherapy, shows further reduction in size and intensity of enhancement of the residual masses. There continues to be regional linear enhancement. **A,** Unsubtracted, enhanced, fat-saturated, axial slice shows susceptibility artifact at the clip site, anterior to the residual index lesion (*arrow*). **B,** Subtracted, enhanced, fat-saturated, axial slice at the same level better shows the residual enhancement. **C,** Sagittal, enhanced, fat-saturated view through the left lateral breast shows the relationship of the residual enhancing masses to each other, aligned in an axis toward the nipple.

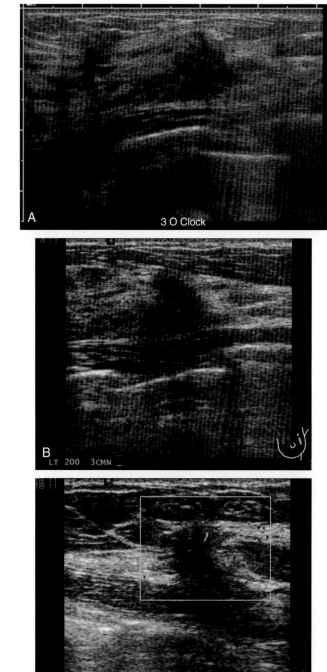

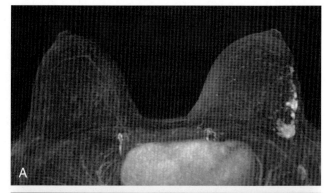

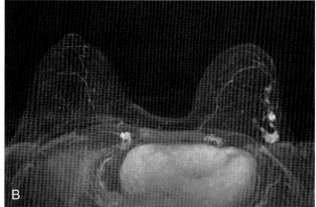

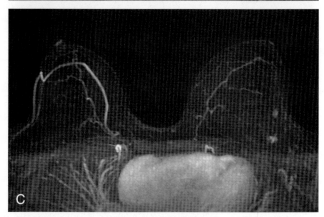

FIGURE 11. Serial ultrasound images of the index ILC mass, for comparison. **A,** At initial diagnosis, before chemotherapy. **B,** Midway through chemotherapy. **C,** Nearing completion of chemotherapy. Hypoechoic, irregularly marginated, taller-than-wide mass persists, with vascularity, although it has declined in size. The more subtle, additional lesion anterior to the index lesion became difficult to identify, although the clip could be visualized (not shown).

FIGURE 12. Serial enhanced, subtracted, axial maximal intensity projection views from the breast MRIs performed before, during, and toward the end of chemotherapy, for comparison. **A,** At initial diagnosis, before chemotherapy. **B,** Midway through chemotherapy. **C,** Nearing completion of chemotherapy. Progressive decline in size and intensity of enhancement, without complete imaging resolution, is demonstrated.

to make the diagnosis, but did not prospectively demonstrate the full extent of involvement.

The role of breast MRI is well established as a valuable adjunct to better local staging of new ILC diagnoses. Not hindered by breast density, breast MRI can also (if performed bilaterally, usually in the axial plane) effectively screen the opposite breast for occult tumor, which occurs up to 10% of the time.

In this case, much more extensive local involvement was convincingly demonstrated. The MRI pattern seen in this case, with multiple lesions, connected by enhancing strands, is among the more common patterns of ILC presentation on MRI. With the MRI in hand as a roadmap, more subtle sonographic correlates may be identifiable as targets for biopsy, allowing confirmation of multifocal disease.

With larger tumors and patients who are highly motivated for breast conservation, and therefore neoadjuvant chemotherapy, clip placement should be considered at the time of staging biopsy. It is difficult to predict the completeness of response of any one patient to neoadjuvant chemotherapy, but it should be anticipated that some patients will have complete imaging responses, which would be difficult to localize for excision without a marker in place. Pre-emptive clip placement in possible neoadjuvant chemotherapy candidates may potentially save the patient from being sent back for another procedure solely for that purpose.

This case also illustrates the propensity of ILC to be less fluorodeoxyglucose (FDG) avid than infiltrating ductal carcinoma (IDC), with even this sizable tumor barely visualized on PET. In such a case, the reassurance that is generally provided by a negative PET scan is considerably tempered.

Another question raised by this case is how best by imaging to monitor responses to neoadjuvant chemotherapy. In general, the modality that best demonstrates the pretreatment extent of disease will be most effective in any one patient in monitoring the response to chemotherapy. Most often, this is MRI, which has been demonstrated to be the most accurate modality in terms of correlating with pathology on lesion size and extent. However, until a consensus emerges, a multipronged approach with combinations of mammography, ultrasound, and MRI will continue to be utilized in most practices.

In the future, dedicated breast PET (positron emission mammography [PEM]) might prove to be useful in such assessments. Clearly, this will be most useful in tumors (such as most IDC) that have high FDG avidity. PEM is a small-field-of-view, high-resolution device, resembling a mammography unit, with detector arrays in compression plates. The patient is injected with FDG, which circulates for an hour (just as in whole-body PET imaging), and tomographic "maps" of the distribution of FDG within the breasts can then be obtained in projections comparable to mammographic views. The principle underlying this is just as in whole-body PET, with many tumors utilizing glucose as a fuel at a higher rate than normal tissues. Validation of this modality is ongoing and at this writing holds out the hope for the future availability of a functionally based modality.

Stage IV ILC; presentation with liver metastases

An 81-year-old woman noted a right breast mass and nipple inversion several months after a fall down stairs. Bilateral mammography at another facility showed a 7-cm spiculated right breast mass. She was assessed initially by a breast surgeon. The clinical impression was of a locally advanced breast cancer with axillary metastases. On physical examination, she had a tethered, shrunken breast compared with opposite side, with a 7-cm palpable upper outer quadrant mass extending centrally. Dimpling of the skin above it was noted. A 2- to 3-cm firm, irregular axillary lymph node was palpated. Palpation-guided core biopsy of the breast mass and fine-needle aspiration (FNA) of the axillary lymph node were performed.

The breast mass histology was invasive lobular carcinoma (ILC), estrogen receptor and progesterone receptor positive and *HER-2/neu* positive. The axillary FNA was nondiagnostic, but subsequent ultrasound-guided FNA did confirm malignant epithelial cells, compatible with metastatic breast carcinoma.

The patient had little in the way of systemic complaints, other than weight loss. Because of the ILC propensity for bilaterality, breast MRI was obtained. Positron emission tomography (PET)/CT was also ordered for systemic staging, given the large size of the tumor and known axillary nodal involvement.

Breast MRI showed an extensive spiculated mass, occupying much of the upper outer quadrant (Figures 1, 2, 3, 4, and 5). A second focus of enhancing tumor at the retroareolar level was connected by an enhancing linear spicule. Multiple such linear tendrils could be seen extending from the dominant mass to the overlying skin, producing the clinically apparent dimpling. The left breast was unremarkable.

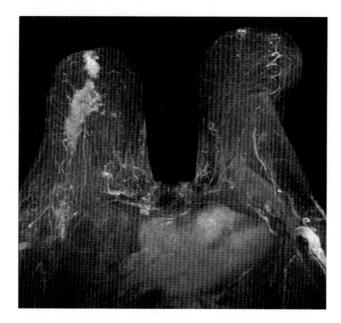

FIGURE 1. Axial maximal intensity projection view from enhanced dynamic breast MRI shows asymmetry in breast size. The left is quite pendulous, whereas the right is comparatively shrunken. Two dominant spiculated enhancing masses are seen on the right, one retroareolar and the other central and lateral. No occult breast cancer is suggested on the left.

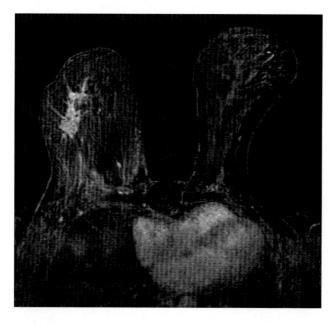

FIGURE 2. Enhanced, subtracted, axial breast MRI shows enhancing linear extensions to the overlying skin from the enhancing lateral mass.

PET/CT showed hypermetabolism in at least four right axillary lymph nodes, as well as modest activity in the right breast mass. Multiple peripherally hypermetabolic, necrotic liver metastases were also identified, indicating that the patient's true

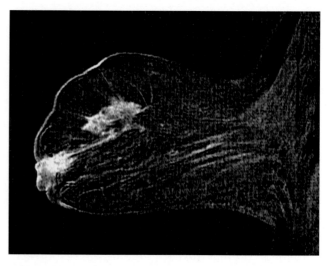

FIGURE 3. Sagittal, enhanced, subtracted breast MRI shows the relationship between the two main tumor masses, with linear enhancement joining them. Thin, enhancing spicules extend superiorly to the skin surface from the dominant mass. The dimpling of the skin surface resulting can be appreciated here.

stage was actually stage IV (Figure 6). These correlated with hypovascular, peripherally enhancing, necrotic-appearing liver metastases on enhanced CT (Figure 7). No hepatomegaly was noted on physical examination, and the patient's liver function tests, other than an elevated alkaline phosphatase, were normal. CT-guided biopsy was performed and confirmed metastatic adenocarcinoma, consistent with breast carcinoma. Planned mastectomy was cancelled, and the patient was begun on letrozole (Femara).

TEACHING POINTS

This case serves to demonstrate many reported features and manifestations of ILC. Classically, ILC grows by infiltration of parenchyma by single-file rows of tumor cells. One of the known presentations of ILC is the "shrinking breast." This can be difficult to recognize on mammography (see Case 8 in this chapter for a bilateral example). In this case, breast asymmetry could be appreciated clinically, and we can appreciate the counterpart findings on MRI. Skin dimpling could also be seen on clinical examination, and the MRI shows the imaging correlate. Multiple, fine, enhancing linear tendrils of presumed tumor could be seen extending to skin surfaces on this MRI.

Another described MRI characteristic of some cases of ILC is slower contrast accumulation and

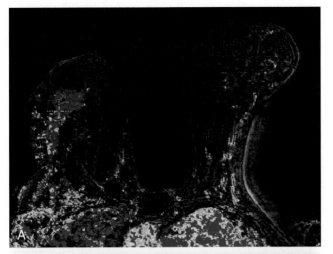

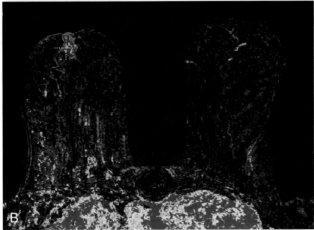

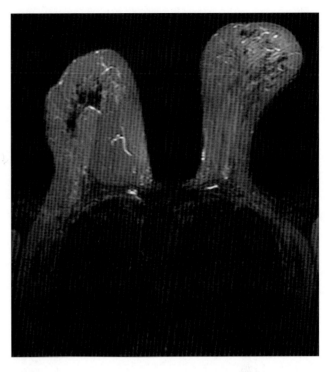

FIGURE 5. STIR axial image of the breasts shows poor detail of the liver. Subsequently demonstrated liver metastases were not suspected based on this study and are difficult to demonstrate even in retrospect.

FIGURE 4. Color-flow kinetics maps (**A,** through the dominant lateral mass; **B,** through the retroareolar component) show most of the enhancement pattern to be plateauing (*blue*). Only a tiny focus of washout was seen (not shown).

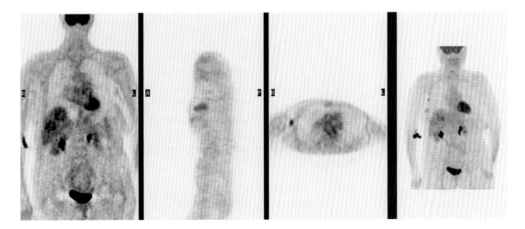

FIGURE 6. PET scan images (left to right: coronal, sagittal, axial, and coronal volume projection) show increased metabolic activity in the primary right breast ILC (sagittal image), in right axillary lymph nodes (the largest and most intense is seen in the axial image), and at the periphery of necrotic liver metastases (coronal image). Note the modest level of metabolic activity of the primary ILC, despite its size.

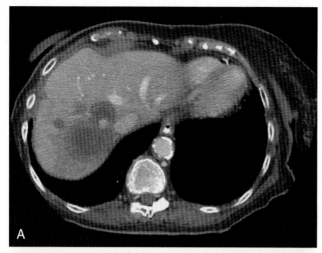

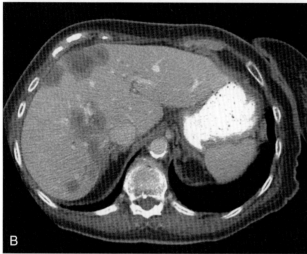

FIGURE 7. Enhanced abdominal CT images (portal venous phase; **A,** near dome, and **B** inferior to **A**) show rim-enhancing, centrally low density, necrotic liver masses, typical in appearance for hypovascular metastases.

lower-level enhancement intensity, also seen in this case. Although the tumor mass is quite sizable, the enhancement intensity is less than that usually seen in comparably sized infiltrating ductal carcinoma (IDC). Most of the mass showed relatively slow wash-in, with eventual plateauing enhancement at 2 to 3 minutes of 200% above baseline. Only a tiny single focus of washout was found.

A characteristic of ILC noted on PET imaging is more modest metabolic activity than IDC. Even this very sizable ILC shows only moderate metabolic activity. In this case, the involved axillary lymph nodes and liver metastases are of higher metabolic activity than the primary tumor.

Depending on the configuration of the breast MRI coil, a portion of the liver is often included in the examination. This should not be relied on to consider the liver adequately imaged for clearance of significant disease, as this case amply illustrates. Even though this patient was demonstrated subsequently to have extensive liver metastases, these were not suspected or clearly identified even in retrospect on the breast MRI. Breast MRI coils are configured to provide maximal signal anteriorly and there is a rapid drop-off in signal posteriorly. The visualized portion of the liver is also often partially obscured by phase artifact from the heart (preferentially set right to left, rather than anterior to posterior, where it would obscure breast tissue). On occasion, a liver cyst will be seen with sufficient clarity on breast MRI to characterize it (bright on STIR or T2, and nonenhancing), but this is the exception (an example is illustrated in Chapter 9, Figure 5). More commonly, the breast imager who suspects or detects a liver lesion on breast MRI (which is not known from prior studies) will need to recommend a dedicated study to characterize it (either triple-phase CT or multiphasic enhanced MRI).

CASE 15

Ultrasound findings of inflammatory cancer

A 78-year-old woman presented to her physician with a swollen and erythematous right breast. Ultrasound of the right breast revealed a suspicious, 13-mm, solid breast mass with microcalcifications (Figure 1). In addition, findings of breast edema and skin thickening were seen, suggesting an inflammatory component (Figure 2). A skin punch biopsy was positive, confirming the diagnosis of inflammatory breast carcinoma. The patient was treated with mastectomy and axillary node dissection, chemotherapy, and radiation therapy.

TEACHING POINTS

Inflammatory breast cancer (IBC) is a rare but very aggressive form of breast cancer, associated with an adverse prognosis. Cancer involvement of the lymphatics of the breast skin is the pathologic hallmark. The diagnosis is usually suspected on clinical exam with the rapid onset of breast edema, erythema, swelling, or the classic peau d'orange skin changes. It can be difficult to distinguish breast infection from inflammatory carcinoma, both clinically and on imaging. Skin punch biopsy can be helpful to confirm a suspected clinical diagnosis of IBC but is not required if the clinical presentation is characteristic and there is biopsy confirmation of cancer from a breast lesion. The constellation of imaging findings in this case, including a suspicious breast mass, breast edema, and skin thickening, are highly suggestive of inflammatory breast carcinoma.

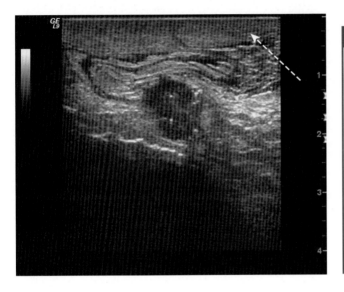

FIGURE 1.   Ultrasound image of the right breast. There is an irregular, hypoechoic, 13-mm mass with spiculated margins. The echogenic foci within the lesion represent microcalcifications. Superficially, abnormal skin thickening is seen (*arrow*), and there is generalized edema.

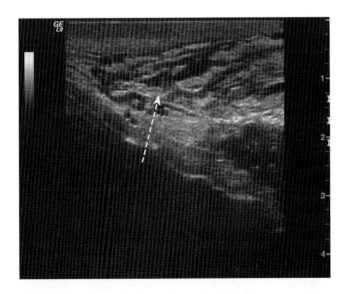

FIGURE 2.   Ultrasound image of the right breast. Multiple anechoic bands are seen in the parenchyma (*arrow*), representing breast edema.

CASE 16

Inflammatory breast cancer in a lactating patient

A 34-year-old lactating woman presented with symptoms of right breast pain, swelling, and erythema. Initially, the findings were thought to be due to breast infection. When the symptoms persisted, MRI was obtained (Figures 1, 2, and 3), a needle biopsy performed, and inflammatory breast cancer diagnosed.

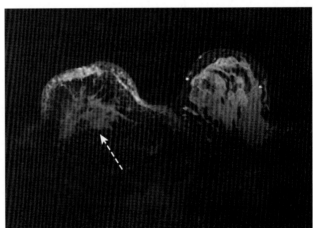

FIGURE 1.   Postcontrast enhanced, axial MRI of both breasts. There is diffuse enhancement of both breasts. However, the right breast demonstrates an area of mass-like enhancement and parenchymal distortion centrally (*arrow*). There is also diffuse skin thickening and enhancement on the right. The constellation of findings is more suspicious for inflammatory carcinoma than breast infection. The left breast shows diffuse enhancement with no mass effect or parenchymal distortion, consistent with benign lactational change.

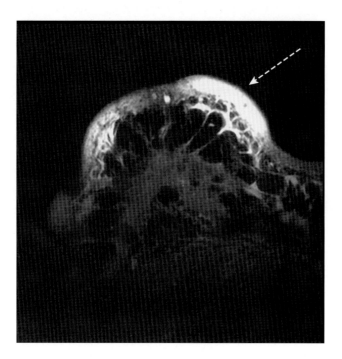

FIGURE 2. Fat-saturated, T2-weighted, spin-echo MRI of the right breast well demonstrates the right breast skin thickening and edema (*arrow*).

TEACHING POINT

This case illustrates the MRI findings of inflammatory breast carcinoma, in contrast to normal lactational changes in the opposite breast. Although any subtype of breast cancer may present as an inflammatory cancer, the definition and classic clinical presentation derive from invasion of dermal lymphatics. Inflammatory breast carcinoma, although uncommon, tends to be very aggressive and to metastasize early. The initial presentation of inflammatory carcinoma may be difficult to distinguish from breast infections, which are common among nursing mothers. Although imaging studies may aid in the diagnosis, the absence of suspicious imaging findings does not exclude inflammatory carcinoma. Ultimately, the diagnosis may have to be made through skin punch biopsy.

SUGGESTED READING

Gunhan-Bilgen I, Ustun EE, Memis A. Inflammatory breast carcinoma: mammographic, ultrasonographic, clinical, and pathologic findings in 142 cases. *Radiology* 2002; 223(3):829–838.

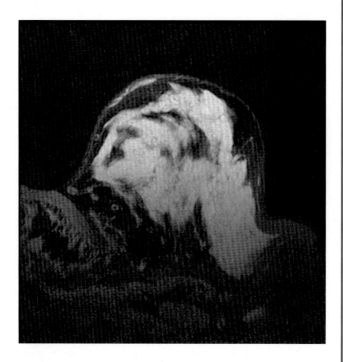

FIGURE 3. Fat-saturated, T2-weighted, spin-echo MRI of the left breast shows diffuse parenchymal engorgement, consistent with benign lactational changes.

CASE 17

Initial identification of breast cancer during breast MRI for implant integrity

A 60-year-old woman with long-standing breast implants noted a left breast lump while lying on her left side. She had been considering implant revision. She had implants initially placed over 20 years before, with the left revised a few years later for encapsulation. A 6-mm, round, mobile mass was palpated by her physician along the medial border of the left implant. She was referred for breast implant MRI.

Because a palpable lump in an implant patient could be either a breast parenchymal mass or related to extracapsular silicone from implant failure, the study was conducted as a hybrid examination. Sequences were obtained both to evaluate the implants and to look for extracapsular silicone, with an enhanced, dynamic subtracted sequence obtained to evaluate the breast parenchyma.

The implants proved to be double-lumen silicone and saline on the right and single lumen silicone on the left (not shown). The implants appeared intact, and no extracapsular silicone was seen. The breast parenchyma showed extensive fibrocystic enhancement, with three discrete sites of more intense mass enhancement (Figures 1 and 2). One was in the left breast at 12 o'clock, with washout. Two were in the right breast, one anteriorly at 8 o'clock and one in the lower inner quadrant at 5 o'clock along the implant margin. Both of these sites showed plateauing enhancement.

Ultrasound correlates were sought. A 1-cm mass with increased vascularity and angular, irregular margins was found on the right at 8 o'clock, correlating with MRI (Figure 3). No ultrasound correlates for either of the two other sites were found. The right 8-o'clock suspicious mass underwent biopsy with ultrasound guidance, confirming infiltrating ductal carcinoma (IDC), estrogen receptor and progesterone receptor positive.

An MRI-guided biopsy was performed on the left 12-o'clock enhancing abnormality. Benign results were obtained, with focal sclerosing adenosis and fibroadenomatous changes.

The patient decided on bilateral mastectomy, with implant removal and bilateral sentinel lymph node sampling. Pathology showed the sampled lymph nodes to be negative, with benign left breast findings and a residual 0.6-cm IDC in the right breast. The margins were negative. No correlate for the second site of concern in the right lower inner breast was found at pathology.

The patient was started on anastrozole (Arimidex) but discontinued it within a year because of intolerance.

TEACHING POINTS

If this patient had elected breast conservation therapy for her biopsy-proven right IDC, the question of what the second site of abnormal enhancement represented in the right lower inner quadrant at 5 o'clock would have had to have been addressed preoperatively. This would have been technically difficult. Its far posterior location in the medial breast and its position against the implant would have made MRI-guided biopsy difficult at best, assuming the lesion could even be reached from a medial approach, which limits how posterior a lesion can be accessed. An MRI-guided clip placement might have been possible, but a vacuum-

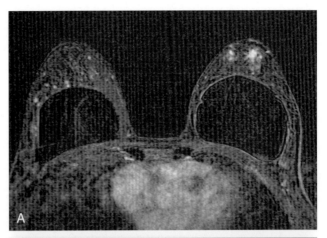
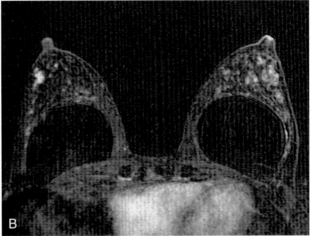
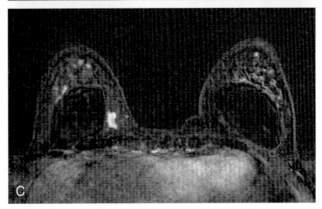

FIGURE 1. Axial enhanced, subtracted, T1-weighted gradient echo images of both breasts from minute 2 of dynamic enhanced series, from above to below (**A** to **C**). **A,** Through the upper breasts: A small, 7-mm enhancing mass is seen on the left at 12 o'clock. Kinetic analysis showed washout (not shown). **B,** Through the level of the nipples: An irregularly marginated mass enhances in the right anterior lateral breast. Kinetic analysis showed a plateauing pattern of enhancement (not shown). **C,** Through the inferior breasts: An irregularly marginated second mass is seen in the posterior medial right breast, against the implant margin. Kinetic analysis showed a plateauing pattern of enhancement (not shown).

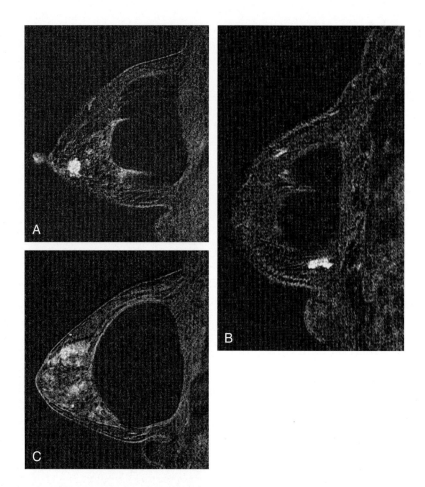

FIGURE 2. Sagittal, enhanced, subtracted, T1-weighted gradient echo images of both breasts, 5 minutes after contrast administration (**A** to **C**). **A,** Through the right lateral breast: The mass seen in Figure 1B at 8 o'clock is depicted. Margins are irregular. **B,** Through the right medial breast: The mass seen in Figure 1C is shown. It has an oblong shape and irregular margins. **C,** Through the left central breast: The early enhancing mass at 12 o'clock with washout now blends into adjacent enhancing breast parenchyma.

assisted biopsy of a lesion against the implant margin runs the risk of rupturing the implant.

The imaging evaluation of palpable breast lumps in patients with implants utilizes the same tools as for women without augmentation. Mammography is the cornerstone, liberally supplemented with ultrasound. Breast MRI is also useful in selected patients and is not hampered either by the presence of breast implants or by increased density. In this case, the patient had had a recent, negative mammogram within a few months before (albeit before the palpable lump was identified). Ultrasound could have been utilized next. In this case, the patient's plastic surgeon thought the palpable finding may have been related to implant rupture and sent the patient for breast MRI. If MRI showed the palpable lump to be related to extracapsular silicone, an enhanced evaluation may not have

been necessary. However, because many facilities do not have the ability to monitor cases in real time, it can be more efficient to design MRI protocols to cover most eventualities. In this case, a "hybrid" protocol was utilized, featuring sequences for breast implant evaluation and enhanced, dynamic imaging for evaluation of the parenchyma. Our protocol for this is not as detailed or high resolution as the dedicated breast implant protocol, but suffices to exclude extravasated silicone as a cause of a palpable breast lump. It consists of a bilateral axial STIR sequence, a bilateral axial STIR sequence with water saturation (on which only silicone is bright), and an enhanced, subtracted, dynamic bilateral axial series for the parenchyma.

In this case, no correlate was found on MRI for the left palpable lump that prompted the MRI evaluation in the first place. Bilateral, suspicious, unsuspected abnormalities were identified, one of which proved to be a small breast cancer. This case points out the nonspecificity of appearance and enhancement characteristics of similar-appearing small MRI lesions. We have histologic diagnoses for two of these three lesions, with one a small IDC, another focal sclerosing adenosis and fibroadenomatous changes, and the other unknown.

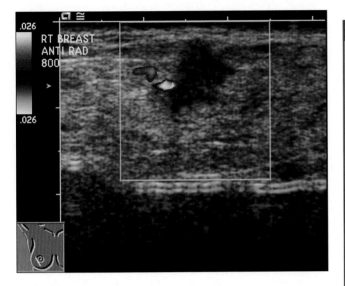

FIGURE 3. Ultrasound of the right breast at 8 o'clock shows a hypoechoic, solid, vascular, taller-than-wide, sonographically suspicious mass with angular margins, which corresponds to the MRI abnormality. Ultrasound-guided biopsy proved it to be an IDC.

CASE 18

Multifocal IDC in a patient with implants and dense breasts

An asymptomatic 71-year-old woman with bilateral subpectoral implants underwent screening mammography and subsequent breast ultrasound at an outside facility, which showed abnormalities suggesting multifocal right breast cancer (Figures 1, 2, 3, and 4). Although the patient had noted no problems, physician examination after the imaging abnormalities were identified found a conglomerate of grape-like masses measuring 2 cm in the right medial retroareolar area. Palpation-guided core needle biopsy of a mass at 3 o'clock identified

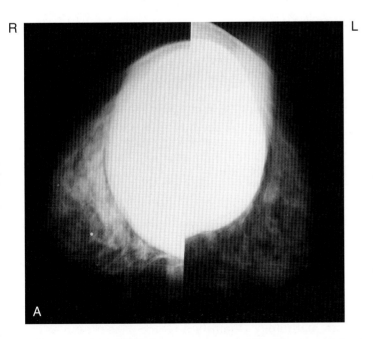

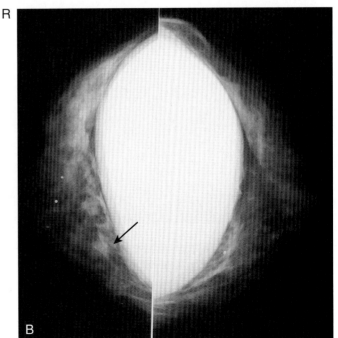

FIGURE 1. MLO (**A**) and CC (**B**) mammograms show heterogeneous increased breast density and bilateral subpectoral implants. Comparison for symmetry shows a mass or mass-like parenchymal focus in the right medial breast on the CC view (*arrow*).

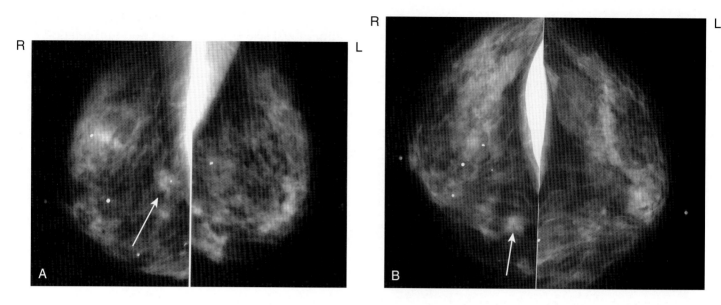

FIGURE 2. MLO (**A**) and CC (**B**) mammographic views with implants displaced suggest asymmetrical nodularity and multiple ill-defined masses in the right posterior medial breast (*arrows*).

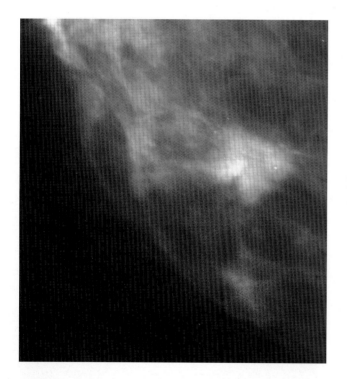

FIGURE 3. Spot compression in the CC projection with implant displacement suggests at least two masses with ill-defined margins.

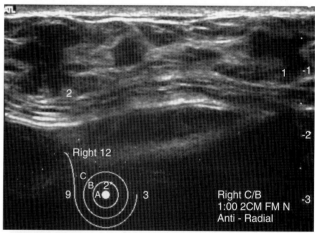

FIGURE 4. Ultrasound of the right upper inner quadrant shows three separate hypoechoic solid masses with angular margins, strongly suggesting multifocal breast cancer. The larger masses are annotated 1 and 2, and the third lesion is in between.

well-differentiated infiltrating ductal carcinoma (IDC). Because of the implants, breast density, and apparent multifocal nature of the patient's disease, local staging was completed with breast MRI. This confirmed multifocal medial right breast cancer, but showed no evidence of disease elsewhere (Figure 5).

Surgical treatment was a right mastectomy, and pathology identified three separate IDC tumor masses, measuring 1.4 cm, 1.3 cm, and 0.7 cm. One of 20 lymph nodes showed metastatic disease.

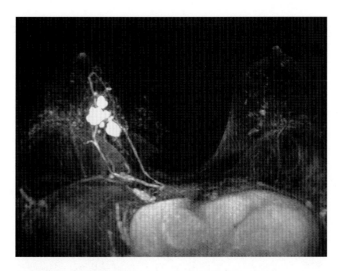

FIGURE 5. Breast MRI (axial maximal intensity projection) confirms multifocal breast cancer, with adjacent intensely enhancing and irregularly marginated masses in the right medial breast. No suspicious abnormality was seen elsewhere in the right breast or on the left.

TEACHING POINTS

This is a difficult-to-image patient by virtue of the presence of implants and breast density. Remarkably, in this case, mammography and ultrasound did a very comprehensive job of locally staging this patient. However, the confidence level that the patient's disease is accurately staged is certainly increased by the use of breast MRI, which is particularly useful in patients who are difficult due to implants, breast density, and prior surgery, radiation, or both.

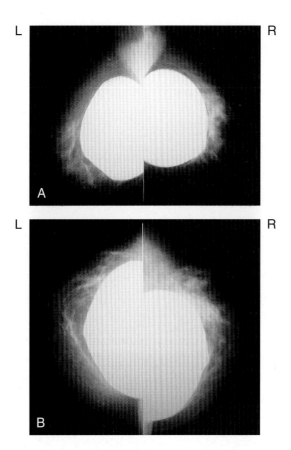

FIGURE 1. MLO (**A**) and CC (**B**) mammographic views show bilateral prepectoral implants. A radiopaque marker was placed at the site of a palpable lump identified by the patient in the right breast. No definite correlate is seen, although some increased tissue density can be seen on the side of concern.   (*continued*)

CASE 19

Large, locally advanced IDC in an implant patient

A 60-year-old woman with long-standing breast implants presented with a large palpable lump in the lower outer quadrant of the right breast, found on monthly breast self-examination. Mam-

mography showed a spiculated mass at the level of the palpable lump on implant-displaced views (Figure 1). Ultrasound demonstrated a large (8 cm) vascular mass with angular and spiculated margins (Figure 2). Sonography of the axilla showed multiple enlarged, rounded, abnormal lymph nodes (Figure 3). Because of the implants, histologic sampling was accomplished with ultrasound guidance, and confirmed poorly differentiated infiltrating ductal carcinoma. Fine-needle aspiration of an axillary lymph node was performed with ultrasound guidance at the same time, and demonstrated malignant cells, consistent with metastatic disease. Breast MRI showed a large dominant tumor mass, with additional satellite lesions (Figures 4 and 5). No evidence of occult disease was seen in the contralateral breast. Because of the large size of the mass, thought to be T3N1, neoadjuvant chemotherapy was given.

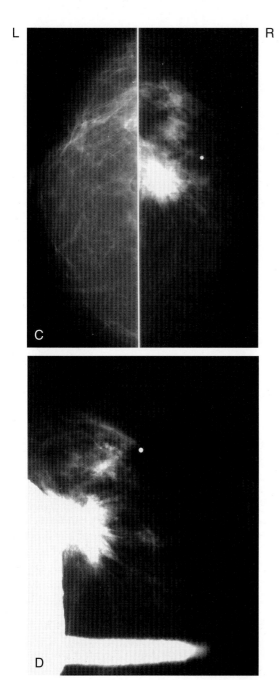

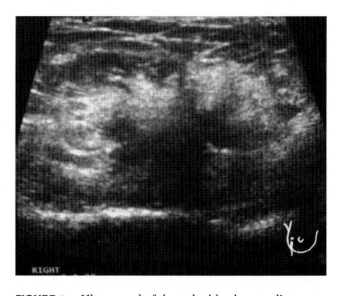

FIGURE 2. Ultrasound of the palpable abnormality shows a large suspicious mass with irregular, angular, and spiculated margins.

FIGURE 1, cont'd **C,** CC implant displaced view shows a dominant right breast mass, at the level of the palpable lump identified by the radiopaque marker. **D,** On spot compression of the palpable lump, with the implant displaced, the spiculated margins of the mass are seen well.

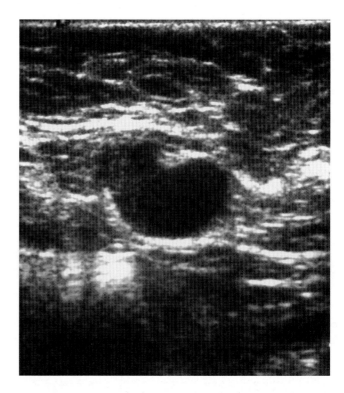

FIGURE 3. Ultrasound of the axilla showed multiple abnormal axillary lymph nodes. One illustrated here is in profile. Although the fatty hilus is preserved, the cortical mantle is abnormally thick.

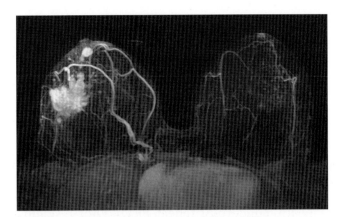

FIGURE 4. Maximal intensity projection of the volumetric data set from minute 1 of the enhanced, subtracted, dynamic acquisition provides an overview of both breasts. In the right breast, an intensely enhancing, dominant, spiculated mass fills the lateral breast. An additional round mass is noted behind the nipple. Right breast vessels are asymmetrically enlarged. The left breast shows only tiny, faint, diffuse stippled foci of enhancement. No pathologic patterns of enhancement were seen in the asymptomatic left side.

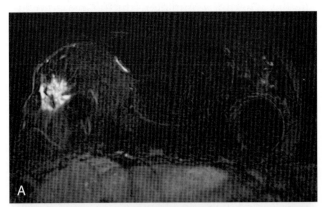

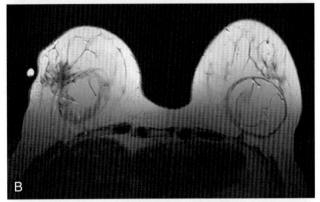

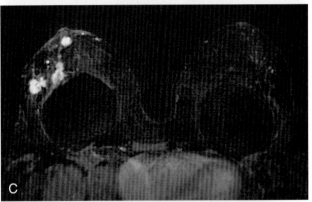

FIGURE 5. **A,** A slice from early in the dynamic enhanced series through the lower outer quadrant palpable abnormality shows a spiculated, dominant, intensely rim-enhancing mass extending to the margin of the breast implant. **B,** A corresponding T2-weighted axial image shows a marker at the level of the palpable lump, with the hypointense spiculated mass immediately subjacent. Most breast cancers (97% has previously been reported) are hypointense on T2-weighted MRI. **C,** A more superior section, through the nipples, shows three separate additional tumor nodules, including one in the retroareolar region. **D,** A sagittal, fat-saturated, enhanced T1-weighted MRI (unsubtracted) through the dominant mass shows clear extension to the implant surface and the nipple.

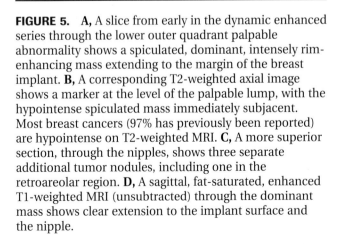

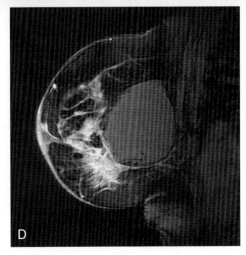

Staging workup, completed during neoadjuvant chemotherapy, included bone scan, chest, abdomen and pelvis CT scans, spine MRI, and positron emission tomography (PET) (Figure 6). These evaluations showed bone metastases. (See Case 1 in Chapter 8 for a discussion of the imaging manifestations of this patient's bony metastatic disease.)

After completion of three cycles of neoadjuvant chemotherapy, the mass and adenopathy decreased. Three months after diagnosis, the patient underwent bilateral mastectomies, right axillary dissection, left sentinel lymph node sampling, and removal of the breast implants. The right mastec-

tomy specimen contained a 3.5-cm invasive ductal carcinoma, with multiple satellite nodules. Nipple involvement was confirmed. The margins were clear. Six of 16 axillary lymph nodes displayed metastases. Left sentinel node sampling was negative.

The preoperative staging workup strongly suggested metastatic disease to bone. A sclerotic T11 vertebral body lesion was initially sampled 2 weeks after the patient's breast surgery, and did not confirm metastatic disease. The needle biopsy was repeated 2 months later, and confirmed metastasis. A nearly concurrent repeat PET/CT for restaging showed normalization.

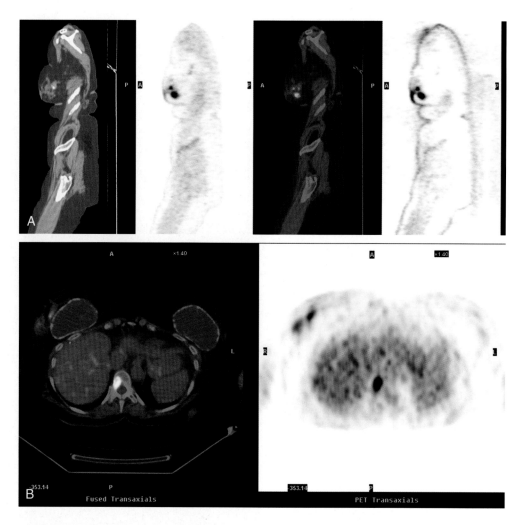

FIGURE 6. Sagittal (**A**) and axial (**B**) PET images show multifocal hypermetabolism in the right lateral breast, corresponding to the MRI findings. The axial section also shows a hypermetabolic focus in a lower thoracic vertebral body, one of several PET findings of bony metastases.

After completion of eight cycles of docetaxel (Taxotere), the patient was started on anastrozole (Arimidex) for her estrogen receptor–positive disease, as well as zoledronic acid (Zometa). She has been essentially asymptomatic on this therapy, with stable imaging studies for 2.5 years since the diagnosis of stage IV breast cancer metastatic to bone.

TEACHING POINT

This sizable tumor was initially thought to be a locally advanced breast cancer. Bone metastases, identified after beginning neoadjuvant chemotherapy, while systemic staging studies were being completed, indicate that the true stage is stage IV.

CHAPTER 5

Locally Advanced Breast Cancer (LABC) and Neoadjuvant Chemotherapy

DEFINITION OF LOCALLY ADVANCED BREAST CANCER

The definition of locally advanced breast cancer (LABC) has continued to evolve since Haagensen and Stout outlined their criteria for operability more than 60 years ago.[1] Their conclusions remain a part of the current American Joint Committee on Cancer Classification System for LABC, as depicted in Table 1. LABC includes large tumors (>5 cm), those (of any size) with involvement of the skin or chest wall, and those with clinically apparent axillary nodal involvement (matted or fixed) or ipsilateral internal mammary, infraclavicular, or supraclavicular nodal disease.

By definition, LABC is nonmetastatic, other than to locoregional nodal basins. This group of patients needs to be carefully evaluated at initial diagnosis because some apparent LABC patients actually have systemic metastases, or stage IV disease.

ASSESSMENT OF PATIENTS SUSPECTED TO HAVE LABC

In recent years, the use of neoadjuvant chemotherapy has played an important role in reducing the number of "inoperable" patients with LABC, as well as providing access to clinical trials. This group of patients, similar to other breast cancer patients, requires an initial diagnosis and assessment of the locoregional extent of disease (typically, with mammography, ultrasound, tissue sampling, and MRI), as well as systemic staging. Systemic assessment generally includes blood studies (e.g., liver function tests, complete blood count, serum tumor markers, lactate dehydrogenase level, and alkaline phosphatase level) and may incorporate imaging modalities such as CT, nuclear medicine bone scintigraphy, MRI of the brain (in symptomatic patients or those with neurologic findings on physical examination), positron emission tomography (PET), and PET/CT. Most often, staging should be completed before initiation of neoadjuvant therapy; it is known that PET may turn negative soon after beginning chemotherapy.

Continued refinement of protocols used to treat LABC has broadened the role of imaging in both neoadjuvant and post-treatment management. Initial diagnosis is routinely accomplished with some combination of physical examination, mammography, ultrasound, and core biopsy. MRI is assuming an ever-increasing role in newly diagnosed patients. Systemic staging is typically performed with CT, bone scintigraphy, and PET. An increasingly important application of imaging in the management of LABC is the monitoring of response to neoadjuvant chemotherapy. This is discussed later with special attention to the emerging role of PET in assessing primary tumor response.

Locoregional staging of breast cancer is covered in depth in Chapter 3, including assessment with mammography, ultrasound, and MRI. The principles outlined in that chapter are identical for the patient who meets the definition of LABC. MRI has proved extremely valuable in accurately estimating tumor size and extent, as well as determining multifocality, multicentricity, and bilaterality (Figure 1). MRI more accurately correlates with tumor size and number of tumors at pathology than mammography or ultrasound. It is the modality of choice for assessment of chest wall invasion (Figure 2).

ASSESSMENT OF RESPONSE TO NEOADJUVANT CHEMOTHERAPY

Assessment of response to neoadjuvant chemotherapy with anatomic imaging modalities can be problematic. On mammography, breast cancers that initially manifest as masses generally decrease in size in response to chemotherapy, but may not completely resolve. Breast cancer manifesting on mammography as microcalcifications is even more difficult to accurately assess in terms of

Table 1   Primary Tumor (T) and Clinical Regional Lymph Node (N) Categories Comprising LABC in the Current American Joint Committee on Cancer Classification System

T3	Tumor >5 cm in greatest diameter
T4	Tumor of any size, with direct extension to chest wall or skin, as described below
T4a	Extension to chest wall, not including pectoralis muscle
T4b	Edema (including peau d'orange) or ulceration of the skin of the breast or satellite nodules confined to same breast
T4c	Both Ta and Tb
T4d	Inflammatory carcinoma
N2	Metastases in ipsilateral axillary nodes fixed or matted, or in clinically apparent ipsilateral internal mammary nodes in the absence of clinically evident axillary node metastases.
N3	Metastases in ipsilateral infraclavicular or supraclavicular lymph nodes or in clinically apparent internal mammary nodes in the presence of clinically evident axillary node metastases.

Data from Greene FL, Page DL, Fleming ID, et al. *AJCC Cancer Staging Manual,* 6th ed. New York, Springer Verlag, 2002.

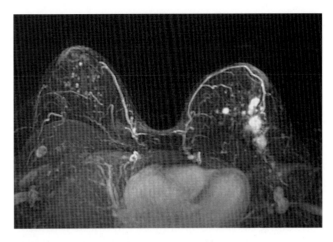

FIGURE 1. Axial maximal intensity projection (MIP) view from contrast-enhanced, subtracted breast MRI of a 52-year-old woman with newly diagnosed left LABC, a multifocal infiltrating ductal carcinoma (IDC), with involvement of 10 of 11 nodes on axillary dissection. Multiple adjacent left lateral breast masses form a large confluent mass. A satellite nodule projects medially. Several enlarged involved left axillary lymph nodes are demonstrated as well.

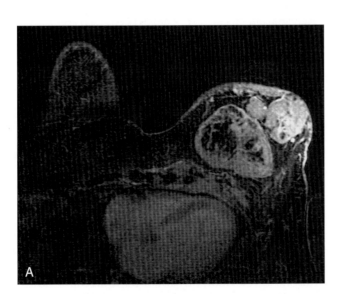
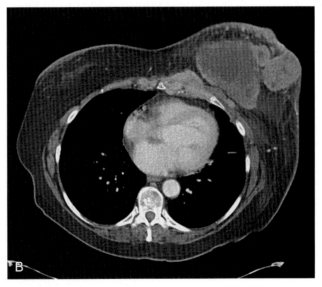

FIGURE 2.   A, Enhanced, subtracted axial breast MRI demonstrates a neglected left LABC. This tumor would be classified as LABC based on size alone, but it demonstrates other criteria as well, including infiltration of the skin and chest wall (note enhancing, thickened skin and chest wall). **B,** Enhanced chest CT of the same patient, for comparison. The bulky left breast tumor masses are well seen, and extension into the thickened skin is shown as well. The bulky chest wall involvement in this case is well seen on CT, but lesser degrees of infiltration are less reliably demonstrated on CT than MRI, owing to the lower inherent soft tissue contrast of CT.

responsiveness to neoadjuvant therapy because microcalcifications may not resolve, even in responders. On ultrasound, responding tumors show a decrease in size and, occasionally, resolution. MRI appears to be the most reliable anatomic imaging modality in common use today for monitoring patients being treated preoperatively.[3–8] In addition to showing decreased tumor size, the enhancement pattern changes in responders. Responding tumors showing intense enhancement and washout initially often show decreased intensity of peak enhancement, as well as more benign patterns of progressive or persistent enhancement (flattening of the enhancement curve). Responding tumors may shrink, retaining a smaller, but still mass-like, morphology, or they can "break apart," manifesting as less intense, smaller foci of enhancement within the distribution of the initial abnormality. Complete response by MRI (complete resolution of all tumor-associated enhancement) does not confirm a complete pathologic response because some patients with complete imaging responses have microscopic disease at pathology. Conversely, some patients with good, but incomplete, responses by MRI (some residual enhancement in the distribution of the original tumor) prove at pathology to have had complete pathologic responses.

Neoadjuvant chemotherapy is being used increasingly to convert some LABC patients with large tumors into breast conservation candidates. Because the degree of response is unknown at the outset of therapy and some patients will have complete imaging resolution of their tumors, it is important to anticipate the need for tumor marking with clip placement. This should be considered at the time of initial diagnostic biopsy of large, highly suspicious abnormalities that appear to be likely candidates for preoperative chemotherapy. Placement of a clip at the time of initial biopsy may save the patient from having to undergo a separate procedure during chemotherapy for just that purpose.

There has been great interest in monitoring the response to chemotherapy in the neoadjuvant setting using molecular imaging with the hope of separate responders from nonresponders. This allows the oncologist to continue effective therapy or change to alternate agents. Although MRI appears to show the best correlation, anatomic imaging modalities (including ultrasound, mammography, and MRI) rely predominantly on change in tumor size or volume to suggest responses. It is known that there may be a significant delay between the initiation of therapy and tumor shrinkage.

Patients may undergo several rounds of chemotherapy to find that they have not responded and need other chemotherapeutic agents. Methods such as MRI and molecular and optical imaging are being studied to determine their ability to predict tumor response earlier, based on functional and metabolic properties other than tumor size. Earlier prediction of response may allow selection of an appropriate chemotherapy regimen sooner, potentially avoiding unnecessary chemotherapy. An ACRIN trial, 6657, is currently under way to study MRI parameters, such as tumor kinetics and choline spectroscopy, to predict breast cancer response to neoadjuvant therapy.

PET and PET/CT are assuming an increasing role in this assessment, and a larger role for breast-specific gamma imaging and positron emission mammography can be anticipated in the future. Quantitative PET assessment, using the standardized uptake value (SUV), has shown early success in separating responders from nonresponders.[10–12] Careful attention must be paid to all the factors influencing SUV measurement, especially region-of-interest assignment and patient glucose level. Flare responses (increased uptake as a manifestation of response), which can be seen on PET with initiation of tamoxifen therapy, are not seen with chemotherapy.

ASSESSMENT OF SENTINEL NODE STATUS IN LABC TREATED NEOADJUVANTLY

A controversial issue in the use of neoadjuvant chemotherapy is whether to assess preoperatively the status of the axilla with sentinel lymph node (SLN) sampling. It has been demonstrated that information from SLN biopsy or axillary dissection performed after completion of chemotherapy correlates well with overall prognosis. The role of SLN sampling and axillary dissection in the postchemotherapy setting was reviewed in a meta-analysis, with an overall accuracy of 95%.[13]

In an attempt to reduce false-negative SLN analysis after neoadjuvant chemotherapy, some surgeons advocate routine SLN sampling before initiation of chemotherapy. Positive SLN biopsy would lead to completion axillary dissection, before or after chemotherapy. Pathology information from prechemotherapy SLN biopsy is used by radiation oncologists in planning radiation field coverage.

ASSESSMENT FOR SYSTEMIC METASTASES (EXCLUSION OF STAGE IV DISEASE)

The most common sites of breast cancer metastasis are bone, lung, and liver, in that order.[14] Evaluation of bone should begin with a careful history to elicit any symptoms or history of recent trauma. Serum alkaline phosphatase and calcium measurements may be helpful if positive and heighten suspicion of bony involvement. Imaging options, discussed in greater depth in Chapter 8, include bone scanning, CT, MRI, and PET. Bone scintigraphy, using a technetium-based agent (e.g., methylene diphosphonate), is exquisitely sensitive to changes in bone metabolism. Localization of these agents into bone is dependent on many factors, with the most important two being blood flow and osteoblastic activity. This results in a very predictable concentration in osteoblastic metastases (Figure 3). Positive findings on scintigraphy antedate findings on plain radiography by weeks to months. Drawbacks of bone scanning include suboptimal specificity, reduced sensitivity in osteo-

lytic metastases, and persistent positivity at sites where active tumor is no longer present. Additionally, the well-recognized flare phenomenon, resulting in apparent worsening on scintigraphy due to treatment response, may mislead the unaware clinician or imager. Specificity is arguably the most problematic feature of whole-body skeletal scintigraphy. Any process that results in an increase in bone remodeling will demonstrate increased uptake of radiopharmaceutical. For this reason and because of the implications of labeling a patient as having bony metastases, correlative imaging (or even tissue sampling) is required. Correlation can be accomplished with plain radiography, CT, or MRI.

Plain radiography is of minimal value as a screening modality, requiring 30% to 50% loss of bone mineral for a metastasis to become visible.[15] Plain radiographic correlation with a scintigraphic abnormality may be of benefit; however, the increased sensitivity and improved anatomic detail (including surrounding soft tissues) are factors favoring CT (Figure 4) or MRI. Although MRI has a higher rate of detection of skeletal metastases than scintigraphy in the spine, pelvis, limbs, sternum,

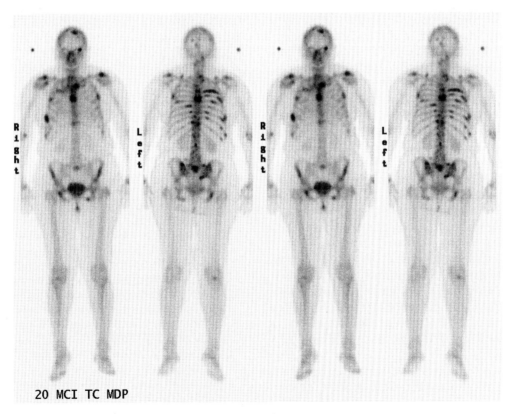

20 MCI TC MDP

FIGURE 3.   Anterior and posterior images from whole-body bone scan in a patient with known breast cancer. Typical bone scan findings of extensive breast cancer bone metastases are demonstrated: multiple lesions in a random distribution, with several rib lesions displaying a particularly suggestive pattern of elongated uptake.

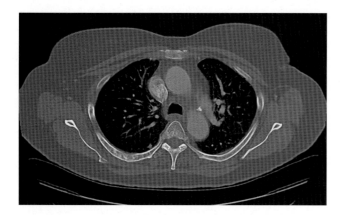

FIGURE 4. Chest CT image, displayed with bone windowing, from the same patient in Figure 3, shows abnormal, mottled, partially blastic bone mineral texture involving a long segment of a right posterior rib, corresponding to the bone scan.

Table 2 Role of Imaging Modalities in Diagnosis (D), Staging (S), Restaging (R), and Monitoring Response to Therapy (M)

	D	S	R	M
Mammography	+	0	0	0
Ultrasound	+	+	0	0
MRI	+	+	+	+
PET	0	++	++	++
Bone scan	+	++	+	+
CT	0	++	+	+

++, Definite value; +, helpful in selected patients; 0, no demonstrated efficacy.

scapulae, and clavicles,[16] the logistics and cost of whole-body MRI give scintigraphy the edge as an initial screening examination.

PET and, more recently, PET/CT have been used to evaluate the entire body for metastases, including bone. An emerging consensus is that PET and scintigraphy have a similar sensitivity for detection of metastases, whereas PET shows a definite increase in specificity.[17–20] There also appears to be a significantly higher sensitivity with fluorodeoxyglucose (FDG) PET for osteolytic metastases. Conversely, bone scintigraphy has shown superiority for demonstration of osteoblastic lesions. Currently, PET and bone scintigraphy are viewed as complementary imaging modalities for the detection of skeletal metastases.

Lung metastases are relatively common in patients with metastatic disease and in those who die from breast cancer. However, lung metastases are very uncommon at initial diagnosis of breast cancer.[21] Many centers still recommend a chest x-ray at initial screening (in part, because of the age of their breast cancer population); however, positive findings on chest x-ray generally necessitate CT correlation. CT is the modality of choice for chest evaluation. PET/CT offers advantages over CT alone in evaluating the mediastinum and as a whole-body survey.[22]

Evaluation of the liver is covered in depth in Chapter 9. In addition to CT, MRI, and PET, ultrasound may be appropriate in selected patients. The number of patients with hepatic metastases at initial presentation is extremely low. Screening, whether using liver enzymes or imaging, is nonspecific and of low diagnostic yield. For symptomatic patients and those with clinical evidence of liver involvement, CT and MRI are considered the imaging modalities of choice.[23] Ultrasound may be useful to help characterize small lesions identified on CT.[24] Finally, FDG PET is best viewed as complementary in the liver; it carries an excellent specificity and will occasionally find lesions not appreciated prospectively on CT or MRI, but it has limited sensitivity for small lesions (<1 cm) and can be difficult to interpret when there is heterogeneous FDG uptake, which can be exacerbated by attenuation correction (Table 2).

REFERENCES

1. Haagensen C, Stout A. Carcinoma of the breast: Criteria of operability. *Ann Surg* 1943; 118:859–868.
2. Greene FL, Page DL, Fleming ID, et al. AJCC Cancer Staging Manual, 6th ed. New York, Springer Verlag, 2002.
3. Rieber A, Brambs HJ, Gabelmann A, et al. Breast MRI for monitoring response of primary breast cancer to neo-adjuvant chemotherapy. *Eur Radiol* 2002; 12(7):1711–1719.
4. Partridge SC, Gibbs JE, Lu Y, et al. Accuracy of MR imaging for revealing residual breast cancer in patients who have undergone neoadjuvant chemotherapy. *AJR Am J Roentgenol* 2002; 179:1193–1199.
5. Rosen EL, Blackwell KL, Baker JA, et al. Accuracy of MRI in the detection of residual breast cancer after neoadjuvant chemotherapy. *AJR Am J Roentgenol* 2003; 181:1275–1282.
6. Londero V, Bazzocchi M, Del Frate C, et al. Locally advanced breast cancer: comparison of mammography, sonography and MR imaging in evaluation of residual disease in women receiving neoadjuvant chemotherapy. *Eur Radiol* 2004; 14(8):1371–1379.
7. Martincich L, Montemurro F, De Rosa G, et al. Monitoring response to primary chemotherapy in breast cancer using dynamic contrast-enhanced magnetic resonance imaging. *Breast Cancer Res Treat* 2004; 83(1):67–76.

8. Yeh E, Slanetz P, Kopans DB, et al. Prospective comparison of mammography, sonography, and MRI in patients undergoing neoadjuvant chemotherapy for palpable breast cancer. *AJR Am J Roentgenol* 2005; 184(3):868–877.

9. Bassa P, Kim EE, Inoue T, et al. Evaluation of preoperative chemotherapy using PET with fluorine-18-fluorodeoxyglucose in breast cancer. *J Nucl Med* 1996; 37(6):931–938.

10. Schelling M, Avril N, Nahrig J, et al. Positron emission tomography using [(18)F]-fluorodeoxyglucose for monitoring primary chemotherapy in breast cancer. *J Clin Oncol* 2000; 18:1689–1695.

11. Biersack HJ, Palmedo H. Locally advanced breast cancer: is PET useful for monitoring primary chemotherapy? *J Nucl Med* 2003; 44(11):1815–1817.

12. Rosen EL, Eubank WB, Mankoff DA. FDG PET, PET/CT, and breast cancer imaging. *RadioGraphics* 2007; 27:S215–S229.

13. Xing Y, Ding M, Ross M, et al. Meta-analysis of sentinel lymph node biopsy following preoperative chemotherapy in patients with operable breast cancer. ASCO Annual Meeting, 2004, New Orleans, LA abstract 561.

14. Huston TL, Osborne MP. Evaluating and staging the patient with breast cancer. In Ross D (ed). Breast Cancer, 2nd ed. Philadelphia, Elsevier Churchill Livingstone, 2005, pp 309–318.

15. Schirrmeister H. Detection of bone metastases in breast cancer by positron emission tomography. *PET Clin* 2006; 1(1):25–32.

16. Chom Y, Chan K, Lam W, et al. Comparison of whole body MRI and radioisotope bone scintigram for skeletal metastases detection. *Chin Med J* (Engl) 1997; 110(6):485–489.

17. Cook GJ, Houston S, Rubens R, et al. Detection of bone metastases in breast cancer by 18 FDG PET: differing metabolic activity in osteoblastic and osteolytic lesions. *J Clin Oncol* 1998; 16(10):375–379.

18. Ohta M, Tokuda Y, Suzuki Y, et al. Whole body PET for the evaluation of bony metastases in patients with breast cancer: comparison with 99 m Tc-MDP bone scintigraphy. *Nucl Med Commun* 2001; 22(8):875–879.

19. Yang SN, Liang JA, Lin FJ, et al. Comparing whole body 18F-2 deoxyglucose positron emission tomography and technetium-99 m methylene diphosphonate bone scan to detect bone metastases in patients with breast cancer. *J Cancer Res Clin Oncol* 2002; 128(6):325–328.

20. Uematsu T, Yuen S, Yukisawa S, et al. Comparison of FDG PET and SPECT for detection of bone metastases in breast cancer. *AJR Am J Roentgenol* 2005; 184(4):1266–1273.

21. Ciatto S, Pacini P, Azzini V, et al. Preoperative staging of primary breast cancer: a multicentric study. *Cancer* 1988; 61(5):1038–1040.

22. Dose J, Bleckmann C, Bachmann S, et al. Comparison of fluorodeoxyglucose positron emission tomography and "conventional diagnostic procedures" for the detection of distant metastases in breast cancer patients. *Nucl Med Commun* 2002; 23(9):857–864.

23. Reinig JW, Dwyer AJ, Miller DL, et al. Liver metastasis detection: comparative sensitivities of MR imaging and CT scanning. *Radiology* 1987; 162:43–47.

24. Eberhardt SC, Choi PH, Bach AM, et al. Utility of sonography for small hepatic lesions found on computed tomography in patients with cancer. *J Ultrasound Med* 2003; 22(4):335–343.

CASE 1

LABC (large tumor size)

A 45-year-old woman was noted on routine physical examination by her physician to have an abnormal left breast examination. Although the patient had not noted any discrete masses, an area of induration and irregularity was palpated in the left upper breast, extending from upper inner to upper outer quadrant.

Breast imaging evaluation showed extremely dense breast parenchyma. New clustered microcalcifications were identified in the upper inner quadrant (UIQ). Sonography showed irregular, hypoechoic parenchymal echotexture in the left upper breast at 11 to 12 o'clock with cysts and shadowing (Figure 1), and the region of the microcalcifications was visualized as well. Ultrasound-guided biopsy confirmed infiltrating ductal carcinoma (IDC) with ductal carcinoma in situ (DCIS).

The patient was evaluated by medical and radiation oncology and surgery for possible breast conservation. All three examiners had difficulty quantifying the size of the palpable abnormality, partly because of the presence of large coexisting cysts. One examiner noted a large area of firm dense tissue extending over 5 to 6 cm at the 12-o'clock level, and was concerned about the true extent of disease, because mammography had shown only a small UIQ microcalcification cluster. A breast MRI was, therefore, ordered to assess the extent of disease.

Breast MRI showed striking asymmetry between the two sides, with findings of a very large, diffusely infiltrating cancer on the left (Figures 2 and 3). The intensely enhancing process, centered at 12 o'clock but spanning 11 to 2 o'clock, showed architectural distortion, with additional extensive clumped enhancement diffusely involving the medial breast. By MRI, the abnormality measured at least 6 cm and involved at least two quadrants extensively, indicating that the patient was not a conservation candidate.

Unfortunately, the surgeon did not become aware of this result until the day of the surgery because the study had been ordered by another physician. Fortunately, the radiologist who scanned the patient for performance of ultrasound-guided needle localization on the day of surgery recognized that the surgeon could not have been aware of the results of the MRI. The patient was subse-

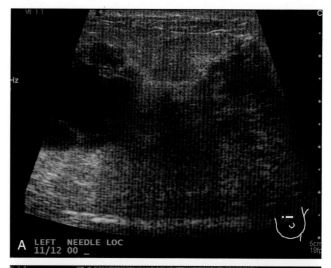

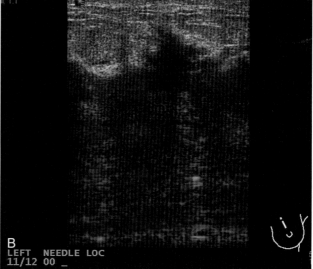

FIGURE 1. **A** and **B,** Representative ultrasound images of the 11 to 12 o'clock region show dense shadowing, with irregular anterior margination. The extent of the process is difficult to define and to differentiate from extreme fibrocystic changes.

quently apprised of the results and the extremely high likelihood of positive margins if lumpectomy was attempted, and therefore underwent mastectomy.

The mastectomy specimen showed an 8-cm IDC of the central breast extending into the upper inner and lower inner quadrants, with a high-grade DCIS component involving 50% of the lesion (extensive intraductal component). Multifocal satellite tumor nodules were noted within the large tumor. Extensive angiolymphatic involvement was seen, and four sentinel lymph nodes showed metastatic carcinoma (Figure 4). Completion axillary dissection showed no additional axillary disease, for a total of 4 of 20 lymph nodes positive for metastatic disease. The deep mastectomy margin was negative.

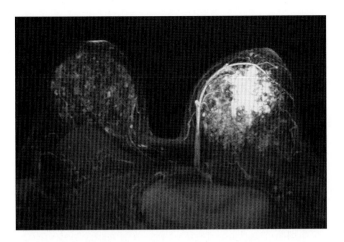

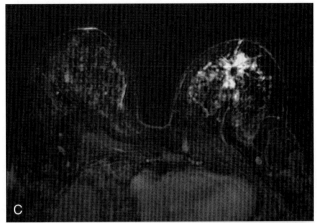

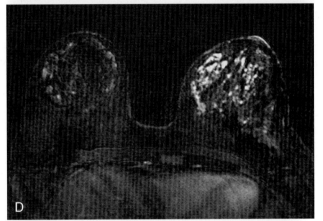

FIGURE 2. Axial enhanced, maximal intensity projection MRI shows extreme asymmetry between sides. The right side shows diffuse low-level, extensive, scattered, tiny fibrocystic foci of enhancement. The left side is dominated by a central mass with architectural distortion, and there is geographic enhancement in the medial breast.

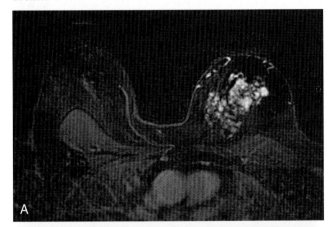

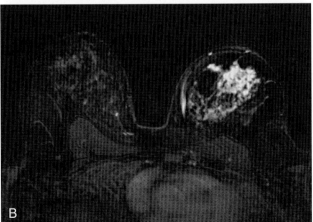

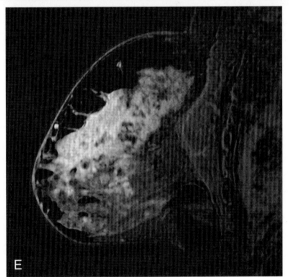

FIGURE 3. Representative axial, subtracted, enhanced images, from above to below. **A,** Clumped enhancement medially with larger central tumor nodules involves both the upper inner and upper outer quadrants at this level. **B,** There is intense central enhancement with distortion and segmental clumped medial enhancement at this level.

FIGURE 3, cont'd   C, The spiculation and distortion of the central enhancing component are well demonstrated on this section. The oval defect within the enhancing spiculated mass represents a cyst, which was surrounded by the enhancing tumor. Clumped segmental medial enhancement, suggesting DCIS, is again seen. **D,** At the level of the nipple, extensive clumped segmental enhancement is seen medially and centrally, suggesting an extensive intraductal component, which was subsequently confirmed. **E,** Sagittal, subtracted, enhanced breast MRI shows how extensively the entire upper half of the breast is infiltrated.

The patient underwent imaging staging post-operatively, with bone scan, CT, and positron emission tomography (PET) (Figures 5 and 6), which showed only postsurgical changes of the axilla and chest wall and no evidence of distant metastatic disease. Final stage was stage IIIA, with T3N1M0 disease, and the tumor was estrogen receptor and progesterone receptor positive.

TEACHING POINTS

The extensive nature of this locally advanced, very large IDC became apparent relatively late in this patient's evaluation and was accurately delineated only by MRI. The clinical examination in this patient confounded multiple examiners. The patient had extremely dense, fibrocystic breasts, with multiple cysts, and examiners found it difficult to delineate the extent of the tumor by palpation. Fortunately, one examiner sensed a discrepancy between the imaging findings and the apparent clinical extent, and breast MRI was ordered. It is not surprising that mammography in a patient with very dense breast tissue and multiple cysts would underestimate the extent of disease. Much of this patient's extensive intraductal disease was noncalcified, with only a small microcalcification cluster noted in the UIQ at mammographic evaluation. The sonogram identified abnormal echotexture in the involved area, accurately guiding core biopsy for a diagnosis, but the size of the process and the full significance of the sonographic findings, with geographic shadowing and poor margin delineation, were not fully appreciated prospectively.

Accurate and timely communication between specialties is a critical part of the care of the newly

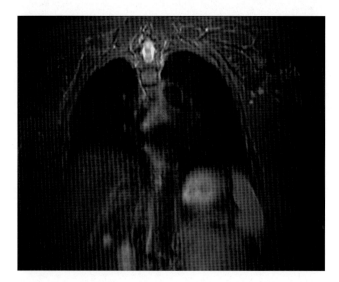

FIGURE 4. Coronal short tau inversion recovery (STIR) image of the thorax (obtained with the body coil at the time of breast MRI) shows three adjacent mildly prominent left axillary lymph nodes. Although not prospectively interpreted as suspicious because no one lymph node is particularly large, in retrospect the asymmetry in number from the opposite side is a clue to the axillary involvement.

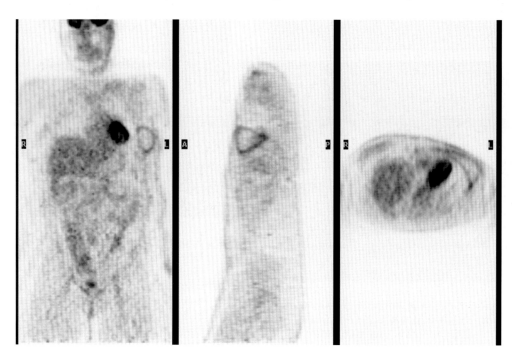

FIGURE 5. PET scan, obtained 2 weeks after left mastectomy, shows a left chest wall photopenic collection with a metabolically active rim, consistent with a postoperative seroma.

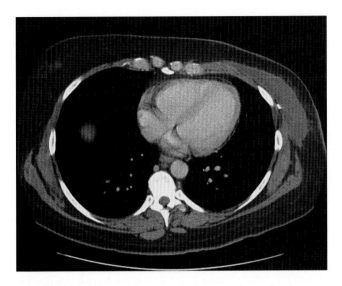

FIGURE 6. Enhanced chest CT image for correlation with PET shows a left chest wall seroma after mastectomy.

diagnosed breast cancer patient, as this case illustrates. Evaluations up to the point of the breast MRI had not shown clear evidence that the patient was not a lumpectomy candidate, and so the treatment planning was proceeding with this expectation. One examiner's concern that there might be a discrepancy between the imaging findings and the clinical examination led to performance of breast MRI, which confirmed a very large, locally advanced tumor. Unfortunately, this was ordered at the last minute and without the knowledge of the surgeon. Fortunately, the radiologist charged with performing the needle localization on the day of surgery was able to rectify the situation, which was precipitously, but satisfactorily, resolved in favor of the patient undergoing mastectomy.

CASE 2

LABC with axillary and internal mammary involvement; staging with whole-body PET and PEM

A 77-year-old woman was noted on routine physical examination by her primary care physician to have a palpable 3-cm mass on the right at 6 o'clock.

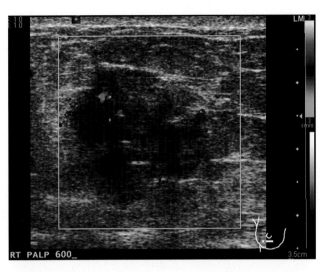

FIGURE 1. Ultrasound of the palpable lump on the right at 6 o'clock shows a very hypoechoic, heterogeneous, vascular mass with lobular and irregular margins, with a highly suspicious sonographic appearance. Biopsy confirmed IDC.

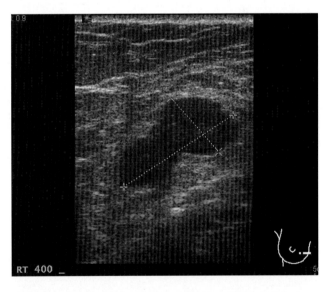

FIGURE 2. Ultrasound of the right 4-o'clock level shows a hypoechoic, bilobed, more smoothly marginated mass, resembling an abnormal lymph node in morphology. Biopsy with ultrasound guidance confirmed IDC.

Breast imaging evaluations confirmed this mass, which was best seen on ultrasound as a 3.2-cm mass with lobular and irregular margins (Figure 1). On ultrasound, a second suspicious mass, which was not seen mammographically, was noted medial to the dominant mass, at 4 o'clock (Figures 2 and 3). This was a bilobed, hypoechoic mass. A highly suspicious axillary lymph node was also found, measuring 2.3 cm, with complete effacement of the fatty hilus (Figure 4).

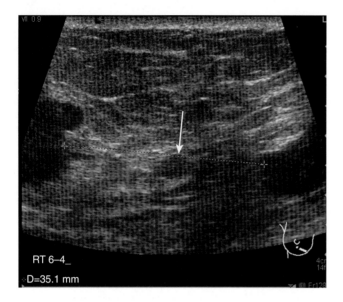

FIGURE 3. Ultrasound shows the relationship between the 4- and 6-o'clock masses, which are 3.5 cm apart by ultrasound. A rounded, sub-centimeter nodule interposed between the two masses (*arrow*) was not noted prospectively. It corresponds to a smaller satellite lesion, which was FDG avid and seen on both whole-body and dedicated breast PET (PEM).

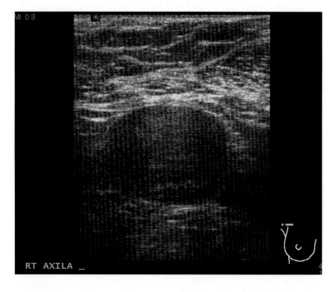

FIGURE 4. Ultrasound of the right axilla shows a round, completely replaced enlarged axillary lymph node. The fatty hilus is completely effaced.

These three abnormalities were biopsied with ultrasound guidance. Both the 4- and 6-o'clock breast masses were poorly differentiated infiltrating ductal carcinomas (IDC), estrogen receptor and progesterone receptor negative, *HER-2/neu* negative, grade 8/9. The axillary lymph node fine-needle

aspiration showed adenocarcinoma, consistent with metastatic breast carcinoma.

Staging evaluations were obtained because of the patient's node-positive status, concurrent complaints of back pain, and concern for possible metastatic disease. The patient had a pacemaker, which limited the options for performing MRI. A bone scan and positron emission tomography (PET)/CT scan were obtained. In addition, a positron emission mammography (PEM) scan was obtained of the breasts, immediately after the PET/CT, using the same dose of fluorodeoxyglucose (FDG).

Bone scan suggested an L1 compression fracture as the etiology of back pain (Figure 5). A band of modest increased metabolic activity was seen at the superior end plate of L1 on PET, and CT showed superior end-plate invagination, confirming the bone scan impression of a compression fracture (Figure 6). Three right lower inner quadrant FDG-avid breast masses were seen on whole-body PET/CT, with a small additional FDG-avid nodule seen between the two known IDC masses at 4 and 6 o'clock. The known involved right axillary lymph node was intensely hypermetabolic and was accompanied by several smaller additional metabolically active axillary lymph nodes. Activity was also seen in two internal mammary lymph nodes, which on CT measured 8 mm (Figures 7 and 8).

A PEM study was also obtained in this patient after completion of PET/CT, using the same FDG dose. The proven multifocality of her tumor would ordinarily have been an indication for breast MRI, but the patient could not readily undergo breast MRI because of her pacemaker. The dominant mass on the right at 6 o'clock was seen with exquisite detail on PEM, with intense heterogeneous uptake of FDG (Figure 9). The 4-o'clock mass was not seen on either view. This result was anticipated because of its far posterior position on the chest wall on CT. The small, intermediately positioned satellite tumor mass was visualized on the mediolateral oblique (MLO) projection, which shows more posterior breast tissue. The PEM also permitted more thorough screening of the left breast.

Modified radical mastectomy and axillary lymph node dissection were performed. At surgery, abutment and adherence of tumor focally to the pectoralis muscle was noted, requiring some excision of muscle.

Pathology showed three IDC tumor masses in the right lower inner quadrant, measuring 4.5 cm each at 4 and 6 o'clock and 1 cm in between. There was angiolymphatic invasion, with the 4-o'clock IDC close (0.09 mm) to the deep margin. Metastatic carcinoma was identified in 7 of 12 axillary lymph nodes, with extreme matting noted by pathology.

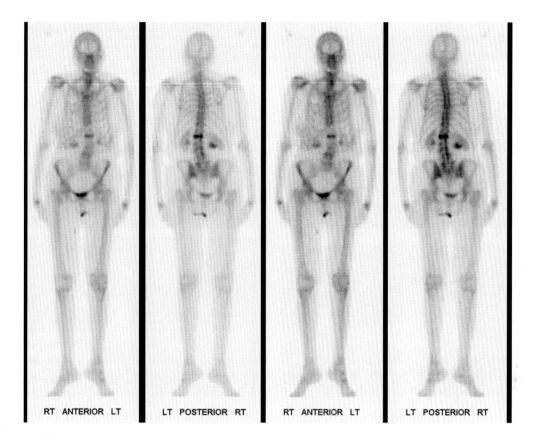

RT ANTERIOR LT   LT POSTERIOR RT   RT ANTERIOR LT   LT POSTERIOR RT

FIGURE 5.   Bone scan images show a band of increased activity at the L1 level. This pattern of activity suggests a compression fracture as the etiology of the patient's back pain.

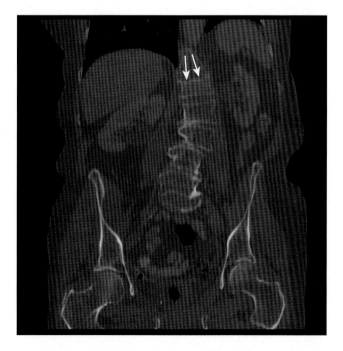

FIGURE 6.   Coronal CT reconstruction of the lumbar spine shows end-plate invagination of the L1 vertebral body, correlating with the bone scan and consistent with a compression fracture (*arrows*). Modest PET scan activity was present at this level. Other lumbar levels show discogenic changes and a levoscoliotic curvature.

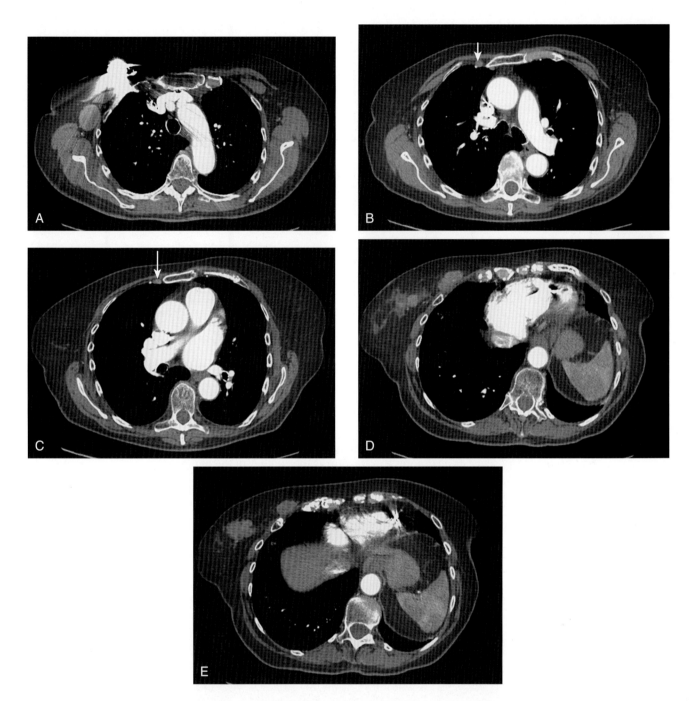

FIGURE 7. Enhanced chest CT images, from above to below. **A,** An oval, markedly enlarged axillary lymph node is seen on the right, corresponding to the ultrasound. Scatter artifact from a right chest wall pacemaker is noted. **B,** A rounded, enlarged right internal mammary lymph node is seen adjacent to the enhanced internal mammary artery (*arrow*). This was hypermetabolic on PET. The vein is seen over the lateral right sternum. **C,** A second right internal mammary (IM) lymph node is seen adjacent to the artery and vein (from right to left: IM artery, IM vein, IM lymph node) (*arrow*). This was also hypermetabolic on PET. **D,** Through the inferior breasts, two right breast masses are seen. The medial one is the same as the 4-o'clock mass on ultrasound. It has a lobulated contour. No fat plane is seen between it and the muscle. A round smaller mass is seen lateral to it. **E,** Further inferior, the dominant right 6-o'clock irregularly marginated mass is seen, as well as the inferior aspect of the 4-o'clock mass.

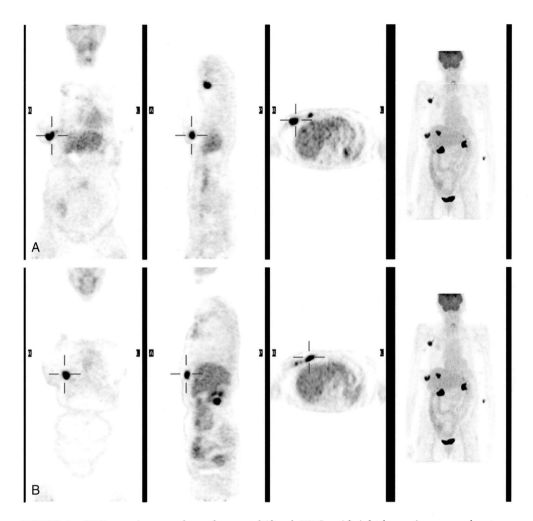

FIGURE 8.   PET scan images show three multifocal, FDG-avid right lower inner quadrant breast masses, as well as FDG-avid axillary lymph nodes and internal mammary nodes (not shown). **A,** Cursors are positioned at the level of the 6-o'clock IDC. A small adjacent FDG-avid nodule is seen on the coronal slice. **B,** Cursors are positioned at the level of the 4-o'clock IDC. The small satellite mass is partially seen on the axial image.

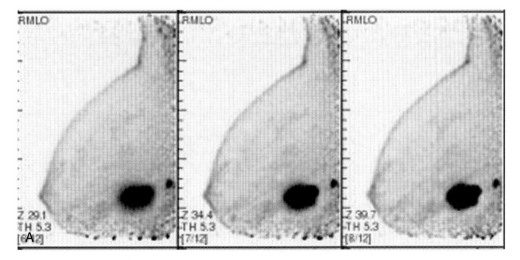

FIGURE 9.   PEM scan images [MLO (**A**) and CC (**B,** next page)] show heterogeneous FDG uptake within the 6-o'clock IDC. The small, adjacent FDG-avid nodule is seen posterior to the 6-o'clock IDC only on the MLO view, which shows more posterior tissue.

Continued

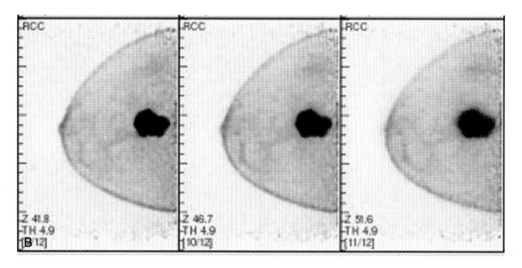

FIGURE 9, cont'd

TEACHING POINTS

This is a locally advanced breast cancer, based on axillary and internal mammary lymph node involvement. This degree of nodal involvement is classified as N3b, making the patient stage IIIC. The internal mammary lymph node involvement does not have to be histologically proven to be considered positive for involvement. In this case, the ease of visualizing these enlarged internal mammary lymph nodes on CT and the FDG avidity seen on PET leave little doubt that they are involved.

This patient's concurrent back pain raised the specter of metastatic disease. Fortunately, the bone scan abnormality is characteristic of a compression fracture and the PET and CT were entirely consistent. Of course, this does not entirely exclude the possibility of a pathologic compression fracture due to a bone metastasis, but without other evidence of osseous metastases, this seems unlikely. An osteoporotic compression fracture is a commonly encountered benign cause of symptoms and bone scan findings in older women.

It is interesting to note the node-like morphology of the 4-o'clock lesion in this case. It strongly resembles an abnormal lymph node and was positioned on the chest wall, suggesting it may be a completely replaced external mammary lymph node.

Normally, with proven multifocal breast cancer, local staging would often be supplemented with breast MRI, which would effectively screen the other breast. In this case, a pacemaker precluded performance of breast MRI. PEM was utilized to screen the other breast. It is interesting to see some of the strengths and weaknesses of PEM displayed by this case. As in mammography, only tissue that is imaged can be evaluated. Far posterior lesions that cannot be positioned between the detector arrays will not be seen, even sizable ones like the 4-o'clock lesion in this case. Design improvements of future PEM devices may improve detectability of posterior lesions. On the other hand, the detail of the heterogeneous FDG uptake of the 6-o'clock IDC is striking in contrast to the whole-body PET depiction.

The role of PEM in the breast imaging armamentarium is currently being assessed by a prospective, multi-institutional clinical trial comparing the performance of PEM to breast MRI in local staging of newly diagnosed breast cancers. Essentially, PEM is a small-field-of-view, high-resolution PET scanner, with in plane resolution on the order of 2 mm. Resembling a mammogram unit, the compression "plates" consist of an array of detectors. Compression is applied to immobilize the breast, but not to the same degree as in mammography. As PEM is a tomographic technique, there is no need to thin the breast to the same degree as in mammography.

CASE 3

LABC with nipple skin involvement

A 56-year-old woman noted new right nipple inversion 4 months before presenting for breast imaging evaluation for a newly developed right palpable axillary lump. Mammography and ultrasound showed a dominant 12-o'clock mass with nipple retraction and localized skin thickening, as well as axillary lymphadenopathy (Figures 1, 2, and 3). Ultrasound-guided biopsy of the dominant mass confirmed invasive ductal carcinoma (IDC), and ultrasound-guided axillary node fine-needle aspiration confirmed metastatic disease. Periareolar dusky erythema was noted, and skin punch biopsy was performed, which was negative. Local staging was completed with breast MRI (Figures 4, 5, 6, 7, and 8).

Systemic staging with positron emission tomography (PET)/CT showed fluorodeoxyglucose (FDG) avidity of the known right breast cancer and axillary lymphadenopathy, but no additional disease. Neoadjuvant chemotherapy was given, consisting of four cycles each of doxorubicin (Adriamycin) and cyclophosphamide (Cytoxan) (AC) and

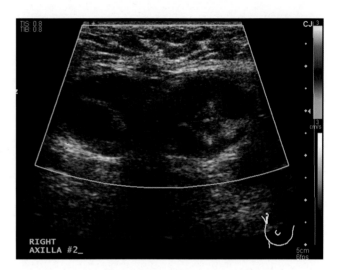

FIGURE 3. Ultrasound of the right axilla shows two adjacent, highly abnormal lymph nodes: both are rounded, with very hypoechoic, thickened cortices. Nodular mass effect is exerted on the echogenic fatty hila, which are partially effaced. No increased vascularity is identified.

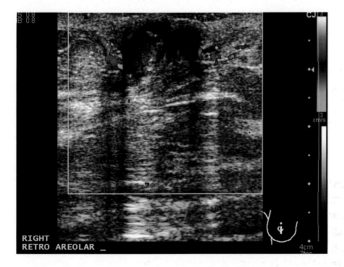

FIGURE 1. Ultrasound of the right upper outer quadrant shows a hypoechoic, taller-than-wide, sonographically suspicious mass with irregular and angular margins.

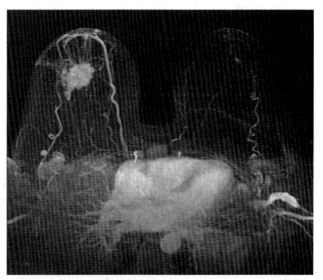

FIGURE 4. Maximal intensity projection of enhanced, subtracted, axial gradient echo data set shows an intensely enhancing, dominant mass in the central right breast. Numerous linear spicules extend anteriorly toward the nipple. There are enlarged, draining veins on the right, and enlarged, enhancing right axillary lymph nodes.

FIGURE 2. Ultrasound of the retracted right nipple shows unusual increased periareolar vascularity.

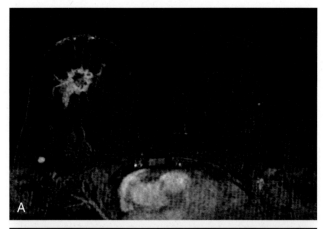

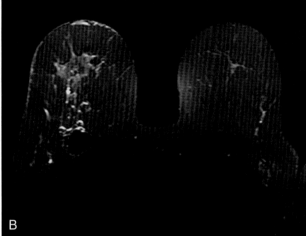

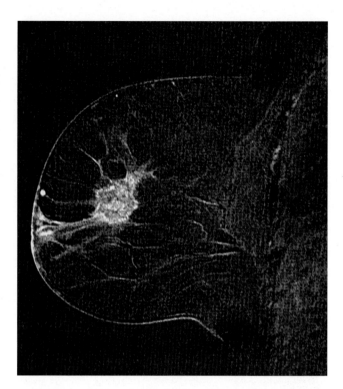

FIGURE 6. Sagittal, subtracted, contrast enhanced MRI of the right breast showing the enhancing linear tendrils extending to the nipple, as well as the periareolar skin enhancement.

FIGURE 5. Axial breast MR images through the dominant right IDC (**A,** enhanced, subtracted, T1-weighted gradient echo; **B,** STIR) show rim enhancement and spiculation of the mass. Linear spicules extend anteriorly toward the nipple and posteriorly toward the pectoral muscle. The periareolar skin is thickened and edematous, and enhances. A rounded, low-lying axillary or intramammary lymph node enhances intensely in the posterolateral right breast.

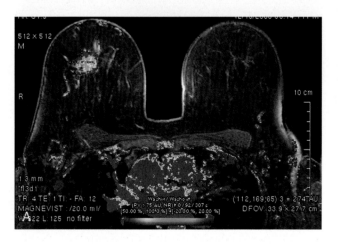

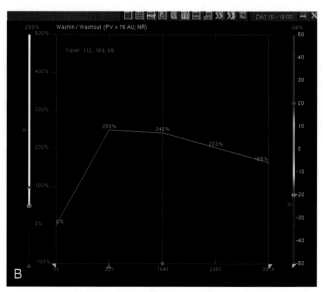

FIGURE 7. Kinetic information (**A,** DynaCAD color map; **B,** enhancement curve) showing washout from portions of the IDC mass.

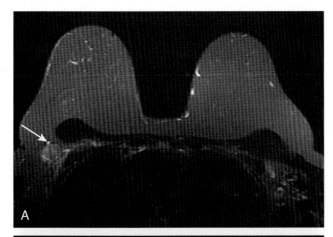

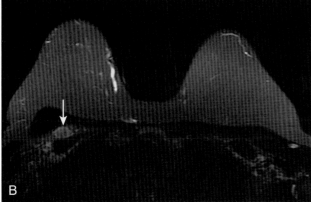

FIGURE 8. Axial STIR images of the axilla. **A,** An enlarged right axillary level I lymph node is seen lateral to the pectoralis major and minor muscles (*arrow*). **B,** An enlarged interpectoral (Rotter's) lymph node is seen on the right, between the pectoralis major muscle in front and pectoralis minor muscle behind (*arrow*).

paclitaxel (Taxol). The nipple inversion resolved, and there was marked clinical regression of the dominant mass. Modified radical mastectomy and axillary dissection were performed. A 4.5-cm residual lesion of admixed IDC and normal breast tissue remained. Margins were negative, and 5 of 13 lymph nodes showed metastatic tumor. Chest wall, supraclavicular, and posterior axillary boost radiation therapy were given, and the patient was placed on anastrozole (Arimidex).

TEACHING POINTS

In this case, the localized periareolar skin thickening, edema, and enhancement probably represented secondary inflammation and involvement by a locally advanced breast cancer (LABC), rather than being a manifestation of primary inflammatory breast cancer.

Natural history of untreated inflammatory breast cancer

A 57-year-old woman noted her right breast to be enlarged and heavier feeling. Mammography showed concerning right upper outer quadrant (UOQ) microcalcifications (Figures 1 and 2). Right breast sonogram showed periareolar skin thickening (Figure 3) and an UOQ 1.5-cm shadowing hypoechoic mass with irregular margins (Figure 4), as well as hypoechoic, rounded, axillary lymph nodes (Figures 5 and 6). Ultrasound-guided core needle biopsy of the UOQ mass confirmed infiltrating ductal carcinoma (IDC), estrogen receptor and progesterone receptor negative, *HER-2/neu* negative. Ultrasound-guided fine-needle aspiration (FNA) of an axillary lymph node confirmed metastatic carcinoma, consistent with breast primary origin. Two skin punch biopsies were performed because of clinical suspicion of inflammatory carcinoma: both were negative. Skin biopsies were subsequently repeated because of persistent high suspicion of inflammatory cancer, and confirmed intralymphatic carcinoma.

Breast MRI showed multiple intensely enhancing right breast masses, as well as enhancement of the skin (Figures 7, 8, 9, 10, and 11). Systemic staging consisted of positron emission tomography (PET)/CT and enhanced body CT scans. Hypermetabolism was identified in the right breast and axillary lymph nodes, but no evidence of distant metastatic disease was found (Figures 12, 13, 14, and 15).

The patient initially declined all conventional therapies and opted against medical advice for a trial of an alternative soy product. After 3 months, she underwent repeat breast MRI and PET/CT to assess her response. The breast MRI showed growth of the multiple breast masses to near confluency (Figures 16 and 17). PET/CT showed progression in the breast and axilla, but no distant metastases. Four cycles of doxorubicin (Adriamycin) and cyclophosphamide (Cytoxan) (AC) neoadjuvant chemotherapy were given, after which the patient underwent a right modified radical mastectomy and axillary lymph node dissection. The mastectomy specimen showed a 5.5-cm IDC with high-grade comedo DCIS and dermal intralymphatic carcinoma. Angiolymphatic invasion was extensive, both peritumoral and distant. The margins showed intralymphatic carcinoma at skin margins.

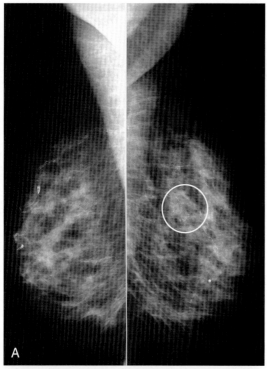

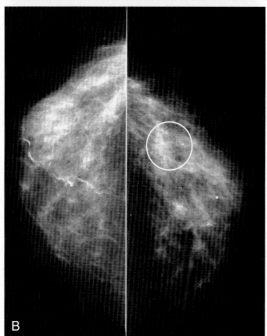

FIGURE 1. MLO (**A**) and CC (**B**) mammograms show heterogeneous breast parenchymal density. No parenchymal changes were detected compared with the prior study, 4 years before. An area containing concerning microcalcifications is *circled* in the UOQ.

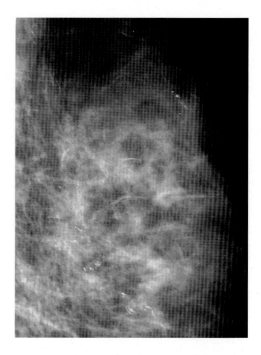

FIGURE 2. Lateral magnification view of the right upper breast shows concerning new microcalcifications.

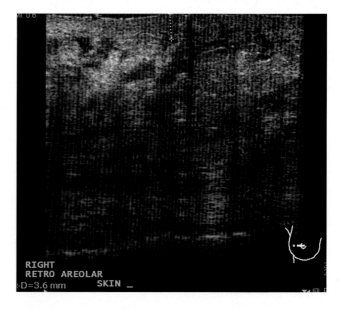

FIGURE 3. Sonographic image of the right periareolar skin is thickened to nearly 4 mm. An edematous appearance of the subjacent tissues is seen, without a discrete mass.

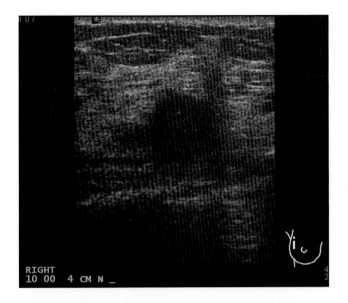

FIGURE 4. A very hypoechoic, highly suspicious mass with angular margins was found in the right UOQ. Ultrasound-guided biopsy confirmed IDC.

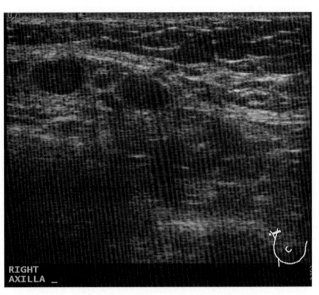

FIGURE 5. Right axillary ultrasound shows two oval, adjacent, very hypoechoic lymph nodes, with no identifiable fatty hila.

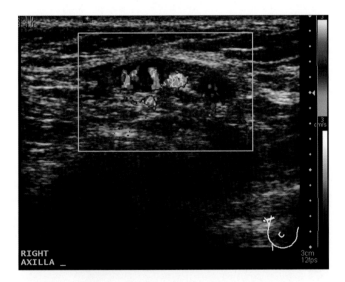

FIGURE 6. Another right axillary lymph node shows cortical mantle thickening, effaced hilus, and abnormally increased vascularity. FNA confirmed metastatic disease.

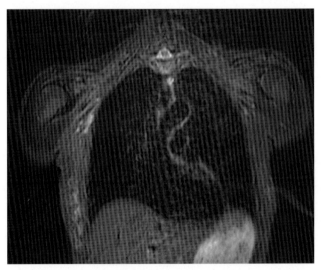

FIGURE 7. Coronal STIR image of the thorax, acquired with the body coil, shows a cluster of small, but asymmetrical, right axillary lymph nodes.

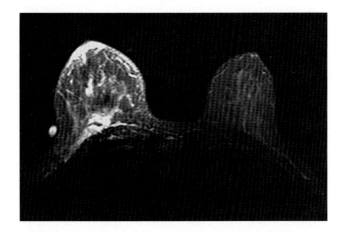

FIGURE 8. Axial STIR MRI shows the right breast to be much larger than the left. The skin is thickened and edematous, and the breast itself shows diffuse increased edema, extending throughout the breast, back to the muscle.

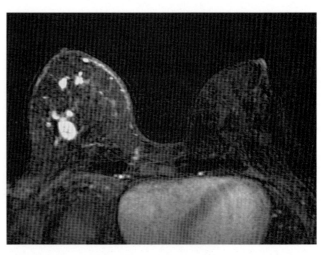

FIGURE 10. Enhanced axial, subtracted image of the breasts shows some of the enhancing right masses. The thickened skin can be seen to enhance as well.

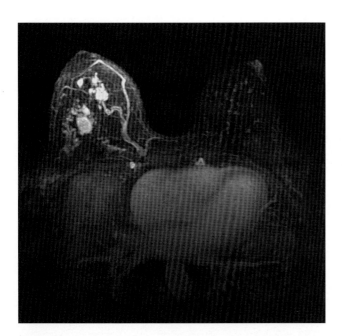

FIGURE 9. Enhanced axial maximal intensity projection view shows multiple intensely enhancing masses in the larger right breast.

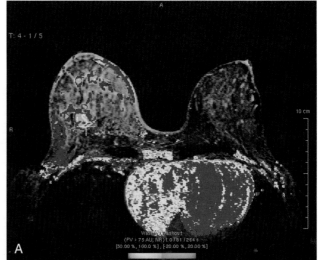

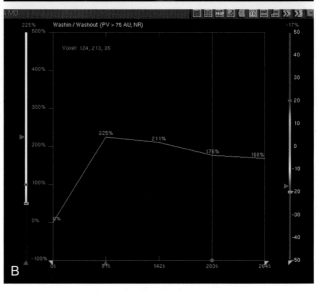

FIGURE 11. Kinetic data from the breast MRI, displayed as a color-coded overlay on the breast MRI data (**A**). A region of interest has been placed, and kinetic data from this is displayed graphically (change in signal intensity versus time) in **B**. There is a sharp and rapid upstroke, reflecting rapid enhancement, and washout, which correlates with angiogenesis.

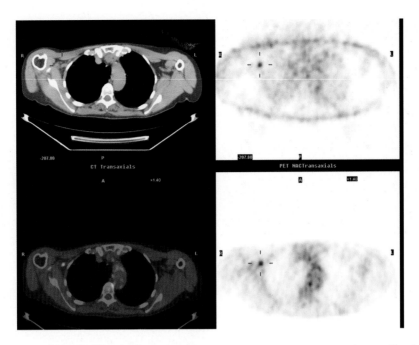

FIGURE 12. Axial PET/CT, through the axilla, shows hypermetabolism of a small right axillary lymph node (*cursors*), suggesting metastatic involvement.

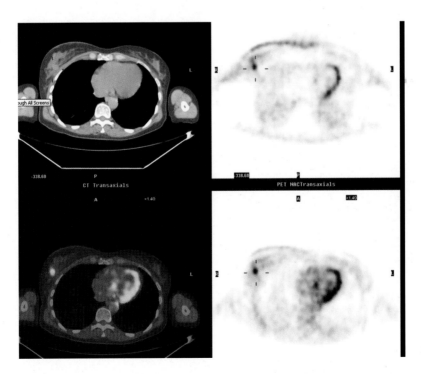

FIGURE 13. Axial PET/CT, through the breasts, shows one of several hypermetabolic masses in the right breast. The entire breast, including the thickened skin, shows mild, generalized increased uptake compared with the left side.

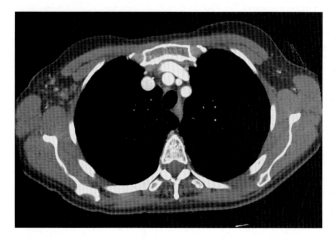

FIGURE 14. Enhanced chest CT image for correlation. The right axilla is filled with asymmetrical, mildly enlarged lymph nodes, and there is diffuse axillary stranding. Although no one of these lymph nodes is markedly enlarged by absolute size criteria, the constellation of findings is highly suspicious, and the stranding is concerning for extranodal extension.

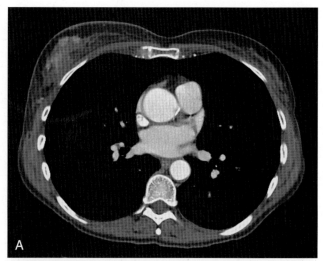

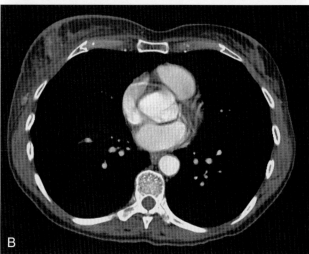

FIGURE 15. Enhanced chest CT images through the breasts (**A** above **B**) show multiple small, enhancing right breast masses, corresponding to the MRI and PET, with several small, enhancing right lateral chest wall lymph nodes. Note the skin thickening on the right.

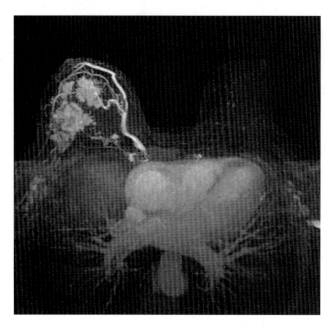

FIGURE 16. Repeat breast MRI, 3 months after diagnosis of right inflammatory breast cancer with no therapy. Axial MIP view shows interval growth of the right breast masses, which now nearly merge together.

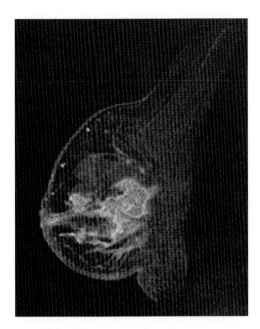

FIGURE 17. Sagittal, subtracted, enhanced right breast MRI from the same study as Figure 16, showing how confluent the diffuse process has become. Skin thickening and enhancement is most pronounced inferiorly.

Fourteen out of 14 lymph nodes showed tumor, with extranodal soft tissue extension and involvement of perinodal lymphatic spaces.

Chemotherapy was resumed postoperatively, with four cycles given of paclitaxel (Taxol). Radiation therapy was then administered to the chest wall and regional lymphatics, including the internal mammary region.

TEACHING POINTS

Inflammatory breast cancer (IBC) is a rare breast cancer, representing about 1% of all breast cancers. This patient presented with clinical features that suggested the diagnosis, which was pursued and confirmed histologically with repeated skin biopsies (two sites sampled on two separate occasions). Multiple examiners noted the patient's right breast to be larger, fuller and firmer than the left, without erythema or discrete masses palpable initially. Subtle edema and a hint of peau d'orange changes were noted by one examiner.

The histologic hallmark of inflammatory breast cancer is involvement of dermal lymphatics with tumor. Skin biopsies, like other biopsies, are subject to sampling error, as demonstrated in this case, and it may take repeated efforts to establish the histologic diagnosis. Multiple imaging studies obtained through the course of this patient's evaluation allow us to review the imaging features of skin involvement and inflammatory breast cancer. Kushwaha and colleagues reviewed a series of 26 cases of primary inflammatory breast cancer to characterize the mammographic findings. They found that the most common mammographic changes were, in descending order, skin thickening (92%), diffuse increased density (81%), trabecular thickening (62%), axillary adenopathy (58%), asymmetrical density or architectural distortion (50%), and nipple retraction (38%). Suspicious microcalcifications and masses were seen in a minority of patients (23% and 15%, respectively). These results differed from other series, in which microcalcifications and masses were found in most patients. The authors emphasized that this likely was due to differing inclusion criteria of their study (only primary inflammatory cancers) compared with other studies, which included locally advanced carcinoma with secondary inflammatory changes. It has been suggested that these are two distinct clinical entities.

The primary mammographic abnormality noted in this patient was suspicious microcalcifications. Although skin thickening was subsequently demonstrated on ultrasound, CT, MRI, and PET, it was not well seen mammographically in this case. Ultrasound was helpful in this case. In addition to showing skin thickening, it identified an irregular mass to target for biopsy, as well as suspicious axillary adenopathy.

The initial breast MRI was the most accurate modality in delineating the extent of breast involvement. In addition to depicting multiple masses, which were not seen on mammography or ultrasound, it showed enhancement of the thickened skin. This finding correlates with tumor involvement of the skin. When seen, it is a helpful imaging clue to differentiate these cases from mastitis, which may also cause breast swelling and edema, with skin thickening and edema.

Breast MRI also gives us a clear imaging window to see how rapidly an untreated inflammatory cancer can progress. This patient progressed clinically over 3 months, from no definite palpable mass to an easily palpable 5- to 6-cm mass. On MRI, individual masses grew to nearly merge with each other.

SUGGESTED READINGS

Gunhan-Bilgen I, Ustun EE, Memis A. Inflammatory breast carcinoma: mammographic, ultrasonographic, clinical, and pathologic findings in 142 cases. *Radiology* 2002; 223(3):829–838.

Kushwaha AC, Whitman GJ, Stelling CB, et al. Primary inflammatory carcinoma of the breast: retrospective review of the mammographic findings. *AJR Am J Roentgenol* 2000; 174:535–538.

Whitman GJ, Kushwaha AC, Christofanilli M, et al. Inflammatory breast cancer: current imaging perspectives. *Semin Breast Dis* 2001; 4(3):122–131.

CASE 5

LABC with secondary inflammation (secondary inflammatory breast cancer)

A 56-year-old woman was noted to have a highly suspicious, spiculated, 1- to 1.5-cm mass in the left breast on screening mammography, for which biopsy was recommended (Figure 1). The patient decided not to undergo a biopsy, on the advice of her chiropractor.

Two and a half years later, the patient noted a change in the left breast, with nipple hardening and aching. The patient also noted an imprint on her lower breast from her underwire bra. Mammography showed an ill-defined spiculated mass at 12 o'clock, which had grown (Figure 2). She was clinically evaluated by a surgeon, who noted skin changes of edema and peau d'orange. A discrete mass was difficult to palpate, being nearly behind the nipple, with generalized thickening and firmness noted. A palpation-guided biopsy was performed, as well as a skin punch biopsy. Infiltrating ductal carcinoma, estrogen receptor and progesterone receptor positive, was identified from both biopsies, with tumor in vascular and lymphatic channels in the skin biopsy.

Staging evaluations were obtained, including bilateral breast ultrasound (Figures 3 and 4); breast MRI (Figure 5); positron emission tomography (PET)/CT (Figure 6); chest, abdomen, and pelvic enhanced CT scans (Figure 7); and bone scan. These studies showed a very extensive left breast cancer, with involvement of the nipple and skin, with evidence on multiple studies of axillary nodal involvement, but no evidence of distant metastatic disease. Neoadjuvant chemotherapy was recommended. The patient decided to pursue alternative and nutritional therapies and declined all conventional therapy. She did agree to periodic laboratory analysis and clinical examination. One year after diagnosis, although the patient's tumor markers continued to rise and there was clear local progression clinically (ulceration of the left nipple and nodularity of the skin), the patient continued to decline conventional therapy.

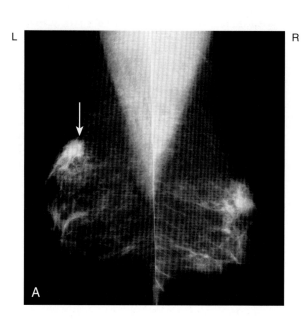
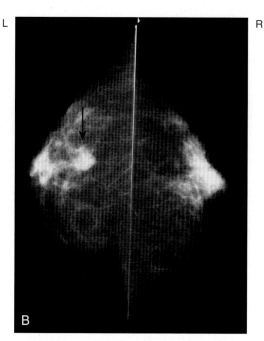

FIGURE 1. Mammogram [MLO (**A**) and CC (**B**)] shows heterogeneous parenchymal density. A dense spiculated mass is seen on the left at 12 o'clock (*arrows*).

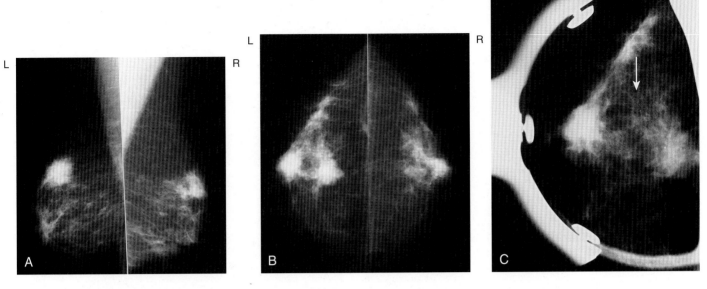

FIGURE 2. Mammogram [MLO (**A**), CC (**B**), and CC spot compression (**C**)], 2.5 years later, after no treatment, shows interval growth of the dense, spiculated, dominant, left 12-o'clock mass. The left retroareolar region appears increasingly dense and mass-like on the CC view, compared with the prior study. The spot compression view shows associated pleomorphic calcifications (*arrow*).

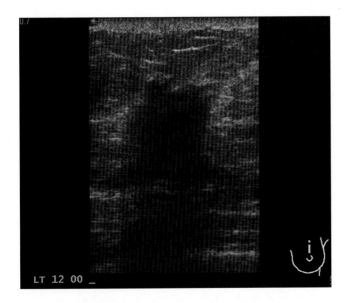

FIGURE 3. Ultrasound of the left breast at 12 o'clock shows a dominant mass, with highly suspicious features. The mass is extremely hypoechoic, with angular and lobular borders and no defined capsule, and shadows intensely. The skin is visibly thickened as well.

TEACHING POINTS

This locally advanced breast cancer (LABC) is essentially a neglected breast cancer. The skin changes of edema and peau d'orange and histologic evidence of dermal lymphatic involvement suggest the diagnosis of inflammatory breast cancer (IBC). However, given the time course, this more likely represents a secondary IBC, namely a locally advanced breast cancer with secondary inflammatory involvement of the skin and nipple, than a primary IBC. Primary IBC is classically notable for a rapid clinical onset of breast swelling, warmth, edema, erythema, and skin changes.

Axillary nodal involvement was never established histologically in this patient, but the imaging evidence of multiple node involvement is compelling. In particular, the PET is strong presumptive evidence of axillary disease, with five fluorodeoxyglucose (FDG)-avid lymph nodes readily visualized. In a large, prospective, multicenter study of 360 women with newly diagnosed invasive breast

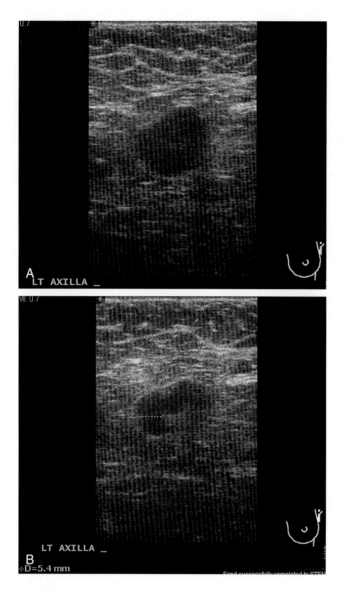

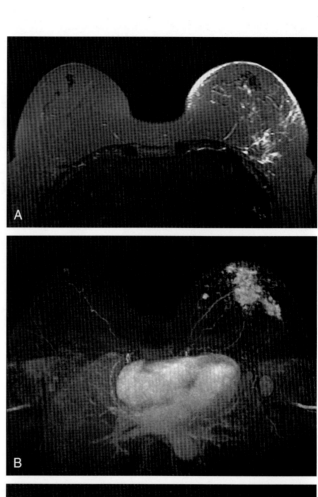

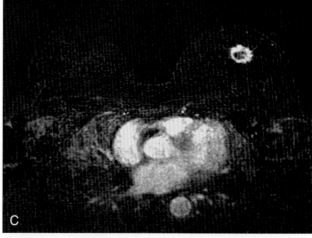

FIGURE 4. Ultrasound of the left axilla shows highly suspicious lymph node findings. **A,** This lymph node is very hypoechoic, with a rounded shape. The cortical thickening is pronounced, with near-complete effacement of the fatty hilus. Only a sliver of the hilus remains visible here. **B,** Another axillary lymph node shows less advanced, but still suspicious findings. The fatty hilum is better preserved, but there is subtle mass effect on it. The hypoechoic cortex is abnormally thick. *Cursors* indicate a dimension of 5 mm.

FIGURE 5. Breast MRI was obtained to better assess the local extent of this neglected, locally advanced cancer. **A,** Axial STIR image shows diffuse left breast skin thickening and edema, as well as asymmetrical edema and reticulation of the left breast compared with the right, especially laterally. **B,** Axial maximal intensity projection view, 1 minute after contrast administration, from the enhanced, dynamic, subtracted series, shows an extensive, intensely enhancing, nearly confluent mass occupying the retroareolar left breast. **C,** A section from the subtracted, enhanced series shows rim enhancement and marginal spiculation of a discrete mass at 12 o'clock, correlating with the mass seen on ultrasound.

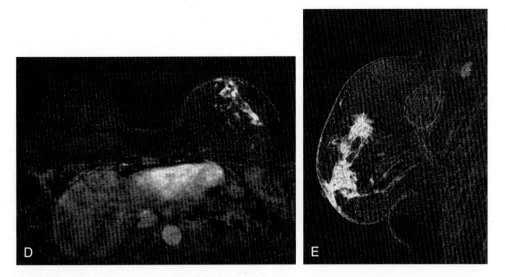

FIGURE 5, cont'd   D, A more inferior section from the subtracted, enhanced MR series shows clumped enhancement in the left lateral breast with a segmental, ductal orientation, extending down to the nipple. **E,** Sagittal, subtracted, enhanced view showing the spiculated 12 o'clock mass seen on ultrasound, connected to confluent retroareolar enhancement. Note the enhancing connecting channels, as well as the nipple skin thickening and enhancement. An enlarged enhancing axillary lymph node is seen at the edge of the field of view.

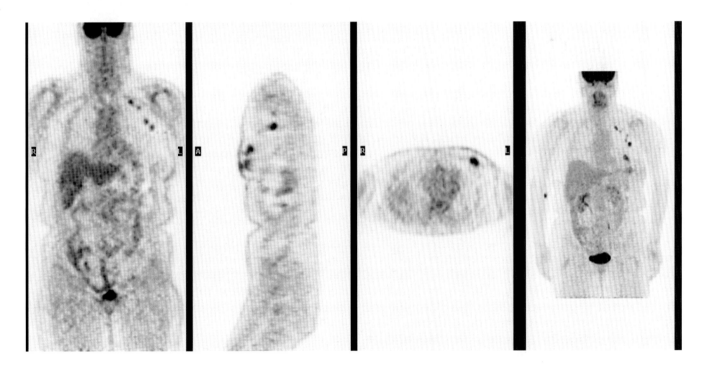

FIGURE 6.   PET scan images (left to right: coronal, axial, sagittal, coronal projection volume image) show intense multifocal hypermetabolism in the left breast (best seen in sagittal and axial projections), as well as a line of hypermetabolic left axillary lymph nodes (best seen in coronal projections). No evidence of distant metastatic disease was seen.

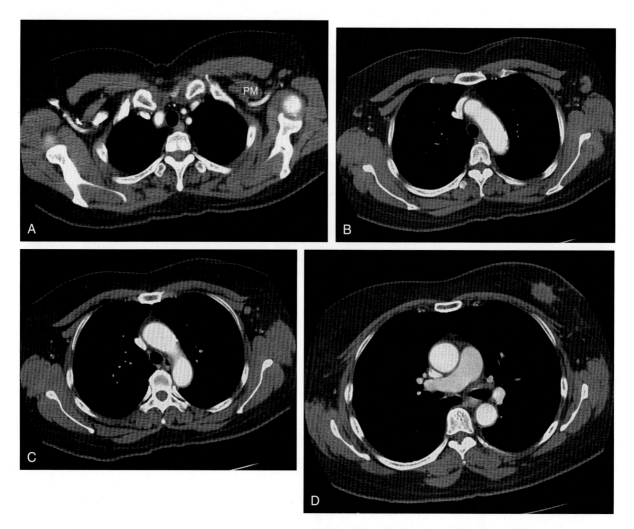

FIGURE 7. Enhanced chest CT images, for correlation. **A,** Through the axilla: two adjacent, abnormally enlarged and rounded left axillary level II lymph nodes are seen beneath the pectoralis minor muscle (PM). **B,** Through the axilla: a clearly abnormal, enlarged left axillary lymph node is seen. Although a sliver of a fatty hilum can still be seen, the cortex is visibly thickened, and the node is rounded and plumper than a normal lymph node. In addition, its margins are fuzzy. Note how sharp the fat is around normal right axillary lymph nodes. **C,** Through the axilla, inferior to **B**: Even without the grossly abnormal lymph node seen in **B,** nodal involvement might still be suspected based on this section. One of the left axillary lymph nodes is round in shape and disproportionate in size compared with other axillary nodes. **D,** Through the left breast cancer at 12 o'clock: the spiculated mass is readily visualized in this case because it is surrounded by fat. Note subtle linear infiltration of breast fat lateral to the mass, as well as skin thickening.

cancer, two or more PET-positive intense axillary foci of uptake were highly predictive of axillary metastases. This would be sufficient evidence of involvement to proceed directly to axillary dissection without sentinel lymph node sampling, if the patient were undergoing surgery. In a patient such as this, who ordinarily would be treated with neo-adjuvant chemotherapy, FDG PET is a reliable indicator of the extent of disease.

The converse is not true; that is, a PET-negative axilla cannot be relied on to avoid sentinel lymph node sampling. Particularly with early-stage disease and small-volume nodal involvement, PET is insufficiently sensitive to be substituted for axillary node sampling (61% in the study by Wahl and colleagues).

SUGGESTED READINGS

Avril N, Adler LP. F-18 fluorodeoxyglucose-positron emission tomography imaging for primary breast cancer and loco-regional staging. *PET Clinics: Breast Cancer* 2006; 1(1):1–13.

Wahl RL, Siegel BA, Coleman E, et al. Prospective multi-center study of axillary nodal staging by positron emission tomography in breast cancer: a report of the staging breast cancer with PET study group. *J Clin Oncol* 2004; 22:277–285.

CASE 6

PABC, treated with neoadjuvant chemotherapy with complete pathologic response

A 33-year-old pregnant patient noted a palpable right breast lump at about 18 weeks of gestation. This was confirmed by her obstetrician, who performed a fine-needle aspiration. No diagnosis or fluid was obtained. Ultrasound identified a suspicious 2.2-cm mass, as well as an abnormal and enlarged axillary lymph node (Figures 1 and 2). Ultrasound-guided core needle biopsy of the breast

mass revealed high-grade infiltrating ductal carcinoma, and fine-needle aspiration (FNA) of the axillary lymph node showed metastatic carcinoma, consistent with breast primary.

On palpation, the mass was large, in the lower outer quadrant, estimated at 6 to 8 cm in size, and thought to be too large to attempt breast conservation. A 2-cm axillary lymph node was also palpable and mobile. The patient was interested in breast preservation and in continuing with her pregnancy, and so neoadjuvant chemotherapy was performed

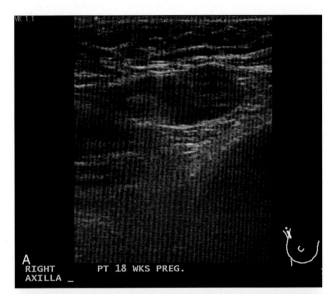

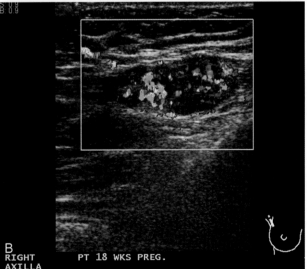

FIGURE 2. Sonography of the axilla [gray scale (**A**) and color Doppler (**B**)] shows abnormal lymph node morphology. A large cortical nodule occupies one half of the lymph node, effacing a portion of the fatty hilus, which remains visible in the other half. Color Doppler shows markedly increased, abnormal vascularity of the cortical nodule. FNA identified metastatic cells.

FIGURE 1. Ultrasound of the right LOQ palpable lump shows highly sinister features of malignancy: extreme hypoechogenicity, taller-than-wide shape; angry-looking, angular margins; and shadowing. Biopsy with ultrasound guidance confirmed IDC.

with four cycles of doxorubicin (Adriamycin) and cyclophosphamide (Cytoxan) (AC).

Breast MRI was obtained to assess the extent of disease, given the discrepancy between physical examination and ultrasound. It showed a large, dominant, irregularly marginated mass occupying most of the lower outer quadrant (LOQ) and measuring 8.1 cm in maximal dimension (Figures 3, 4, 5, 6, and 7). Clinical stage was stage III, T3N1, estrogen receptor and progesterone receptor low positive, *HER-2/neu* positive.

The patient was treated with four cycles of AC, with delivery of the baby planned for 36 weeks' gestation, with paclitaxel (Taxol) and trastuzumab (Herceptin) therapy afterward for *HER-2/neu*-positive disease. After the four AC cycles, the mass

was no longer palpable. The patient was induced and delivered a healthy baby at about 33 weeks' gestation.

Her chemotherapy was resumed after delivery, with weekly Taxol and Herceptin for 12 weeks, with Herceptin planned weekly for 40 additional weeks (1 year total). Mid-chemotherapy restaging studies were obtained, showing a smaller ultrasound residual mass, now 1.2 cm, and resolution of the abnormal axillary findings (Figure 8). Given the marked imaging regression of the tumor, the patient underwent ultrasound-guided clip placement into the residual for future localization (Figure 9). Repeat breast MRI showed marked regression of the mass, reduced to a linear residual (Figure 10).

Staging studies were repeated 2 months later, after completion of Taxol therapy, and showed further regression, with only minimal residuals on both ultrasound and MRI (Figures 11 and 12). The patient was treated surgically with a partial mastectomy, which showed no invasive carcinoma and negative margins. A limited axillary dissection removing six lymph nodes was performed, and there was no evidence of metastatic tumor in the sampled nodes. Radiation therapy was subsequently administered to the breast and supraclavicular region.

TEACHING POINTS

This case well illustrates the typical features of breast cancers diagnosed during pregnancy, which tend to be large and node-positive and may be inoperable. Pregnancy-associated breast cancer

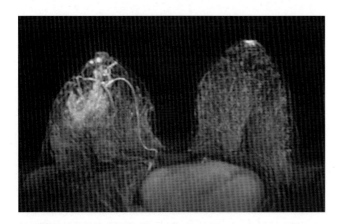

FIGURE 3. Axial maximal intensity projection view from enhanced, dynamic, subtracted breast MRI series shows marked asymmetry, with diffuse increased enhancement in the right lateral breast. Generalized lower-level enhancement of both breasts is attributable to the hormonal effects of pregnancy.

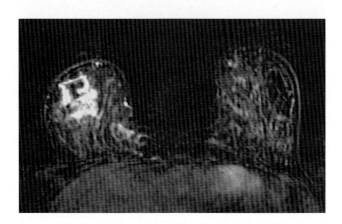

FIGURE 4. Enhanced, subtracted, axial MRI through the inferior breasts shows irregular mass enhancement occupying much of the right LOQ.

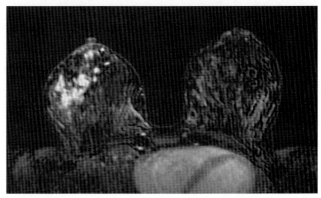

FIGURE 5. A more superior slice, through the nipple, shows that the clumped and multifocal mass enhancement is extensive. No focal or concerning left breast enhancement is seen.

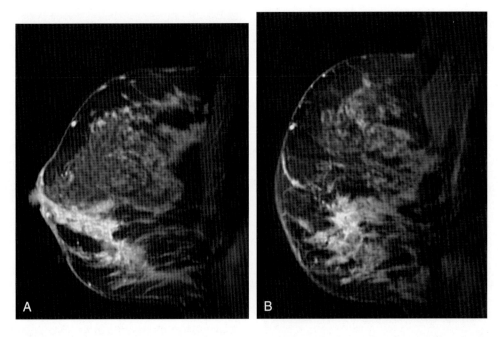

FIGURE 6. Sagittal, enhanced, subtracted images of the right breast (**A,** through the nipple; **B,** laterally) obtained about 5 to 6 minutes after contrast administration show the extensive process as nearly confluent enhancement.

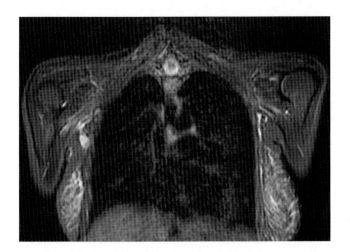

FIGURE 7. Coronal STIR image of the thorax (obtained with the body coil) shows both breasts to be very engorged and fluid in signal intensity. An enlarged axillary lymph node is seen on the right.

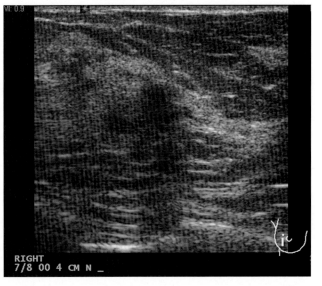

FIGURE 8. Repeat breast ultrasound, after completion of four cycles of chemotherapy with AC, shows evidence of a response. The sonographically visible component of the mass is smaller.

(PABC) is generally defined as breast cancer diagnosed during pregnancy or within a year of delivery. PABC tends to be advanced at diagnosis, with contributions from physician and patient-related delays in diagnosis. The difficulty of physical examination in pregnancy and lactation-engorged breasts is thought to contribute to delayed diagnosis.

Although PABC is generally regarded as rare, complicating 1 in 3000 pregnancies in the United States, the actual number of PABCs is about what would be predicted based on the incidence of breast cancer in women of reproductive age and the expected pregnancy rate in these women.

Ultrasound is an excellent first imaging choice in assessing a palpable mass in a pregnant patient. If ultrasound did not identify a mass or satisfactory

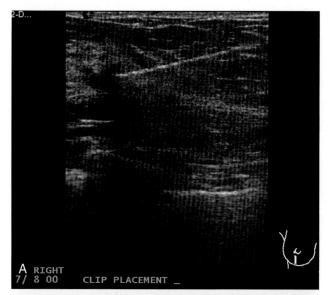

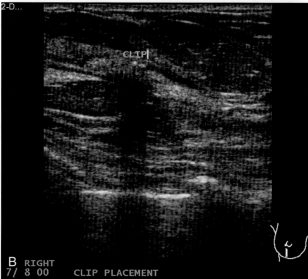

FIGURE 9. Sonographic images from ultrasound-guided clip placement (**A,** with needle in place; **B,** final image, with clip deployed). A clip was placed because of the marked regression of the tumor in response to neoadjuvant chemotherapy, to ensure the region could be localized in case complete imaging resolution were to ensue.

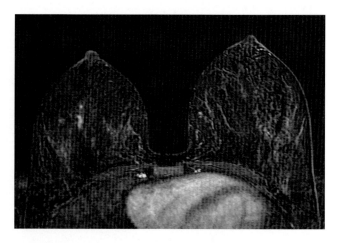

FIGURE 10. Repeat breast MRI, after four cycles of chemotherapy with AC, shows only a minimal linear residual at the site.

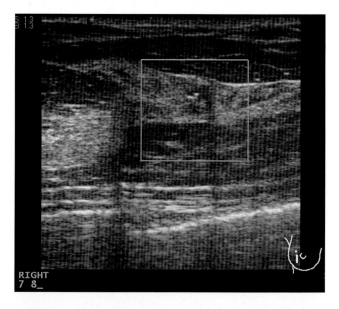

FIGURE 11. Final breast ultrasound, 2 months later, after completion of neoadjuvant chemotherapy with four cycles of AC and 12 weekly doses of Taxol and Herceptin, shows no residual mass. A minimal hypoechoic collar outlines the clip (*in box*).

explanation for a palpable lump, the imaging evaluation could safely be extended to include mammography, based on an estimated fetal dose of 500 μGy from two-view film screen mammography with abdominal shielding.

Breast MRI is another viable imaging option for use during pregnancy, preferably after the first trimester. Particularly in such a case as this, when a diagnosis of breast cancer is established, breast MRI can be considered for local staging and assessment of the extent of disease. Although hormonal

engorgement of the breasts is expected, as seen in this case, in general such changes and increased density are not an issue for breast MRI.

In formulating a treatment plan for a pregnant patient with breast cancer, the usual approach is to treat the cancer while allowing the pregnancy to proceed. Both surgery and chemotherapy can be safely performed during pregnancy, whereas radiation is preferentially given after delivery. In this case, the patient was initially considered for mastectomy while pregnant, but her excellent response

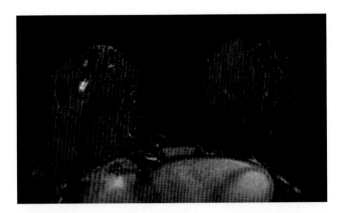

FIGURE 12. Final breast MRI, 2 months later, after completion of neoadjuvant chemotherapy with four cycles of AC and 12 weekly doses of Taxol and Herceptin, shows linear enhancement at the site, in a slightly different pattern than that seen previously. The sharp definition of the edges suggests an iatrogenic etiology, namely enhancement around the clip placed since the prior MRI.

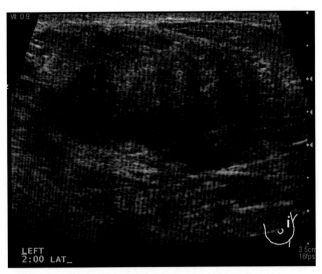

FIGURE 1. Ultrasound of the left UOQ shows heterogeneous, hypoechoic echotexture, which differed in appearance from other regions.

to neoadjuvant chemotherapy during pregnancy enabled successful lumpectomy, performed after induced delivery.

This patient had a dramatic imaging response to neoadjuvant chemotherapy, with virtually complete resolution by imaging of what had been a very sizable tumor. Although this correlates well in this case with the complete pathologic response that was obtained, it has been well documented in the literature that a complete response by imaging does not exclude microscopic residual disease on pathology.

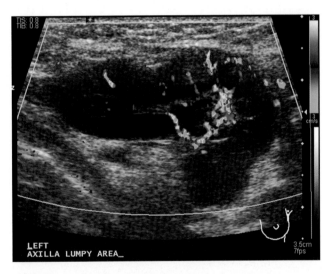

FIGURE 2. Ultrasound of the palpable left axillary lump shows a massively enlarged and vascular lymph node, with dramatic cortical thickening.

CASE 7

Postpartum LABC, with multiple axillary nodes involved; excellent response to neoadjuvant chemotherapy

A 41-year-old woman, 4 months postpartum and tapering breast-feeding, noted a left axillary lump. She also noted left breast tenderness and swelling. A massively enlarged and vascular axillary lymph

node was found on ultrasound, which also showed a region in the left upper outer quadrant (UOQ) of parenchymal hypoechogenicity (Figures 1, 2, 3, and 4). Core needle biopsy with ultrasound guidance of the left UOQ showed infiltrating ductal carcinoma (IDC), estrogen receptor negative, progesterone receptor weakly positive, *HER-2/neu* negative. Ultrasound-guided fine-needle aspiration (FNA) of the axillary lymph node showed a mixed population of lymphocytes, but no malignant cells. Clinically and morphologically, the axilla was suspected to be involved, despite the negative

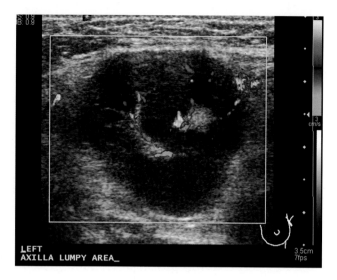

FIGURE 3. Transverse view of the same lymph node shows nearly complete effacement of the echogenic fatty hilum. Abnormal (nonhilar) vascularity is demonstrated, and the cortex is massively thickened.

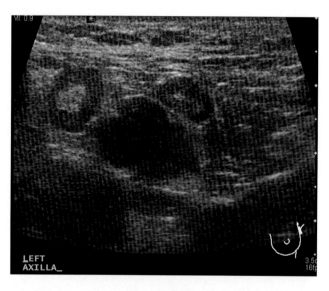

FIGURE 4. Additional sonographic view of the left axilla shows multiple additional, abnormal lymph nodes. One is very hypoechoic, is rounded and lobular in shape, and shows complete hilar loss. Even the two more normal-appearing lymph nodes shown here are more subtly abnormal. Although their fatty hila remain, their cortices are abnormally thickened.

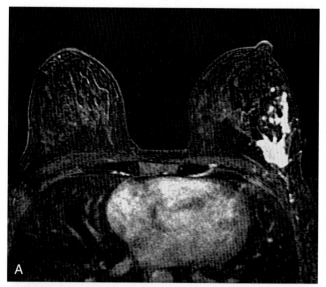

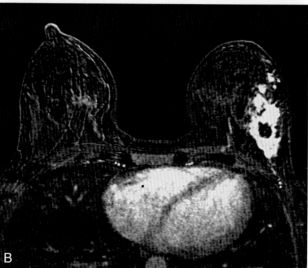

FIGURE 5. Dynamic contrast-enhanced, subtracted views of both breasts (**A** above **B**) show intense, multifocal enhancement in the left lateral breast, with a large, irregularly shaped posterior mass, and multiple smaller masses and clumped linear and ductal enhancement extending in a ductal ray anteriorly. Note also the fine linear enhancement at the posterior and lateral aspects of the dominant mass. No abnormalities are seen in the right breast.

FNA. Physical examination of the breast noted a large area of nodularity and induration, estimated at 5 cm in size, but difficult to precisely define.

Breast MRI was obtained to better define the extent of the tumor (Figures 5 and 6). It showed a much larger area of involvement, spanning 8 cm in the left lateral breast. This consisted of multiple intensely enhancing masses, with clumped, linear, and ductal enhancement, oriented along a ductal ray.

Positron emission tomography (PET)/CT and enhanced CT scans were obtained to systemically stage the patient. These showed intense multifocal hypermetabolism in the left lateral breast and in multiple left axillary enlarged lymph nodes (Figures 7, 8, 9, 10, and 11). No evidence of stage IV disease was seen.

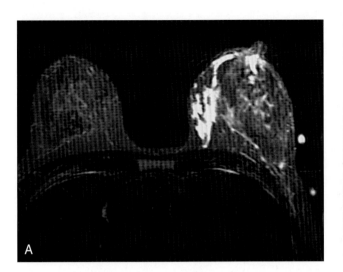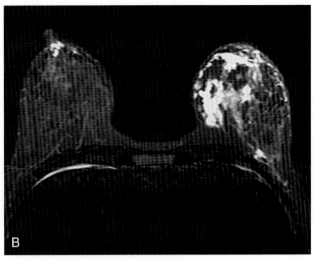

FIGURE 6.   Axial STIR images (**A** above **B,** at the same levels as Figure 5) show the lateral region of the left breast to be hypointense compared with the edematous, engorged appearance of the remainder of the breast. The appearance is in striking contrast to the right breast, which shows localized retroareolar ductal ectasia only. The lateral left breast skin is thickened and edematous, but showed no abnormal enhancement.

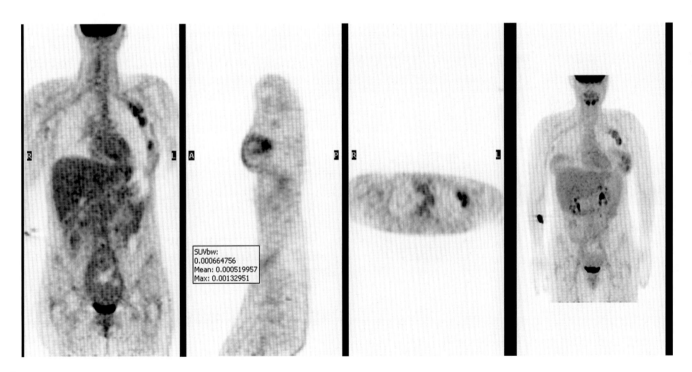

FIGURE 7.   PET scan images show intense hypermetabolism in the lateral left breast, as well as in multiple left axillary lymph nodes. Normal, low-level, physiologic uptake is seen in the right breast.

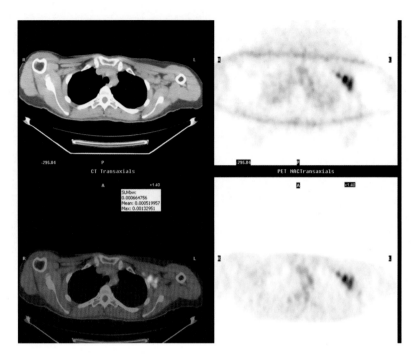

FIGURE 8.   Axial PET/CT images through the axilla show multiple enlarged and hypermetabolic left axillary nodes.

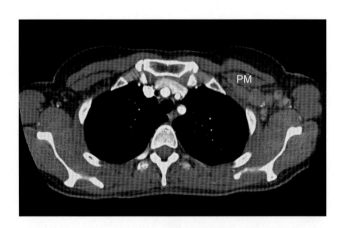

FIGURE 9.   The corresponding enhanced chest CT shows enlarged, nearly confluent left level I (lateral to the pectoralis minor [PM] muscle) and II (under the muscle) axillary lymph nodes.

Neoadjuvant chemotherapy was recommended, owing to the large size of the tumor. Four cycles each of doxorubicin (Adriamycin) and cyclophosphamide (Cytoxan) (AC) and docetaxel (Taxotere) were given. Restaging with breast ultrasound and MRI (Figures 12, 13, and 14) and PET/CT was performed after four cycles of AC and again after 4 cycles of Taxotere (Figures 15 and 16). Restaging showed an excellent imaging response, with dramatic shrinkage and decreased enhancement of

the tumor and axillary lymph nodes, and resolution of the PET uptake.

The left UOQ residual was needle-localized for surgery with two wires, and a residual, mildly abnormal-appearing left axillary lymph node was also needle-localized with ultrasound guidance. Pathology showed multifocal microscopic foci of atypical cells, consistent with residual carcinoma. The anterior margin was close (<1 mm). The extent of the residual tumor was estimated at 1.5 cm. The localized axillary lymph node was enlarged and fibrotic, with no evidence of neoplasm. A wide breast re-excision specimen showed no residual malignancy.

The patient began tamoxifen, and radiation therapy to the breast and peripheral lymphatics was given.

TEACHING POINTS

These axillary lymph nodes were so enlarged at presentation, a "plumbing problem" can be suspected to underlie the unusual pattern of edema and engorgement seen in the remainder of the left breast. The linear enhancing strands seen extending from the multifocal breast neoplasm toward the axilla suggest tumor-engorged lymphatics. The skin thickening and edema in the left lateral breast,

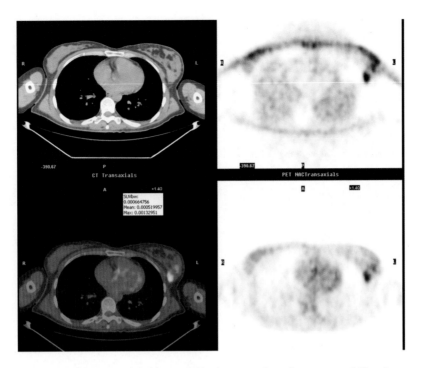

FIGURE 10. Axial PET/CT images through the breasts show intense, multifocal hypermetabolic activity in the left lateral breast.

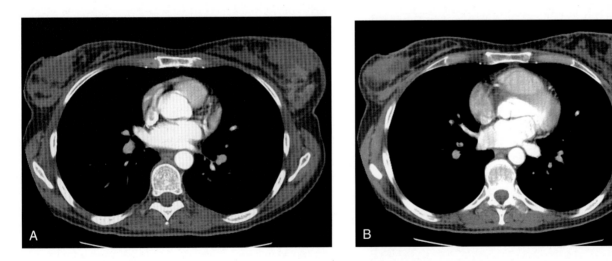

FIGURE 11. Contrast-enhanced chest CT images of the breasts (**A** above **B**) show multifocal, ill-defined enhancement in the left lateral breast, poorly delineated from normal parenchyma. The left lateral breast skin is thickened.

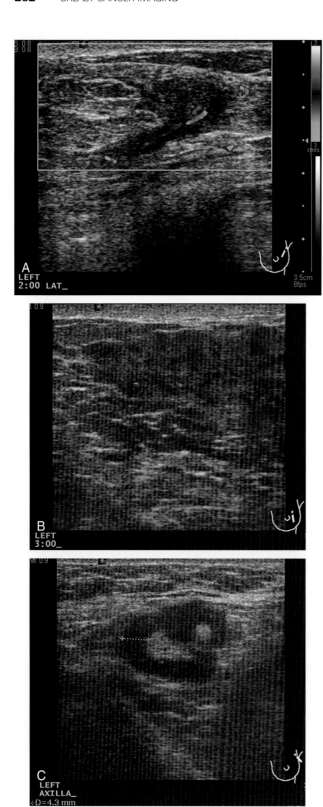

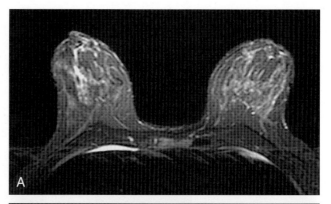

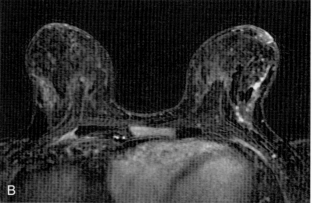

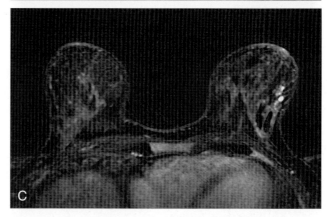

FIGURE 13. Restaging breast MRI, 3 months later, after four cycles of AC chemotherapy. **A,** Axial STIR shows a much more normal and symmetrical pattern of signal intensity. **B,** Axial, dynamic, enhanced, subtracted MRI shows dramatic improvement. A linear array of enhancing foci is seen in the lateral left breast where the extensive multifocal masses were previously. **C,** A more inferior image from the same series.

FIGURE 12. Restaging lateral left breast ultrasound, 3 months later after four cycles of AC chemotherapy. **A,** At 2 o'clock, there is a vascular hypoechoic residual mass. **B,** Persistent hypoechoic echotexture is seen at 3 o'clock. **C,** The axillary lymph node, which was massively enlarged previously, is markedly improved but shows persistent cortical thickening (4 mm).

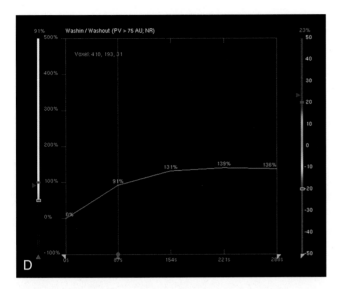

FIGURE 13, cont'd **D,** No washout is now seen. The curve shows slow uptake, with plateauing enhancement.

best seen on STIR MRI and on chest CT, is not accompanied by enhancement, and so probably is part of the generalized engorgement and edema. Skin thickening with enhancement would be concerning for an inflammatory component.

Another potentially contributory factor to the markedly engorged appearance of the left breast at presentation was the patient's lactational status. She was 4 months postpartum and had been breast-feeding; at presentation she was actively weaning her child (breast-feeding one-half of the day). However, the marked asymmetry between breasts argues for obstructed lymphatics as the dominant factor.

This patient had a very extensive tumor. This is a locally advanced breast cancer (LABC), based both on size (>5 cm) and the extensive axillary involvement. The only imaging modality that accurately delineated the true extent of this LABC was MRI. This tumor can also be considered a pregnancy-associated breast cancer (PABC), defined as breast cancer diagnosed during pregnancy or within the first year after delivery. In the developed world, PABC constitutes about 1% of all breast cancers.

By both imaging and pathology, this patient had a good response to primary systemic chemotherapy. At presentation, she had been inclined to undergo a mastectomy, but was persuaded that preoperative chemotherapy was advisable because of the size of the tumor. Downsizing of the tumor to a degree at which breast conservation became a viable option was an unexpected benefit of neoadjuvant therapy in this case.

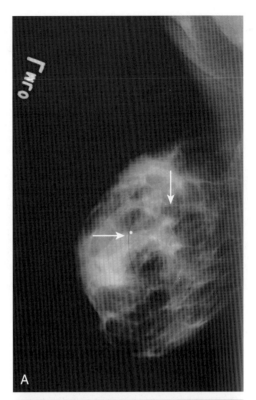

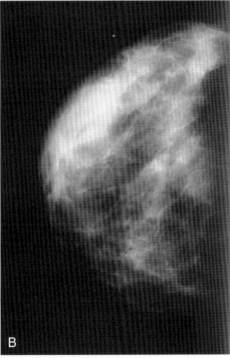

FIGURE 14. Mammogram, after four cycles of AC chemotherapy, shows heterogeneously dense breast parenchyma [MLO (**A**) and CC (**B**)]. There is a suggestion of architectural distortion (*arrows*) on the MLO view. A marker has been placed at the site of palpable induration.

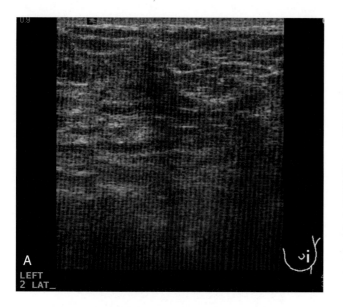
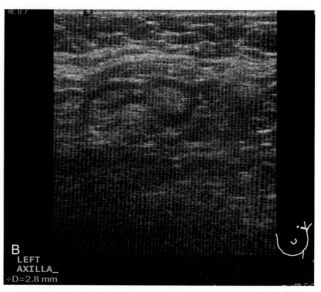

FIGURE 15. Restaging lateral left breast ultrasound, 6 months after diagnosis and after four cycles each of AC and Taxotere chemotherapy. **A,** An ill-defined hypoechoic residual mass is seen at 2 o'clock. **B,** The axillary lymph node has further normalized in appearance. Cortical thickness is now borderline.

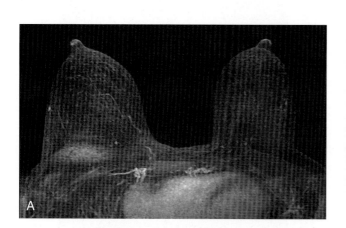
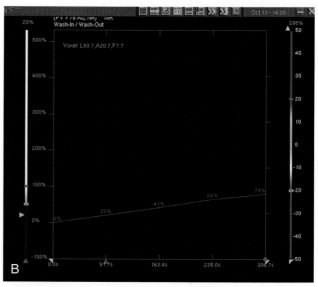

FIGURE 16. Restaging breast MRI, 6 months after diagnosis and after four cycles each of AC and Taxotere chemotherapy. **A,** Axial maximal intensity projection (3 minutes after contrast injection) shows only a few foci of enhancement at the lateral left breast site of treated IDC. **B,** Only slow, persistent enhancement can now be identified.

IDC treated with neoadjuvant chemotherapy with incomplete imaging response, but complete pathologic response

A 47-year-old woman presented with a growing palpable lump, noted initially a year before evaluation. Mammographic evaluation showed development since the prior year of a new upper outer quadrant (UOQ) right breast mass, which was 4 cm, spiculated, and associated with pleomorphic calcifications (Figure 1). Additional suspicious microcalcifications were seen medial and caudal to the dominant mass. Palpation-guided biopsy by a breast surgeon was suspicious with atypia, but not conclusive. Subsequently, ultrasound demonstrated a 2.9-cm mass (Figure 2), with highly suspicious features, and core needle biopsy with ultrasound guidance confirmed moderately differentiated infiltrating ductal carcinoma (IDC), estrogen receptor and progesterone receptor positive, *HER-2/neu* negative.

Breast MRI showed the mass to be larger than previously suspected, measuring 5 cm (Figures 3 and 4). The patient opted for neoadjuvant chemotherapy to downsize the tumor. The mass shrank in response, as assessed on follow-up mammograms and MRI (Figures 5 and 6). By MRI, the dominant mass declined in size from 5 cm pretreatment to 3 cm post-treatment, with an adjacent 1-cm mass inferomedially. Mammography showed a decline in size of the visible mass from 4 cm to 1.5 cm. However, sampling of the unchanged microcalcifications was now recommended, because of their location in the lower outer quadrant (LOQ), separate from the known IDC in the UOQ. Stereotactic biopsy confirmed the calcifications represented ductal carcinoma in situ (DCIS), and with two quadrants involved, the patient was deemed unsuitable for breast conservation.

Accordingly, the patient underwent a mastectomy and sentinel lymph node sampling. No residual IDC was found in the mastectomy specimen. There was residual cribriform and solid DCIS in the LOQ measuring 1.8 cm. The margins were negative, and one lymph node was negative as well.

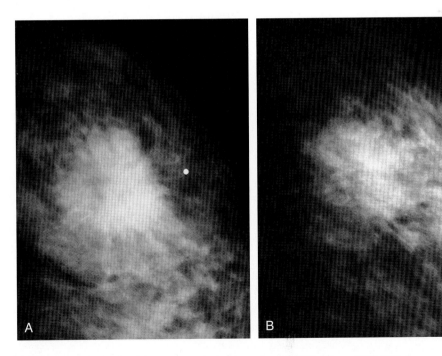

FIGURE 1. Mammographic spot compression views [MLO (**A**) and CC (**B**)] show a dominant, dense mass with spiculated margins, which was palpable. (Note adjacent marker on the MLO projection.)

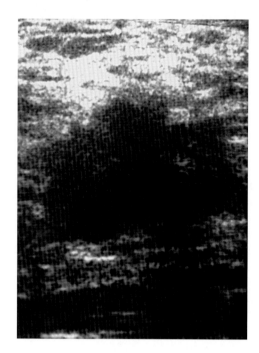

FIGURE 2. Ultrasound of the palpable lump in the right UOQ shows a highly suspicious appearance, being very hypoechoic, with shadowing and irregular, angular margins.

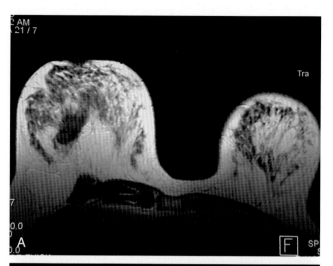

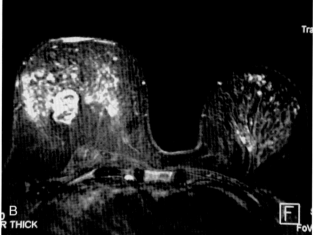

FIGURE 3. Staging breast MRI axial images (**A,** T2-weighted; **B,** enhanced, subtracted T1-weighted gradient echo) show the right breast to be larger than the left. The dominant mass in the right lateral breast is hypointense on T2-weighted images and shows rim enhancement on subtracted enhanced images.

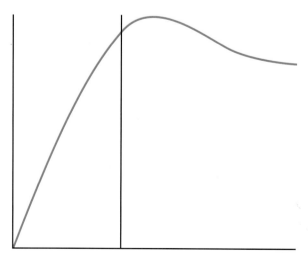

FIGURE 4. Signal intensity–time enhancement curve shows a suspicious pattern, with rapid uptake of contrast, and washout, indicating angiogenesis.

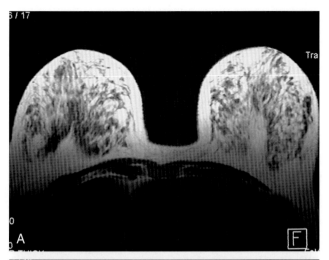

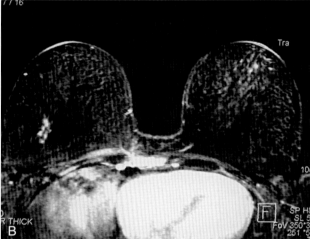

FIGURE 5. Restaging breast MRI images (**A,** T2-weighted; **B,** enhanced, subtracted T1-weighted gradient echo), after neoadjuvant chemotherapy, show shrinkage of the mass, which is still visible as a contracted residual on both views.

Additional therapy given included radiation therapy to the chest wall and supraclavicular fossa, and the patient was started on tamoxifen.

TEACHING POINTS

Good responses to neoadjuvant chemotherapy may convert a nonoperable patient into operability with mastectomy, or can convert a mastectomy candidate to eligibility for breast-conserving lumpectomy. However, as this case shows, even a good response to neoadjuvant chemotherapy may still necessitate treatment with a mastectomy. This tumor was considered a locally advanced breast cancer based on the large size of lesion (>5 cm). It

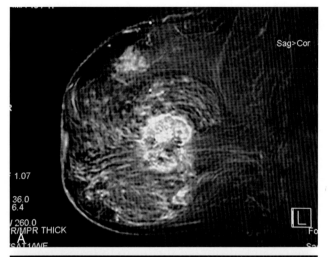

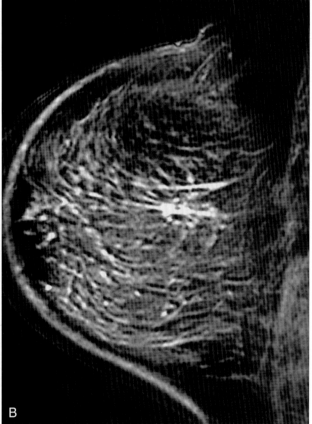

FIGURE 6. Sagittal enhanced, subtracted, T1-weighted gradient echo views. **A,** Before neoadjuvant chemotherapy. **B,** After chemotherapy, for comparison.

can be easier to perform mastectomy with clear margins after shrinking a tumor with neoadjuvant chemotherapy, and no difference in recurrence rates has been demonstrated for administration of chemotherapy preoperatively compared with postoperatively.

CASE 9

LABC, responsive to neoadjuvant chemotherapy; splenic activation on PET with G-CSF therapy

A 55-year-old woman saw a new primary care physician, who found on physical examination a large, firm, mobile, nontender right lateral breast mass. The patient attributed the lump to breast trauma in the same region 3 years before, and had noted no interval change since first identifying it.

Mammography confirmed a large spiculated new UOQ mass (Figure 1). Ultrasound confirmed a 6.6-cm mass at 9 o'clock with a separate 1.5-cm lesion at 12 o'clock and an enlarged and suspicious right axillary lymph node (Figures 2, 3, and 4). The surgeon noted right lateral breast skin indentation, with an easily palpable 6-cm mass with possible fixation. Palpation-guided core needle biopsy by the surgeon confirmed infiltrating ductal carcinoma (IDC), estrogen receptor and progesterone receptor positive. Breast MRI was requested to evaluate the question of fixation.

Breast MRI showed the dominant tumor to be a 5-cm, multilobulated, heterogeneously and rim-enhancing mass with washout. An additional, 7-mm enhancing mass at 12 o'clock, 3.5 cm away from the dominant IDC, showed washout as well and seemed to correlate with the separate abnormality seen on ultrasound (Figures 5, 6, 7, and 8).

Under ultrasound guidance, a clip was placed into the dominant 9-o'clock mass in anticipation of primary systemic chemotherapy. The satellite mass at 12 o'clock was marked with a clip at the time of biopsy, also confirming IDC. The largest axillary lymph node was sampled with fine-needle aspira-

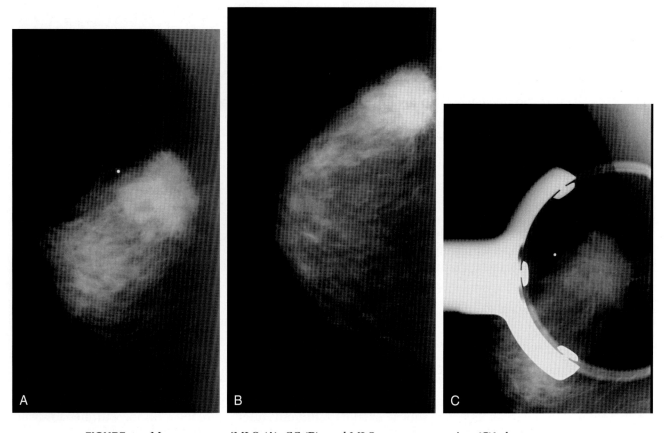

FIGURE 1. Mammograms [MLO (**A**), CC (**B**), and MLO spot compression (**C**)] show very dense breast parenchyma. A radiopaque marker has been placed at the UOQ level of a palpable mass. A large, dense, spiculated mass is posterior in position. Anteriorly, its margins merge with the dense breast tissue.

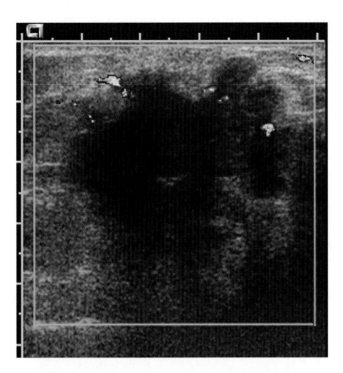

FIGURE 2. Right breast ultrasound of the lateral palpable lump at 9 o'clock shows a large, malignant-appearing hypoechoic mass with angular margins, posterior shadowing, and peripheral vascularity. Ultrasound-guided biopsy confirmed IDC.

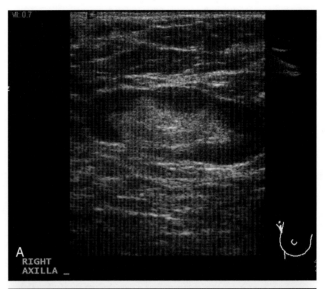

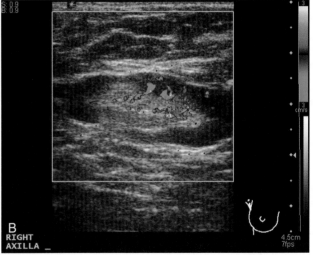

FIGURE 4. Right axillary lymph node ultrasound, without (**A**) and with (**B**) color Doppler, shows highly suspicious morphology. The cortex is very hypoechoic, as well as abnormally thickened and nodular. Note the "rat bite," scalloped appearance of mass effect on the echogenic fatty hilus, best seen without color Doppler. Increased and abnormal vascularity is seen with color Doppler applied. Normal lymph node vascularity is seen only at the hilus.

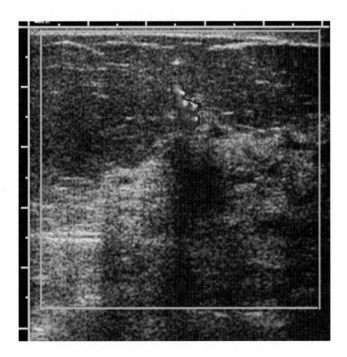

FIGURE 3. Right breast ultrasound at 12 o'clock identified a second mass with multiple suspicious features: hypoechoic, taller-than-wide, ill-defined margins and increased local vascularity. Ultrasound-guided core needle biopsy showed IDC.

tion (FNA) technique, identifying malignant cells, consistent with metastatic adenocarcinoma.

Systemic staging studies were undertaken, owing to the large tumor size and axillary involvement. Bone scan, positron emission tomography (PET)/CT, and enhanced body CT scans were obtained. The bone scan showed uptake of the radiopharmaceutical in the known right breast cancer, but no suspicious osseous findings (Figure 9). The PET scan showed intense hypermetabolism of the right

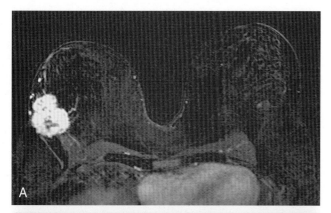

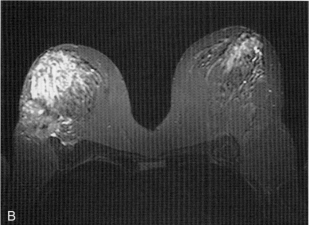

FIGURE 5. Axial breast MRIs [dynamic, enhanced, subtracted (**A**) and STIR (**B**)] show the dominant known IDC on the right laterally. Irregular, spiculated margins and intense and rim enhancement are all characteristic features of malignancy. Distortion of the underlying pectoralis muscle is seen, presumably reflecting tumor desmoplasia. No enhancement within the muscle is seen to suggest it is invaded.

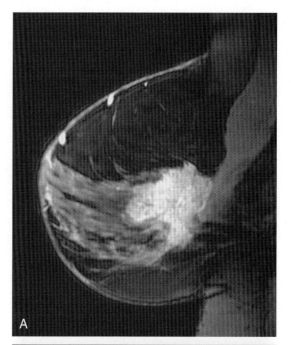

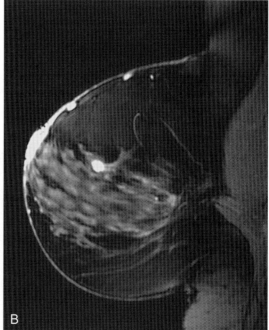

FIGURE 7. Sagittal, enhanced, fat-saturated, T1-weighted gradient echo images (**A,** through the lateral right breast 9-o'clock IDC; **B,** through the right 12-o'clock IDC) show extension of the 9-o'clock IDC down to the level of the pectoralis fascia (no intervening fat plane is visible here), but without actual muscle enhancement to suggest invasion.

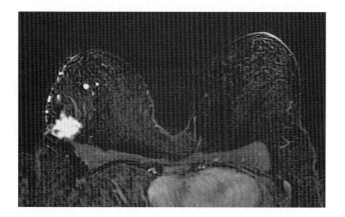

FIGURE 6. At a higher level, a second, small, separate small mass is seen at 12 o'clock, corresponding in location to the separate 12-o'clock IDC known from ultrasound. The top of the 9-o'clock IDC is also included in this slice.

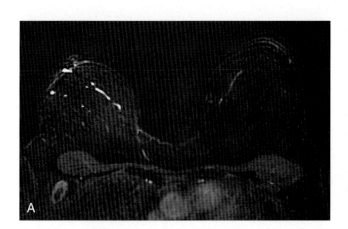
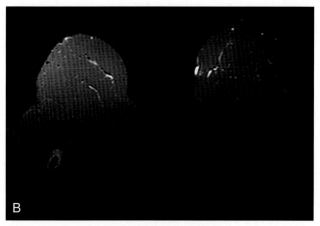

FIGURE 8.   Axial breast MRIs through the axilla [enhanced, subtracted (**A**) and STIR (**B**)] show the MRI counterpart to the abnormal right axillary lymph node seen on ultrasound and confirmed by FNA to be involved with metastatic disease.

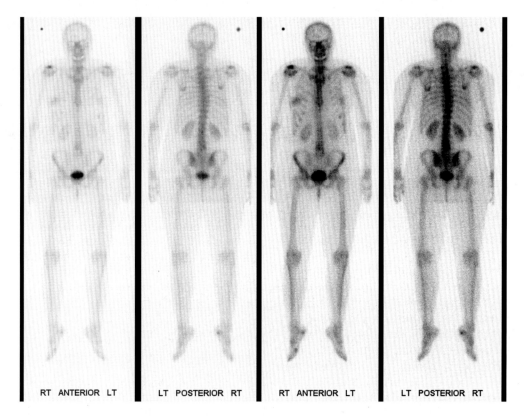

RT ANTERIOR LT   LT POSTERIOR RT   RT ANTERIOR LT   LT POSTERIOR RT

FIGURE 9.   Anterior and posterior whole-body bone scan images. Bone scan showed no findings to suggest bone metastases, but did show abnormal increased uptake in the right breast, corresponding to the LABC. Low-level, physiologic activity in left breast tissue is also seen.

lateral IDC, as well as of four right axillary level I and II lymph nodes, which were enlarged by CT (Figures 10 and 11). No distant metastases were seen on CT or PET. Because of the size of the tumor, neoadjuvant chemotherapy was recommended.

Four cycles of doxorubicin (Adriamycin) and cyclophosphamide (Cytoxan) (AC) were given, after which restaging studies of the breast were obtained. Clinically, there was a good response, with the palpable mass much less distinct and resolution of palpable adenopathy. Breast imaging with mammography, ultrasound, and MRI confirmed improvement, with decrease in size and enhancement of the dominant IDC and resolution on ultra-

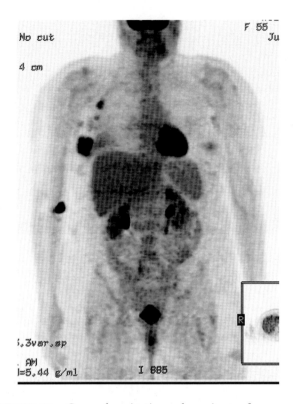

FIGURE 10. Coronal projection volume image from the PET scan at initial staging shows intense hypermetabolism in the right lateral breast cancer, as well as in multiple axillary lymph nodes. The left breast activity is physiologic uptake in the nipple. Right elbow–level activity is retained at the intravenous site.

sound and MRI of the 12-o'clock mass (Figures 12, 13, and 14).

After these restaging studies, additional chemotherapy was given with four cycles of docetaxel (Taxotere). Repeat breast imaging was obtained after completion of chemotherapy (Figures 15 and 16). The patient received granulocyte colony-stimulating factor (G-CSF) with later cycles of chemotherapy after developing an infection and borderline white blood cell levels. Repeat PET scan after completion of chemotherapy showed complete resolution of the axillary nodal uptake, with nearly complete resolution of uptake in the breast. Marrow activation changes of bone were noted, and new increased activity was seen in the spleen as well (Figure 17).

A right modified radical mastectomy was performed, with en bloc removal of the axillary contents. The pathology showed extensive fibrosis and sclerosis at the site of the treated 9-o'clock IDC, with residual nests of IDC tumor cells extending over about 2.5 cm. The deep margin was close (<2 mm), and all others were clear. No residual tumor was identified at the 12-o'clock clip site.

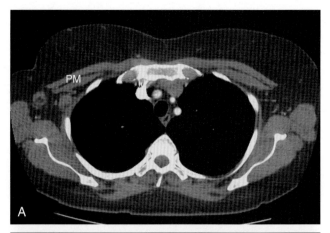

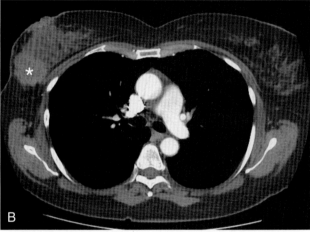

FIGURE 11. Enhanced chest CT images. **A,** Through the axilla: Two enlarged right axillary lymph nodes are seen at this level, one lateral to the pectoralis minor (PM) muscle (level I) and one beneath the muscle (level II). **B,** Through the breasts: the large right lateral breast cancer is irregularly marginated and more solid in appearance than the rest of the breast tissue (*asterisk*).

There were 11 benign lymph nodes in the specimen.

TEACHING POINTS

This is a large, at least multifocal, node-positive, locally advanced breast cancer (LABC) treated initially with primary systemic (neoadjuvant) chemotherapy, with a good clinical and imaging response. The smaller IDC mass at 12 o'clock, never evident on mammography, completely resolved with chemotherapy by ultrasound and MRI. Fortunately, neoadjuvant chemotherapy had been anticipated, and a clip was placed to mark the site of the lesion at the time of biopsy. The center of the dominant

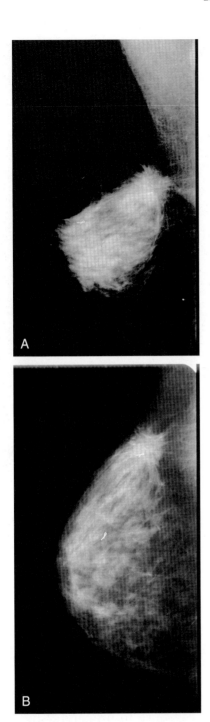

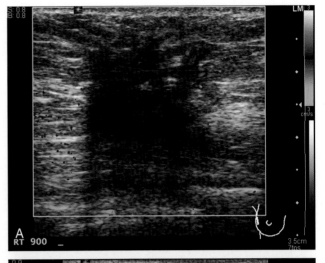

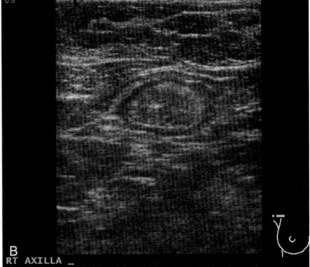

FIGURE 13.   Restaging ultrasound, 3 months after initial diagnosis, after four cycles of AC chemotherapy. **A,** The right 9-o'clock IDC mass has shrunk. It still is clearly seen, with highly malignant features as before. The 12-o'clock second IDC was no longer seen by ultrasound. **B,** The axillary lymph node has normalized. The cortex is now thin.

FIGURE 12.   Restaging mammogram, 3 months later, after four cycles of AC chemotherapy. **A,** Lateral mammogram. **B,** Exaggerated CC view. The UOQ spiculated mass has shrunk. A clip has been placed within it to mark its position, a hedge against it resolving with neoadjuvant therapy. A more anterior clip at 12 o'clock was placed at the second IDC site at the time of ultrasound biopsy.

9-o'clock IDC was also marked. It is difficult to predict how complete a response any one patient or lesion will have to chemotherapy. To keep the patient's choices open in case breast conservation therapy becomes a viable option, it is advisable to mark disease sites for subsequent localization in case a complete imaging response to chemotherapy ensues.

Imaging changes that successful neoadjuvant chemotherapy induces in a breast cancer are well demonstrated by this example. A responding mass can decrease in size, retaining the same basic

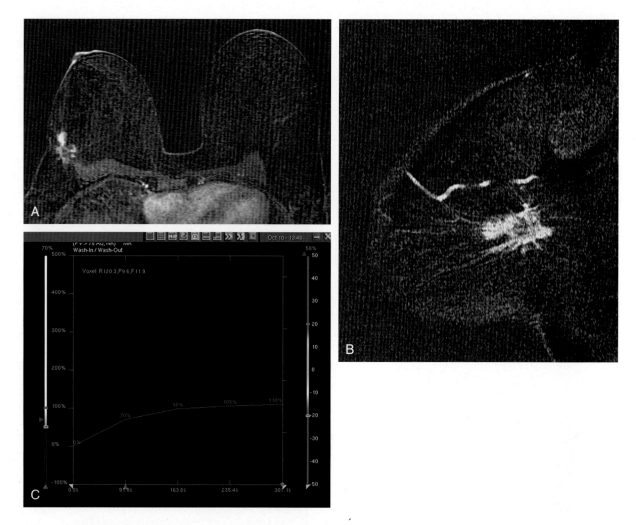

FIGURE 14. Restaging MRI, 3 months after initial diagnosis, after four cycles of AC chemotherapy. **A,** Axial enhanced, subtracted view of the right 9-o'clock IDC, 3 minutes after contrast injection. **B,** Sagittal, enhanced, subtracted view of the right 9-o'clock IDC, 5 to 6 minutes after contrast injection. **C,** Kinetic curve shows slow uptake of contrast, which plateaus. The dominant IDC mass has markedly decreased in size. The contrast enhancement has markedly diminished, and the pattern has changed. No washout is seen. The 12-o'clock lesion is no longer seen.

shape, or can "break up" into smaller residual components. The intensity and pattern of enhancement change. The rapid uptake of contrast and washout demonstrated by this tumor on initial breast MRI changed to a pattern of slow, plateauing contrast accumulation.

As shown here, the response to neoadjuvant chemotherapy can be assessed with mammography and ultrasound, if the disease was initially well seen on those modalities. However, it is well established that MRI most accurately depicts the initial extent of untreated disease as compared with mammography and ultrasound. Similarly, breast MRI is the most reliable anatomic imaging modality to

assess the response to primary systemic chemotherapy. Functional imaging, with fluorodeoxyglucose (FDG) PET, is an alternative means of assessing a chemotherapy response. This is seen in this case with whole-body FDG PET, which showed normalization of the pretreatment findings. In addition, whole-body PET provides reassurance that the patient's disease has not metastasized before undergoing surgery.

At this writing, small-field-of-view, higher-resolution, molecular breast imaging and breast-specific gamma imaging units are becoming available. Positron emission mammography may prove to be useful alternative functional means of

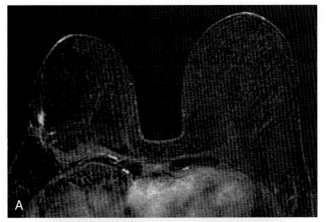

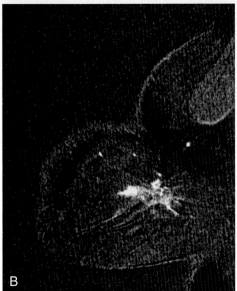

FIGURE 15.   Restaging MRI, 6 months after initial diagnosis, after four cycles of AC and four cycles of Taxotere chemotherapy. **A,** Axial enhanced subtracted view of the right 9-o'clock IDC, 3 minutes after contrast injection. **B,** Sagittal, enhanced, subtracted view of the right 9-o'clock IDC, 5 to 6 minutes after contrast injection. There has been further improvement, with more interval decrease in size and enhancement.

assessing chemotherapy responses, although this validation process is currently ongoing.

This case also illustrates the imaging features of a common chemotherapy "side effect." Many chemotherapeutic agents are myelosuppressive and may result in depressed white blood cell counts (neutropenia), predisposing patients to infection. This may result in hospitalization, delays in treatment or dose adjustments, potentially affecting the efficacy of treatment. To counteract these myelosuppressive effects, a patient may be treated with G-CSF, given with each cycle as necessary. This is a

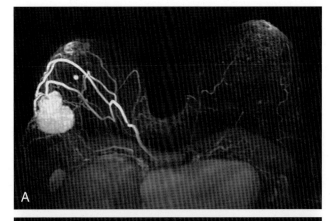

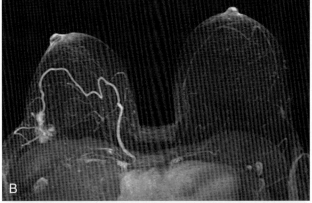

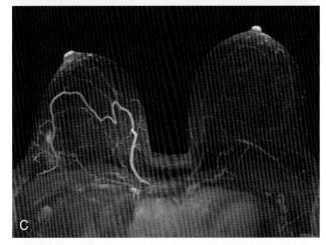

FIGURE 16.   Axial maximal intensity projection views from the dynamic enhanced portions of the breast MRIs obtained before (**A**), during (**B**), and after (**C**) chemotherapy. **A,** Initial staging study, minute 1 of dynamic enhanced series. Both the dominant IDC mass and the small 12-o'clock second IDC enhance intensely. The enlarged right axillary lymph node also enhances strongly. **B,** Three months later, after four cycles of AC, minute 3 of dynamic enhanced series. The 12-o'clock IDC is no longer seen. The right 9-o'clock dominant IDC has markedly shrunk and enhances more slowly and much less intensely. **C,** Six months after initial diagnosis, after four cycles of AC and four cycles of Taxotere, minute 3 of dynamic enhanced series. The right 9-o'clock IDC enhances slowly, and there has been a further decline in size of the mass.

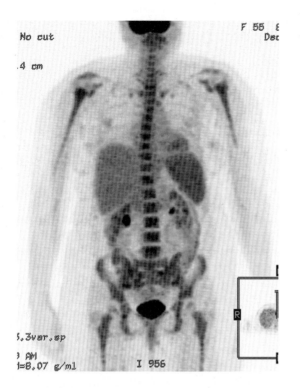

FIGURE 17. Restaging PET scan, coronal volumetric projection image, after completion of chemotherapy. The patient required G-CSF because of reduced white cell counts. The right IDC and axillary uptake are no longer seen. Changes attributable to G-CSF are seen, with diffuse increase in marrow and splenic activity.

CASE 10

Complete imaging response to neoadjuvant chemotherapy

A 54-year-old postmenopausal woman with a family history of breast cancer underwent routine screening mammography, which identified developing asymmetrical density and possible architectural distortion in the right upper outer quadrant (UOQ). Mammographic spot compression confirmed the suspected abnormality, and ultrasound showed corresponding ill-defined shadowing in the 9- to 10-o'clock region (Figure 1). Stereotactic biopsy was recommended because the abnormality seemed to be better visualized mammographically than sonographically. However, the lesion could not be satisfactorily visualized for stereotactic biopsy, presumably because of the less effective compression achievable with stereotactic procedures. The hypoechoic shadowing correlate was biopsied with ultrasound guidance, confirming infiltrating ductal carcinoma (IDC).

On surgical, medical oncology, and radiation oncology evaluations, no palpable mass was identified. Because the size of the lesion and true extent

growth factor that primarily stimulates neutrophils and neutrophil precursors. Increased FDG uptake in bone marrow in patients receiving G-CSF with chemotherapy is a frequently observed PET phenomenon. This is well demonstrated in this case. A less commonly observed G-CSF–induced change is also illustrated here. The spleen displays increased FDG uptake on the postchemotherapy PET scan. This phenomenon was initially described by Sugawara and associates in a study of LABC patients undergoing chemotherapy who were evaluated before, during, and after G-CSF treatment. The increased FDG uptake in the spleen was thought to reflect changes of extramedullary hematopoiesis. These bone marrow and splenic changes regress with cessation of G-CSF treatment.

SUGGESTED READING

Sugawara Y, Zasadny KR, Kison PV, et al. splenic fluoro-deoxyglucose uptake increased by granulocyte colony-stimulating factor therapy: PET imaging results. *J Nucl Med* 1999; 40:1456–1462.

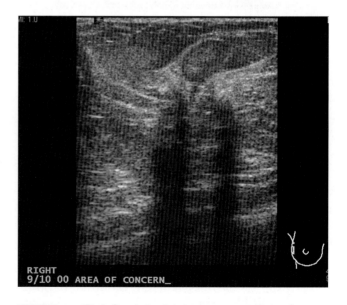

FIGURE 1. Ill-defined shadowing emanates from the right lateral breast, in the region of the mammographic abnormality. The margins and precise dimensions are difficult to delineate. The process distorts the normal breast tissue planes. Biopsy with ultrasound guidance confirmed IDC.

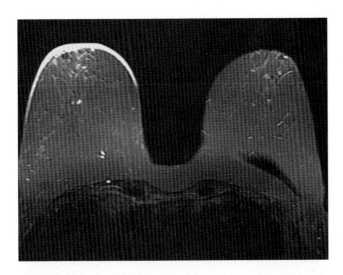

FIGURE 2.   Axial STIR breast MRI shows marked skin asymmetry. The right breast skin is thick and edematous. However, little increased edema is seen within the breast itself.

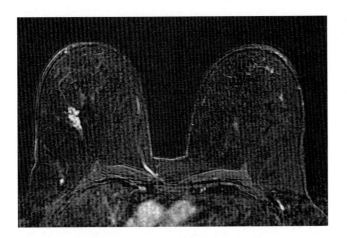

FIGURE 3.   Axial enhanced, subtracted, T1-weighted, gradient echo images show irregularly marginated, intense enhancement in the right lateral breast, corresponding to the known IDC. In this plane, the size correlated fairly well with the ultrasound estimate of index lesion size.

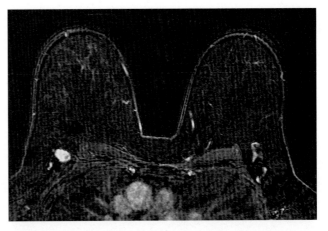

FIGURE 4.   Another section, through the axilla, shows an intensely enhancing and enlarged right axillary lymph node.

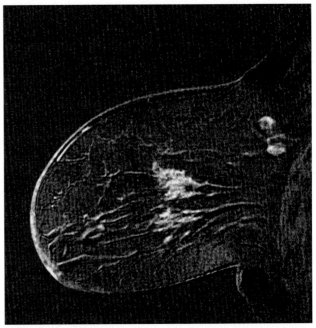

FIGURE 5.   Sagittal, subtracted breast MRI of the right lateral breast shows the craniocaudal extent of disease. The process appears more extensive and larger than previously suspected. Enhancing right axillary lymph nodes are also depicted. The thickened supra-areolar skin shows enhancement, suggesting a possible inflammatory component.

of disease were difficult to estimate accurately based on clinical breast exam, mammography, and ultrasound, breast MRI was requested.

MRI suggested more advanced disease than suspected to that point (Figures 2, 3, 4, and 5). Multiple intensely enhancing right axillary lymph nodes were identified, which were up to 1.1 × 1.8 cm in size. The index lesion was larger than previously demonstrated, with maximal dimension estimated to be 4 cm (prior estimate by ultrasound was 2 cm). The skin of the right breast was noted to be asymmetrically thickened and edematous, with en-

hancement. Nearly concurrent with this, the patient noted new faint erythema of the right breast, and a tender right axillary lymph node was now palpable. She was placed on antibiotics for a possible infection. The erythema persisted, but no peau d'orange changes were ever noted. A punch skin biopsy was performed to assess for a possible inflammatory

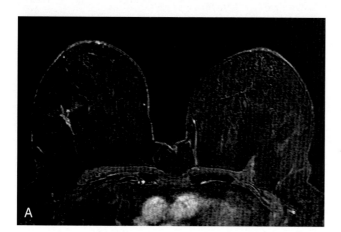
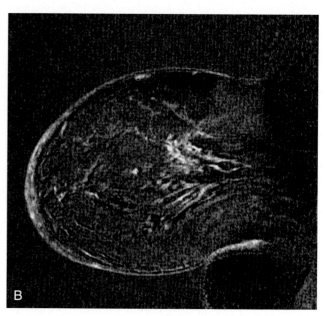

FIGURE 6. Repeat breast MRI, 3 months later, after four cycles of AC chemotherapy, shows decreased size of the enhancing mass [axial (**A**) and sagittal (**B**)], with a contracted, strandy residual remaining. The enhancement is much less intense. These findings completely resolved on repeat breast MRI, performed after completion of chemotherapy (not shown).

component, but showed only perivascular inflammation, with no dermal or intralymphatic carcinoma seen.

Although the patient had initially been interested in breast conservation therapy, the more extensive nature of her tumor suggested by these evaluations led to a decision to begin neoadjuvant chemotherapy after clip placement (under ultrasound guidance) into the mass. While undergoing this, the patient had *BRCA* gene testing and was confirmed to be *BRCA2* positive. Her family history of breast cancer included a sister diagnosed at age 48 and mother diagnosed at age 65, with death at age 67 from metastatic breast cancer. After this information became available, the patient decided to undergo bilateral mastectomies after completing neoadjuvant chemotherapy.

After four cycles of chemotherapy with doxorubicin (Adriamycin) and cyclophosphamide (Cytoxan) (AC), breast MRI was repeated (Figures 6 and 7). This showed a response, with the enhancing tumor reduced in size and a marked decline in intensity of enhancement. Only slow progressive enhancement was now identified. The enhancing axillary lymph nodes also resolved.

After four cycles of docetaxel (Taxotere), restaging breast studies were obtained. By MRI, there was a complete response, with no residual enhancement identified. The patient's right breast skin was noted to be persistently thickened and edematous,

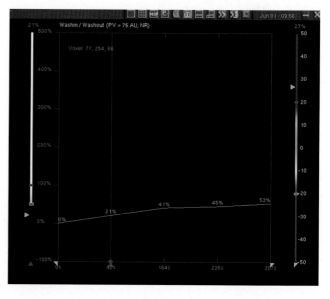

FIGURE 7. The signal intensity–time curve shows only slow, progressive, low-level enhancement now. These minimal findings were completely resolved on the next follow-up, after four cycles of Taxotere.

but without abnormal enhancement. No residual disease was demonstrable by mammography or ultrasound.

The patient elected surgical treatment with bilateral mastectomies. On the right, a sentinel lymph node was positive for malignancy, and so axillary dissection was performed. Two of four axillary lymph nodes showed tumor. The right mastectomy specimen contained residual IDC, spread over a 1.3-cm expanse. There was angiolymphatic invasion. The skin and margins were uninvolved. The left mastectomy specimen showed fibrocystic changes only.

Right chest wall, supraclavicular, and posterior axillary boost radiation was given, and the patient was started on anastrozole (Arimidex).

TEACHING POINTS

This case reminds us that complete imaging responses to neoadjuvant chemotherapy are not equivalent to complete pathologic response. Although no imaging evidence of disease remained after chemotherapy, there was microscopic residual IDC. The converse can also occur: Complete pathologic responses can be seen in patients whose tumorous imaging findings do not completely resolve.

CASE 11

IDC with cystic component; mixed response to neoadjuvant chemotherapy

A 28-year-old woman noted a palpable left breast lump while in the shower, which was subsequently confirmed by her primary care physician's physical examination in the upper outer quadrant (UOQ). Ultrasound showed a 2.9-cm complex mass with cystic and solid components (Figure 1). Biopsy was recommended and accomplished with ultrasound guidance. The solid component was sampled with 14-gauge core needle biopsy technique and the cystic component aspirated, with the bloody aspirate sent for cytologic analysis. Pathology showed poorly differentiated invasive ductal carcinoma

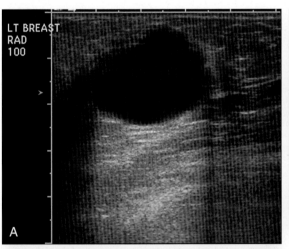

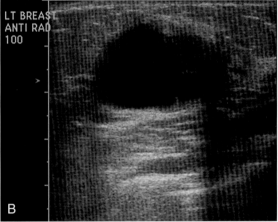

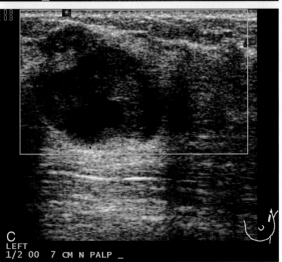

FIGURE 1. Ultrasound images of the palpable left upper outer quadrant mass. **A,** Anechoic cystic component shows a sharp back wall and enhanced through-transmission, with a deceptively benign appearance at first glance. **B,** Another ultrasound section shows mural thickening and a solid component on the right side of the cystic portion. **C,** This image, through the solid component, does not look innocent. Although the margins are lobular and relatively circumscribed, there is no well-defined capsule. The solid component is heterogeneous in echotexture, and there is peripheral vascularity, all features suggesting this needs to be sampled. Biopsy confirmed high-grade IDC.

(IDC), estrogen receptor and progesterone receptor negative, *HER-2/neu* negative, and the fluid cytology showed malignant cells.

Breast MRI was obtained next and showed the left UOQ known IDC to be partially cystic (Figure 2). By MRI, the maximal dimension was 3.7 cm. An unsuspected 1-cm, intensely enhancing, circumscribed mass was found in the posterior right lateral breast (Figure 3). Subsequent workup with diagnostic mammography and ultrasound was performed. On the right, ultrasound found a 1.0- × 0.3-cm hypoechoic, oval, benign-appearing mass against the chest wall, which seemed to correspond to the MRI finding (Figure 4). Subsequent right ultrasound-guided core needle biopsy confirmed a diagnosis of fibroadenoma.

Initial consultations with surgery, medical oncology, and radiation oncology noted the tumor to be large relative to the patient's breast size. The patient desired breast conservation, and so neoadjuvant chemotherapy with four cycles of doxorubicin (Adriamycin) and cyclophosphamide (Cytoxan) (AC) and four cycles of docetaxel (Taxotere) was elected. Preliminary staging studies with positron emission tomography (PET)/CT and enhanced body CT scans showed hypermetabolism of the peripheral solid left IDC components, but no evidence of nodal or distant metastatic disease (Figure 5). Ultrasound and breast MRI studies obtained during and at the conclusion of neoadjuvant chemotherapy showed a waxing and waning response, with improvement midway through therapy (after four cycles of AC), but partial

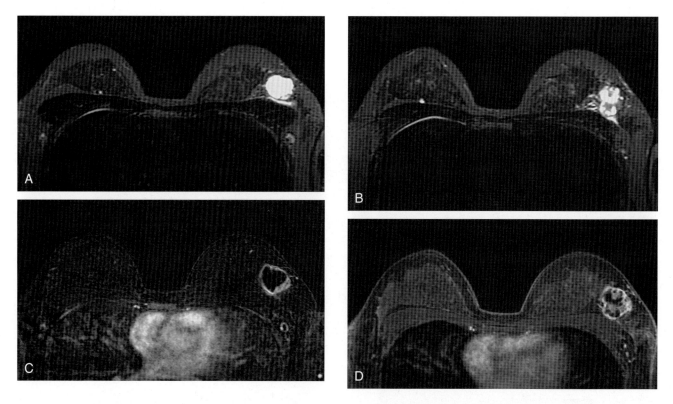

FIGURE 2. MRIs of the known left UOQ IDC mass. **A,** Axial STIR shows a cystic mass in the left lateral breast. A septation or focal mural thickening is seen within this cystic component posterolaterally. Fluid between the mass and the pectoral muscle may be related to the preceding biopsy. A mildly prominent left axillary lymph node with suggestive cortical mantle thickening is seen. Ultrasound-guided left axillary fine-needle aspiration was negative for malignancy, as was sentinel node evaluation after neoadjuvant chemotherapy. **B,** A more inferior axial STIR image shows a more heterogeneous, multilocular cystic and solid appearance of the left lateral IDC. **C,** Enhanced, subtracted image of the left IDC shows peripheral, thick-walled enhancement of the cystic component, with solid mural components, particularly posterolaterally. **D,** Unsubtracted, enhanced, T1-weighted, gradient echo image through the inferior portion of the left IDC shows papillary peripheral enhancement of the partially cystic mass.

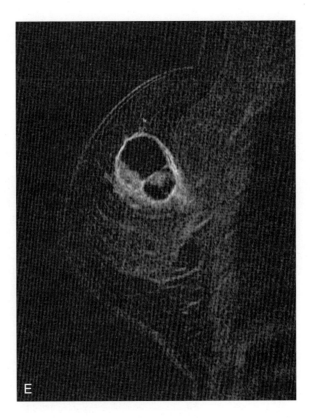

FIGURE 2, cont'd   E, Enhanced, subtracted, sagittal image shows the solid mural components projecting into the lumen of the partially cystic mass.

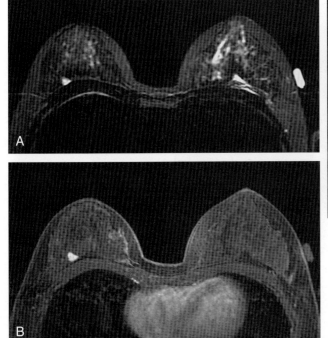

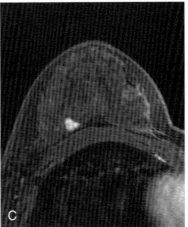

FIGURE 3. MRIs of a previously unsuspected right breast mass. **A,** A small (about 1 cm) hyperintense mass is seen against the posterior chest wall in the right lateral breast on axial STIR. **B,** Unsubtracted, enhanced, fat-saturated, T1-weighted, gradient echo image of the right mass shows smooth lobular contours. **C,** Detail of the right mass shows faint, nonenhancing internal septa within.

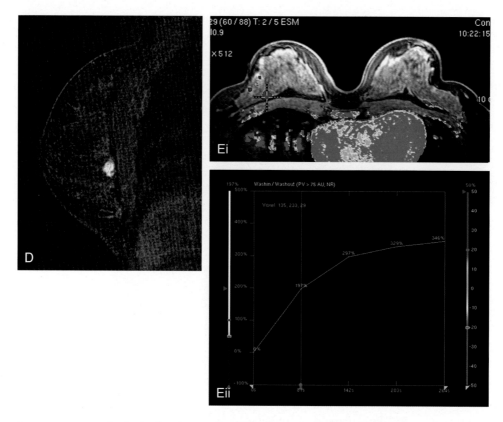

FIGURE 3, cont'd   D, Sagittal, subtracted, enhanced view of the same right mass. **E,** Kinetic analysis shows progressive enhancement of the mass. These characteristics suggest this represents a benign fibroadenoma, which was confirmed by subsequent ultrasound-guided core biopsy. **i,** Color map. **ii,** Signal intensity change–time curve.

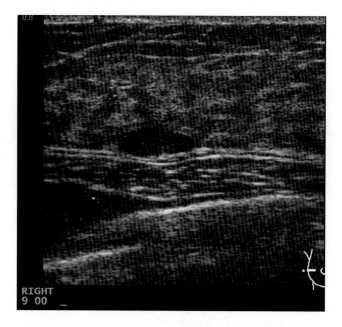

FIGURE 4.   Ultrasound of the right breast shows an oval, circumscribed, benign-appearing mass against the pectoral muscle, corresponding to the enhancing abnormality on MRI. This was confirmed by ultrasound core needle biopsy to be a fibroadenoma.

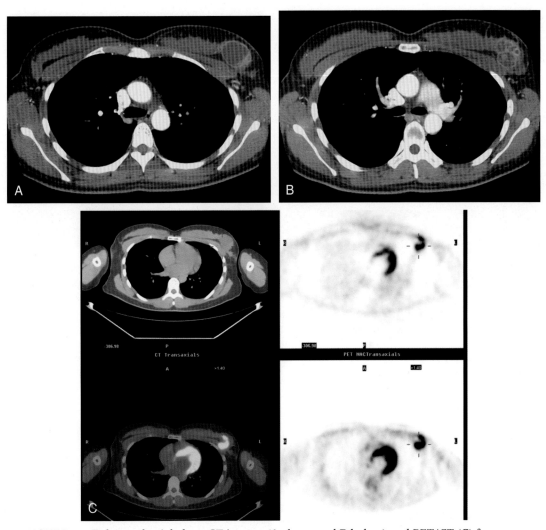

FIGURE 5. Enhanced axial chest CT images (**A** above and **B** below) and PET/CT (**C**) for correlation with MRI. **A,** At this level, the mass is complex cystic in appearance with thick and irregular solid enhancement posterolaterally. **B,** An even more suspicious appearance is seen at the inferior margin of the mass, with multilocularity, enhancing septa, and papillary projections. **C,** Axial PET/CT images show a C-shaped rim of intense hypermetabolism corresponding to the solid rim component of this multiloculated cystic neoplasm. No nodal or distant metastatic disease was identified on these studies.

regrowth after four cycles of Taxotere (Figures 6, 7, 8, 9, and 10). The final imaging evaluations did show overall improvement in comparison with the staging studies, despite the partial regression of the response demonstrated midway through therapy.

The patient was successfully treated with a lumpectomy, followed by radiation therapy to the breast and supraclavicular region (owing to the high position of the index lesion). Final pathology of the partial mastectomy specimen showed a 1.8-cm residual high-grade (grade 9/9) IDC, with negative margins. One sentinel lymph node was negative for tumor. Final stage was stage II, T2N0M0.

TEACHING POINTS

This case is interesting from multiple vantage points. Because of the patient's youth, the workup of the palpable mass started with ultrasound, as is appropriate. At first glance with ultrasound, the cystic portions of this mass are deceptively innocent looking. However, the identification of solid components mandates further evaluation. The sonographic differential includes malignancies (intracystic carcinoma, papillary carcinoma) and benign diagnoses (post-traumatic resolving hematoma or seroma, abscess, papilloma and complex cyst). How best to sample such a complex mass,

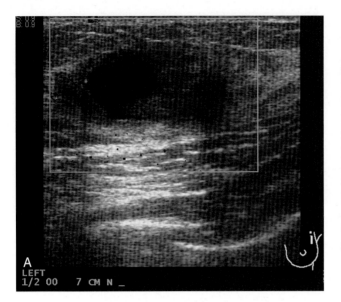 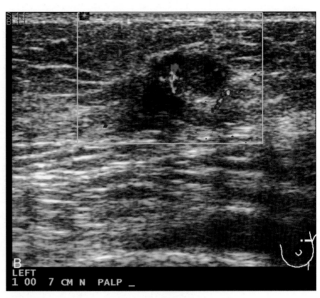

FIGURE 6.   Interim ultrasound (US) examinations, obtained during chemotherapy to assess the response. **A,** After two cycles of AC chemotherapy, the mass contracted, with decrease in the size of the cystic component. **B,** After four cycles of AC, further contraction is seen. The cystic component resolved. The residual solid component is irregularly marginated and vascular.

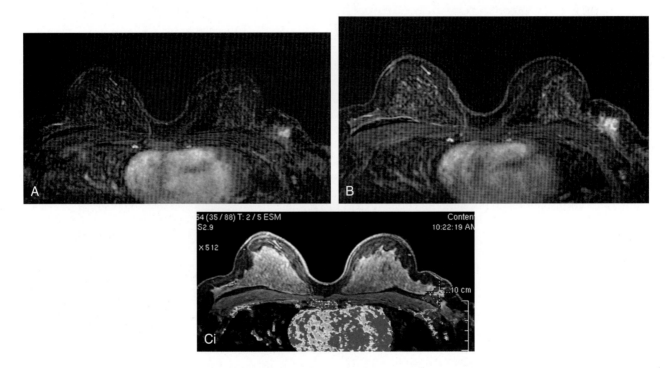

FIGURE 7.   Repeat breast MRI, after completion of four cycles of AC neoadjuvant chemotherapy. **A,** Enhanced, subtracted axial image from minute 1 of the dynamic series shows early enhancement of a smaller solid component. The cystic component of the mass was no longer evident on this examination. **B,** Enhanced, subtracted axial image from minute 3 of the dynamic series shows less intense, more delayed plateauing enhancement of the rest of the solid residual. Overall size has decreased to 2 cm in maximal dimension. **C,** DynaCAD kinetic color map (**i**) showing the differential enhancement of the residual solid mass. A 1-cm component anteriorly (*red* and *yellow*) shows washout, whereas the larger posterior component shows a plateauing enhancement pattern.

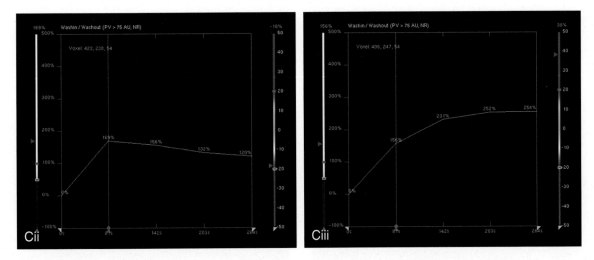

FIGURE 7, cont'd   ii, Graph (signal intensity–time curve) from the early enhancing 1-cm anterior component (in *red* on color map). **iii,** Graph (signal intensity–time curve) from the delayed, plateauing posterior enhancing component (in *blue* on color map).

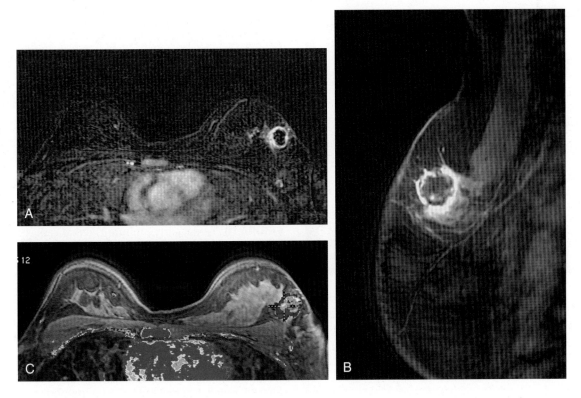

FIGURE 8.   Third breast MRI, obtained at the conclusion of neoadjuvant chemotherapy (four cycles of AC and four cycles of Taxotere), shows a waxing and waning, mixed response. Despite improvement seen after the four cycles of AC, this study shows recurrence of the cystic component, with overall increase in size resulting. In addition, angiogenesis is demonstrable from the nodular rim of the mass. **A,** Axial enhanced, subtracted view of the left IDC shows a change in appearance, with reaccumulation of cyst fluid. The rim is thick, nodular, and irregular. **B,** Sagittal, enhanced, subtracted view of the same for correlation. The enhancing rim is not smooth, but nodular and variable in thickness. **C,** Color kinetic map also shows interval change. A region of interest has been placed on the nodular medial component (colored *yellow*).

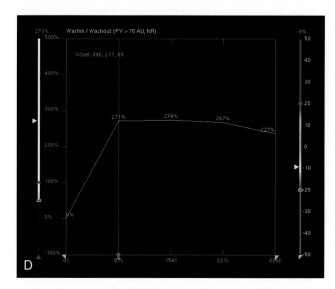

FIGURE 8, cont'd   D, Curve (signal intensity–time curve) shows intense early enhancement with plateauing.

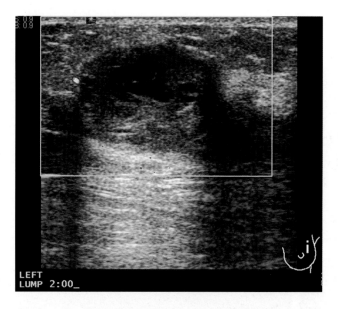

FIGURE 9.   Final ultrasound, obtained at the conclusion of neoadjuvant chemotherapy, also reflects the waxing and waning variable appearance of this tumor. Partial reaccumulation of a cystic component is seen, with persistent solid tissue peripherally and vascularity.

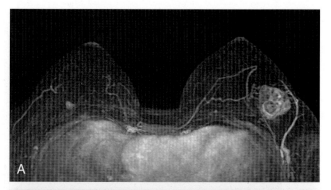

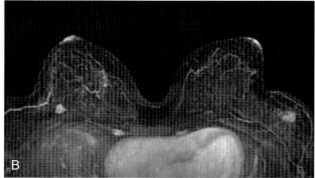

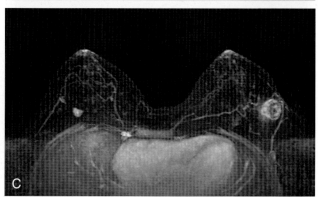

FIGURE 10.   Axial early (minute 1) enhanced, subtracted, maximal intensity projection images from the dynamic series of three breast MRIs, for comparison. **A,** At initial diagnosis, before neoadjuvant chemotherapy. The dominant left lateral IDC is large relative to the patient's overall breast size. A lobular, biopsy-proven fibroadenoma is seen in the posterior right lateral breast against the pectoral muscle. **B,** Midway through chemotherapy, after four cycles of AC, the left breast IDC appears considerably improved. An early, enhancing 1-cm component is seen, with a stable appearance of the known right breast fibroadenoma. **C,** Final breast MRI, after four cycles of AC and four cycles of Taxotere, shows regrowth of the left IDC on Taxotere, partly because of reaccumulation of cyst fluid. The overall mass is still smaller than the pretreatment baseline. The right fibroadenoma is unchanged.

with both cystic and solid components? Options to consider include excision, cyst aspiration under ultrasound guidance, core needle biopsy with ultrasound guidance or some combination, as was performed here. Considerations at the time of image-guided sampling include whether and in which order to sample the fluid and the solid components. In this case, the solid component was sampled with 14-gauge core needle biopsy technique, followed by aspiration of the fluid, which was bloody. If aspiration was performed first, many advocate stopping the aspiration before completion if bloody fluid is obtained, with consideration of placing a marker clip if there is no visible residual. Aspiration alone with cytologic evaluation of the fluid runs the risk of a false-negative result, indicating the need for sampling of the solid component.

Performance of bilateral breast MRI effectively screens the opposite breast for cancer, but as in this case, runs the risk of identifying additional findings that may or may not be significant and that may engender additional workups and biopsies. Here, the right breast MRI findings were suggestive of a fibroadenoma, and an ultrasound correlate with a corresponding appearance is also consistent with that diagnosis, as was subsequently proved by biopsy.

This case also demonstrated a waxing and waning response to neoadjuvant chemotherapy. The initial response to AC was encouraging, but repeat imaging after completion of four cycles of Taxotere showed evidence of regrowth. There was nevertheless an overall decline in the size of the mass, making the patient a better candidate for breast conservation, which was successfully achieved with lumpectomy to clear margins.

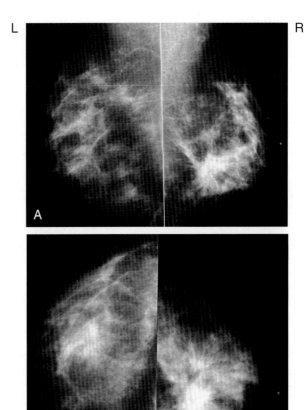

FIGURE 1. Mammograms [MLO (**A**) and CC (**B**)] obtained for evaluation of a palpable lump and nipple retraction on the right (marked) show a spiculated dominant mass behind the nipple.

CASE 12

LABC, unresponsive to neoadjuvant chemotherapy

A 46-year-old premenopausal woman presented with a palpable periareolar lump for 1 month, with nipple retraction. Mammography identified a 2- to 3-cm spiculated mass at 6 o'clock (Figure 1), and ultrasound showed a corresponding shadowing 2.1-cm mass (Figure 2). Ultrasound-guided core needle biopsy confirmed invasive carcinoma with tubular and lobular features.

Breast MRI showed the mass to be even larger than previously suspected, with the maximal dimension estimated to be 6 cm (Figure 3). Initial surgical assessment was that the patient was probably not a suitable breast conservation candidate because of the size of the palpable lump and prox-

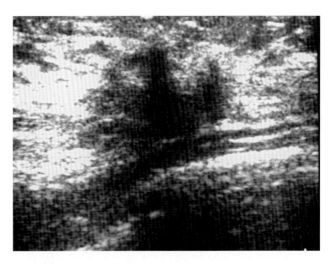

FIGURE 2. Ultrasound of the right palpable lump shows a highly suspicious corresponding mass: shadowing, hypoechoic, with irregular margins and disruption of the normal breast architecture.

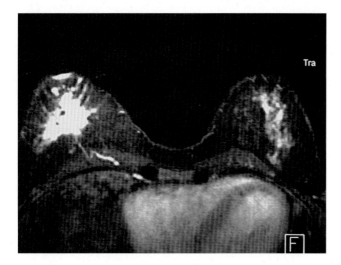

FIGURE 3.   Prechemotherapy breast MRI shows a large, dominant, intensely enhancing spiculated central right breast mass.

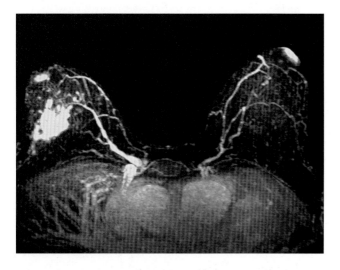

FIGURE 4.   Repeat breast MRI (maximal intensity projection view), 5 months later after neoadjuvant chemotherapy, shows little change, with a persistent, large, intensely enhancing residual mass.

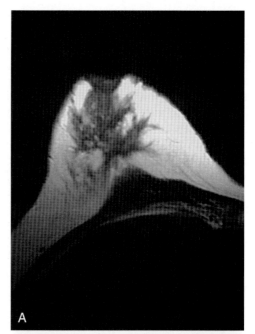

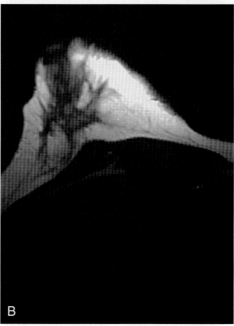

FIGURE 5.   Axial T2-weighted images from the prechemotherapy (**A**) and postchemotherapy (**B**) breast MRI show hypointense architectural distortion and mass, little changed over the two examinations.

imity to the nipple. However, the patient desired an attempt at lumpectomy, and opted for neo-adjuvant chemotherapy. After four cycles of chemotherapy with doxorubicin (Adriamycin) and cyclophosphamide (Cytoxan) (AC), imaging re-evaluation with breast MRI was obtained. Only a modest response was noted, with the maximal dimension of the persistent spiculated mass esti-mated at 4.5 cm. Repeat breast MRI, 2 months later after three cycles of docetaxel (Taxotere), showed no change, with a persistent, intensely enhancing residual 4.5-cm mass (Figures 4, 5, and 6). By phy-sical examination, the mass size was estimated at 2 cm. Mastectomy was again recommended,

and declined. Following ultrasound-guided needle localization, a lumpectomy was performed. The specimen contained a 3.3-cm mixed infiltrating ductal carcinoma (IDC) with ductal and lobular features, estrogen receptor positive, progesterone receptor negative, and *HER-2/neu* negative. The medial margin was positive, and multiple addi-tional margins were close. One of two lymph nodes was positive, with a 2-mm focus of tumor.

Subsequent mastectomy showed two microscopic foci of IDC (largest, 2 mm) and negative margins. Right chest wall, supraclavicular, and peripheral lymphatics were radiated subsequently. The patient was started on tamoxifen, which was not well tolerated, and switched to anastrozole (Arimidex) and subsequently to exemestane (Aromasin). No evidence of recurrence has been identified 2.5 years after diagnosis.

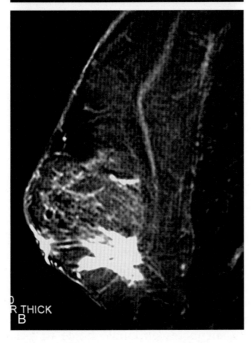

FIGURE 6. Enhanced subtracted sagittal views, prechemotherapy (**A**) and postchemotherapy (**B**), show little change.

TEACHING POINTS

Not every patient responds to neoadjuvant chemotherapy with significant tumor shrinkage, as this case illustrates. Approximately 70% to 75% of patients do respond. There is prognostic information portended by the response to chemotherapy, with patients with large residual masses like this having significantly poorer prognoses than those who respond well.

CASE 13

Rapidly progressive inflammatory breast cancer, unresponsive to chemotherapy

A 79-year-old woman with a prior history of recurrent renal cell carcinoma (RCC) noted a left breast mass while traveling abroad. She had a breast ultrasound while overseas, which confirmed a breast mass. Biopsy was recommended, which the patient deferred until after her trip. On her return, she underwent an abdominal and pelvic CT scan for surveillance for recurrent RCC (she had had two recurrences previously resected).

The CT scan showed a large, dominant, enhancing, irregularly marginated mass in the left breast, which was a dramatic change from a CT scan performed 4 months before (Figures 1 and 2). Palpation-guided core needle biopsy confirmed an infiltrating ductal carcinoma (IDC), estrogen receptor and progesterone receptor negative, *HER-2/neu* negative. Periareolar erythema was noted, as well as palpable axillary lymph nodes. Chemotherapy was started. While receiving chemotherapy, a bone scan was obtained to evaluate right shoulder and forearm pain. Although no findings particularly suggestive of bony metastases were seen, the large left breast cancer was visualized (Figure 3).

Three months later, after four cycles of doxorubicin (Adriamycin) and cyclophosphamide (Cytoxan) (AC) with little clinical improvement, a repeat CT scan was obtained (Figure 4). This showed the left breast mass to be little changed,

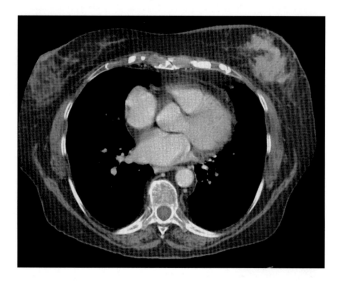

FIGURE 1. Enhanced abdominal CT image shows a large, dominant, irregularly shaped, enhancing mass in the left breast. Left breast skin is thickened as well.

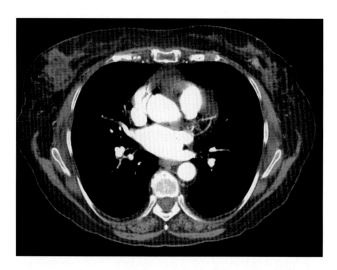

FIGURE 2. Comparison with a chest CT from 4 months before shows dramatic interval change. In retrospect, a small enhancing mass can be suspected in the same region. The skin appears normal.

with worsening of skin thickening and enhancement. Progressive axillary and internal mammary adenopathy was noted.

Docetaxel (Taxotere) was administered. After three cycles, worsened erythema and induration were noted. A breast MRI was obtained to more accurately assess the extent of disease (Figures 5 and 6). A skin biopsy was obtained, showing multifocal intralymphatic carcinoma. Palliative radiation therapy was administered for local control.

Toward the end of radiation, the patient developed right upper quadrant pain. CT scan showed innumerable new hypovascular liver metastases (Figure 7). The patient died less than a month later, 7 months after the inflammatory breast cancer (IBC) diagnosis.

TEACHING POINTS

Inflammatory breast cancers (IBCs) are rare and represent about 1% of breast cancers. Primary IBC is aggressive, with a poor prognosis, and should be differentiated from locally advanced breast cancers secondarily involving the skin and inducing inflammatory changes. In this case, we have a rare imaging window through which we can see just how rapidly such an aggressive tumor can grow. Over a 4-month period, we have CT documentation of dramatic growth of a dominant mass and development of skin thickening. A rapid onset of the characteristic clinical features of swelling, warmth, edema, and erythema has been emphasized in many descriptions of IBC. If the clinical features are suggestive enough, the diagnosis is made clinically. Skin biopsy will usually confirm tumor in dermal lymphatics, the pathologic hallmark of IBC, although demonstration of this is not required to make the diagnosis. The American Joint Committee on Cancer (AJCC) *Staging Manual* classifies IBC as a T4d tumor (involving the skin), which is stage III. The patient should display the clinical features of IBC and have biopsy-proven breast cancer either in the breast parenchyma or dermal lymphatics.

The underlying tumor is most commonly a poorly differentiated IDC, but the clinical syndrome of IBC can be associated with any histologic subtype of invasive breast cancer. There may or may not be an identifiable tumor mass on imaging. In some cases, the breast is diffusely infiltrated by tumor without forming a discrete mass.

Once the diagnosis is established, systemic staging studies should be obtained to survey for metastatic disease. In this case, body CT and bone scans were obtained. PET (especially PET/CT) is probably the single best modality choice for whole-body assessment for distant metastases, but ideally is used to complement information derived from enhanced body CT and bone scans.

CT is an unconventional choice to assess the response to neoadjuvant chemotherapy for breast cancer. In this case, this patient had a long-standing history of an indolent, multiply recurrent

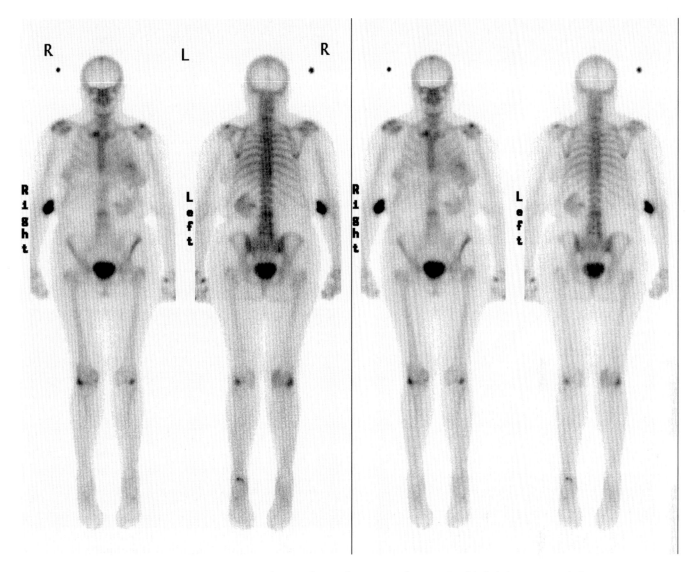

FIGURE 3.   Bone scan images show right nephrectomy changes. Multiple joint-centered sites of arthritic and degenerative change are seen. An upper lumbar band of activity correlated with discogenic changes on x-ray and CT. The left breast shows a diffuse increase in activity, whereas the right shows a physiologic pattern of mild breast tissue uptake.

RCC, for which she was regularly followed with CT. (Her initial diagnosis of RCC was 15 years before, with surgically resected regional recurrences 5 and 2 years before.) The choice of CT to follow this patient's chemotherapy response presumably reflects her oncologist's familiarity with CT, as well as that the IBC was large and well seen on CT. CT does allow evaluation of regional nodal basins well, with the evaluation directed to detection of interval change and the presence or absence of nodes, and assessment of their size, shape, and density. In some nodal basins, like the internal mammaries, normal lymph nodes are not routinely seen, and so

visualization of any lymph nodes is suspicious. In other regions, such as the axilla, normal lymph nodes are routinely visualized, and so the assessment is based more on comparison with the opposite side for asymmetry, such as an abnormally increased number of visualized nodes, disproportionately sized nodes (even if not clearly "enlarged"), or nodes with abnormal morphology (rounded, enlarged, effaced fatty hilus, fuzzy margins).

IBC is aggressive and confers a poor prognosis. This patient had no appreciable response to chemotherapy, and clinically progressed while receiv-

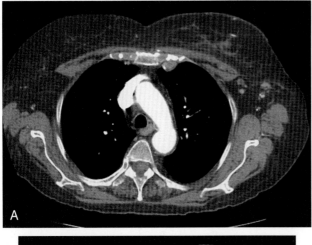

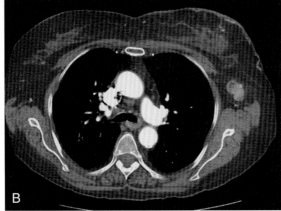

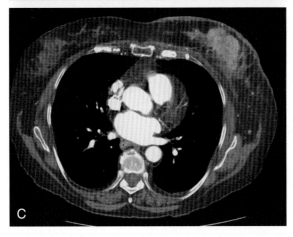

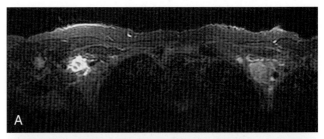

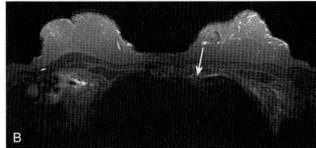

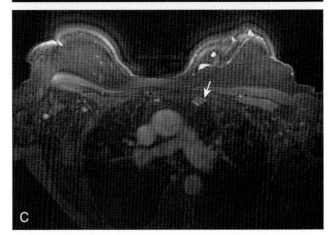

FIGURE 5.   Breast MRI showed multiple abnormally enlarged lymph nodes. **A,** Axial STIR through the axilla shows a markedly enlarged, rounded, 3-cm left axillary level II (under the pectoralis minor muscle) lymph node. **B,** Axial STIR image shows a left internal mammary lymph node, which displaces the internal mammary vessels posteriorly (*arrow*). **C,** Fat-saturated, enhanced, T1-weighted, gradient echo image (unsubtracted) also shows the enlarged left internal mammary lymph node, posteriorly displacing the vessels (*arrow*).

FIGURE 4.   Repeat CT scan, 3 months after Figure 1 and after four cycles of AC chemotherapy (**A** to **C,** from above to below). **A,** Four mildly prominent (more notable for increased number and asymmetry than size) left axillary lymph nodes are seen, as well as a pathologically enlarged left internal mammary lymph node. **B,** A pathologically enlarged left axillary lymph node is seen at this level. Note diffuse increase in reticulation and density of the left breast and left breast skin thickening. **C,** The dominant enhancing left breast mass is still bulky, and there is pronounced increased skin thickening and enhancement.

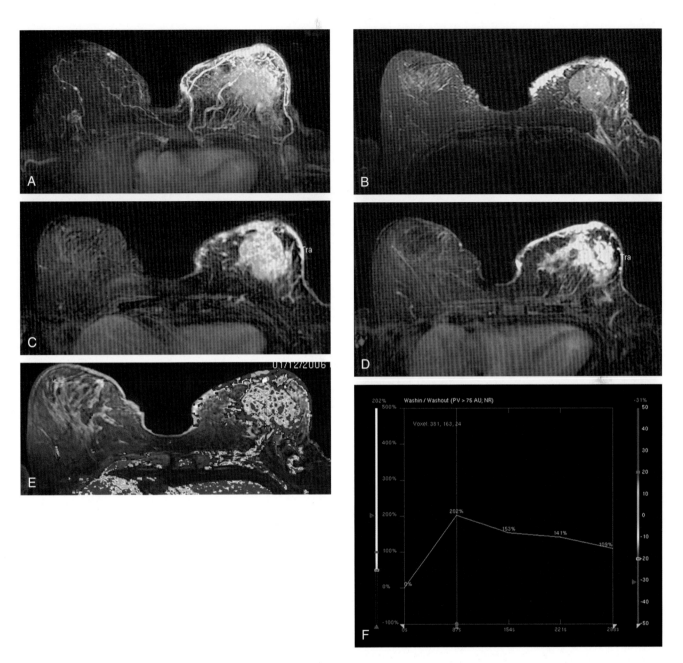

FIGURE 6. Breast MRIs show the extensive left IBC. **A,** Axial enhanced subtracted maximal intensity projection view. The left breast is occupied by an intensely enhancing dominant mass, with diffuse skin enhancement and multiple enlarged draining veins. **B,** Axial STIR through the dominant mass, showing the marked skin thickening and edema, as well as the diffuse reticulation and edema of the breast, especially laterally. **C,** Enhanced, subtracted, dynamic, T1-weighted, gradient echo image showing the intense enhancement of the round, more discrete mass component of this IBC. The thickened skin also enhanced intensely. **D,** Inferior to **C,** the mass is less well defined. The skin thickening and enhancement are even more pronounced in the inferior breast. **E,** DynaCAD color map of the enhancement shows multiple regions colored *red,* indicating washout. **F,** Accompanying graph (signal intensity change–time curve) shows rapid uptake, and subsequent decline, reflecting arteriovenous shunting (washout).

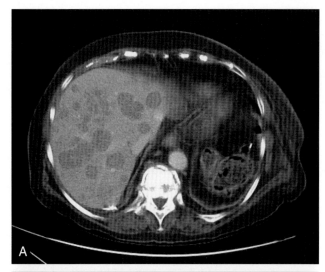

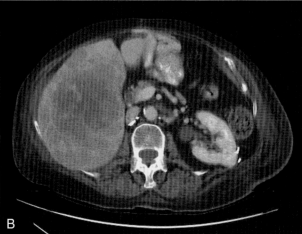

FIGURE 7.   Enhanced abdominal CT scans (**A** above **B**), obtained to evaluate new right upper quadrant pain, show innumerable hypovascular liver metastases, new from a CT scan 4 months before.

ing it. Liver metastases were a late, terminal development in the rapid course of this patient's disease. IBC patients who do respond to primary systemic therapy (neoadjuvant chemotherapy) are generally then treated with mastectomy and postoperative radiation therapy to the chest wall and regional node basins.

SUGGESTED READING

Cristofanilli M, Buzdar AU, Hortobágyi GN. Update on the management of inflammatory breast cancer. *Oncologist* 2003; 8:141–148.

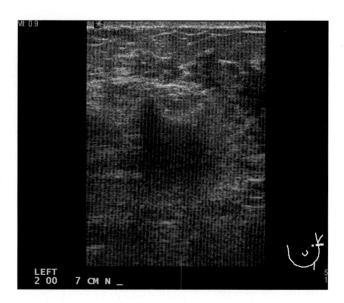

FIGURE 1.   Sonography of the left upper outer quadrant at the site of the palpable lump shows a highly suspicious mass: very hypoechoic, with angular margins.

CASE 14

LABC, good response by imaging to neoadjuvant chemotherapy, but significant residual pathologic disease; imaging-guided tailored lumpectomy

A 41-year-old woman noted a left breast lump after rolling over in bed. A palpable mass was confirmed by her primary care physician. Clinical estimates of the size of the mass were on the order of 4 cm, or a T2 lesion. Palpation-guided sampling of the abnormality by surgery did not yield a definitive diagnosis. Subsequent breast imaging workup with mammography and ultrasound confirmed a highly suspicious mass on both, accompanied by suspicious, enlarged axillary lymph nodes (Figures 1, 2, and 3). By ultrasound, the mass measured up to 3.5 cm. Ultrasound-guided biopsy of the breast mass proved the lesion to be grade 6/9 invasive ductal carcinoma (IDC), estrogen receptor and progesterone receptor positive, *HER-2/neu* negative. Sonogram-guided axillary node fine-needle aspiration showed cancer of breast primary origin.

The patient desired breast conservation. Because of the large size of her mass, neoadjuvant chemotherapy was planned in hopes of shrinking the tumor and improving the cosmetic outcome. Her staging evaluation was completed with enhanced body CT scans, positron emission tomography (PET)/CT, and breast MRI. The breast MRI showed a much larger lesion than suspected previously, measuring 9.5 × 4 cm, occupying much of left lateral breast (Figure 4). The dominant mass

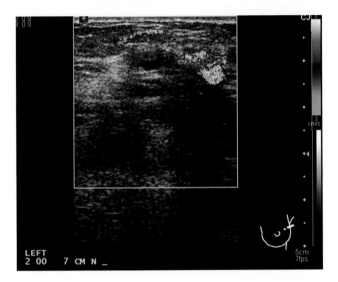

FIGURE 2. Adjacent to the discrete mass depicted in Figure 1 was a less well-defined area of abnormal echotexture with shadowing and increased vascularity.

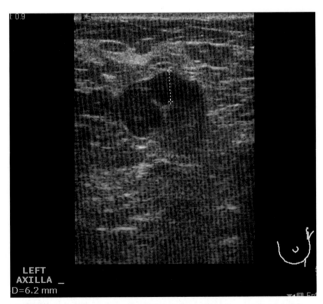

FIGURE 3. Ultrasound of the left axilla showed a highly suspicious appearance of this lymph node: the fatty hilus is partially effaced, with mass effect on it from cortical nodules. The cortical thickness is abnormal, measuring 6 mm.

consisted of multiple contiguous components, which enhanced intensely, with washout.

PET scans showed the dominant left breast cancer to be hypermetabolic and accompanied by multiple metabolically active axillary lymph nodes, as well as subtle evidence of probable supraclavicular uptake in small lymph nodes (Figures 5, 6, and 7). No distant metastases were found by CT or PET.

Neoadjuvant chemotherapy, consisting of four cycles of doxorubicin (Adriamycin) plus cyclophosphamide (Cytoxan) (AC) and four cycles of docetaxel (Taxotere), was given. The patient's response was assessed halfway through chemotherapy with repeat breast MRI (Figure 8). A response to chemotherapy was seen, with shrinkage of the tumor to 6.2 × 2.9 cm, with less intense enhancement. The

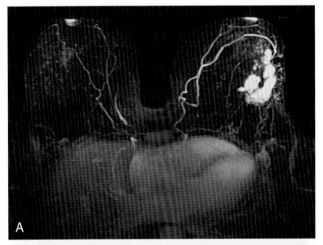

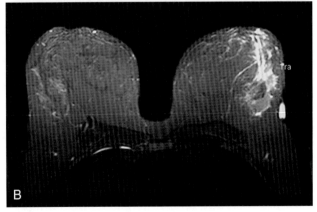

FIGURE 4. Breast MRI was obtained to assess the local extent at initial diagnosis. **A,** Axial maximal intensity projection (MIP) view of the enhanced data set shows an intensely enhancing, large left lateral breast cancer, with contiguous irregular masses. **B,** Axial STIR shows the largest, posterior palpable component to be minimally hyperintense, with brighter peritumoral edema extending anteriorly in a segmental distribution toward the nipple.

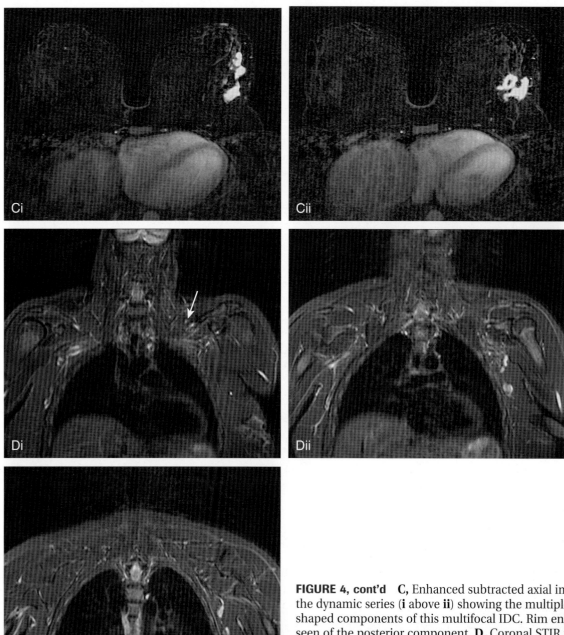

FIGURE 4, cont'd **C,** Enhanced subtracted axial images from the dynamic series (**i** above **ii**) showing the multiple irregularly shaped components of this multifocal IDC. Rim enhancement is seen of the posterior component. **D,** Coronal STIR images of the thorax, obtained with the body coil (**i** to **iii,** from anterior to posterior), showing: **i,** a small, sub-centimeter left supraclavicular lymph node (*arrow*); **ii,** mildly enlarged, asymmetrical left axillary adenopathy; and **iii,** additional suspicious left axillary nodes.

pattern of enhancement also changed, with no washout seen and an overall plateauing enhancement pattern. Restaging studies with ultrasound and breast MRI at the conclusion of chemotherapy showed further improvement (Figures 9 and 10A). On ultrasound, a residual 7-mm mass could be identified. On MRI, there was further contraction of the mass. It still showed an elongated configuration, and now measured 5.8 × 1 cm. The intensity and quality of the enhancement also had improved,

with progressive and less intense enhancement only.

Breast conservation had been planned. A clip was placed into the small residual mass seen by ultrasound (see Figures 10B and C). Based on correlation with MRI, it seemed unlikely that localization of this one component would result in clear margins without additional guidance. Accordingly, clips were placed under MRI guidance at the anterior and posterior extremes of the residual enhance-

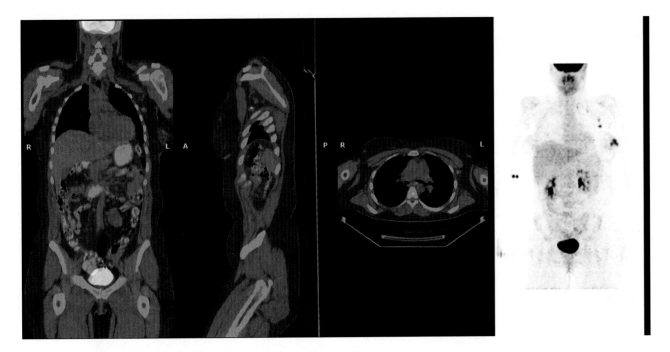

FIGURE 5.   PET/CT images in three planes, with volumetric data on the right displayed in the coronal projection, show the left breast IDC to be hypermetabolic. Hypermetabolism is also seen in axillary lymph nodes.

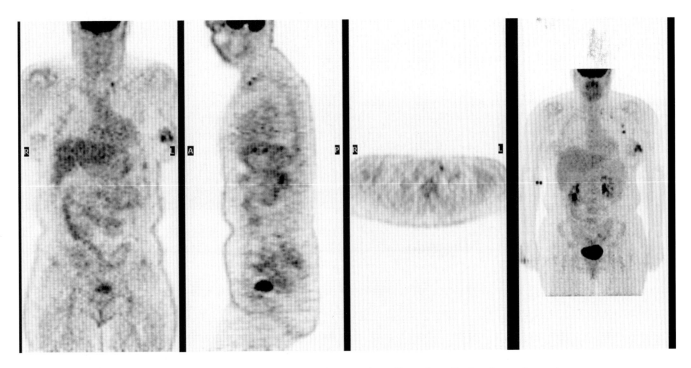

FIGURE 6.   PET scans in three planes, with intensity adjusted to display fluorodeoxyglucose (FDG) uptake in a small left supraclavicular lymph node, as well as in the left breast and axilla.

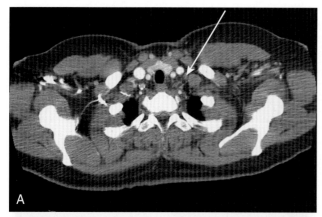

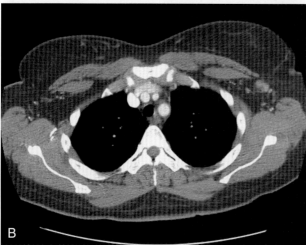

FIGURE 7. Enhanced chest CT scans for correlation with PET. **A,** A sub-centimeter left supraclavicular lymph node is seen posterolateral to the jugular vein (*arrow*). **B,** An enlarged enhancing left axillary lymph node has too many "normal"-sized companion nodes.

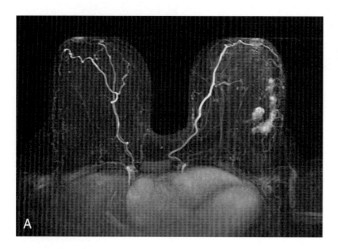

FIGURE 8. Repeat breast MRI, 3 months after diagnosis, after four cycles of AC chemotherapy. **A,** Axial MIP (compare to Figure 4A) shows marked reduction in volume and intensity of enhancement of the multifocal IDC.

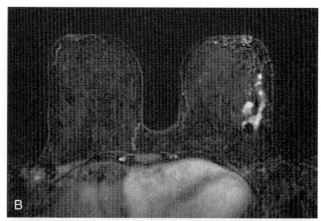

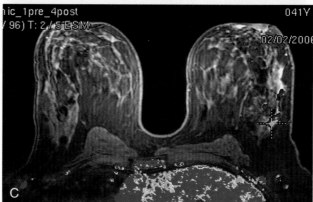

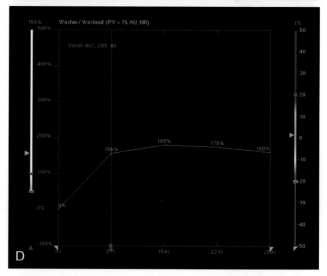

FIGURE 8, cont'd **B,** Enhanced, subtracted, axial image from the dynamic series (compare with Figure 4C) shows contraction of the mass, which is reduced to a beaded irregularly shaped residual. **C,** DynaCAD color map of the enhancement, with a region of interest placed on the posterior enhancing component. **D,** Graphical display of this kinetic data (change in signal intensity–time curve) shows a plateauing pattern of enhancement.

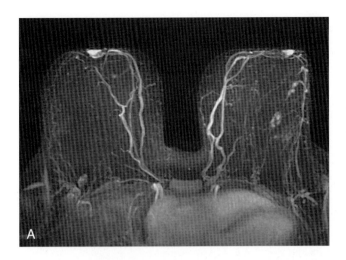
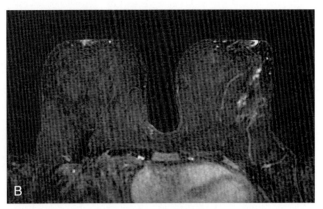

FIGURE 9. Third breast MRI, obtained two additional months later, after completion of four cycles of Taxotere: **A,** Axial MIP view (compare with Figures 4A and 8A) shows clumped residual foci of enhancement in the left lateral breast. The MRI appearance is much improved. **B,** Enhanced, subtracted, axial image from the dynamic series (compare with Figures 4C and 8B) shows clusters of clumped foci of enhancement. Only progressive enhancement was now identified.

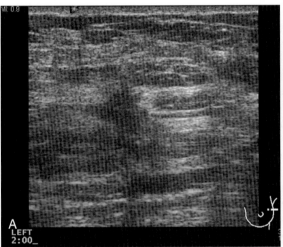
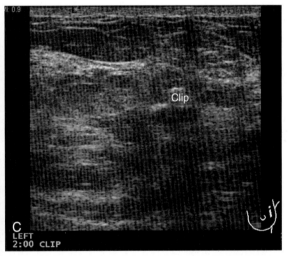

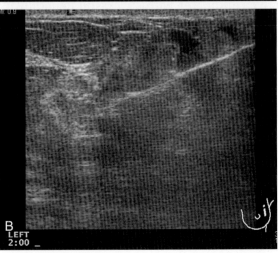

FIGURE 10. Breast ultrasound, after completion of neoadjuvant chemotherapy, 6 months after the study in Figure 1. **A,** The smaller, hypoechoic residual mass, now measuring 7 mm, continues to show angular margination. **B,** Under ultrasound guidance, a clip is placed to mark the residual mass. The needle can be seen traversing the mass from the right. **C,** After clip deployment, the hyperechoic clip can be seen against the background of the hypoechoic residual mass. Care needs to be taken to try to deploy ultrasound-placed clips where they will contrast with more hypoechoic tissue to aid in their visualization.

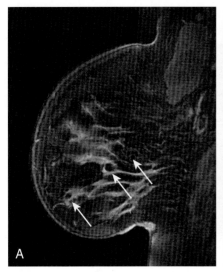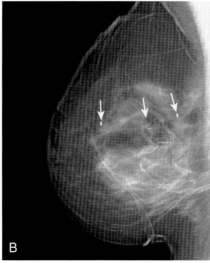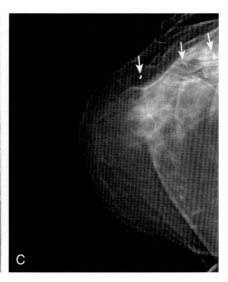

FIGURE 11.   Images after MRI-guided clip placement. **A,** Sagittal, fat-saturated, enhanced image shows three foci of susceptibility in a line (*arrows*). The largest, in the middle, is from the ultrasound-placed clip. Anterior and posterior to it are seen smaller foci of susceptibility demarcating the anteroposterior extent of the residual enhancement. **B,** Post-MRI clip placement digital mammogram in the lateral projection shows a line of three clips in the upper breast (*arrows*). **C,** CC view of the three clips in the lateral breast, confirming successful clip deployment.

ment (Figure 11). These were needle-localized by placement of two localizing wires in proximity to the MRI-placed clips (Figure 12).

The pathology showed a greater than 5 cm IDC with extensive angiolymphatic invasion at multiple positive margins. By gross, the residual mass measured 4.5 cm in maximal dimension. Numerous small clusters of malignant cells were noted to extend distant from the main mass, including at the margins, but there was no gross tumor involvement of margins. Six of 12 lymph nodes contained metastatic carcinoma, with several foci larger than 2 mm. Additional surgery was considered, but because the positive margins were due to lymphangitic tumor, it seemed unlikely there would be benefit from additional surgery.

Radiation therapy to the breast and peripheral lymphatics was administered subsequently, and the patient began tamoxifen.

TEACHING POINTS

Clinical breast exam, mammography, and ultrasound all have known limitations in accurately predicting the size and extent of breast cancers. In a correlation study with mastectomy specimens by Boetes and colleagues, MRI was demonstrated to be more accurate than mammography or ultrasound in predicting extent of breast cancer.

This IDC mass was much bigger than suspected based on clinical exam or conventional breast imaging. It clearly meets the criteria to be classified as a locally advanced breast cancer (LABC), based on size greater than 5 cm and also by suspected supraclavicular node involvement. LABC is advanced, nonmetastatic breast cancer, based on any of these criteria: size greater than 5 cm, skin or chest wall involvement, fixed or matted axillary lymphadenopathy, or ipsilateral supraclavicular, infraclavicular, or internal mammary adenopathy.

Patients with LABC may be candidates for neoadjuvant chemotherapy given preoperatively to reduce their tumor size. Patients who are initially inoperable, even by mastectomy, may become operative candidates with successful neoadjuvant chemotherapy. Some patients who would be mastectomy candidates may be converted into suitable breast conservation candidates.

Not all breast cancers respond to neoadjuvant chemotherapy. To identify those patients who are not responding and may benefit from a change in therapeutic approach, both clinical and imaging monitoring is performed periodically during neoadjuvant chemotherapy. Here again, breast MRI has been shown to be the most accurate of the current breast imaging techniques in assessing responses to treatment. Although better than mammography and ultrasound, breast MRI is not perfect and can both under- and overestimate the amount of residual disease. Even patients with complete

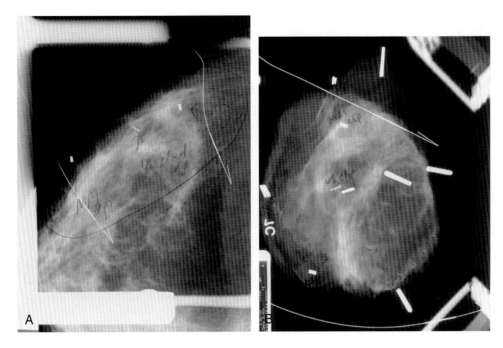

FIGURE 12. Images from the needle localization procedure. **A,** CC view. Two hook wires have been placed from a lateral approach on either side of the clips placed under MRI guidance. The ultrasound-placed clip projects in the center of the localized area. **B,** Specimen radiography shows all three clips. A spiculated mass is in the center, with the ultrasound-placed clip adjacent.

imaging responses may have microscopic disease at histology. Patients like this, with what appeared to be an excellent response by MRI, can still have a significant disease burden. In this case, the actual dimension of the measured residual enhancement correlated fairly well with the maximal dimension of the residual mass at partial mastectomy.

Neoadjuvant chemotherapy can in some patients produce complete resolution of the imaging findings. For this reason, clip placement should be considered during biopsy of large masses, which might be considered for neoadjuvant treatment. This could save a patient a return visit for just this purpose.

In this case, it is clear that ultrasound severely underestimated the extent of this patient's cancer and that localization of the small residual mass seen by ultrasound would have been doomed to positive margins. As it happens, even the valiant attempt made to obtain clear margins with MRI-guided clip placement was also doomed, owing to extensive angiolymphatic involvement, which clearly was underestimated by MRI. This result is not surprising, given that this is essentially microscopic disease.

Clearly, this patient is at high risk for recurrence, and the hope is that radiation therapy will treat the microscopic disease that remains. Fortunately, the tumor is strongly estrogen receptor positive, so hormonal therapy with tamoxifen will be an important line of defense for this high-risk patient.

SUGGESTED READINGS

Boetes C, Mus RD, Holland R, et al. Breast tumors: comparative accuracy of MR imaging relative to mammography and US for demonstrating extent. *Radiology* 1995; 197:743–747.

Dash N, Chafin SH, Johnson RR, et al. Usefulness of tissue marker clips in patients undergoing neoadjuvant chemotherapy for breast cancer. *AJR Am J Roentgenol* 1999; 173:911–917.

Rosen EL, Blackwell KL, Baker JA, et al. Accuracy of MRI in the detection of residual breast cancer after neoadjuvant chemotherapy. *AJR Am J Roentgenol* 2003; 181:1275–1282.

Yeh E, Slanetz P, Kopans DB, et al. Prospective comparison of mammography, sonography, and MRI in patients undergoing neoadjuvant chemotherapy for palpable breast cancer. *AJR Am J Roentgenol* 2005; 184:868–877.

Imaging Surveillance for Locally Recurrent Disease

Effective palliative, as well as curative, treatment is now available for patients with recurrent breast cancer. Optimal therapy is dependent on an accurate assessment of the location and extent of recurrent disease, which dramatically influences treatment decision making. Gene expression analysis has been used to identify patients at increased risk for distant recurrence.[1,2] There is also the suggestion that expression profiling may be helpful in identifying patients at greater risk for local recurrence.[3] This information can potentially be used to tailor the frequency and types of imaging modalities used to monitor these patients.

Most often, the imaging assessment of recurrent disease extent requires use of both anatomic modalities, such as mammography, ultrasound, CT, and MRI, and molecular or metabolic imaging, utilizing positron emission tomography (PET) or combination PET/CT. While fluorodeoxyglucose (FDG) PET is a highly accurate method for evaluating the whole body for recurrence (both local and distant), anatomic and molecular imaging should be viewed as complementary. Hathaway and associates demonstrated the value of combining PET with MRI nearly a decade ago.[4]

The superb spatial resolution of CT and MRI is of great value in defining the size, shape, and precise location of suspected metastases, whether locoregional or distant. However, anatomically based imaging modalities may be suboptimal in separating active tumor from treatment-related changes. FDG PET can be very helpful in this situation. Additionally, whole-body PET can often change a patient's stage; confirmation of local recurrence only may direct the treating physician toward a more aggressive, curative-intent approach (e.g., surgery, localized radiation, or both). One study showed that FDG PET changed the clinical stage in 36% of patients and led to a change in therapy in 58%.[5]

As with any tumor, knowledge of the typical biologic behavior and predictable sites of recurrence is helpful in focusing attention on specific regions. In patients treated with mastectomy, axillary node dissection, and chemotherapy, the most frequent sites of locoregional recurrence are the chest wall and supraclavicular nodes.[6] Remote sites may include the mediastinum, internal mammary nodes, and most commonly, the skeleton.[7]

The following sites deserve comment with respect to appropriate imaging modalities for identification and characterization of disease recurrences: locoregional, brachial plexus, chest, bone, and distant metastases.

LOCOREGIONAL

Locoregional recurrence may occur in up to 22% of patients undergoing breast conservation surgery and radiation.[8] Breast cancer 10-year local recurrence rates in women with negative surgical margins who undergo lumpectomy and radiotherapy may be as low as 10% or less.[9–12] Although overall recurrence rates are low, higher recurrence rates have been reported in select patient groups, such as those with high-grade ductal carcinoma in situ (DCIS).[13] In addition, recurrence rates in younger women and in women who do not undergo radiation therapy have been reported as high as 35%.[14]

Despite the increasing utilization of accelerated partial breast irradiation, the long-term impact on recurrence rate for these newer techniques compared with whole breast irradiation is currently unknown. These techniques include interstitial radiotherapy with a multicatheter approach, intraoperative radiotherapy (IORT), using either electrons produced by linear accelerators or 50-kV x-rays (Intrabeam), the balloon-catheter technique (MammoSite), or three-dimensional conformal external-beam radiotherapy.

Serial surveillance mammography, as well as diagnostic mammography when there is clinical suspicion of breast recurrence, remains the cornerstone of the imaging approach to previously treated breast cancer patients (Figure 1). Complementary studies include breast ultrasound and MRI, as discussed in Chapter 3 (Figures 2 and 3). Cases presented in this chapter illustrate the spectrum of imaging manifestations of locally recurrent breast cancer.

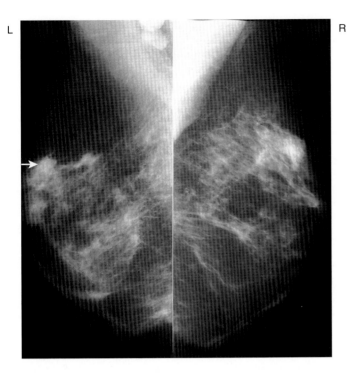

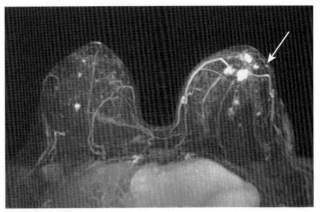

FIGURE 3. Contrast-enhanced axial breast MRI maximal intensity projection view of the same patient shows multiple intensely enhancing masses in the left subareolar region (*arrow*). Multifocal infiltrating ductal carcinoma was confirmed at subsequent mastectomy.

FIGURE 1. Bilateral mediolateral oblique (MLO) mammograms, obtained in a 57-year-old woman 9 months after a pathologic diagnosis of DCIS was made from the right side of bilateral reduction mammoplasty specimens. New left supra-areolar masses are indicated by the *arrow*, and increased size and density were noted of left axillary lymph nodes.

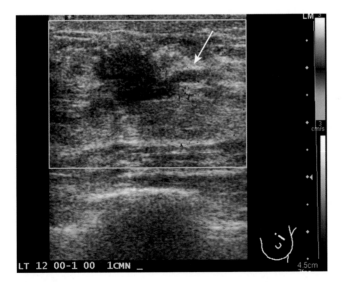

FIGURE 2. Ultrasound of the same patient in Figure 1 shows one of multiple solid masses identified by ultrasound. This mass has particularly suspicious sonographic features: it is solid and irregularly marginated with no definable capsule, and a tail of suspected ductal extension can be seen extending to the right (*arrow*).

Local failure most commonly occurs in or near the lumpectomy bed, in the same quadrant, and may manifest in a manner similar to the initial presentation (e.g., microcalcifications developing where calcified DCIS has previously been treated). Such changes arising in a lumpectomy bed under surveillance need careful analysis, such as with magnification views, to differentiate from similar-appearing, treatment-related changes (e.g., calcification due to fat necrosis). In some cases, differentiation based on morphology may not be possible, and tissue sampling will be required.

In general, surgical scars are expected to contract over time. Post–partial mastectomy scars should be carefully scrutinized on follow-up mammograms for increased size or density, which may signify recurrent disease. Scar enhancement can be expected on MRI in the first year after surgery and radiation therapy, but should decline in intensity over time, and little enhancement should be seen by about 18 months after treatment. More than 18 months after breast conservation therapy, MRI can be very helpful in differentiating postoperative scarring from recurrence, with scars expected to show little, if any, enhancement, unlike most recurrent tumor masses.

Palpable lumps developing in the breast, axilla, or chest wall of a patient previously treated for breast cancer raise the specter of recurrent disease, but not infrequently are due to treatment-related mimics, such as fat necrosis masses. Depending on location, these can be evaluated with some combination of mammography, ultrasound, and tissue sampling. At times, such mimics are sufficiently characteristic that imaging alone can make the diagnosis, but histologic sampling may be necessary for confirmation.

Mammographic follow-up is warranted in patients who have undergone subcutaneous mastectomy because of the considerable amount of remaining breast tissue. The yield from mammographic surveillance of the breast after standard mastectomy or skin-sparing mastectomy and reconstruction has been questioned. Because most recurrences occur in the skin and subcutaneous tissues, they can usually be detected on physical examination. The overall annual recurrence rate of T1 or T2 tumors following mastectomy has been reported to be 1% to 2% during the first 5 years.[15] Annual mammographic evaluation following mastectomy and transverse rectus abdominis musculocutaneous (TRAM) flap reconstruction has been advocated to screen for any residual breast tissue and to detect recurrences before they are palpable.[16]

The timing for mammographic follow-up after breast conserving therapy has not been standardized. At a minimum, a 6-month follow-up mammogram should be performed to establish the patient's baseline after surgery. The incidence of a recurrence in the ipsilateral breast 20 years after surgery is 14.3% among women who undergo irradiation after lumpectomy and 39.2% among those who undergo lumpectomy without irradiation.[17]

Larger-field-of-view anatomic modalities, such as CT and MRI, are often more suitable to assess suspected chest wall or supraclavicular abnormalities. Because a growing number of patients with locally recurrent disease are being treated with curative intent, whole-body PET is recommended to confirm active tumor at sites identified as abnormal or suspicious with CT or MRI, and to search for distant metastases. Upstaging or downstaging may influence the choice of therapy.

BRACHIAL PLEXUS

Symptoms in the distribution of the brachial radial plexus may be due to recurrent tumor or the effects of therapy. MRI, combined with PET, offers the highest diagnostic yield. Whereas MRI provides exquisite anatomic detail, it may be unable to separate scarring and postoperative changes from tumor. PET, and more recently, PET/CT, improves specificity and, again, allows for a whole-body examination.

CHEST

Pathologic involvement of the internal mammary lymph nodes and mediastinal lymph nodes is best determined by PET.[18] Although both areas are evaluable by CT, reliance on size alone has been shown to be inferior to assessment of metabolic activity in patients with non–small cell lung cancer (histologic gold standard).[19] In one series of 73 patients, FDG PET was found to be twice as accurate as CT in identifying involved internal mammary or mediastinal nodes.[20]

BONE

Bone metastases are covered in depth in Chapter 8. Imaging options include plain radiographs, CT, MRI, nuclear medicine bone scans, and PET. Plain radiographs are readily available, are relatively inexpensive, expose the patient to a low level of radiation, require no patient preparation, and are completed rapidly. Typically, a minimum 30% reduction in bone mineralization is necessary before a radiograph becomes abnormal. Additionally, radiographs provide limited coverage. These factors reduce sensitivity both at the site of concern and for distant disease. Most commonly, bone radiographs are performed in an effort to improve the specificity of a nuclear bone scan. Even this function is being replaced by the utilization of CT or MRI for scintigraphic correlation. Both of these modalities dramatically improve diagnostic accuracy, compared with plain radiographs, in bone and surrounding soft tissue. However, the screening method of choice remains the nuclear medicine bone scan. It is a whole-body scan, delivers low radiation, and is exquisitely sensitive to changes in bone metabolism. PET and PET/CT utilizing F-18 FDG and sodium fluoride (NaF), are covered in greater detail in Chapter 8. Preliminary data suggest an advantage for PET over bone scintigraphy in the identification of skeletal metastases (especially lytic metastases). NaF, also a positron-emitting pharmaceutical, is a bone-specific agent, whereas FDG PET allows a whole-body (bone and soft tissue) evaluation.

DISTANT METASTASES

The confirmation and quantitation of distant metastases has both therapeutic and prognostic implications. Imagers are often asked to provide answers to the following questions: (1) Are distant metastases present? (2) Is the disease focal or widespread? (3) What are the prognostic implications? (4) In the absence of symptoms, with elevated serum tumor markers, where is the disease? Since the answers to questions 1 to 3 are applicable to most patients under investigation for recurrence, in many centers, PET has become the modality of choice to search for breast cancer metastases following initial therapy. Whole-body surveys have shown FDG PET to be both sensitive and specific for detection of distant disease.[19–22]

REFERENCES

1. van de Vijver MJ, He YD, van 't Veer LJ, et al. A gene-expression signature as a predictor of survival in breast cancer. *N Engl J Med* 2002; 347:1999–2009.

2. Paik S, Shak S, Tang G, et al. A multigene assay to predict recurrence of tamoxifen-treated, node-negative breast cancer. *N Engl J Med* 2004; 351:2817–2826.

3. Mamounas E, Tang G, Bryant J, et al. Association between the 21-gene recurrence score assay (RS) and risk of locoregional failure in node-negative, ER-positive breast cancer: results from NSABP B-14 and NSABP B-20 [abstract]. Presented at the San Antonio Breast Cancer Symposium 28th Annual Meeting, December 10, 2005.

4. Hathaway PB, Mankoff DA, Maravilla KR, et al. The value of combined FDG-PET and magnetic resonance imaging in the evaluation of suspected recurrent local-regional breast cancer: preliminary experience. *Radiology* 1998; 210(3):807–814.

5. Yap CS, Seltzer MA, Schiepers C, et al. Impact of whole-body 18-FDG PET on staging and managing patients with breast cancer; the referring physician's perspective. *J Nucl Med* 2001; 42(9):1334–1337.

6. Katz A, Strom EA, Bucholz TA, et al. Locoregional recurrence patterns after mastectomy and doxorubicin-based chemotherapy: implications for postoperative irradiation. *J Clin Oncol* 2000; 18:2817–2827.

7. Eubank WB, Mankoff DA. Current and future uses of positron emission tomography in breast cancer imaging. *Semin Nucl Med* 2004; 34(3):224–240.

8. Huston TL, Simmons RM. Locally recurrent breast cancer after conservation therapy. *Am J Surg* 2005; 189(2):229–235.

9. Smitt MC, Nowels KW, Zdeblick MJ, et al. The importance of the lumpectomy surgical margin status in long-term results of breast conservation. *Cancer* 1995; 76:259–267.

10. Neuschatz AC, DiPetrillo T, Safaii H, et al. Long-term follow-up of a prospective policy of margin-directed radiation dose escalation in breast-conserving therapy. *Cancer* 2003; 97:30–39.

11. Obedian E, Haffty BG. Negative margin status improves local control in conservatively managed breast cancer patients. *Cancer J Sci Am* 2000; 6:28–33.

12. Provenzano E, Hopper JL, Giles GG, et al. Histological markers that predict clinical recurrence in ductal carcinoma in situ of the breast: an Australian population-based study. *Pathology* 2004; 36:221–229.

13. Borg MF. Breast-conserving therapy in young women with invasive carcinoma of the breast. *Australas Radiol* 2004; 48:376–382.

14. Scott WJ, Gobar LS, Terry JD, et al. Mediastinal lymph node staging of nonsmall cell lung cancer: a prospective comparison of computed tomography and positron emission tomography. *J Thorac Cardiovasc Surg* 1996; 111(3):642–648.

15. Kroll SS, Schusterman MA, Tadjalli HE, et al. Risk of recurrence after treatment of early breast cancer with skin-sparing mastectomy. *Ann Surg Oncol* 1997; 4:193–197.

16. Helvie MA, Bailey JE, Roubidoux MA, et al. Mammographic screening of TRAM flap breast reconstructions for detection of nonpalpable recurrent cancer. *Radiology* 2002; 224:211–216.

17. Fisher B, Anderson S, Bryant J, et al. Twenty-year follow up of a randomized trial comparing total mastectomy, lumpectomy, and lumpectomy plus irradiation for the treatment of invasive breast cancer. *N Engl J Med* 2002; 347:1233–1241.

18. Eubank WB, Mankoff DA, Takasugi J, et al. [18]Fluorodeoxyglucose positron emission tomography to detect mediastinal or internal mammary metastases in breast cancer. *J Clin Oncol* 2001; 19(15):3516–3523.

19. Lonneux M, Borbath 1, Berliere M, et al. The place of whole-body PET/FDG for the diagnosis of distant recurrence of breast cancer. *Clin Positron Imaging* 2000; 3:45–49.

20. Hubner KF, Smith GT, Thie JA, et al. The potential of F-18-FDG/PET in breast cancer: detection of primary lesions, axillary lymph node metastases, or distant metastases. *Clin Positron Imaging* 2000; 3:197–205.

21. Gallowitsch HJ, Kresnik E, Gasser J, et al. F-18 fluorodeoxyglucose positron-emission tomography in the diagnosis of tumor recurrence and metastases in the follow-up of patients with breast carcinoma: a comparison to conventional imaging. *Invest Radiol* 2003; 38:250–256.

22. Kamel EM, Wyss MT, Fehr MK, et al. [18F]-fluorodeoxyglucose positron emission tomography in patients with suspected recurrence of breast cancer. *J Cancer Res Clin Oncol* 2003; 129(3):147–153.

CASE 1

Postoperative scar with hematoma on MRI

A 47-year-old woman with dense breasts was evaluated with a breast MRI 1 year after being treated for stage I, T1N0M0 right breast cancer. Her tumor was a 1.5-cm infiltrating ductal carcinoma (IDC) with mucinous and clear cell features, without angiolymphatic invasion, estrogen receptor and progesterone receptor positive, with margins clear for invasion and notable only for a focal close (1 mm) inferior medial margin for ductal carcinoma in situ (DCIS). Five sentinel lymph nodes were negative. She had been treated with partial mastectomy, four cycles of doxorubicin (Adriamycin) and cyclophosphamide (Cytoxan) (AC) chemotherapy, and radiation therapy, with a boost to the lumpectomy bed, and was taking tamoxifen. See Case 8 in Chapter 1 for the imaging features of this patient's breast cancer at initial diagnosis.

Because of her extreme breast density, surveillance breast MRI and ultrasound were obtained 1 year after breast cancer treatment. At the lumpectomy level, findings of a small residual hematoma were seen at the scar level on MRI (Figures 1, 2, and 3). The ultrasound correlate is seen in Figure 4.

TEACHING POINT

Most postoperative fluid collections are seromas, which display fluid signal on MRI (low on T1 and high signal on short tau inversion recovery (STIR) and T2). Hematomas may be differentiated from seromas by recognition of blood product signal intensity. In this example, bright signal seen on unenhanced T1-weighted sequences is methemo-

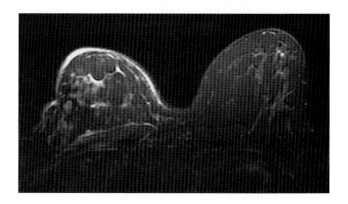

FIGURE 2. Axial STIR image shows thickening and edema of the skin and generalized reticulation and edema of the breast from radiation therapy. The postoperative collection in the right lateral breast shows a hypointense rim and central hyperintensity.

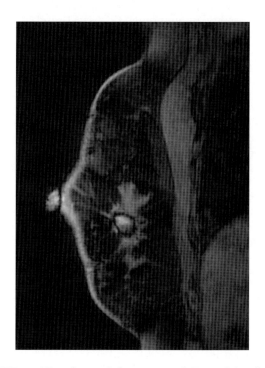

FIGURE 3. Unenhanced, fat-saturated, T1-weighted, gradient echo, sagittal view of the right lateral breast at the level of the scar shows hyperintensity centrally and a hypointense rim of hemosiderin.

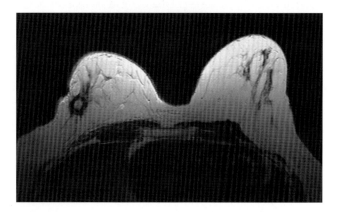

FIGURE 1. Axial T2-weighted breast MRI shows a postsurgical scar in the right posterior lateral breast. The center is relatively bright in signal intensity/ and there is a hypointense surrounding rim.

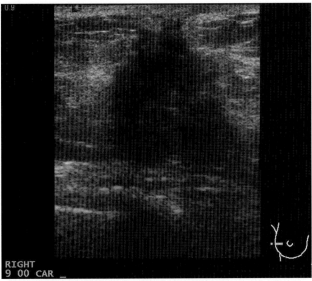

FIGURE 4. Ultrasound correlate, through the scar. The hypoechoic, irregularly marginated shadowing scar extends superficially toward the skin.

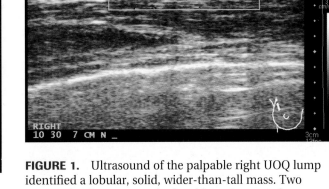

FIGURE 1. Ultrasound of the palpable right UOQ lump identified a lobular, solid, wider-than-tall mass. Two concerning features are depicted here: increased vascularity and angular margins (note upper right border of the mass, the morphology of which suggests ductal extension).

globin, and the hypointense rim, best seen on gradient echo sequences, is characteristic of hemosiderin.

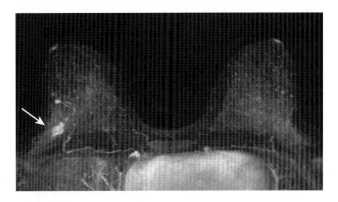

FIGURE 2. Axial maximal intensity projection (MIP) from enhanced, dynamic breast MRI series, 1 minute after contrast injection, shows three early enhancing right breast nodules. Two are adjacent in the posterior lateral breast and correspond to the ultrasound. The separate, more anterior lateral focus was hyperintense on STIR, suggesting a possible small intramammary lymph node or fibroadenoma.

CASE 2

Changes from recent bilateral mastectomy and tissue expander placement

A 36-year-old woman noted a palpable right upper outer quadrant (UOQ) breast mass. Breast imaging evaluations showed a corresponding 1-cm hypoechoic, solid, vascular, sonographically indeterminate breast mass. Ultrasound-guided biopsy identified infiltrating ductal carcinoma (IDC) (Figure 1).

The past medical history was notable for prior mantle radiation for Hodgkin's disease 12 years before. Preoperative breast MRI evaluation showed the known IDC as a 1.1-cm, early enhancing mass with washout, with a 4-mm suspected satellite nodule adjacent. A separate, lobular 5 × 3-mm pos-

sible intramammary lymph node was noted in the lateral breast. The left breast showed no focal or concerning findings (Figures 2 and 3).

The patient elected to undergo bilateral mastectomies, with tissue expanders placed. The right mastectomy specimen contained a 0.9-cm IDC, with high-grade ductal carcinoma in situ (DCIS) extending 5 mm beyond the invasive carcinoma, estrogen receptor negative, *HER-2/neu* negative. Atypical ductal hyperplasia was identified in multiple quadrants, as well as found in the left mastectomy specimen. The margins were negative. Four right axillary lymph nodes showed no evidence of disease.

Staging evaluations with positron emission tomography (PET) and CT obtained before chemotherapy showed chest wall changes attributable to surgery, as well as normal variant endometrial activity (Figures 4, 5, and 6).

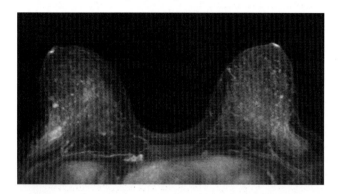

FIGURE 3. Axial MIP from enhanced dynamic breast MRI series, 2 minutes after contrast injection, shows washout of the largest mass. There is also loss of conspicuity due to progressive breast parenchymal enhancement.

TEACHING POINTS

Younger patients treated for lymphoma with mantle radiation are at increased risk for a second malignancy (the incidence is 10% to 20% at 20 years of follow-up). Mantle radiation includes the neck, supraclavicular, infraclavicular, axillary, mediastinal, and hilar regions (Figure 7). The unshielded upper outer quadrants of the breasts receive the highest doses.

In women, if a second malignancy develops, it is most commonly breast cancer.

Travis and colleagues found 105 cases of breast cancer in a series of 3817 females treated for Hodgkin's disease before the age of 30 years. The risk is dose dependent, and the highest risk is in those treated in adolescence (ages 10 to 20 years). Presumably, the breast tissue is most susceptible to radiation injury during earlier development.

In such patients, breast conservation therapy is often not an option because repeat radiation may not be possible.

The normal, early postoperative findings of mastectomy with tissue expander placement are demonstrated here. A described, normal variant source of fluorodeoxyglucose (FDG) activity on whole-body PET is also seen here in the pelvis. Endometrial activity is most commonly seen in premenopausal patients during the first (menstruation) or third (ovulation) week of the menstrual cycle. If endometrial activity is identified on PET in

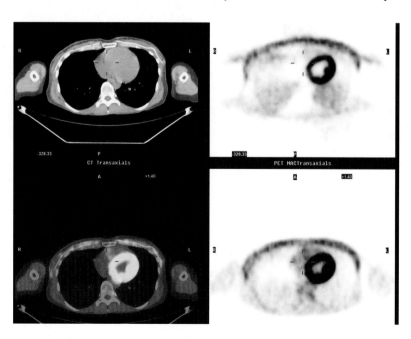

FIGURE 4. Axial PET/CT images, obtained for systemic staging after bilateral mastectomy (left prophylactic) and tissue expander placements, show symmetrical increased anterior chest wall uptake.

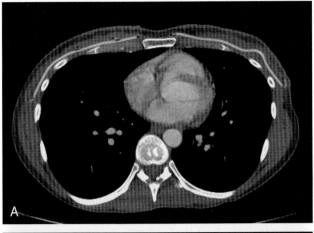

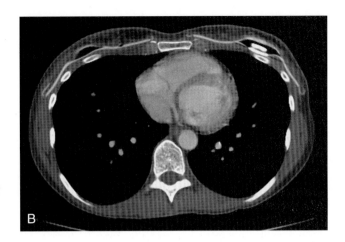

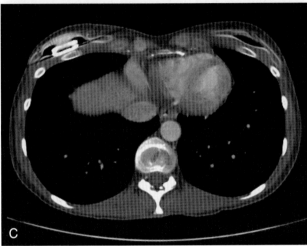

FIGURE 5. Corresponding enhanced chest CT images (**A** to **C**, from above to below), for correlation with PET, showing postoperative changes from recent bilateral mastectomy, with tissue expander placements. Symmetrical skin thickening and induration are noted of the anterior chest wall. Tissue expanders are usually positioned so that the upper two thirds are below the pectoral muscle. The integrated port can be seen on the left in **B**, and on the right in **C**.

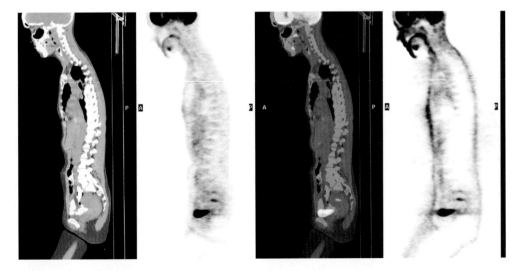

FIGURE 6. Sagittal PET/CT images show linear increased metabolic activity in the pelvis, localizing to the endometrial lining.

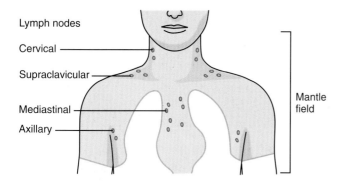

FIGURE 7. Mantle field radiation encompasses the nodal basins in the neck, supraclavicular and infraclavicular regions, axilla, mediastinum, and hila. *From Estabrook A, Giron G. Treatment of unusual malignant neoplasias and clinical presentations. In Roses DF (ed): Breast Cancer, 2nd ed. Philadelphia: Churchill Livingstone, 2005, p 705.*

a postmenopausal patient, this warrants further investigation, because endometrial carcinoma can manifest this way.

SUGGESTED READINGS

Estabrook A, Giron G. Treatment of unusual malignant neoplasias and clinical presentations. In Roses DF (ed): *Breast Cancer*, 2nd ed. Philadelphia: Churchill Livingstone, 2005, pp 705–706.

Lerman H, Metser U, Grisaru D, et al. Normal and abnormal 18F-FDG endometrial and ovarian uptake in pre- and postmenopausal patients: assessment by PET/CT. *J Nucl Med* 2004; 45:266–271.

Travis LB, Hill DA, Dores GM, et al. Breast cancer following radiotherapy and chemotherapy among young women with Hodgkin disease. *JAMA* 2003; 290 (4):465–475.

CASE 3

Normal CT appearance of bilateral TRAM flap reconstruction and post–TRAM flap abdominal complications

A 38-year-old woman elected to undergo prophylactic left mastectomy and bilateral transverse rectus abdominis musculocutaneous (TRAM) flap reconstruction 10 months after finishing radiation therapy for a right stage II, T2N1, 3-cm infiltrating ductal carcinoma (IDC), estrogen receptor and progesterone receptor negative, and *HER-2/neu* negative-, with 3 of 22 involved axillary lymph nodes. She had been treated with right mastectomy with clear margins, chemotherapy with four cycles of doxorubicin (Adriamycin) and cyclophosphamide (Cytoxan) (AC) and four cycles of paclitaxel (Taxol), and right chest wall, supraclavicular, and posterior axillary boost radiation therapy (see Case 18 in Chapter 3 for the presenting imaging features and initial staging of this patient).

The patient had undergone genetic testing subsequent to her diagnosis and treatment and proved to be *BRCA-1* positive. Her family history was of premenopausal breast cancer in a maternal aunt. As a consequence, she decided to undergo hysterectomy and oophorectomy, which was performed at the same time as prophylactic left mastectomy and bilateral TRAM flap reconstruction (Figures 1, 2, and 3). Her left breast mastectomy specimen was benign.

The patient's postoperative course was complicated by development of abdominal wound infection (Figure 4), requiring débridement twice of infected, necrotic tissue and intravenous antibiotic therapy, as well as anticoagulation for pulmonary embolism.

TEACHING POINTS

This patient had a protracted recovery from surgery. In the same procedure, she underwent hysterectomy, bilateral oophorectomy, and prophylactic left mastectomy, as well as bilateral breast reconstruction using myocutaneous abdominal wall flaps (TRAM flaps). In this procedure, a portion of the abdominal wall, including the rectus abdominis muscle and abdominal wall fat and skin, is transposed to the chest as a pedicle or free flap to reconstruct the breast. In a pedicle procedure, as was performed here, the flap, a large ellipse of lower abdominal fat and skin obtained with a transverse abdominal incision, is tunneled underneath the anterior chest wall into position. The flap remains attached to the rectus muscle, which provides the blood supply. The imaging findings seen here show the typical CT features of such reconstructed breasts, and findings compatible with the abdominal wound infection and necrosis complicating this procedure.

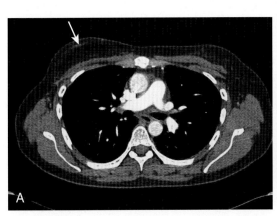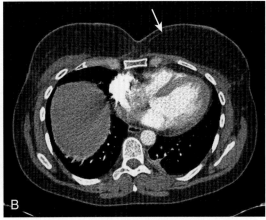

FIGURE 1. Enhanced chest CT images (**A**, above; **B**, below) show typical changes of bilateral TRAM flap reconstruction after bilateral mastectomy. This study was obtained 3 weeks after surgery. The reconstructed breasts are fatty. Thin, soft tissue density, curvilinear bands can be seen underneath and parallel to the skin surface of the reconstructed breasts. On the right, this is best seen in **A**, and on the left, in **B** (*arrows*). This thin line represents the de-epithelialized abdominal wall skin of the flap, which has been tunneled up into position from the abdomen. The fat overlying this thin line is part of the native chest wall, and the fat deep to this line is abdominal wall fat transposed with the flap.

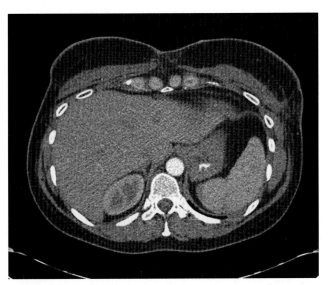

FIGURE 2. At the level of the epigastrium, usually at the level of the fifth, sixth, or seventh costal cartilages, the tunneled rectus muscles are visualized paralleling the costal margin. They can be expected to atrophy with time.

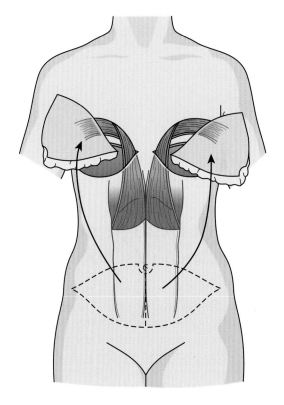

FIGURE 3. Drawing illustrates bilateral ipsilateral TRAM flap breast reconstruction. In this procedure, a large ellipse of lower abdominal fat and skin, including the rectus abdominis muscle, is obtained with a transverse abdominal incision. This flap is transposed to the chest by tunneling underneath the anterior chest wall. The flap remains attached to the rectus muscle, which provides the blood supply.

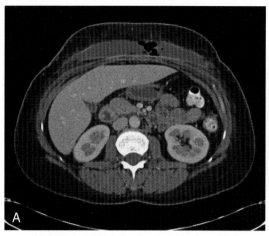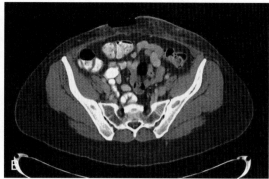

FIGURE 4.   Enhanced abdominal CT images (**A**, above; **B**, below), 3 weeks after surgery, show changes from infection and necrosis of the abdominal wound. At this point, the patient's abdominal wall wound was 3 days post débridement of infected necrotic tissue. Air and an elliptical abdominal wall fluid collection are seen in **A**, with strandy induration of the anterior abdominal wall and an open wound seen more inferiorly in **B**. Note absence of the rectus muscles in **B**.

SUGGESTED READING

LePage MA, Kazerooni EA, Helvie MA, et al. Breast reconstruction with TRAM flaps: normal and abnormal appearances at CT. *RadioGraphics* 1999; (19)1593–1603.

CASE 4

Recurrent DCIS presenting as new microcalcifications

A 53-year-old woman, 2 years postmenopausal, underwent routine mammographic screening. A small cluster of faint, new, indeterminate microcalcifications was identified on the left (Figure 1), in the lower inner quadrant. The patient was unable to tolerate stereotactic biopsy and underwent surgical excision after needle localization. Pathology showed a 1-cm ductal carcinoma in situ (DCIS) lesion (with necrosis, cribriform, solid, and focal micropapillary forms), estrogen receptor negative, *HER-2/neu* positive, with a focal (0.2 cm) microinvasive component. The margins were close.

She underwent re-excision and sentinel node sampling. Two lymph nodes were negative. No additional DCIS was found. Additional treatment for this stage I, T1aN0 tumor was with radiation.

Eleven months after radiation therapy, routine mammographic surveillance showed new clustered left microcalcifications, which had developed since a prior study 6 months before (Figures 2 and 3). These were sampled stereotactically, and identified as DCIS.

Mastectomy was performed. The histology showed a 6-mm focus of high-grade DCIS with comedo necrosis and negative margins. One examined axillary lymph node was negative. Breast MRI was obtained 1 month postoperatively to evaluate the opposite side, given the patient's unusual clinical course (Figure 4). No concerning findings were seen.

Clinically, the patient was doing well 22 months after mastectomy.

TEACHING POINTS

This patient had an unusual clinical course, with rapid development of calcified DCIS only 11 months after undergoing treatment for DCIS with lumpectomy and radiation. In retrospect, perhaps breast MRI might have been useful in the initial evaluation of this patient's extent of disease. The use of breast MRI with DCIS diagnoses, to look for invasive disease or to assess the extent of DCIS, is considered controversial and is far from universal in practice. However, because it is known that DCIS

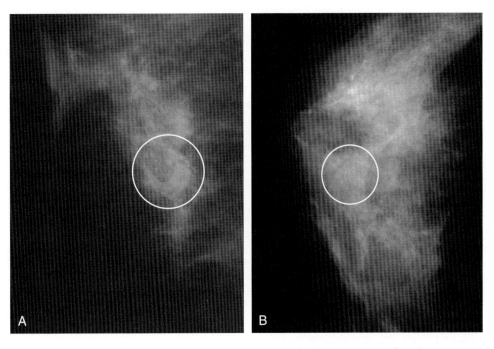

FIGURE 1.   Magnification views of the left breast [lateral (**A**) and CC (**B**)] show a new, faint, indeterminate cluster of microcalcifications (*circled*) in dense breast tissue.

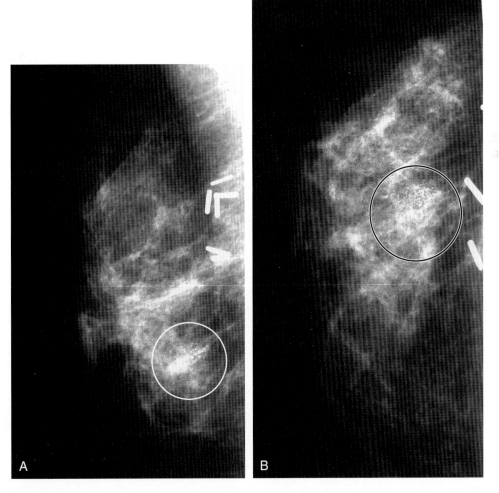

FIGURE 2.   Postlumpectomy and radiation therapy mammograms [MLO (**A**) and CC (**B**)] show clips from the prior surgery 11 months before and new indeterminate clustered microcalcifications in the 6-o'clock position (*circled*).

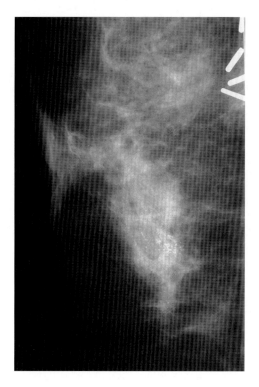

FIGURE 3. Lateral magnification view of the new microcalcifications show indeterminate morphology. The microcalcifications were new from a prior post-treatment mammogram obtained 6 months before.

is often noncalcified, and not accurately mapped by mammography when noncalcified, and because DCIS on core biopsy is not infrequently upstaged on excision to micro or frank invasion, cogent arguments can be made to consider the use of breast MRI in initial staging of DCIS as well as invasive cancer.

CASE 5

Recurrent DCIS detected on surveillance MRI

A 51-year-old woman, with prior left breast ductal carcinoma in situ (DCIS) treated with lumpectomy only, underwent annual screening MRI. The MRI demonstrated a developing 1.2-cm focal area of enhancement in the left breast, lateral to the patient's prior lumpectomy site (Figures 1 and 2). Mammography showed no abnormality. Ultrasound demonstrated a small area of altered echotexture that appeared to correspond to the abnormal finding on MRI (Figure 3). Ultrasound-guided core needle biopsy identified intermediate-grade DCIS. The patient was treated with surgical excision and radiation therapy.

TEACHING POINTS

This case demonstrates the ability of MRI to detect in-breast recurrence that is occult on mammogra-

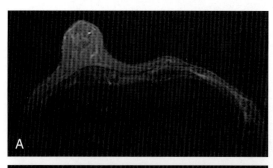

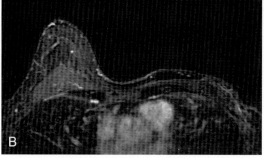

FIGURE 4. Axial breast MRIs (**A**, STIR; **B** enhanced, subtracted, T1-weighted), 1 month after left mastectomy, show typical early postmastectomy changes. Edema and mild enhancement is seen of the left pectoralis muscles and axilla.

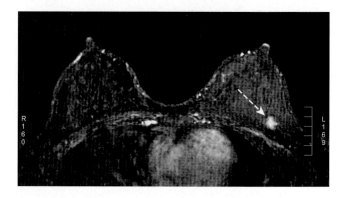

FIGURE 1. Postcontrast, subtracted, axial MRI demonstrates a developing 1.2-cm area of abnormal, irregularly marginated mass enhancement in the left breast, lateral to the patient's prior lumpectomy (*arrow*).

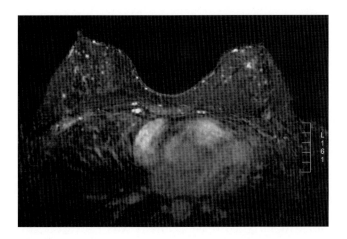

FIGURE 2. Postcontrast, subtracted, axial MRI, 1 year before, for comparison. No suspicious areas of enhancement are seen. There are a few tiny, benign-appearing, scattered foci of enhancement. Vague, low-level focal enhancement is seen on the left laterally, where the suspicious abnormality developed on the following year's exam.

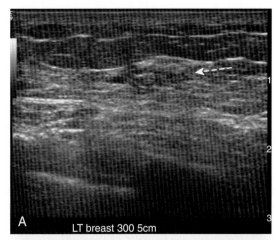

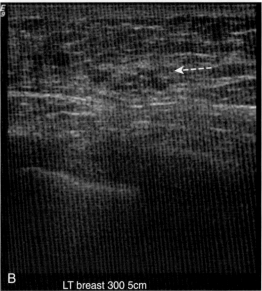

FIGURE 3. Ultrasound images (**A** and **B**) of the lateral left breast demonstrate a subtle area of altered echotexture (*arrows*). This appeared to correspond in size, shape, and location to the enhancing mass seen on MRI. This finding was just lateral to the scar from prior lumpectomy. Ultrasound-guided core needle biopsy confirmed intermediate grade DCIS.

phy and nearly occult on ultrasound. Without the level of suspicion generated by the MRI finding or the MRIs to guide directed ultrasound evaluation, it is unlikely that the cancer recurrence in this patient would have been detected on whole-breast survey ultrasound. The 10-year local recurrence rates in patients who undergo lumpectomy with negative margins and radiation therapy have been reported to be as low as 10% or less. However, some patients are at increased risk for local recurrence. These include younger patients, patients with an extensive intraductal component, and patients with close or positive surgical margins. MRI may be a useful adjuvant to screening mammography in these patients. In addition, MRI aids in surveillance of patients who undergo no radiation therapy or partial- rather than whole-breast irradiation.

SUGGESTED READINGS

Neuschatz AC, DiPetrillo T, Safaii H, et al. Long-term follow-up of a prospective policy of margin-directed radiation dose escalation in breast-conserving therapy. *Cancer* 2003; 97:30–39.

Obedian E, Haffty BG. Negative margin status improves local control in conservatively managed breast cancer patients. *Cancer J Sci Am* 2000; 6:28–33.

Smitt MC, Nowels KW, Zdeblick MJ, et al. The importance of the lumpectomy surgical margin status in long-term results of breast conservation. *Cancer* 1995; 76:259–267.

CASE 6

ADH/DCIS found on breast MRI obtained to evaluate silicone implant integrity in a breast conservation therapy (BCT) patient

A 62-year-old woman, with a prior history of T1cN0M0 right breast cancer 13 years earlier, underwent surveillance mammography. She had silicone implants, which had been placed 9 years before, which replaced earlier implants. Her breast cancer had been treated with partial mastectomy, radiation, and chemotherapy. She had only been able to tolerate tamoxifen for 1 year.

Her mammogram suggested possible implant rupture, with new findings of a right suspected silicone granuloma and new increased density of left axillary lymph nodes. Breast implant MRI was performed to assess implant integrity. Because of her prior history of breast cancer, a hybrid protocol was performed to assess for implant rupture and to evaluate the parenchyma with enhanced, subtracted, dynamic technique. Enlarged left axillary and internal mammary lymph nodes were identified (Figure 1). They were bright on a "silicone-only" sequence (STIR with water saturation), indicating the lymph nodes contained silicone. Rupture of the right breast implant was noted, and postsurgical distortion was seen of the right breast. No abnormal enhancement was seen on the right, but the left breast showed a large (6 cm), lateral expanse of multinodular, clumped, morphologically concerning enhancement (Figure 2). Breast ultrasound was performed to see if a correlate could be identified for biopsy, but none was seen.

The left axilla was evaluated and showed "snowstorm" shadowing from an enlarged lymph node, characteristic of silicone (Figure 3).

An MRI-guided biopsy was performed of the left breast, targeting the anterior extent of the nodular enhancement, avoiding the implant. Low-grade ductal carcinoma in situ (DCIS), estrogen receptor and progesterone receptor positive, was obtained.

The patient was evaluated for possible left breast conservation therapy. However, because of the 6-cm extent of disease suggested by MRI, it seemed likely that clear margins might not be attained. Since her right breast implant was ruptured, the patient elected to undergo removal of both implants, with bilateral skin-sparing mastectomies and placement of tissue expanders. A left sentinel lymph node sampling and limited axillary dissection was performed, with 5 nodes obtained containing silicone, but no malignancy. No malignancy was found in either breast. In the left lateral breast, fibrocystic changes with sclerosing adenosis, intraductal papilloma, and focal areas of atypical ductal hyperplasia were identified. A chest CT obtained postoperatively showed enlarged internal mammary and pericardial lymph nodes, as well as the appearance of tissue expanders (Figure 4).

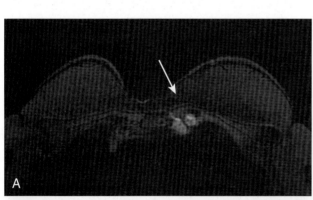

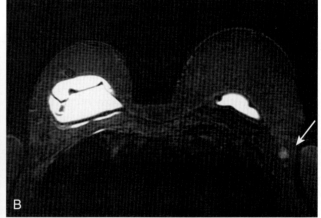

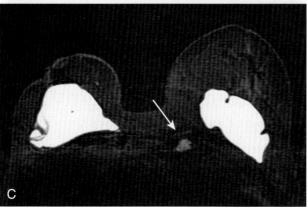

FIGURE 1. Axial STIR with water saturation images of breasts and implants (**A** to **C**, from above to below) shows bright, enlarged left axillary and internal mammary lymph nodes (*arrows*). The right breast is smaller than the left, with lateral postsurgical distortion. On this sequence, only silicone should be bright. The fat signal is by definition nulled on a STIR sequence, and the water signal has been suppressed with a saturation pulse. In general, silicone in lymph nodes or in the tissues will not be as bright as silicone within an implant, as seen here.

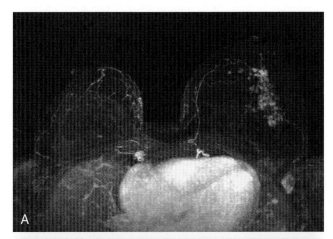

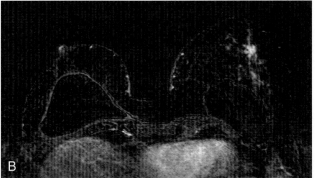

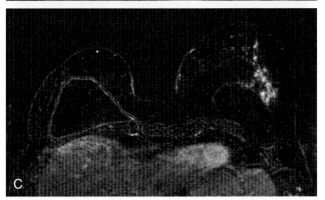

FIGURE 2. Axial, enhanced, subtracted breast MRIs from the dynamic series for parenchymal evaluation (**A**, maximal intensity projection, minute 1; **B**, minute 2 subtraction, above; **C**, minute 2 subtraction, below) show bilateral breast implants and postsurgical change in the size and shape of the previously treated right breast. No abnormal enhancement is seen on the right. On the left, a clumped, multinodular band of enhancement extends through the lateral breast over a 6-cm expanse, back to the level of the implant.

TEACHING POINTS

Breast cancer patients who have undergone reconstruction with silicone implants may present with imaging findings that result from implant failure, but mimic breast cancer recurrence. In this example,

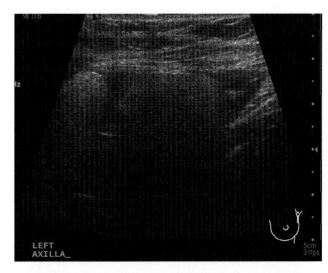

FIGURE 3. Left axillary ultrasound shows ill-defined, hyperechoic foci of dirty shadowing emanating from an enlarged lymph node, portions of which can be seen. This appearance is characteristic of silicone. Ultrasound of the breast showed no correlate for the MRI findings.

routine mammographic surveillance of a patient previously treated with breast conservation raised the question of loss of implant integrity. Breast implant MRI is performed unenhanced, and does not generally provide diagnostic information about the breast parenchyma. Breast implant protocols rely on high-resolution, sagittal and axial, T2-weighted sequences to assess for intracapsular rupture. The presence of extracapsular silicone is sought using a sequence in which only silicone is bright, such as the STIR with water saturation sequence used here. Silicone-containing lymph nodes within the field of view will be bright, as demonstrated here. In this case, characteristic ultrasound findings confirming silicone in the left axilla were found subsequently. Presumably, even the enlarged pericardial lymph node seen on chest CT is due to uptake of silicone. Unfortunately, only time (longitudinal follow-up) or histologic sampling can confirm that the nodal enlargement is due to silicone. PET imaging in this circumstance could potentially be misleading because silicone-containing lymph nodes may well be hypermetabolic, owing to the intense granulomatous response silicone incites (see Case 10 in Chapter 10).

Because this patient had a known history of breast cancer, and because the presence of implants hampers mammographic evaluation, a "hybrid" breast MRI protocol was utilized, with sequences obtained for evaluation of the implants, as well as enhanced, subtracted, dynamic breast parenchymal imaging. The enhanced portion of the study

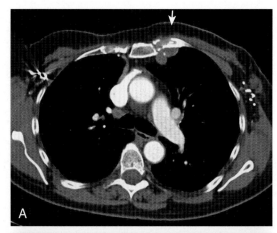

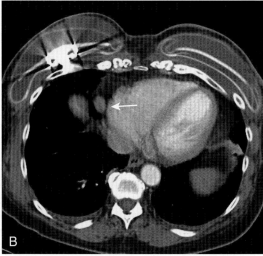

FIGURE 4.   Images from a contrast-enhanced chest CT (**A**, above; **B**, below) show surgical clips in both axilla. Soft tissue density at the left axillary level is postoperative. Adjacent enlarged left internal mammary lymph nodes correspond to those seen in Figure 1A on MRI. In **B**, small pleural effusions are seen. Bilateral tissue expanders are in place. An enlarged pericardial lymph node is seen in **B** (*arrow*).

showed unexpectedly intense and segmental clumped enhancement. The pattern is morphologically concerning, with a segmental distribution of tiny enhancing nodules. The MRI differential includes infiltrating lobular carcinoma, DCIS, and atypical ductal hyperplasia (ADH). When no sonographic correlate was identified, MRI-guided biopsy was performed. This could be safely performed because most of the enhancement extends anterior to the implant. The histology of DCIS fit the morphologic features of the abnormality, which appeared extensive by MRI. Complete excision of the area of enhancement with a satisfactory cosmetic result and clear margins would be difficult. Because the patient now had confirmation of

implant failure as well, bilateral skin-sparing mastectomy and implant removal were performed. Not surprisingly, the right mastectomy specimen was negative for malignancy. Surprisingly, no additional malignancy was found in the left mastectomy specimen, only ADH.

Could this case have been handled differently? If ADH had been obtained on initial MRI-guided sampling, that would also have required excision because there is a known incidence of undersampling and upgrading of ADH lesions to DCIS between core and excisional biopsies. Excision of such an extensive area of enhancement would have been technically difficult to accomplish with a good cosmetic result. This case does reaffirm that MRI findings need histologic proof before being acted on, but difficulty can arise from the inherent limitations of sampling. See Case 16 in Chapter 3 for a similar case of a "borderlands" breast lesion.

CASE 7

New palpable chest wall lump postmastectomy with implant reconstruction, excisional biopsy–proven recurrent IDC

A 48-year-old woman, 3 years post-mastectomy and chemotherapy for a right stage I invasive ductal breast cancer, developed a small, 0.5-cm, firm nodule lateral to the nipple tattoo of her reconstructed breast. Her original tumor was a T1N0 lesion, estrogen receptor positive and *HER-2/neu* negative. She had been treated with four cycles of doxorubicin (Adriamycin) plus cyclophosphamide (Cytoxan) (AC), and had been taking tamoxifen since.

Ultrasound showed a 6-mm, irregularly marginated mass, disrupting the normal architecture planes (Figure 1). This was surgically excised, identifying recurrent infiltrating ductal carcinoma (IDC), estrogen receptor and progesterone receptor positive and *HER-2/neu* negative, involving the subcutaneous adipose tissue and skeletal muscle of the chest wall.

Staging evaluations with positron emission tomography (PET)/CT and bone scan showed no additional sites of recurrent breast cancer. The patient underwent excision, with removal of the implant, and axillary dissection. No residual cancer was found in the breast, and 1 of 11 lymph nodes showed involvement (largest focus was 0.8 cm).

Chemotherapy with docetaxel (Taxotere) and capecitabine (Xeloda) was given, and the patient was treated additionally with right chest wall, supraclavicular, and posterior axillary boost radiation.

TEACHING POINTS

Implants hamper mammographic evaluation of breast tissue. However, the stretching and thinning of breast tissue over an implant can actually make lumps more easily palpable and can aid sonographic evaluation as well (Figure 2).

The sonographic appearance of this small mass was certainly suspicious: it is as tall as wide, with irregular margins and disruption of tissue planes. Of course, not every new, suspicious sonographic mass developing in a patient with previous breast cancer represents recurrent breast cancer. See Figure 3 (Case 9 in Chapter 7) for a very similar-appearing finding that proved to be fibrosis and foreign body giant cell reaction in a previously treated breast cancer patient with recently placed implants.

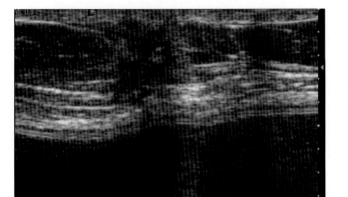

FIGURE 1. Ultrasound of the palpable lump shows a superficial, sonographically suspicious mass with irregular margins and disruption of tissue planes (*arrow*). The patient is post-mastectomy, with implant reconstruction. The sonolucent implant is seen beneath the mass.

SUGGESTED READING

Handel N, Silverstein MJ. Breast cancer detection in women with implants. *Semin Breast Dis* 2004; 7:172–181.

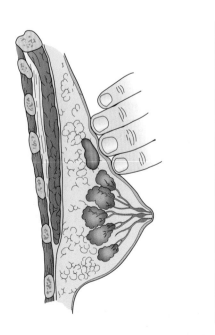
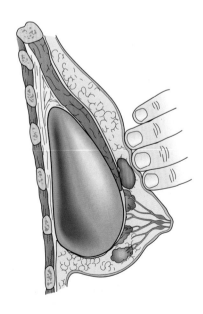

FIGURE 2. Comparison of palpation of a lump in a non-augmented breast *(left)* vs. in an augmented breast *(right)*: The presence of an implant thins the overlying tissue and may make a lump more readily palpable.

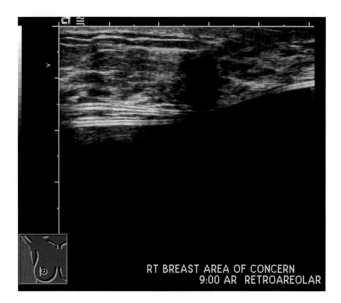

RT BREAST AREA OF CONCERN
9:00 AR RETROAREOLAR

FIGURE 3. Ultrasound of a palpable periareolar mass in another patient, a 54-year-old woman, treated 10 years before with partial mastectomy, radiation therapy, six courses of Cytoxan, methotrexate, 5-fluorouracil (CMF) chemotherapy, and 5 years of tamoxifen, for T1cN1M0, left breast IDC. Bilateral, subpectoral implants had been placed in the past year. A very hypoechoic, taller-than-wide, irregularly marginated mass was biopsied with ultrasound guidance, with 14-gauge core biopsy technique. Pathology showed no carcinoma, with sclerosis, fibrosis, and foreign body giant cell reaction found.

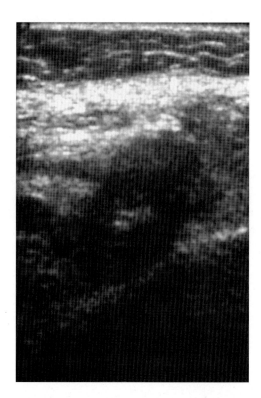

FIGURE 1. Ultrasound of the left axilla shows an irregularly marginated, hypoechoic mass with hyperechoic foci within. The patient presented with no imaging studies or supporting documents, with only a history of a recent abnormal PET scan showing axillary recurrence.

CASE 8

Axillary recurrence, presentation with pain

A 50-year-old woman presented with a 6-month history of progressive left axillary and shoulder pain, and suspicion of recurrent breast cancer. She had undergone a left modified radical mastectomy 13 years before, with subsequent reconstruction with an implant. She was also treated at the time of initial diagnosis with Cytoxan, methotrexate, 5-fluorouracil (CMF) chemotherapy for node-positive disease, with 6 of 25 lymph nodes involved. She reportedly had undergone a positron emission tomography (PET)/CT scan at an outside facility showing left axillary and supraclavicular hypermetabolism, but no films were available initially to substantiate this. She had been advised at the outside facility to undergo radiation and begin tamoxifen based on the PET/CT evidence of recurrence, but was transferring care. She had no tissue diagnosis of recurrence at the time of transfer of care. She was referred for ultrasound-guided biopsy following a diagnostic ultrasound.

On ultrasound, an ill-defined, deep, hypoechoic mass was seen in the axilla (Figure 1). Hyperechoic foci were noted within this, suggesting coarse calcifications or metal. Because the patient presented without any supporting imaging or reports, she was sent for a contrast-enhanced chest CT scan to better define the nature of the axillary findings and her anatomy. Contrast enhanced CT of the chest showed clips from prior lymphadenectomy in the left axilla, surrounded by mass-like soft tissue (Figure 2), which seemed to correlate with the sonographic findings. Based on this, a 14-gauge ultrasound-guided core needle biopsy was performed, confirming infiltrating ductal carcinoma (IDC), estrogen receptor positive, progesterone receptor negative.

Subsequently, images from her outside PET scan became available, showing hypermetabolism in

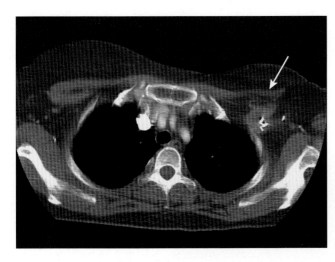

FIGURE 2.   To better define this patient's anatomy, a contrast-enhanced chest CT scan was obtained. Surgical clips from prior left axillary dissection are surrounded by soft tissue. These findings seemed to correlate with the ultrasound. Ultrasound-guided core biopsy was performed, and confirmed IDC, estrogen receptor positive.

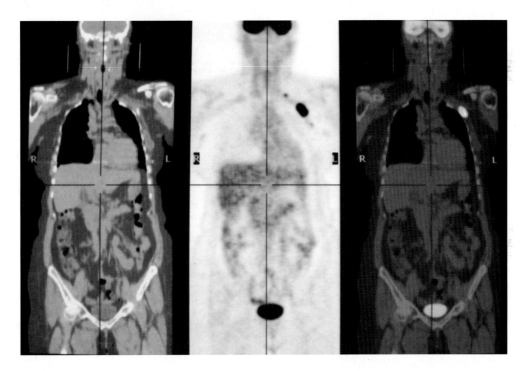

FIGURE 3.   Images from PET/CT (performed 2 months before at another facility, but not available at the time of presentation for biopsy) show a line of hypermetabolic foci in the left axilla, including a larger focus that corresponds with the ultrasound and CT abnormality.

the left axilla, corresponding to the ultrasound and CT abnormalities (Figure 3).

The patient was treated with radiation therapy, with relief of her pain, and started on anastrozole (Arimidex). Repeat PET/CT showed resolution of the abnormalities noted previously (Figures 4 and 5).

TEACHING POINTS

It is always easier to find your way if you have a map. In this case, the patient presented for biopsy without any supporting documents or images. She gave a history of an abnormal recent PET scan, but

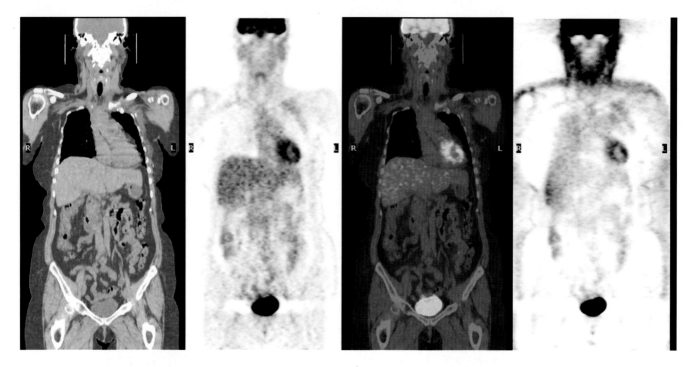

FIGURE 4.   Repeat PET/CT, 11 months after PET/CT in Figure 3 and 6 months after left axillary radiation therapy, shows resolution of the hypermetabolism present before. In its stead is seen a band of low-level activity, compatible with radiation therapy effect.

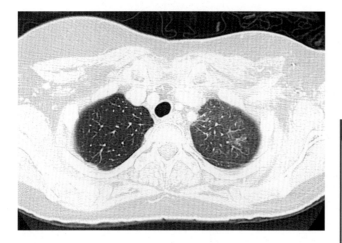

FIGURE 5.   Lung windows from a chest CT, obtained 2 months after completion of left axillary radiation therapy, for correlation with the PET/CT in Figure 4. New ground-glass opacity is seen of left apical lung parenchyma, from the interval radiation.

no images were then available. Evaluation with ultrasound showed concerning but difficult to define axillary findings. Chest CT was obtained to better delineate her anatomy, and made clearer the significance of the ultrasound findings. The echogenic foci were surgical clips from prior lymphad-enectomy, making the surrounding soft tissue bulk highly suspicious for recurrence.

CASE 9

Parasternal recurrence, draining to contralateral axilla (role of lymphoscintigraphy)*

A 43-year-old woman with a history of treated left breast cancer 3 years before developed a growing palpable and tender left parasternal nodule, which on physical examination was noted to be firm and fixed to the chest wall. Excisional biopsy confirmed infiltrating ductal carcinoma (IDC), thought to be

*Case courtesy of Dr. Eva Lean, Tri-City Medical Center, Oceanside, CA.

recurrent disease in a lower internal mammary lymph node.

Her prior breast cancer manifested as extensive suspicious microcalcifications in the left upper breast. After stereotactic confirmation of high-grade ductal carcinoma in situ (DCIS), the patient underwent mastectomy with immediate TRAM flap reconstruction. The mastectomy specimen showed diffuse high-grade DCIS, with Paget's disease of the nipple and a 6-mm focus of IDC, estrogen receptor positive. Margins were focally close (the invasive component was within 1 mm of an inked circumferential margin), and six examined axillary lymph nodes were negative for tumor. The patient had been taking tamoxifen in the interval.

The recurrence at the left lower inner quadrant parasternal level had been operatively excised because of its fixation to the chest wall, and margins of this excision were involved. Before re-excising the proven recurrence, lymphoscintigraphy was obtained to assess the drainage pattern, and showed drainage to the contralateral axilla (Figure 1). Right axillary sentinel lymph node sampling showed several foci of subcapsular metastatic ductal carcinoma, measuring up to 2 mm. The re-excised proven recurrence site contained a 1-cm poorly differentiated IDC, as well as several areas of intramammary metastases.

The patient was treated with chemotherapy—four cycles of doxorubicin (Adriamycin) plus cyclophosphamide (Cytoxan) (AC), followed by paclitaxel (Taxol)—and radiation to bilateral axilla and supraclavicular regions, and the left chest wall, encompassing the internal mammary region.

TEACHING POINTS

Lymphoscintigraphy at the time of injection for breast cancer sentinel lymph node identification is not universal practice, in contrast with nuclear medicine practice with other types of neoplasms, such as melanoma. Arguments for performing lymphoscintigraphy include the ability to mark skin sites where sentinel nodes are identified on scintigraphy, potentially shortening the surgeon's time spent identifying the lymph nodes. Drainage surprises, such as depicted by this case, are encountered occasionally, and can direct sampling to sites that might otherwise be undetected. Demonstration of drainage to sites that are not readily sampled, such as internal mammary or infraclavicular, can provide information that could be incorporated in design of radiation therapy fields. Arguments against routine imaging after sentinel lymph node injection are that it is time-consuming, occupying gamma cameras and requiring radiologist's input, with a low yield, and that surgeons can successfully identify sentinel nodes intraoperatively without skin marker guidance.

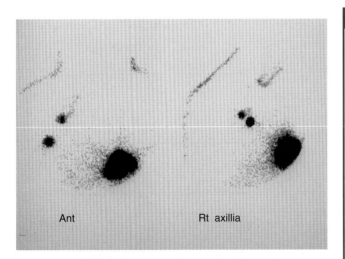

FIGURE 1. Views from lymphoscintigraphy, obtained at the time of detection of the left parasternal recurrence, show drainage to the contralateral (right) axilla, where two lymph nodes are depicted. Subsequent histologic evaluation of a right axillary sentinel node showed foci of subcapsular metastases up to 2 mm in size.

CASE 10

Multicentric recurrent breast cancer with skin involvement

A 54-year-old woman was noted to have skin induration 3 years after left lumpectomy and radiation therapy for breast cancer. Her original tumor presented as a small cluster of microcalcifications (Figure 1). Stereotactic biopsy established the diagnosis of infiltrating ductal carcinoma (IDC), with extensive high-grade ductal carcinoma in situ (DCIS). Her tumor was stage IIB, T2N1, with one of nine lymph nodes involved.

The patient underwent mammographic evaluation to assess the clinically noted skin thickening (Figure 2). Postsurgical scarring was noted, but no concerning change was seen on mammography.

Breast MRI was obtained to evaluate for clinically suspected recurrence (Figures 3, 4, and 5). At surgery, an initial excisional biopsy was performed. Frozen section showed carcinoma in the specimen and overlying skin. A simple mastectomy was per-formed. The specimens showed a 1.6-cm, high-grade invasive carcinoma with multiple additional small foci of tumor and extensive vascular invasion, as well as involvement of the upper dermis of the skin. The tumor was estrogen receptor negative, progesterone receptor positive, and *HER-2/neu* positive.

TEACHING POINTS

Even fairly bulky local recurrences such as this can be difficult to identify on mammography. The mammogram shows prominent, but not atypical, postsurgical scarring and architectural distortion. Change from a prior study, such as increased density or size of a scar, could signify a recurrence, but no such change was seen in this case. Breast MRI can be very helpful in this setting. More than 18 months after breast conservation treatment, normal surgical scars will show no or minimal enhancement. Some of the MRI findings noted here can be ascribed to radiation therapy effects (skin thickening, parenchymal reticulation, and skin, parenchymal, and muscular edema), but the degree of skin thickening seen here would be unusual for radiation. The enhancement of the nipple, skin, and scar is much too intense and too remote from treatment to be considered other than highly suspicious for recurrent tumor.

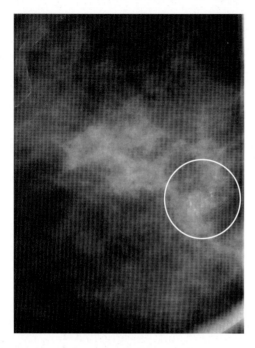

FIGURE 1. CC magnification view of the left breast shows clustered microcalcifications, which vary in shape and density from one another (*circled*).

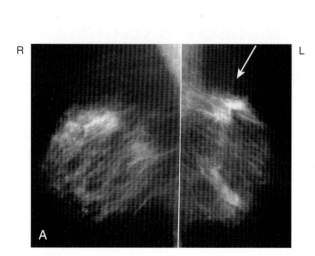
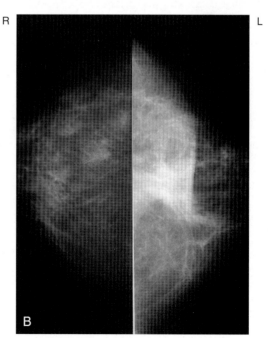

FIGURE 2. MLO (**A**) and CC (**B**) mammograms 3 years after left lumpectomy and radiation therapy for IDC show pronounced scarring and architectural distortion at 12 o'clock on the left, which was not clearly changed from prior studies.

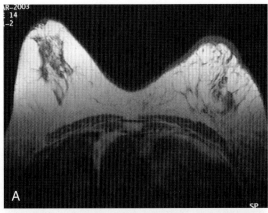

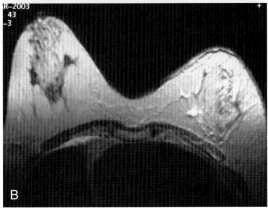

FIGURE 3. Axial MRIs (**A**, T1-weighted; **B**, T2-weighted) at the same level show marked left breast skin thickening and edema. There is also asymmetrical left breast reticulation and edema, as well as edema of the left chest wall musculature.

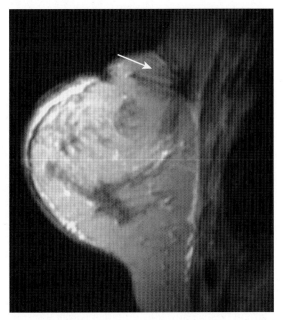

FIGURE 4. Sagittal T2-weighted image through the left breast scar, seen as a hypointense spiculated focus producing skin retraction in the upper posterior breast at 12 o'clock.

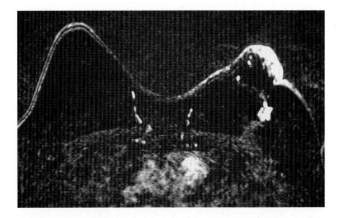

FIGURE 5. Axial subtracted, enhanced breast MRI acquired dynamically shows intense enhancement of a stellate mass in the posterior 12-o'clock left breast, as well as marked enhancement and thickening of the nipple and adjacent skin.

CASE 11

Physical examination change and abnormal enhancement of a 4-year-old lumpectomy scar; pathology-proven fat necrosis mimicking tumor bed recurrence

A 70-year-old woman developed scar retraction and induration 4 years after treatment for a T1bN0M0 right breast infiltrating ductal carcinoma (IDC). Clinically, the change was concerning for recurrence. Her prior treatment was with a lumpectomy and radiation therapy for a 0.9-cm IDC, and she had been taking tamoxifen since.

Ultrasound showed no definite abnormality, and mammography 3 months before had been stable (Figure 1). MRI was requested to evaluate for possible recurrence. It showed a spiculated, progressively enhancing, 3-cm mass in the lumpectomy bed, suspicious for recurrence (Figures 2 and 3).

Palpation-guided biopsy by the surgeon showed only fatty fibrous breast tissue.

Subsequent surgical excision removed an elliptical, 5-cm specimen consisting of skin and the underlying fibrofatty tissue and containing a stellate scar. The pathology showed fat necrosis,

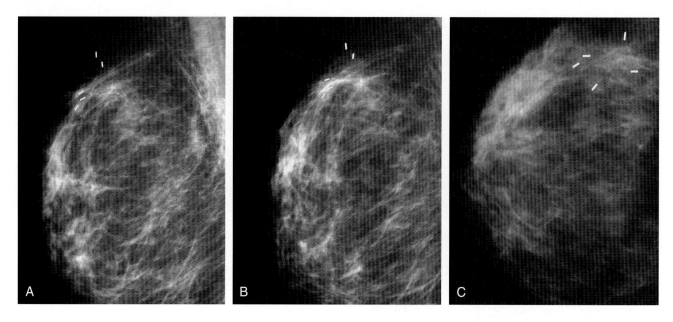

FIGURE 1. MLO (**A**), 90-degree lateral (**B**), and CC (**C**) mammograms show clips at the lumpectomy site in the upper outer quadrant (UOQ). Density at the scar level was stable compared with prior mammograms.

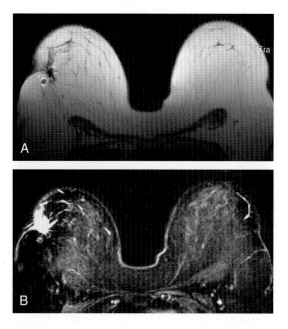

FIGURE 2. Axial bilateral breast MRIs from the same level (**A**, T2-weighted; **B**, enhanced, subtracted T1-weighted gradient echo) show susceptibility artifact and skin puckering at the right UOQ scar site. An irregularly marginated, spiculated, intensely enhancing mass in the lumpectomy bed is suspicious for malignancy, given that the patient is 4 years out from prior surgery and radiation therapy for IDC.

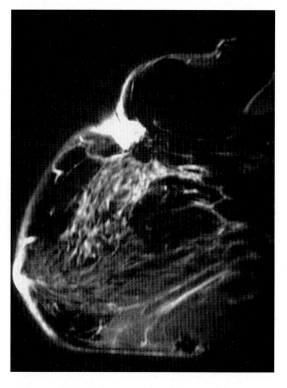

FIGURE 3. Sagittal, enhanced, subtracted image of the right lateral breast shows the enhancing scar site retracting the skin.

reactive inflammation and fibrosis, and no carcinoma. Postoperative healing was complicated by development of a chronic draining open wound. Six months later, with the wound continuing to drain and failing to heal completely, the patient underwent completion mastectomy. Pathology of the specimen showed no invasive or in situ carcinoma. A healing, inflamed biopsy cavity with metaplastic squamous epithelial lining and a cutaneous fistula was found, as well as fat necrosis, fibrosis, and active inflammation at the prior biopsy site.

TEACHING POINTS

Fat necrosis can perfectly mimic recurrent breast cancer, as it did in this case. A normal 4-year-old surgical scar should be "silent" on enhanced breast MRI, with minimal if any enhancement. Given the clinical change and the abnormal MRI findings, concern that this represented a local recurrence was certainly appropriate.

Unfortunately, the inconclusive palpation-guided biopsy led to the scar being excised surgically. Because of poor wound healing of the previously radiated tissue, this led ultimately to the patient undergoing a completion mastectomy. This was necessary from a quality-of-life and wound management standpoint, but not necessary from a histologic standpoint. Arguably, if a confident benign diagnosis of fat necrosis had been obtained using an image-guided biopsy, perhaps this patient could have been followed, rather than undergo the surgery that led ultimately to mastectomy for poor wound healing. This case certainly illustrates the heightened risk in tissue exposed to prior radiation of what is generally thought of as "minor surgery." After radiation therapy, any intervention has to be done with as little trauma to the tissues as possible.

This is an unusual chain of events, but certainly not unique. Factors contributing to delayed and complicated healing after breast preservation therapy could be patient related. It is interesting to review details of the radiation therapy itself, as well as the technique of surgical scar excision. Potentially significant patient risk factors include diabetes, smoking, and obesity. In this case, there was no history of either smoking or diabetes. The patient was at least 30 pounds overweight and had a history of hypertension and nonalcoholic steatohepatitis. Her radiation therapy consisted of opposed medial and lateral tangential fields to the breast and cone-down electron boost to the tumor bed. The external-beam dose to the breast was 5040 cGy, given with 6 MV photons, with the boost dose to the tumor bed of 1440 cGy using 15 MeV electrons. The surgical intervention, preceded by biopsy, resulted in a nonhealing fistula. Careful surgical technique and occasionally use of hyperbaric oxygen can enhance the healing of tissue exposed to prior radiation.

CASE 12

Enhancing scar, suspicious for recurrence; contralateral axillary nodal presentation of new occult breast primary

A 61-year-old woman underwent periodic breast MRI for surveillance. She had been treated with lumpectomy and radiation therapy 14 years before for right breast ductal carcinoma in situ (DCIS).

Breast MRI identified concerning findings bilaterally, including progressive enhancement of the right lumpectomy scar and enlargement of a left axillary lymph node (Figures 1, 2, and 3).

Ultrasound was obtained for correlation. At the level of the right lumpectomy scar site, dense shadowing was noted. There was a very hypoechoic mass–like component with vascularity, which was targeted for ultrasound-guided core biopsy (Figure 4). Pathology showed dense collagenous stroma and no carcinoma.

Left axillary lymph node ultrasound-guided fine-needle aspiration of a lymph node with cortical mantle thickening (Figure 5) showed rare atypical cells. It was repeated, with atypical ductal epithelial cells obtained. Surgical excision was recommended.

Needle localizations were performed bilaterally. The left axillary node contained metastatic adenocarcinoma, consistent with a breast primary. The right excised scar site showed focal atypical ductal hyperplasia and dense hyalinized and sclerotic stroma associated with cystic fat necrosis and chronic inflammation.

The assessment was that this was a new axillary presentation of left breast cancer. Breast MRI was repeated to look for a primary but did not identify one (Figure 6). Bilateral diagnostic mammograms

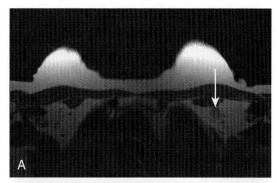

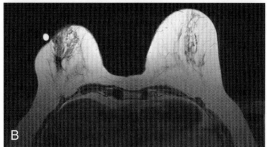

FIGURE 1.   Axial T2-weighted breast MRIs (**A**, through axilla; **B**, through right scar level) show a mildly enlarged left axillary lymph node (*arrow*). The right lumpectomy scar (*marked*) is hypointense and spiculated.

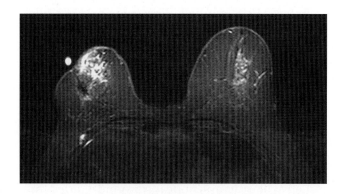

FIGURE 2.   Axial STIR at the same right lumpectomy scar level (*marked*). The scar is hypointense.

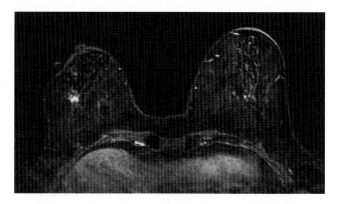

FIGURE 3.   Enhanced, subtracted, axial section at the level of the scar shows the scar to be enhancing. The enhancement was progressive and new from a prior study. This image is from 3 minutes after contrast injection.

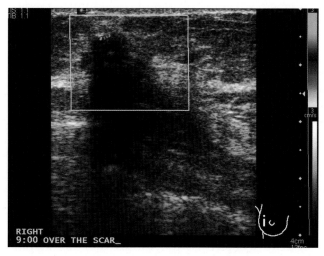

FIGURE 4.   Ultrasound of the right lateral scar site shows a component (*in box*) that is mass-like, with irregular margins and vascularity. Dense shadowing is seen as well.

were also negative (Figure 7). Positron emission tomography (PET)/CT was also negative.

Left axillary dissection was subsequently accomplished, and metastatic adenocarcinoma was found in a total of 3 of 8 lymph nodes.

The patient was treated with six cycles of Taxotere, Adriamycin, Cytoxan (TAC) chemotherapy and radiation therapy to the left breast and peripheral lymphatics (supraclavicular and posterior axillary boost). Repeat breast MRI 4 months after completion of radiation therapy shows expected left breast radiation changes, and evolution of the right breast postsurgical changes (Figure 8).

TEACHING POINTS

A normal scar, especially a 14-year-old one, should not enhance. Enhancement of postsurgical scars is expected to largely resolve by 18 months, so new enhancement at a lumpectomy scar (a change from a previous MRI) appropriately raises concern for recurrence. Of course, not all new enhancement represents recurrent breast cancer. Fat necrosis and inflammation at areas of prior tissue trauma from surgery or radiation can develop years after treatment, and raise the question of recurrence.

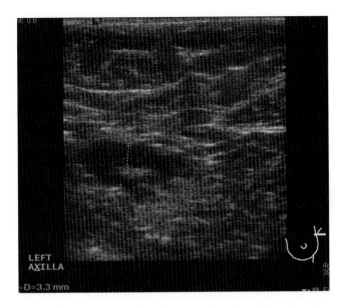

FIGURE 5. Ultrasound of the left axilla identifies a lymph node with an abnormally thick cortical mantle of 3 mm (*cursors*).

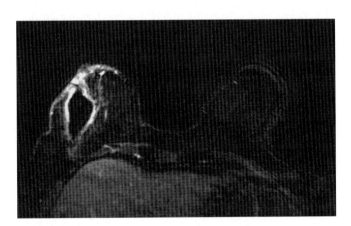

FIGURE 6. Repeat breast MRI, 5 months after breast MRI in Figures 1 to 3 and 3 weeks after surgery to excise the right lumpectomy scar and sample a left axillary lymph node. Enhanced, subtracted, axial image at the level of the excised scar shows 3-week-old postsurgical changes, including a large seroma at the surgical site, with a thin, enhancing rim and generalized skin enhancement.

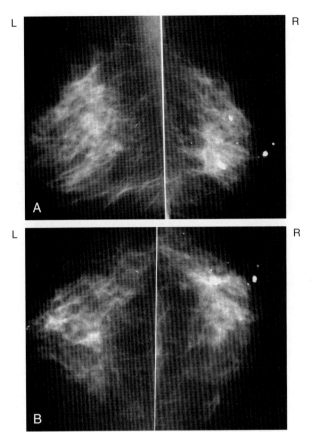

FIGURE 7. Bilateral MLO (**A**) and CC (**B**) mammograms show heterogeneously dense breast parenchyma. Coarse, fat necrosis–type calcifications are seen on the right. A marker (*BB*) has been placed at the right lateral lumpectomy level. No mammographic evidence of malignancy was seen.

Histologic sampling with imaging guidance is appropriate. If the results do not indicate malignancy and the sampling was thorough, a benign result offering a reasonable alternative diagnosis may allow the patient to be followed. Additional tissue injury from sending a patient to surgery has to be carefully considered in a previously radiated field. Histologic proof of recurrent malignancy is a clear indication for a more aggressive approach. If there is not proof of malignancy, the risk-to-benefit ratio has to be carefully weighed. In this case, the

patient's scar was excised, and she healed uneventfully. See Case 11 in this chapter, a similar case in which fat necrosis complicating a scar led to a patient having to undergo a histologically unnecessary mastectomy for wound management.

Although breast MRI is the most sensitive breast imaging modality to search for an occult breast cancer in the case of axillary node presentation, it succeeds only about half of the time. Even in pathology series of mastectomies performed for axillary node presentation, the primary is not found in up to one third of specimens.

Typical early (first 3 to 6 months after treatment) postradiation therapy findings are demonstrated here. They include skin thickening, edema, and enhancement, as well as parenchymal edema and reticulation. These findings are well seen on fluid-sensitive sequences (STIR or fat-saturated, T2-weighted), and peak at 3 to 6 months. Mild generalized increased parenchymal enhancement compared with the untreated opposite side can be

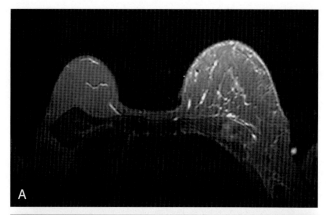

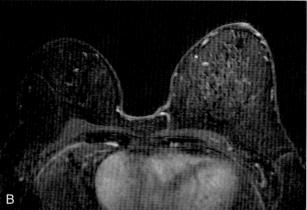

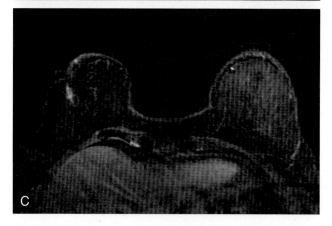

FIGURE 8. Breast MRI, 4 months after completion of left breast radiation therapy and 1 year after breast MRI in Figure 6. **A**, Axial STIR shows the left breast to be larger than the right. There is a diffuse increase in high signal reticulation and skin thickening on the left from radiation therapy. Note also the increased signal of the pectoralis and chest wall musculature. **B**, Enhanced subtracted view of both breasts shows low-level increased diffuse enhancement of the left breast compared with the right, also attributable to radiation. **C**, Enhanced, subtracted view of both breasts at the level of the previously excised right lumpectomy scar. The seroma present previously has resorbed, leaving only an enhancing linear scar.

detected in the first months after treatment and is demonstrated here. This low-level enhancement is not sufficiently intense to interfere with detection of clinically relevant disease. These changes are the result of acute tissue reaction to the ionizing radiation.

Proven multicentric fat necrosis mimicking multicentric recurrence

A 73-year-old woman with a previous stage I, T1N0M0, well-differentiated right infiltrating ductal carcinoma presented 3 years after treatment with a palpable abnormality in the right upper outer quadrant near the lumpectomy site. Her prior treatment consisted of lumpectomy with clear margins and radiation therapy, and the patient was taking anastrozole (Arimidex).

Mammographic evaluations showed postsurgical changes, with increasing density with associated coarse dystrophic calcifications (Figures 1 and 2). MRI was recommended for evaluation of the palpable abnormality. This was interpreted as suspicious for multifocal recurrence in the same quadrant as the prior lumpectomy (Figures 3, 4, 5, and 6). Ultrasound-guided biopsy was recommended.

Ultrasound showed multiple sites of intense shadowing (Figure 7). Core needle biopsy of a representative region returned benign histology of fat necrosis with fibrosis and microcalcification. Subsequent mammographic and clinical follow-up has been stable, with no evidence of recurrence 2 years after biopsy.

TEACHING POINTS

Not everything that enhances intensely in a lumpectomy bed is a recurrence. As on other breast imaging modalities, fat necrosis can be a perfect mimic of breast cancer on MRI (see Case 8 in Chapter 7 and Case 11 in this chapter). In this case, the mammographic changes are well within

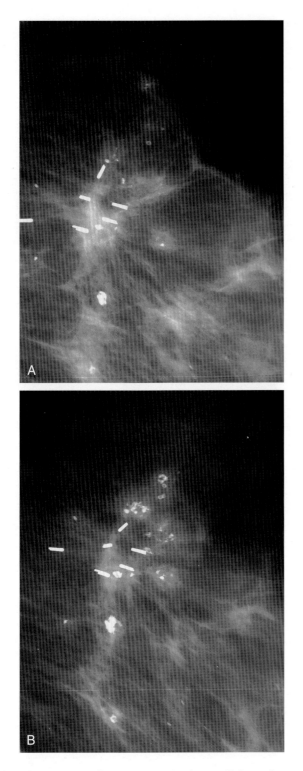

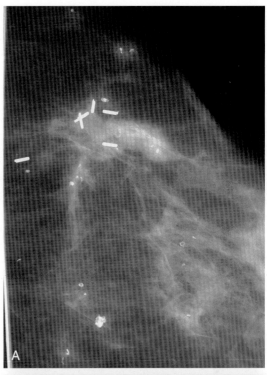

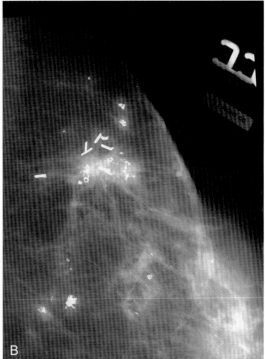

FIGURE 1. Magnification views in the mediolateral projection of the lumpectomy scar in the right upper outer quadrant (UOQ), 6 months apart. **A**, Architectural distortion and density are seen at the level of the surgically placed clips. Coarse dystrophic calcification is developing. **B**, Six months later, increased coalescence of nodular densities is noted, with increased coarse and dystrophic calcification.

FIGURE 2. **A** and **B**, Craniocaudal magnification views of the lumpectomy scar, 6 months apart, performed at the same time as in Figure 1. Contracting density at the level of the clips is seen developing between the two exams, with coarse associated calcification. More peripheral small nodular densities also display coarse, chunky, progressive calcification.

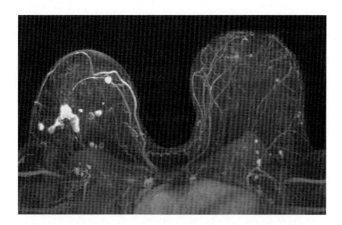

FIGURE 3. Axial maximal intensity projection, enhanced, subtracted breast MRI shows the previously treated right breast to be smaller. Multiple sites of intense mass enhancement are seen on the right, mostly within the UOQ near the prior lumpectomy.

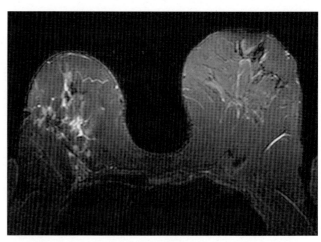

FIGURE 4. Axial STIR breast MRI through the lumpectomy level shows localized edema in the UOQ, extending back to the pectoral muscle level.

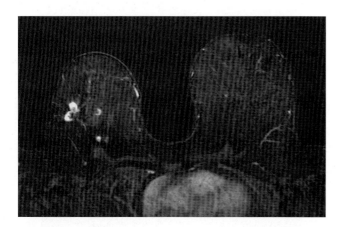

FIGURE 5. Axial enhanced, subtracted breast MRI shows many of the small enhancing masses to be of similar morphology, with partial rings of rim enhancement.

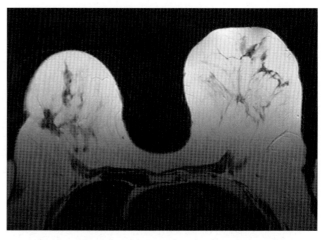

FIGURE 6. Axial T2-weighted image through the same level for correlation.

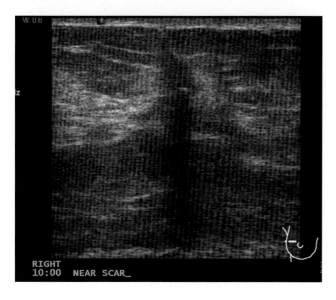

FIGURE 7. Representative ultrasound image through the UOQ shows dense shadowing. Multiple such foci were seen throughout the UOQ.

the described spectrum of fat necrosis changes in the setting of a radiated postlumpectomy scar. The scar shows contraction and increased density over time. Small nodular opacities in the vicinity show progressive coarse, dystrophic calcifications. The MRI findings are clearly abnormal, but correlation with the mammographic findings does suggest fat necrosis as a potential diagnosis. Of course, histologic sampling is required before consideration of the next course of action. In this case, the original breast MRI interpretation of the findings as highly suspicious for recurrent malignancy (without offering any additional differential possibilities) led to concern for possible sampling error when the ultrasound-guided histology of fat necrosis was obtained.

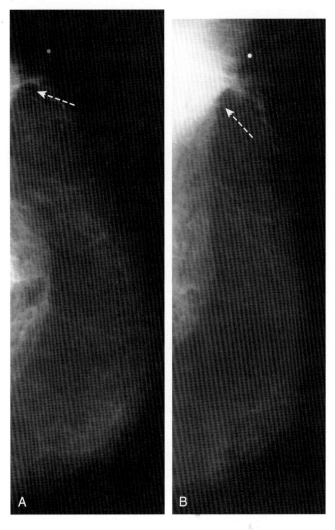

FIGURE 1.   CC (**A**) and laterally exaggerated CC (**B**) mammographic views demonstrate an ill-defined dense mass involving the posterior lateral aspect of the left neobreast (*arrows*). This corresponded to the patient's palpable finding.

CASE 14

TRAM flap recurrence on mammography

A 68-year-old woman, 5 years after left breast mastectomy and transverse rectus abdominis musculocutaneous (TRAM) flap reconstruction, presented with a palpable mass at the lateral aspect of the left TRAM reconstruction (Figure 1). Subsequent core needle biopsy confirmed recurrent infiltrating ductal carcinoma.

TEACHING POINTS

Even when complete mastectomy is performed, a small amount of residual breast tissue remains. TRAM flap recurrence is relatively uncommon, occurring in about 4% to 11% of patients. Many cases present as a palpable mass on clinical exam. Annual mammographic evaluation of the TRAM reconstruction has been advocated to screen any residual breast tissue and to detect recurrences before they are palpable.

SUGGESTED READING

Helvie MA, Bailey JE, Roubidoux MA, et al. Mammographic screening of TRAM flap breast reconstructions for detection of nonpalpable recurrent cancer. *Radiology* 2002; 224:211–216.

CASE 15

Residual carcinoma in TRAM flap–reconstructed neobreast

A 54-year-old woman presented with a palpable mass within the upper outer right breast. The patient was referred to a surgeon for evaluation. Needle biopsy of the palpable mass revealed ductal carcinoma in situ (DCIS). The patient underwent a preoperative MRI, which demonstrated an exten-

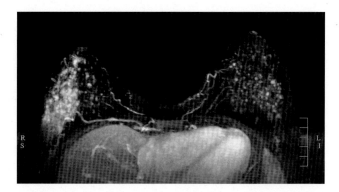

FIGURE 1. Postcontrast subtracted, maximum intensity projection MRI. MRI demonstrates a diffuse segmental area of enhancement involving a large portion of the lateral right breast. In a patient with known right DCIS, these findings are highly suspicious for extensive intraductal carcinoma. Extensive background fibrocystic enhancement is noted bilaterally.

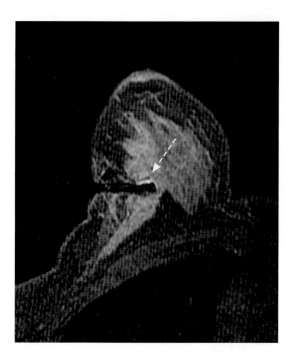

FIGURE 2. Postcontrast axial biopsy MRI of the right breast. MRI-guided biopsy was performed to confirm the extent of the patient's disease. The tip of the biopsy needle (*arrow*) is seen traversing the area of enhancement from a lateral approach. Following the biopsy, a metallic marker clip was placed in the biopsy cavity.

sive area of enhancement in the lateral right breast, suggesting extensive intraductal disease (Figure 1). Mammography and ultrasound failed to demonstrate with certainty the extensive findings seen on MRI. Therefore, MRI-guided biopsy was performed for surgical planning to establish the extent of disease (Figure 2). The MRI-guided biopsy of a site distant to the known right DCIS confirmed additional DCIS. Because of this, the patient underwent right mastectomy with transverse rectus abdominis musculocutaneous (TRAM) flap reconstruction. Pathology showed close margins for the mastectomy specimen. Six months later, the patient had a follow-up MRI that was interpreted as normal (Figure 3). On mammography 1 year after mastectomy, the small marker clip from MRI biopsy was noted in the lateral aspect of the TRAM flap (Figure 4). Ultrasound evaluation of the area of the clip demonstrated multiple small nodules (Figure 5). Core needle biopsy revealed both DCIS and invasive ductal carcinoma. The patient was treated with surgical resection and radiation therapy.

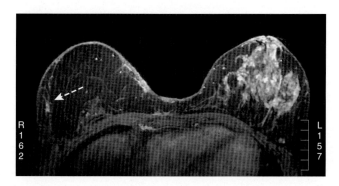

FIGURE 3. Fat-saturated, postcontrast delayed MRI obtained 6 months after the patient's right mastectomy and TRAM flap reconstruction was interpreted at the time as normal. However, in retrospect, a small area of enhancement is seen in the lateral aspect of the TRAM flap reconstructed right breast (*arrow*).

TEACHING POINTS

This case illustrates the role of mammography in surveillance for residual or recurrent disease in patients who undergo mastectomy and TRAM flap reconstruction. This recurrence was not initially detected on follow-up MRI. This case also highlights the fact that even with complete mastectomy, some breast tissue or carcinoma may be left behind, despite negative surgical margins. For that reason, mammographic surveillance of the mastectomy

side may be beneficial. The presence of the MRI-guided biopsy marker clip on the postmastectomy mammogram, from a biopsy positive for DCIS, indicated the patient's disease had not been completely excised. Ultrasound showed suspicious findings for residual disease and served for biopsy guidance. MRI should be used as an adjuvant to mammography for surveillance rather than a

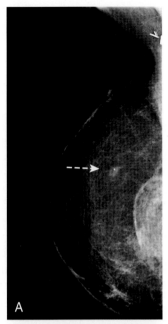

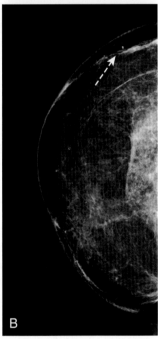

FIGURE 4. Right MLO (**A**) and CC (**B**) mammographic views. The right breast demonstrates changes consistent with mastectomy and TRAM reconstruction. However, a small metallic marker clip is seen in the upper outer neobreast (*arrows*). This is the marker clip from the prior MRI-guided biopsy, performed at the time of initial diagnosis of DCIS.

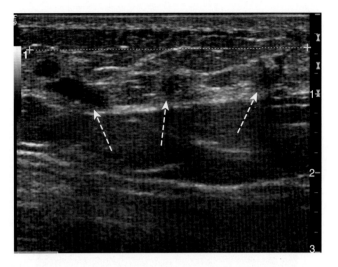

FIGURE 5. Ultrasound image of the TRAM flap. Within the area of the clip, in the lateral TRAM flap reconstructed breast, are demonstrated several small hypoechoic nodules aligned in a ductal orientation (*arrows*).

On both mammography and MRI, the muscular pedicle is seen posteriorly, and the neo-breast is fatty.

SUGGESTED READING

Helvie MA, Bailey JE, Roubidoux MA, et al. Mammographic screening of TRAM flap breast reconstructions for detection of nonpalpable recurrent cancer. *Radiology* 2002; 224:211–216.

replacement. In cases with close or positive surgical margins, MRI cannot exclude small or microscopic foci of residual disease.

The typical imaging features of a TRAM-flap reconstructed breast are well demonstrated here.

CASE 16

TRAM flap reconstruction with fat necrosis and supraclavicular lymphadenopathy, simulating recurrent disease

A 57-year-old woman was suspected to have recurrent breast cancer, based on palpable left supraclavicular adenopathy, 2 years after left mastectomy and TRAM flap reconstruction for recurrent left breast cancer. Her original cancer had been a poorly

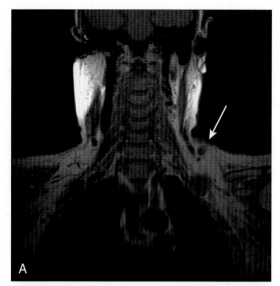

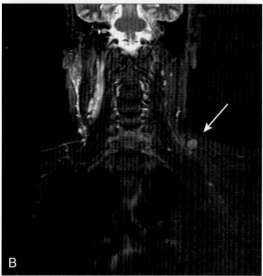

FIGURE 1. T1-weighted (**A**) and STIR (**B**) coronal images from an MRI of the neck soft tissues show a small round left supraclavicular lymph node (*arrow*), which was initially detected by palpation.

later referred for CT-guided biopsy. This obtained a fragment of a benign lymph node, with no morphologic evidence of metastatic carcinoma. The patient was followed clinically, and underwent positron emission tomography (PET)/CT about 1.5 years after the lymph node was first noted. Two hypermetabolic foci were identified on PET/CT, one in the reconstructed neo-breast and one corresponding with the left supraclavicular node (Figures 2, 3, 4, and 5). The findings were interpreted as consistent with recurrent breast malignancy. Breast MRI was obtained subsequently and showed a rim-enhancing mass with fatty and soft tissue elements at the posterior aspect of the reconstructed breast (Figure 6). This was thought to be secondary to the TRAM flap surgery, with fat necrosis. The patient had not had a mammogram since the surgery, so mammography was obtained for correlation (Figures 7 and 8). This showed rim and coarse fat necrosis–type calcifications (CT images provided for correlation, Figures 9 and 10). Subsequent ultrasound-guided biopsy confirmed fat necrosis with dense fibrosis and calcification (Figure 11). The left supraclavicular lymph node was excised, was benign, with nonspecific granulomatous lymphadenitis, and presumably was reactive and secondary to the breast process.

TEACHING POINTS

Development of palpable lymphadenopathy and thoracic foci of hypermetabolism on PET are certainly ominous in patients who have been previously treated for breast cancer, particularly a patient like this with a prior recurrence. This case reminds us that not all hypermetabolic foci on PET are due to neoplasia, and it requires careful correlation with the clinical data and other imaging studies to draw the correct conclusions. Often, as in this case, alternative, benign diagnoses may be suggested by other information and may require histologic proof or longitudinal follow-up for differentiation.

The fat necrosis findings in this case are a florid, dramatic example, but nonetheless display many of the typical features of fat necrosis lesions. Fat necrosis is a nonsuppurative, inflammatory process of aseptic saponification of fat, induced by blood and tissue lipase after trauma. The trauma can be surgical, as in this case; and surgery, especially extensive surgery, is the most common cause of fat necrosis. Other commonly encountered etiologies are blunt or penetrating trauma and radiation therapy. Other insults, such as breast infection or

differentiated, stage 1, node-negative, estrogen receptor– and progesterone receptor–negative tumor, which was treated with lumpectomy, four cycles of doxorubicin (Adriamycin) plus cyclophosphamide (Cytoxan) (AC) and radiation therapy 2.5 years before recurring.

Two years after undergoing mastectomy and TRAM flap reconstruction, the patient was noted on physical examination to have a 2-cm firm left supraclavicular lymph node. It was confirmed by MRI (Figure 1). Referral to an ear, nose, and throat specialist for fine-needle aspiration (FNA) resulted in development of arm paresthesias during the procedure, which was stopped. The patient was

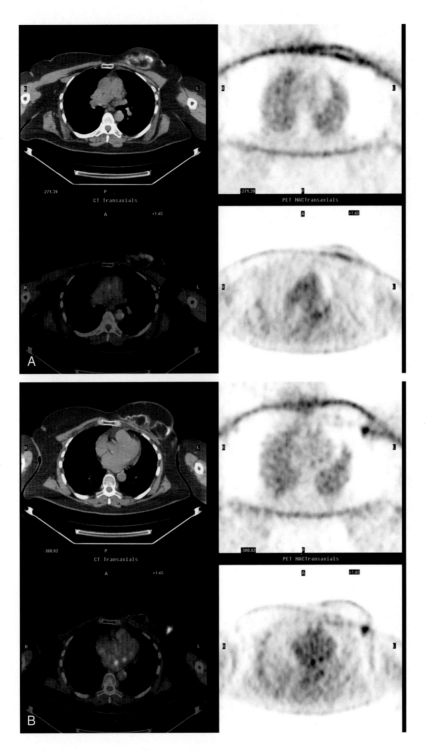

FIGURE 2.   Axial images (two levels, **A** and **B**) from PET/CT (*upper left*: CT; *upper right*: non-attenuation-corrected (NAC) PET; *lower left*: fused PET/CT; *lower right*: CT attenuation-corrected PET) through the breasts. The left breast has been reconstructed postmastectomy, using a TRAM flap. At the posterior aspect of the neo-breast, a whorl of fat with surrounding soft tissue rind and coarse calcifications is seen. Hypermetabolism is seen, which localizes to the coarsely calcifying components. This appears more linear in (**A**) and more focal below (**B**).

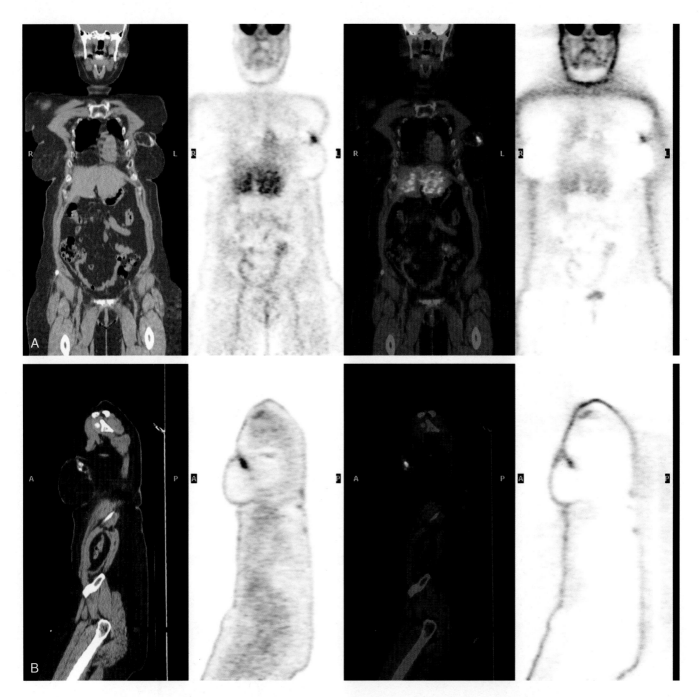

FIGURE 3.   Coronal (**A**) and sagittal (**B**) views through the focal activity within the left neo-breast (*from left to right*: CT, PET, fused PET/CT, NAC PET).

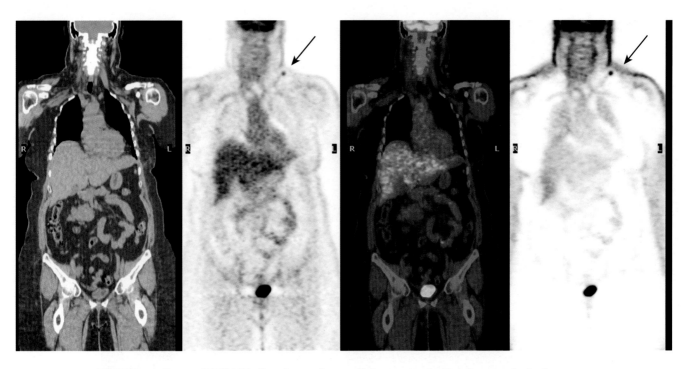

FIGURE 4. Coronal PET/CT slice shows the small, hypermetabolic left supraclavicular lymph node.

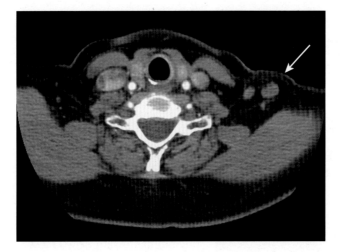

FIGURE 5. Axial section from a contrast-enhanced CT scan at the supraclavicular level shows two adjacent, mildly enlarged lymph nodes.

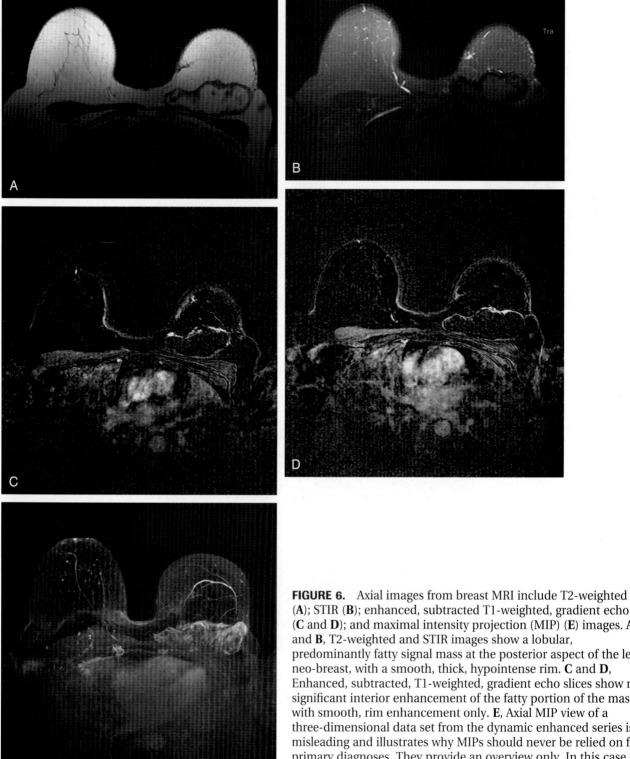

FIGURE 6.   Axial images from breast MRI include T2-weighted
(**A**); STIR (**B**); enhanced, subtracted T1-weighted, gradient echo
(**C** and **D**); and maximal intensity projection (MIP) (**E**) images. **A**
and **B**, T2-weighted and STIR images show a lobular,
predominantly fatty signal mass at the posterior aspect of the left
neo-breast, with a smooth, thick, hypointense rim. **C** and **D**,
Enhanced, subtracted, T1-weighted, gradient echo slices show no
significant interior enhancement of the fatty portion of the mass,
with smooth, rim enhancement only. **E**, Axial MIP view of a
three-dimensional data set from the dynamic enhanced series is
misleading and illustrates why MIPs should never be relied on for
primary diagnoses. They provide an overview only. In this case,
the rim-enhancing fat necrosis mass is summated, and it appears
here as a more extensively enhancing mass.

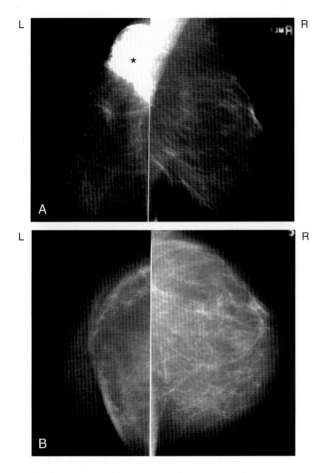

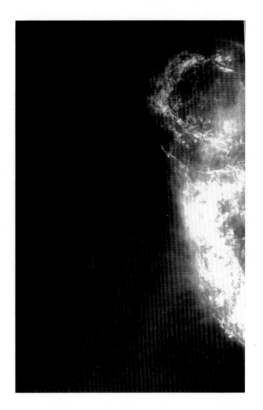

FIGURE 8.   Detail view (exaggerated CC view) of the left breast calcification shows it to be coarse, shell-like, and dystrophic.

FIGURE 7.   MLO (**A**) and CC (**B**) mammograms show the fatty composition of the reconstructed left neo-breast. Dense calcification is mass-like overlying the pectoral muscle on the left, posteriorly and superiorly on the MLO view (*asterisk*).

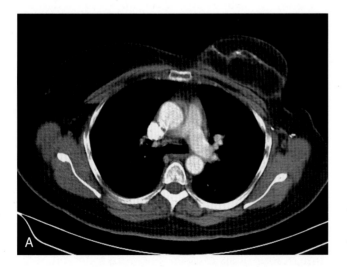

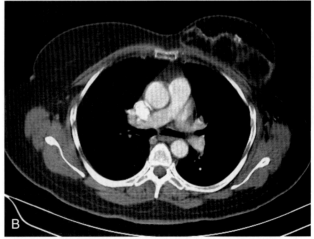

FIGURE 9.   Corresponding CT images (**A** and **B**) show a lobular, centrally fatty mass in the upper reconstructed left breast, with thick soft tissue density rim and coarse peripheral calcifications.

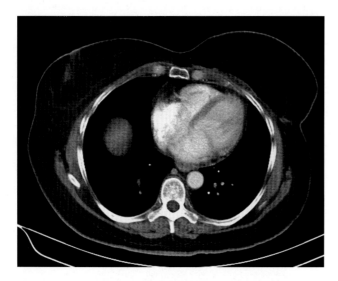

FIGURE 10. A section through the inferior left neo-breast shows a more typical, uncomplicated TRAM flap appearance, being essentially completely fatty, with the atrophied rectus muscle flap against the chest wall, with minimal asymmetry compared with the native right chest wall.

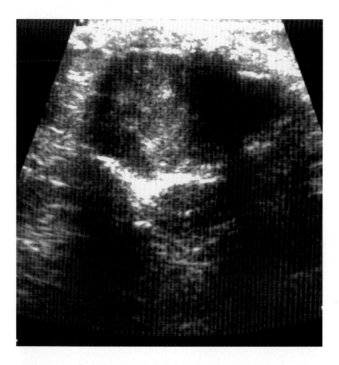

FIGURE 11. Sonography of the fat necrosis mass in the left neo-breast shows it to be lobular, solid, and very heterogeneous, with hyperechoic and hypoechoic components.

spontaneous subareolar duct rupture, are less common causes of fat necrosis. When symptomatic, fat necrosis most commonly is detected clinically as a painless, palpable breast mass. The imaging appearance ranges from characteristically

benign (oil cysts) to confounding. On both clinical and imaging grounds, fat necrosis can be indistinguishable from malignancy and may require sampling for differentiation. Fat necrosis can be considered the "great mimic" of breast cancer because it can present as calcifications, spiculated masses, or architectural distortion. See Cases 11 and 13 in this chapter and Case 8 in Chapter 7 for additional examples. The most reliable mammographic finding for the diagnosis is an oil cyst, resulting from liquefaction of fat. Calcifications forming in response to fat necrosis can be fairly characteristic when mature, being coarse and dystrophic and forming eggshell or rim-like forms, often on the margins of oil cysts. Of course, developing fat necrosis calcifications can often be indeterminate when first detected. The decision to biopsy newly identified calcifications forming in a surgical bed depends on numerous factors, including how the prior cancer manifested (mass versus microcalcifications), the morphology of the calcifications, and the time course since surgery, with fat necrosis most commonly developing within 3 years after completion of therapy. Histologically, fat necrosis lesions show fat cell death, with vacuole formation, with surrounding fibroblasts, lipid-laden macrophages, and multinucleated giant cells.

Review of the imaging features of this lesion delineates many of the imaging manifestations of fat necrosis. The mass is fatty centrally, with characteristic density on CT and signal intensity on MRI. The soft tissue component is peripheral and rim-like, and the calcifications are coarse and dystrophic. The enhancement associated with the mass on MRI corresponds to the peripheral fibrosis component. The sonographic appearance is of a complex and heterogeneous solid mass but is well within the spectrum described as potential ultrasound appearances of fat necrosis masses in a series by Soo and colleagues. The ultrasound findings in this study ranged from cystic to complex to solid-appearing masses, with circumscribed or irregular margins, often with distortion of the normal adjacent breast anatomy. The ultrasound appearances of 31 fat necrosis masses in 23 patients analyzed in this report categorized them as solid in 15, complex with mural nodules in 7, complex with echogenic bands in 4, anechoic with posterior acoustic enhancement in 2, anechoic with shadowing in 2, and without a visible mass in 1. Evolution of the sonographic appearance was noted over time of four of six masses that were followed, with complex lesions either becoming increasingly solid in three or increasingly cystic in one. These six fat necrosis masses, which were followed with ultrasound, either stayed unchanged in size over time (two cases) or decreased in size (four cases).

The inflammation associated with fat necrosis presumably accounts for the PET positivity noted in this case. Inflammatory cells, namely leukocytes and macrophages, utilize glucose and take up fluorodeoxyglucose (FDG), and so active inflammatory processes can be expected to be visualized on FDG PET. In general, the degree of activity is less intense than in most neoplastic processes, but there is overlap. In this case, the large size and extent of the fat necrosis are presumed to be responsible for the supraclavicular nodal reaction that ultimately led to this extensive evaluation.

SUGGESTED READINGS

Devon RK, Rosen MA, Mies C, et al. Breast reconstruction with a transverse rectus abdominis myocutaneous flap: spectrum of normal and abnormal MR imaging findings. *RadioGraphics* 2004; 24(5):1287–1299.

LePage MA, Kazerooni EA, Helvie MA, et al. Breast reconstruction with TRAM flaps: normal and abnormal appearances at CT. *RadioGraphics* 1999; 19:1593–1603.

Soo MS, Kornguth PJ, Hertzberg BS, et al. Fat necrosis in the breast: sonographic features. *Radiology* 1998; 206:261–269.

CASE 17

Chest wall recurrence detected on surveillance MRI

A 72-year-old woman, 7 years after treatment with lumpectomy and radiation therapy for left breast infiltrating ductal carcinoma, underwent annual screening MRI. The MRI demonstrated an abnormal area of enhancement involving the anterior chest wall, suspicious for chest wall recurrence (Figure 1). CT and positron emission tomography (PET) scans were performed to further evaluate the finding. The CT scan confirmed the findings (Figure 2), and the PET scan showed increased uptake of the abnormality (Figure 3). Subsequent needle biopsy confirmed the suspected diagnosis of chest wall recurrence, and the patient was treated with radiation therapy.

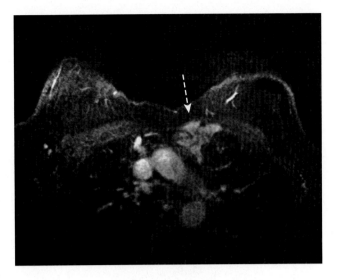

FIGURE 1. Postcontrast, subtracted, axial MRI demonstrates an ill-defined geographic area of enhancement in the left anterior chest wall, extending into the anterior mediastinum (*arrow*).

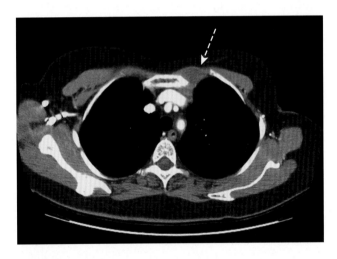

FIGURE 2. Postcontrast CT confirms an abnormal area of soft tissue density in the left anterior mediastinum, involving the anterior chest wall (*arrow*), corresponding to the finding on MRI.

TEACHING POINTS

This case illustrates the ability of MRI to detect recurrent disease in patients treated for breast carcinoma. In addition to in-breast recurrences, the anterior chest wall, mediastinum, and axilla can be evaluated on MRI. PET/CT may help to improve diagnostic confidence and accuracy in evaluating the extent of recurrent disease. It

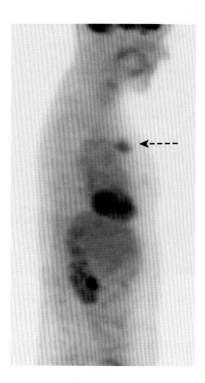

FIGURE 3. Sagittal projection PET volume image. Within the anterior chest wall is an area of focally increased uptake (*arrow*) that corresponds to the area seen on MRI and CT. Together, the findings are highly suspicious for chest wall recurrence.

also plays an important role in the diagnosis of bone metastases, providing information regarding the presence or absence of structural skeletal lesions on CT as well as their degree of metabolic activity.

SUGGESTED READINGS

Fueger BJ, Weber WA, Quon A, et al. Performance of 2-deoxy-2-[F-18]fluoro-D glucose positron emission tomography and integrated PET/CT in restaged breast cancer patients. *Mol Imaging Biol* 2005; 7:369–376.

Isasi CR, Moadel R, Blaufox MD. A meta-analysis of FDG-PET for the evaluation of breast cancer recurrence and metastases. *Breast Cancer Res Treat* 2005; 90:105–112.

Tastumi M, Cohade C, Mourtzikos M, et al. Initial experience with FDG-PET/CT in the evaluation of breast cancer. *Eur J Nucl Med Mol Imaging* 2006; 33:254–262.

CASE 18

Recurrent IDC and radiation-induced pleomorphic sarcoma, with chest wall invasion*

A 79-year-old woman noted a change in the appearance of her right breast for several months. She was 5 years post–breast conservation therapy for a stage I, T1N0, 1.2-cm poorly differentiated infiltrating ductal carcinoma (IDC), estrogen receptor and progesterone receptor positive, *HER-2/neu* negative, with five negative lymph nodes. She had been taking tamoxifen and later anastrozole (Arimidex).

On physical examination, the right lateral breast was indurated and fixed to the chest wall. Her mammogram showed suspicious increased density deep to the level of her scar (Figures 1, 2, and 3). Ultrasound showed a corresponding, heterogeneous, hypoechoic mass with irregular margins (Figure 4). Ultrasound-guided core needle biopsy showed recurrent ductal carcinoma and a very atypical spindle cell proliferation, with atypia in excess of that expected from radiation damage. This component was thought to be a pleomorphic sarcoma, probably radiation induced.

Subsequent evaluations included breast MRI; chest, abdomen, and pelvis CT scans; and positron emission tomography (PET)/CT. The breast MRI showed the mass to be large, with rim enhancement and washout. The mass penetrated and invaded the chest wall and was accompanied by a large internal mammary lymph node (Figures 5, 6, 7, and 8). Both the mass and the internal mammary lymph node were intensely hypermetabolic on PET, as was a right lower lobe nodule (Figure 9).

TEACHING POINTS

Locally recurrent breast cancer may be heralded by a change in physical examination or may be first identified by a change on imaging. Local recurrences in patients previously treated with breast conservation most commonly occur within the lumpectomy bed. Contraction of a postsurgical

*Case courtesy of Dr. Eva Cean, Tri-City Medical Center, Oceanside, CA.

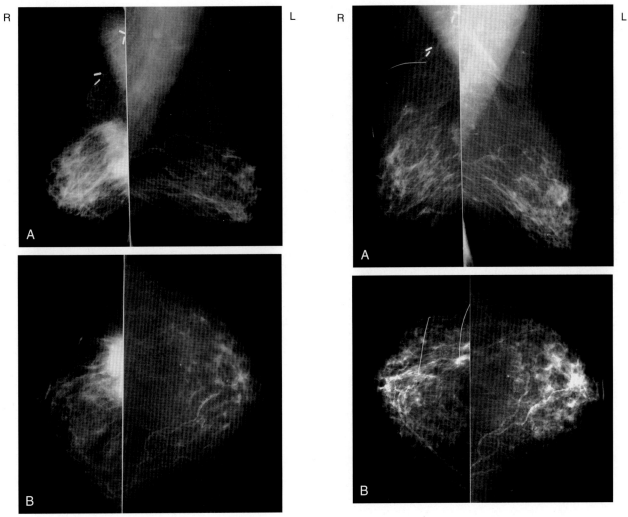

FIGURE 1. MLO (**A**) and CC (**B**) mammograms show the previously treated right breast to be smaller than the left. New increased density seen in the deep lateral right breast, subjacent to the scar level, is not visualized in its entirety. Right axillary surgical clips from prior dissection are noted.

FIGURE 2. MLO (**A**) and CC (**B**) mammograms from 2 years earlier with scar markers delineating the area of prior lumpectomy.

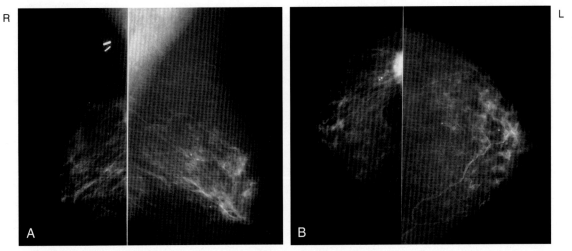

FIGURE 3. MLO (**A**) and CC (**B**) comparison mammograms from 1 year earlier show developing density in the right posterior lateral breast, included only on the CC view.

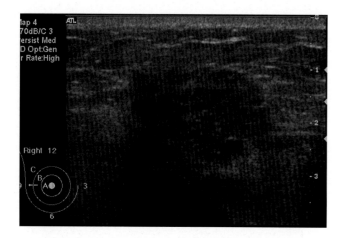

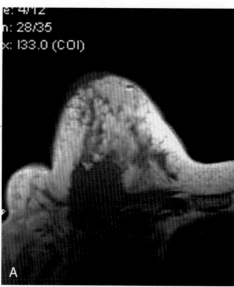

FIGURE 4. Breast sonogram shows a hypoechoic mass with posterior shadowing and irregular margins in the right lateral breast, corresponding to the mammographic abnormality.

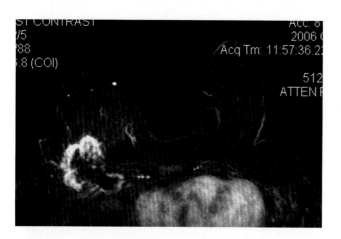

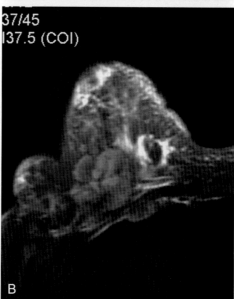

FIGURE 5. Enhanced, subtracted, axial breast MRI view of both breasts shows a lobular mass in the right posterior lateral breast, with intense rim enhancement. The mass traverses the chest wall and extends into the chest.

FIGURE 6. Axial T1-weighted (**A**) and STIR (**B**) views of the mass show it to be hypointense on T1 and mildly hyperintense on STIR. The right breast skin is thickened, and there is diffuse edema and reticulation of the breast. Although these findings are expected with prior radiation, the changes are more than generally seen 5 years after treatment. This suggests lymphedema from obstructed lymphatics as a potential alternative explanation.

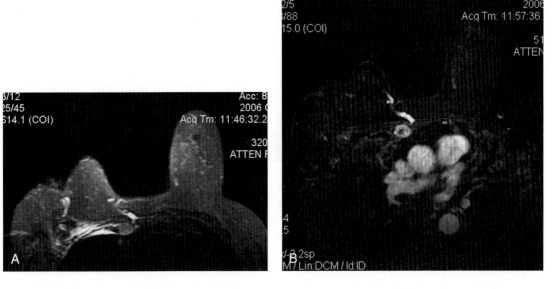

FIGURE 7. Axial STIR (**A**) and enhanced, subtracted, T1-weighted gradient echo (**B**) MRI views show an enlarged right internal mammary lymph node. Its enhancement is peripheral, similar to the primary, suggesting central necrosis.

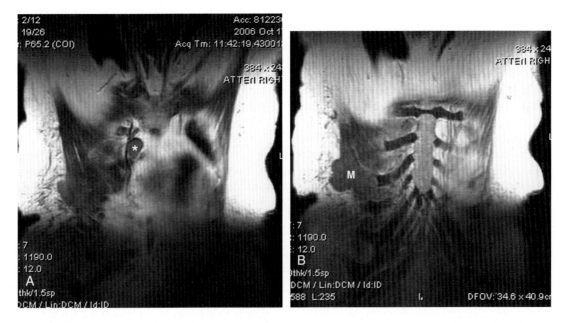

FIGURE 8. Adjacent T1-weighted, coronal MRIs of the thorax (**A** anterior to **B**) show the enlarged right internal mammary (IM) lymph node adjacent to the IM vessels (*asterisk*). The lobular primary mass (M) infiltrates chest wall muscle.

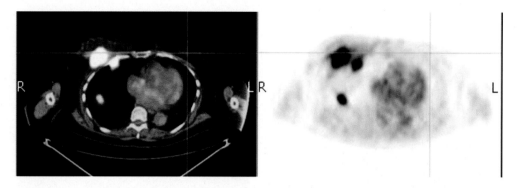

FIGURE 9. Axial fused PET/CT and PET images show intense hypermetabolism of the right breast mass, extending through the chest wall, and in a right lower lobe lung metastasis.

scar can be expected as a normal evolution in the appearance of a previously treated breast. However, increased size or density of a scar should be cause for concern and further evaluation. Enhanced breast MRI can be very helpful in differentiating between a scar and recurrent disease, although occasionally, a complicated scar, such as by fat necrosis, can convincingly mimic recurrent disease (see Case 11 in this chapter).

In this case, there is a dramatic change on mammography to correlate with the concerning change on physical examination. The mass is posterior, but the true extent of its posterior involvement is difficult to assess based on mammography and ultrasound. On mammography, the posterior margin is never visualized, and on ultrasound, there is intense posterior shadowing. The clinical fixation is highly concerning. Before any therapeutic decisions can be made, the issue of chest wall invasion has to be addressed. The best modality available is breast MRI, with its high soft tissue contrast and high sensitivity to contrast enhancement. Morris and colleagues have shown that abutment of muscle or obscuration of the intervening fat plane by a posterior breast mass does not imply involvement. Actual enhancement within muscle is necessary to predict muscular invasion.

Breast MRI can accurately depict whether the pectoralis muscle (considered part of the breast) or chest wall (ribs, intercostal muscles, serratus anterior muscle) is involved. The degree of involvement has important surgical implications. If only superficial enhancement of the pectoralis muscle is identified, a portion of the muscle will have to be excised to obtain a negative posterior margin. If more extensive pectoralis muscle involvement is

evident, radical mastectomy, with excision of the muscle, may be necessary. If chest wall involvement is found, surgical treatment will need to include chest wall reconstruction. Chest wall involvement signifies a T4 lesion (any size, skin or chest wall involved), making the patient's stage at least stage IIIB.

In this case, the degree of chest wall involvement is such that there is penetration into the thorax, forming a lobular pleural-based component. This degree of involvement is so extensive that it can be readily appreciated on both CT and PET, but lesser degrees of chest wall involvement cannot reliably be detected by CT or PET. Surgery is not indicated at this point in this patient because there is evidence of metastases (right lower lobe lung nodule).

The dual histology in this case is also unusual. The ultrasound-guided core biopsy specimens were compared with the original breast primary and were morphologically similar, representing recurrent invasive poorly differentiated ductal carcinoma. However, a component with atypical spindle cell proliferation was noted, in excess of that expected in a radiation-damaged field, which was interpreted by outside consultation as a postirradiation pleomorphic sarcoma. Radiation-induced sarcomas are a rare, but recognized, late potential complication of radiation therapy in breast conservation patients. See Case 9 in Chapter 13 for an additional example and discussion of this issue.

SUGGESTED READING

Morris EA, Schwartz LH, Drotman MB, et al. Evaluation of pectoralis major muscle in patients with posterior breast tumors on breast MR images: early experience. *Radiology* 2000; 214:67–72.

CHAPTER 7

Breast Cancer Mimics

A variety of processes, both benign and malignant, may mimic primary breast carcinoma.[1-4] Many of these can be distinguished from breast cancer on the basis of imaging findings alone. However, some may ultimately require histopathologic confirmation. The most common benign causes of masses in women are fibroadenomas and breast cysts.[5] High-quality imaging, including diagnostic mammography and high-resolution ultrasound and strict adherence to interpretive criteria can, for the most part, distinguish fibroadenomas and cysts from breast cancer. However, because there is sufficient overlap in the appearance of benign and malignant lesions, a new or enlarging solid mass that is not classically benign (e.g., hamartoma or lipoma) requires biopsy. In addition to lesions related to the duct-lobular system, mimics of primary breast cancer may also be caused by a wide spectrum of pathologic disorders arising in mesenchymal structures of the mammary gland. These include tumors arising in the stroma of the breast that are breast specific, such as pseudoangiomatous stromal hyperplasia (PASH) and phyllodes tumors, as well as tumors arising from non-breast-specific stromal structures, including fibrous tissue, vascular structures, lymphoid tissue, nerves, and skin. These non-breast-specific tumors include focal fibrosis, fibromatosis, malignant fibrohistiocytomas, vascular malformations, angiosarcomas, neurofibromas, lymphomas, and liposarcomas. In addition, cancer mimics may also be caused by inflammatory processes (foreign body reaction, mastitis, and abscess), trauma (hematoma, fat necrosis), lactational changes, and metastasis from extramammary malignancies.

EPITHELIAL BREAST LESIONS

Fibroadenomas

Fibroadenomas, the most common benign tumors in the breast, are fibroepithelial tumors that develop in the lobules at the ends of mammary gland ducts. On mammography, fibroadenomas appear as well-defined round, oval, or lobulated masses. They may be calcified, initially with small peripheral calcifications that later coalesce over time into coarser popcorn-shaped features. Classic calcified fibroadenomas require no further workup or biopsy. On ultrasound, fibroadenomas appear as well-circumscribed elliptic masses that are either hypoechoic or isoechoic and have uniform echogenicity. In 15% of cases, multiple fibroadenomas are present. Fibroadenomas occasionally develop into very large masses, particularly in adolescent girls and young women; such masses are called juvenile giant fibroadenomas. Other special varieties of fibroadenomas include lactating adenomas and tubular adenomas.

Sclerosing Adenosis

Although most breast calcifications are benign, clustered microcalcifications that do not appear classically benign on mammography (e.g., milk of calcium, vascular or rim calcifications), usually require biopsy. Sclerosing adenosis, a form of fibrocystic change, is a frequent mimicker of breast carcinoma. The mammographic findings of sclerosing adenosis include microcalcifications, a circumscribed mass, an ill-defined mass, a spiculated mass, focal asymmetry, and focal architectural distortion.[6-8]

Papillomas

Benign papillomas are another common breast lesion that can mimic carcinoma. Typically they present with bloody nipple discharge and occur in perimenopausal women. Mammographically, they present as single or multiple circumscribed or irregular masses, with or without microcalcifications. Sonographically, they may present as a complex intracystic lesion, intraductal lesion, or a homogeneous solid lesion. Because papillomas cannot be distinguished from papillary carcinoma or ductal carcinoma on the basis of clinical features or imaging features, biopsy is necessary.[9]

Radial Scars

Radial scar (RS), also known as a complex sclerosing lesion, is a benign lesion that is often mistaken

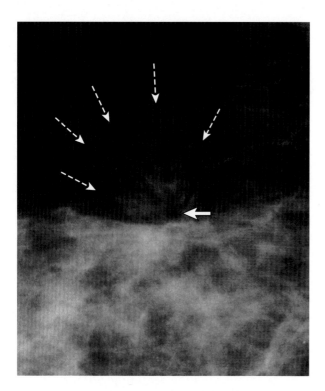

FIGURE 1. Close-up mammographic view of a radial scar. The thin spicules (*small arrows*) and lucent center (*large arrow*) are suggestive of a radial scar. However, biopsy is necessary to exclude malignancy.

for carcinoma because of its spiculated appearance (Figure 1).

The pathogenesis of RS remains obscure. It has been postulated that these lesions arise as a result of unknown injury, leading to fibrosis and retraction of surrounding breast tissue. Although imaging features such as lack of a central mass and long, thin, radiating spicules help to suggest the diagnosis of RS, because they are commonly associated with atypia and malignancy, biopsy is necessary.[10–11]

LESIONS OF THE BREAST STROMA (BREAST SPECIFIC)

Pseudoangiomatous Stromal Hyperplasia
Pseudoangiomatous stromal hyperplasia is a mesenchymal lesion composed of myofibroblasts, which sometimes includes glandular components. It is frequently a microscopic incidental finding in breast biopsies but may occasionally present as a round or oval circumscribed or partially circumscribed mass mammographically.[12–15] The sonographic appearance may be variable, with most presenting as a solid, hypoechoic mass without

posterior acoustic shadowing. They typically occur in premenopausal women and pathologically may be mistaken for angiosarcoma.

Phyllodes Tumor
Phyllodes tumor, also called *cystosarcoma phyllodes*, are unusual fibroepithelial tumors composed of epithelium and a spindle cell stroma and can exhibit a wide range of clinical behavior. Radiographically they present as a rapidly growing, hypoechoic, circumscribed mass.[16] They are classified as benign, borderline, or malignant based on histopathologic features. However, histologic classification does not always predict outcome. The prognosis of phyllodes tumors is favorable, with local recurrence in about 15% of patients overall and distant recurrence in about 5% to 10%.

LESIONS OF THE BREAST STROMA (NONBREAST–SPECIFIC)

Focal Fibrosis
Focal fibrosis, also known as fibrous mastopathy, is similar to pseudoangiomatous stromal hyperplasia. These lesions typically occur in premenopausal women and present as a circumscribed mass, irregular mass, or focal asymmetry and are hypoechoic on ultrasound. They are composed of dense collagenous stroma with sparse glandular and vascular elements.[17–18]

Fibromatosis
Fibromatosis, also known as extra-abdominal desmoid tumor, is an extremely rare low-grade infiltrative tumor composed of well-differentiated fibroblasts. The lesions tend to develop in the pectoralis fascia and may be fixed, causing retraction of the pectoralis muscle, skin, or nipple. On mammography, fibromatosis usually appears as a spiculated mass simulating carcinoma.[19] On ultrasound, the lesions manifest as an irregular hypoechoic mass with posterior acoustic shadowing (Figure 2). Biopsy is necessary for diagnosis. Although fibromatosis does not metastasize, there is a high rate of local recurrence.

Diabetic Fibrous Mastopathy
Diabetic mastopathy is an unusual form of stromal fibrosis with lymphocytic infiltration, which typically occurs in premenopausal women with juvenile-onset insulin-dependent diabetes (type 1). Patients present with solitary or multiple nontender, hard masses. Mammography shows generalized dense tissue, and ultrasound shows an

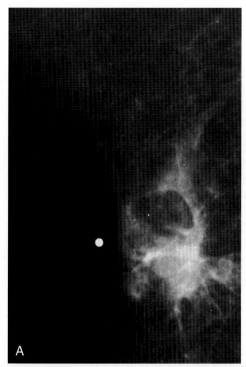

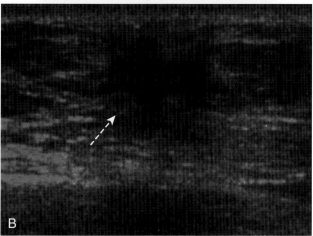

FIGURE 2. Fibromatosis (extra-abdominal desmoid). **A,** Close-up mammographic view demonstrates a spiculated mass in the inframammary fold of the right breast. **B,** Ultrasound demonstrates an irregular hypoechoic solid mass (*arrow*).

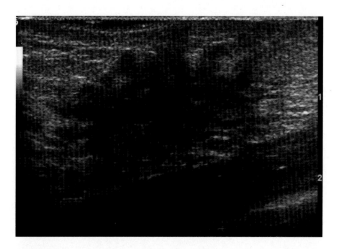

FIGURE 3. Diabetic fibrous mastopathy. Ultrasound evaluation of a 38-year-old woman with a history of diabetes who presented with a palpable mass reveals an irregular hypoechoic mass with posterior acoustic shadowing. Biopsy revealed diabetic fibrous mastopathy.

irregular hypoechoic mass with posterior acoustic shadowing (Figure 3).

Vascular Tumors

Vascular tumors of the breast are uncommon and include hemangiomas and angiosarcomas.[20] Hemangiomas are extremely rare, are usually smaller than 2 cm, and can be differentiated from dermal hemangiomas by their distinct separation from the epidermis. Mammographically, breast hemangio-mas are small, well-defined, lobulated masses. On ultrasound, their appearance may be variable, being either circumscribed hypoechoic masses, mixed echogenicity masses, or ill-defined hypere-choic masses (Figure 4). Angiosarcomas of the breast are more common than hemangiomas and are usually larger in size. Radiographically, they present as an ill-defined calcified or noncalcified hypoechoic mass. They may occur in the chest wall as a rare complication following radiation therapy for primary breast cancer.

Neural Tumors

Breast tumors of neural origin are rare and include granular cell tumors and neurofibromas. Granular cell tumors are uncommon benign tumors of prob-able Schwann cell origin that occasionally present as a breast mass. They occur more frequently in the upper inner quadrant, corresponding to the cuta-neous sensory territory of the supraclavicular nerve. Granular cell tumors occur in middle-aged, premenopausal women, usually as an irregular or spiculated hypoechoic mass with posterior acous-tic shadowing. Wide local excision is generally the preferred treatment because these tend to recur if incompletely excised. Neurofibromas are benign peripheral nerve sheath tumors, usually occurring in the subcutaneous tissue and occasionally are found in the breast. Mammographically they appear as multiple, well-defined, benign-appearing cuta-neous masses. On ultrasound, they appear as well-defined hypoechoic masses with posterior acoustic enhancement, located in the subcutaneous tissue. Clinical history usually makes the diagnosis

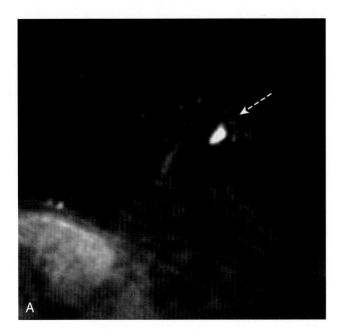 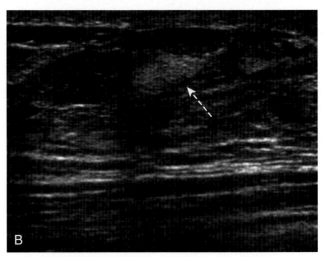

FIGURE 4.   Capillary hemangioma. **A,** Postcontrast subtracted axial MRI demonstrates a smooth, oval, enhancing mass in the superior left breast (*arrow*). **B,** Ultrasound demonstrates a corresponding superficial hyperechoic mass (*arrow*).

obvious. Neurofibromas occurring in the breast are rare, are usually associated with neurofibromatosis type 1 in the pediatric patient and occur in a peri-areolar location.

INFECTION AND INFLAMMATION

Mastitis

Mastitis is a focal or diffuse infection of the breast and can present as a swollen, red, and tender breast with or without axillary adenopathy. *Staphylococcus aureus* and streptococcal bacteria are the most common agents, and occasionally mastitis may develop into an abscess. It may be difficult to distinguish breast infection from inflammatory carcinoma. Ultimately, skin punch biopsy may be necessary in cases of persistent infections to exclude carcinoma.

Granulomatous Mastitis

Granulomatous mastitis of the breast is a rare entity that often presents as a palpable mass. The clinical and imaging findings may be confused with inflammatory carcinoma of the breast. The diagnosis should be suspected in patients from endemic regions. In addition to infectious causes such as tuberculosis and fungus, granulomatous mastitis

may also be due to autoimmune diseases, such as sarcoidosis, or it may be idiopathic in nature.[21-23]

MISCELLANEOUS BREAST LESIONS

Fat Necrosis

Fat necrosis is a benign, nonsuppurative process related to breast trauma, usually from prior surgical procedures. On mammography, fat necrosis can produce changes that are similar in appearance to malignancy (Figure 5). It can appear as a hypoechoic, shadowing mass with spiculated margins that may contain indeterminate microcalcifications and can cause skin retraction.[24-25] The presence of central fat or dystrophic rim calcifications is usually diagnostic. Correlation of the imaging finding with the clinical history can aid in the diagnosis.

Metastasis

Metastatic disease should be considered when there is bilateral axillary adenopathy or multiple bilateral irregular solid masses. The most common metastatic lesions in the breast, in order of frequency, are due to lymphoma; melanoma (Figure 6); lung, ovarian, renal cell, and cervical carcinoma; and leukemia.[26]

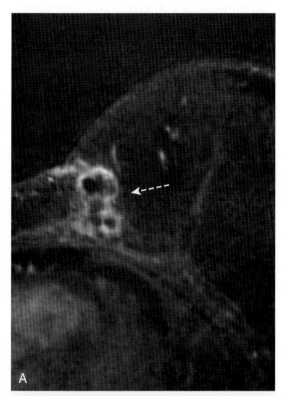

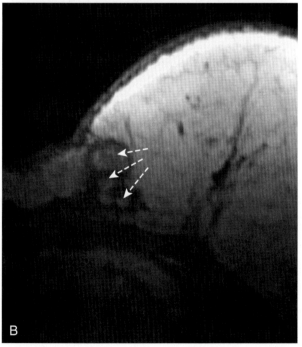

FIGURE 5. Fat necrosis. **A,** Postcontrast axial MRI of a 65-year-old woman after left mastectomy and transverse rectus abdominis myocutaneous (TRAM) flap reconstruction who presented with a palpable mass. Within the medial aspect of the TRAM flap, corresponding to the palpable mass, is an irregular, rim-enhancing lesion (*arrow*). **B,** The precontrast non-fat-saturated axial T1-weighted MRI demonstrates several areas of fat signal intensity (*arrows*) within the lesion, characteristic of fat necrosis.

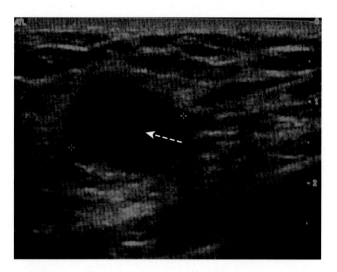

FIGURE 6. Metastatic melanoma to the breast. Ultrasound demonstrates an irregular hypoechoic solid mass with posterior acoustic enhancement. Although this could be mistaken for a cyst, its irregular margins and internal echoes (*arrow*) are suspicious for a solid mass. Biopsy revealed metastatic melanoma.

Metastatic involvement of the breast from an extramammary malignancy is uncommon, with an incidence of between 0.8% and 6.6%. Rhabdomyosarcoma is the most common extramammary malignancy to metastasize to the breast in the pediatric age group but is rare in adults.

REFERENCES

1. Iglesias A, Arias M, Santiago P, et al. Benign breast lesions that simulate malignancy: magnetic resonance imaging with radiologic-pathologic correlation. *Curr Probl Diagn Radiol* 2007; 36(2):66–82.
2. Porter GJ, Evans AJ, Lee AH, et al. Unusual benign breast lesions [review]. *Clin Radiol* 2006; 61(7):562–569.
3. Harvey JA. Unusual breast cancers: useful clues to expanding the differential diagnosis. *Radiology* 2007; 242(3):683–694.
4. Pojchamarnwiputh S, Muttarak M, Na-Chiangmai W, et al. Benign breast lesions mimicking carcinoma at mammography. *Singapore Med J* 2007; 48(10):958–968.
5. Foster ME, Garrahan N, Williams S. Fibroadenoma of the breast: a clinical and pathological study. *J R Coll Surg Edinb* 1998; 33:16–19.
6. Cyrlak D, Carpenter PM, Rawal NB. Breast imaging case of the day: florid sclerosing adenosis. *RadioGraphics* 1999; 19:245–247.
7. Nielsen NS, Nielsen BB. Mammographic features of sclerosing adenosis presenting as a tumour. *Clin Radiol* 1986; 37:371–373.

8. Günhan-Bilgen I, Memis A, Ustün EE, et al. Sclerosing adenosis: mammographic and ultrasonographic findings with clinical and histopathological correlation. *Eur J Radiol* 2002; 44:232–238.

9. Lam WW, Chu WC, Tang AP, et al. Role of radiologic features in the management of papillary lesions of the breast. *AJR Am J Roentgenol* 2006; 186(5): 1322–1327.

10. Ciatto S, Morrone D, Catarzi S, et al. Radial scars of the breast: review of 38 consecutive mammographic diagnoses. *Radiology* 1993; 187:757–760.

11. Kennedy M, Masterson AV, Kerin M, et al. Pathology and clinical relevance of radial scars: a review. *J Clin Pathol* 2003; 56(10):721–724.

12. Powell CM, Cranor ML, Rosen PP. Pseudoangiomatous stromal hyperplasia: a mammary stromal tumor with myofibroblastic differentiation. *Am J Surg Pathol* 1995; 19:270–277.

13. Polger MR, Denison CM, Lester S, et al. Pseudoangiomatous stromal hyperplasia: mammographic and sonographic appearances. *AJR Am J Roentgenol* 1996; 166:349–352.

14. Cohen MA, Morris EA, Rosen PP, et al. Pseudoangiomatous stromal hyperplasia: mammographic, sonographic, and clinical patterns. *Radiology* 1996; 198:117–120.

15. Mercado CL, Naidrich SA, Hamele-Bena D: Pseudoangiomatous stromal hyperplasia of the breast: sonographic features with histopathologic correlation. *Breast J* 2004; 10:427–432.

16. Telli ML, Horst KC, Guardino AE, et al. Phyllodes tumors of the breast: natural history, diagnosis, and treatment [review]. *J Natl Compr Cancer Netw* 2007; 5(3):324–330.

17. Venta LA, Wiley EL, Gabriel H, et al. Imaging features of focal breast fibrosis: mammographic-pathologic correlation of noncalcified breast lesions. *AJR Am J Roentgenol* 1999; 173(2):309–316.

18. Goel NB, Knight TE, Pandey S, et al. Fibrous lesions of the breast: imaging-pathologic correlation. *RadioGraphics* 2005; 25(6):1547–1559.

19. Schwarz GS, Drotman M, Rosenblatt R, et al. Fibromatosis of the breast: case report and current concepts in the management of an uncommon lesion [review]. *Breast J* 2006; 12(1):66–71.

20. Glazebrook KN, Morton MJ, Reynolds C. Vascular tumors of the breast: mammographic, sonographic, and MRI appearances. *AJR Am J Roentgenol* 2005; 184:331–338.

21. Schelfout K, Tjalma WA, Cooremans ID, et al. Observations of an idiopathic granulomatous mastitis [review]. *Eur J Obstet Gynecol Reprod Biol* 2001; 97(2):260–262.

22. Bakaris S, Yuksel M, Ciragil P, et al. Granulomatous mastitis including breast tuberculosis and idiopathic lobular granulomatous mastitis. *Can J Surg* 2006; 49(6):427–430.

23. Ozturk M, Mavili E, Kahriman G, et al. Granulomatous mastitis: radiological findings. *Acta Radiol* 2007; 48(2):150–155.

24. Hogge JP, Robinson RE, Magnant CM, et al. The mammographic spectrum of fat necrosis, *RadioGraphics* 1995; 15:1347–1356.

25. Soo MS. Fat necrosis in the breast: sonographic features. *Radiology* 1998; 206:261–296.

26. Mihai R, Christie-Brown J, Bristol J. Breast metastases from colorectal carcinoma. *Breast* 2004; 13: 155–158.

Papilloma presenting with bloody nipple discharge; ductogram and ultrasound

A 72-year-old woman presented with intermittent spontaneous right breast bloody nipple discharge for 2 weeks. A ductogram revealed an intraductal filling defect in the subareolar right breast (Figure 1). The intraductal mass was also demonstrated on ultrasound (Figure 2). Ultrasound-guided core needle biopsy yielded a diagnosis of benign papilloma. Subsequent needle localization and excisional biopsy confirmed the diagnosis of benign intraductal papilloma.

TEACHING POINTS

This case illustrates a clinical mimic of breast carcinoma, the benign papilloma. Evaluation is war-

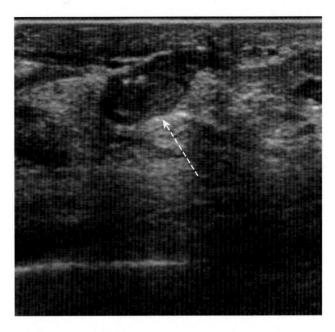

FIGURE 2. Retroareolar ultrasound. Corresponding to the filling defect on ductography is a hypoechoic intraductal solid mass (*arrow*).

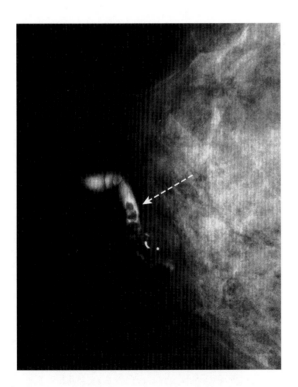

FIGURE 1. Ductogram CC mammographic view. Image performed after injection of contrast into the symptomatic duct. There is a filling defect outlined by contrast (*arrow*). Distally, associated coarse calcifications are seen.

ranted for single duct spontaneous clear or bloody nipple discharge. Although papillomas are the most common cause of bloody nipple discharge, because they cannot be distinguished from ductal carcinoma on the basis of clinical or imaging features, histologic diagnosis is necessary. Although papillomas with malignant or atypical features require surgical excision, the management of benign papillomas diagnosed at core needle biopsy has not been standardized. Prior studies have reported upgrade rates of about 5% at excisional biopsy of papillomas to carcinoma. However, more recent studies have suggested upgrade rates in a range acceptable for follow-up rather than excision (<2%). The use of larger-gauge vacuum-assisted biopsy devices may obviate the need for surgical excision in the diagnosis of benign papillomas.

SUGGESTED READINGS

Mercado CL, Hamele-Bena D, Oken SM, et al. Papillary lesions of the breast at percutaneous core-needle biopsy. *Radiology* 2006; 238(3):801–808.

Sohn V, Keylock J, Arthurs Z, et al. Breast papillomas in the era of percutaneous needle biopsy. *Ann Surg Oncol* 2007; 14(10):2979–2984.

CASE 2

Multiple papillomas

A 69-year-old woman with a right breast nipple discharge underwent MRI evaluation. The MRI showed multiple enhancing masses in the superior right breast that were oriented in a ductal pattern (Figures 1 and 2). Correlation with the patient's mammogram revealed that the masses seen on MRI corresponded to multiple masses in the superior right breast on mammography (Figure 3). The masses had slowly increased in size over several years. The appearance on ultrasound suggested that these were intraductal masses (Figure 4). Needle localization and excisional biopsy were performed (Figures 5 and 6). Pathology revealed multiple benign papillomas.

TEACHING POINTS

This case illustrates that benign papillomas may exhibit malignant features on MRI. In this example,

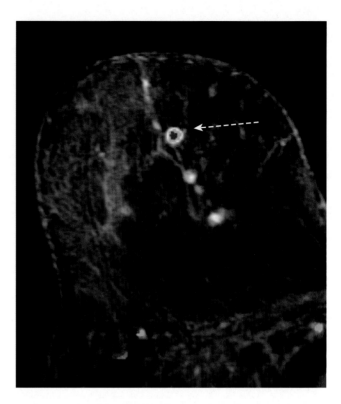

FIGURE 2. Postcontrast, subtracted, axial MRI with kinetic color overlay. The more anterior mass demonstrates central washout kinetics as denoted by the red area (*arrow*).

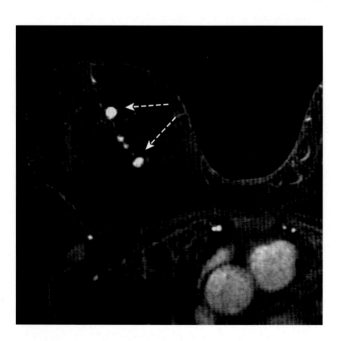

FIGURE 1. Postcontrast, subtracted, axial MRI demonstrates multiple, small, enhancing masses in the superior central right breast (*arrows*). The masses are aligned in a ductal orientation.

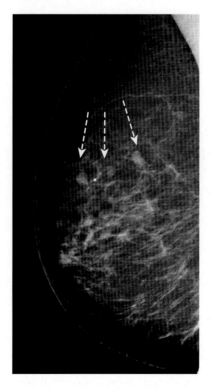

FIGURE 3. Right breast mediolateral oblique (MLO) mammographic view demonstrates multiple masses in the superior right breast, corresponding to the lesions seen on MRI (*arrows*).

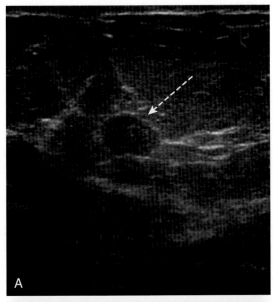

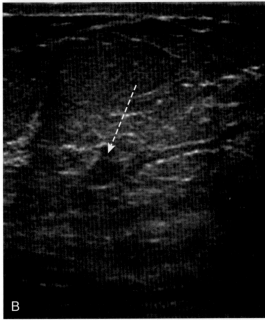

FIGURE 4. Ultrasound images of the superior right breast (**A** and **B**) demonstrate multiple solid masses (*arrows*) corresponding to the MRI and mammographic findings. Adjacent fluid-filled ducts (seen in **B**) suggest that the masses are intraductal.

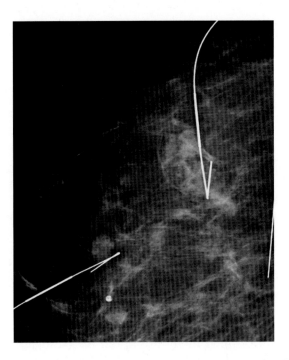

FIGURE 5. Needle localization mammogram, Two hook wires are seen bracketing the targeted masses.

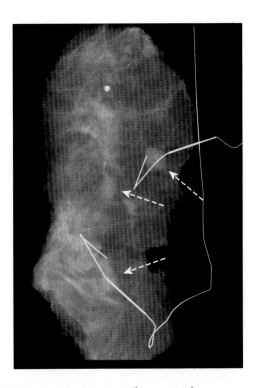

FIGURE 6. Specimen x-ray. The targeted masses are identified in the right breast surgical specimen (*arrows*).

multiple masses are seen in a ductal orientation, mimicking DCIS. In addition, papillomas may display a suspicious washout kinetic pattern, concerning for invasive carcinoma. Because of the overlap in the imaging appearance of papillomas and carcinoma, biopsy is required to establish the diagnosis.

CASE 3

Large phyllodes tumor (ultrasound)

A 39-year-old woman was evaluated for an enlarging right breast lump. This had initially developed about 8 months before, as a golf ball–sized mass that had been noted a month after breast trauma. The findings were thought to be post-traumatic, and the patient was reassured. No imaging was performed.

The mass never resolved. At the time of imaging evaluation, the patient noted an increase in size of the mass over the preceding 2 months. On physical examination, a mobile, tender, palpable, 8-cm mass occupied the entire upper breast, distorting the breast and stretching the overlying skin. Sonographic evaluation showed a 10-cm, solid, vascular mass with circumscribed margins (Figures 1, 2, and 3). Biopsy with ultrasound guidance obtained a pathologic result of biphasic neoplasm with cellular stroma, with differential diagnosis of cellular fibroadenoma versus phyllodes tumor.

Surgical treatment was with a skin-sparing simple mastectomy, with tissue expander placement. The pathology showed a benign phyllodes tumor, 11 cm, with negative surgical margins.

TEACHING POINTS

Phyllodes tumors are uncommon, representing less than 1% of breast neoplasms. They take their name from "leaf-like" in Greek, referring to the histologic feature of papillary growths of epithelial-lined stroma protruding as leaf-like masses. The typical clinical course is as in this example with a large, rapidly growing, circumscribed mass. The pathologic spectrum ranges from benign to borderline to malignant; most are benign. In a single institution series of 335 phyllodes tumors, 75% were benign, with 16% borderline and 9% malignant. The treatment of choice is wide excision.

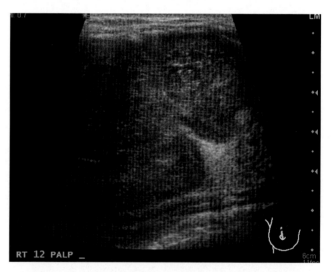

FIGURE 2. Another margin is lobulated.

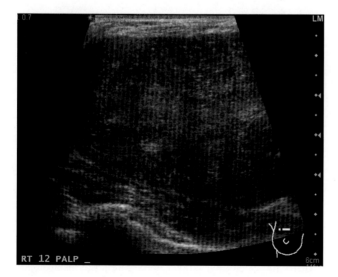

FIGURE 1. Ultrasound of the palpable lump shows it to be solid. It is sufficiently large that it could not be encompassed in a single view. The posterior margin visualized here is circumscribed, with a thin, echogenic capsule visible.

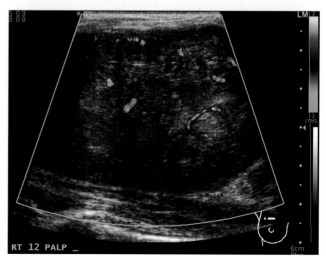

FIGURE 3. Color Doppler demonstrates the internal vascularity of the mass.

SUGGESTED READING

Liberman L, Bonaccio E, Hamele-Bena D, et al. Benign and malignant phyllodes tumors: mammographic and sonographic findings. *Radiology* 1996; 198:121–124.

CASE 4

Large phyllodes tumor

A 70-year-old woman presented with a large palpable mass replacing much of her left breast (Figure 1). Ultrasound showed a corresponding hypoechoic solid mass (Figure 2). Core biopsy yielded a diagnosis of a benign phyllodes tumor. Because of the size of the lesion, the patient underwent left mastectomy.

TEACHING POINTS

This case illustrates an example of a large phyllodes tumor. Phyllodes tumor should be suspected in patients with large or rapidly growing masses. In this example, although the tumor replaces much of the left breast, there is no significant breast edema or distortion, as might be expected with an invasive breast carcinoma of this size.

Phyllodes tumors of the breast are unusual fibroepithelial tumors composed of epithelium and a spindle cell stroma and can exhibit a wide range of clinical behavior. They are classified as benign, borderline, or malignant, based on histopathologic features. However, histologic classification does not always predict outcome. Immunohistochemical features of phyllodes tumors may help in predicting their clinical outcome. The prognosis of phyllodes tumors is favorable, with local recurrence in about 15% of patients overall and distant recurrence in about 5% to 10%. It may be difficult to distinguish a phyllodes tumor from a fibroadenoma on core needle biopsy. When a rapidly growing mass is detected and core biopsy reveals a

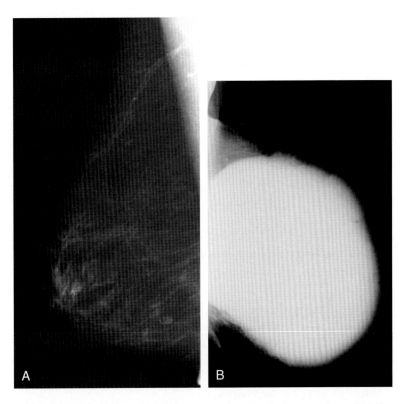

FIGURE 1. Bilateral MLO mammographic views (**A,** right, for comparison; **B,** left) demonstrate a large, mostly circumscribed, dense mass expanding the left breast.

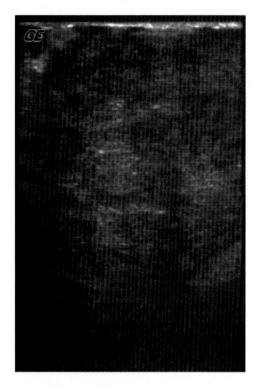

FIGURE 2. Ultrasound shows a corresponding large, heterogeneously hypoechoic, solid mass.

cellular fibroadenoma, phyllodes tumor should be suspected. Wide excision, which may require mastectomy, is the definitive primary therapy for phyllodes tumors.

SUGGESTED READING

Telli ML, Horst KC, Guardino AE, et al. Phyllodes tumors of the breast: natural history, diagnosis, and treatment [review]. *J Natl Compr Canc Netw* 2007; 5(3):324–330.

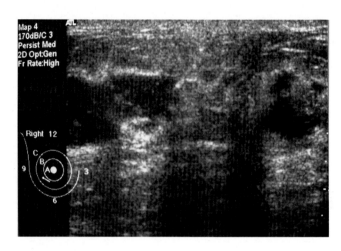

FIGURE 1. Ultrasound of the right lower outer quadrant (LOQ) shows two similar-appearing, hypoechoic, irregularly marginated masses, a few centimeters apart. Both show enhanced through-transmission.

quadrant mass. Ultrasound showed two hypoechoic, similar-appearing masses with angular, irregular margins (Figure 1). Ultrasound-guided core needle biopsies of both masses returned diagnoses of acute mastitis, with acute neutrophilic infiltrate, edema, and focal chronic inflammation. There was no evidence of malignancy.

TEACHING POINTS

Inflammatory processes can mimic neoplasms perfectly in their imaging features. The clinical history usually allows differentiation. These "masses" are actually complex fluid collections, or abscesses. Other than the enhanced through-transmission, which suggests a homogeneous or fluid consistency, the sonographic features are those of malignancy.

CASE 5

Multifocal breast abscesses

A 37-year-old woman developed two right palpable breast masses, which were exquisitely tender. There was no erythema. Mammographic and sonographic evaluations were performed. Mammography showed a dense, ill-defined lower outer

CASE 6

Granulomatous mastitis

A 61-year-old woman presented from South America, with a history of chronic left breast pain, swelling, and erythema. An MRI showed diffuse enhancement of the left lateral breast (Figures 1 and 2). Subsequent biopsy and cytologic evaluations confirmed a diagnosis of granulomatous mastitis from tuberculosis (TB) of the breast.

TEACHING POINTS

Granulomatous mastitis of the breast is a rare entity that often presents as a palpable mass. The clinical and imaging findings may be confused with inflammatory carcinoma of the breast. The diagnosis should be suspected in patients from endemic regions. However, in addition to sarcoid and infectious causes such as TB, granulomatous mastitis may be idiopathic in nature. Fine-needle aspiration cytology may be nondiagnostic; therefore, biopsy and polymerase chain reaction testing may be necessary for diagnosis.

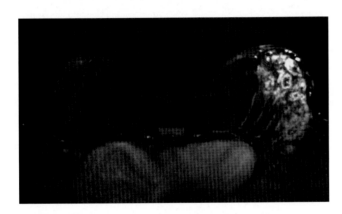

FIGURE 1.   Postcontrast, subtracted, axial MRI demonstrates diffuse irregular enhancement involving the left breast. There are areas of ring-like, nodular, and clumped enhancement.

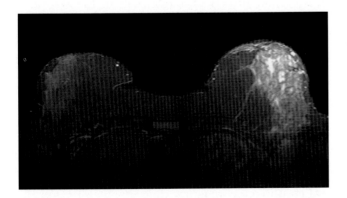

FIGURE 2.   T2-weighted axial image shows corresponding diffuse edema of the left lateral breast.

SUGGESTED READING

Bakaris S, Yuksel M, Ciragil P, et al. Granulomatous mastitis including breast tuberculosis and idiopathic lobular granulomatous mastitis. *Can J Surg* 2006; 49(6):427–430.

CASE 7

Lymphocytic mastitis

A 47-year-old healthy woman developed a left retroareolar tender mass and a palpable 2-cm lump. She was sent for ultrasound for a suspected cyst. Ultrasound showed increased vascularity in the para-areolar region, but no discrete mass. No mammographic abnormality or change was seen (Figure 1). The surgeon's physical examination noted tender induration without a discrete mass of the upper areola, extending 1 to 2 cm beyond the areola. A core needle biopsy was obtained in the office, and a 1-week trial of antibiotics was given. The needle biopsy specimen showed acute and chronic inflammation. A mixed inflammatory infiltrate of neutrophils, plasma cells, and lymphocytes was noted. Improvement was noted on antibiotics, but the tenderness subsequently recurred and antibiotics were restarted, without complete resolution.

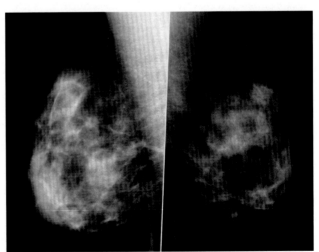

FIGURE 1.   MLO mammograms show heterogeneous, increased parenchymal density. The left retroareolar region is asymmetrically increased in density.

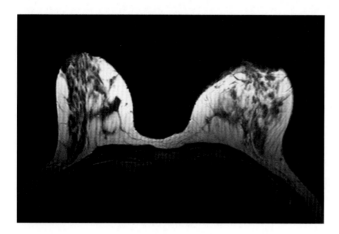

FIGURE 2. Axial T2-weighted breast MRI shows thickening of the left medial breast skin, extending to the nipple, which is retracted.

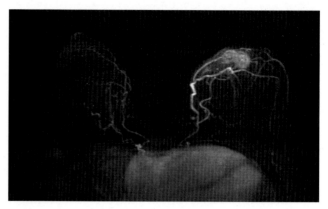

FIGURE 4. Maximal intensity projection view of both breasts from enhanced, subtracted dynamic series shows a superficial, intensely enhancing, mass-like process involving the left medial breast.

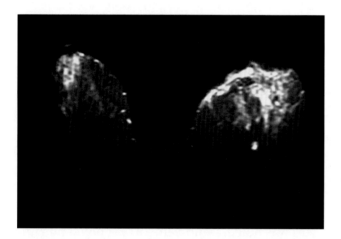

FIGURE 3. Axial short tau inversion recovery (STIR) image shows marked thickening and edema of the left medial breast skin. There is a diffuse increase in edema of the central retroareolar left breast compared with the right. A small cyst is seen on the left posteriorly.

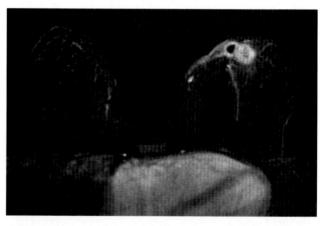

FIGURE 5. Enhanced, subtracted view from the dynamic series shows intense, mass-like enhancement of the thickened left medial breast skin and retroareolar region. A fluid collection is outlined by the enhancing tissue.

Breast MRI was obtained to better define the extent of the process (Figures 2, 3, 4, 5, 6, and 7). Intense mass-like enhancement of the medial left breast skin and retroareolar region was found, surrounding a fluid collection. Excisional biopsy removed a region of apparent granulation tissue and surrounding induration. The specimen showed chronically inflamed granulation tissue with adjacent fibrosis. Varying degrees of periductal, perilobular, and perivascular lymphocytic inflammation were noted, consistent with lymphocytic mastitis.

TEACHING POINTS

Inflammatory processes can mimic the imaging features of breast cancers. Compare the MRI findings in this case to those of Case 10 in Chapter 6, in which similar enhancement of the skin and nipple are due to recurrent breast cancer. Generally, the clinical features allow differentiation. This patient had a waxing and waning clinical course of recurrent tenderness, without fluctuation or drainage, which did not resolve with multiple courses of antibiotics. On initial imaging with ultrasound, no drainable fluid collection was seen. Breast MRI showed a fluid collection, which was small relative to the impressive, sheet-like confluent enhancement of the medial skin, subjacent breast parenchyma, and retroareolar region.

Lymphocytic mastitis has been reported in patients with diabetes and in autoimmune disease. This patient had no known risk factors.

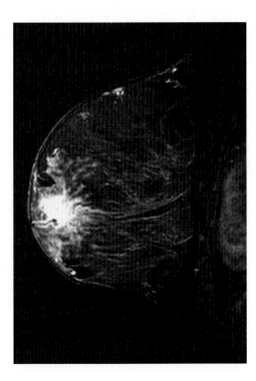

FIGURE 6. Sagittal subtracted view of the left retroareolar level shows an intensely enhancing, poorly marginated mass. Periductal enhancement is seen.

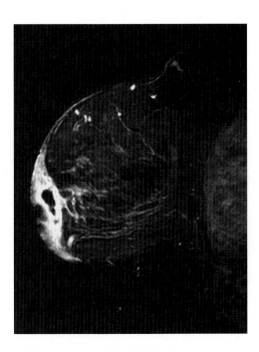

FIGURE 7. More medial sagittal, subtracted view shows the confluent skin and subjacent enhancement, surrounding a fluid collection.

CASE 8

New fat necrosis mass mimicking recurrence

A 73-year-old woman, previously treated for bilateral breast cancer with lumpectomies and radiation therapy, underwent routine mammographic surveillance. This was 11 years after treatment for right breast cancer and 3 years after treatment for the left, a T1N0, estrogen receptor–positive tumor. Mammography showed a new 8-mm mass with indistinct margins in the upper outer left breast (Figure 1). Sonography identified a corresponding abnormality, a 6-mm hypoechoic, shadowing mass with spiculated margins (Figure 2). Recurrent breast cancer was suspected, and the lesion was biopsied with ultrasound guidance (Figure 3).

Pathology demonstrated benign fat necrosis with hyalinized sclerosis. Subsequent evaluations have shown postbiopsy changes and stable postoperative findings (Figures 4 and 5); no evidence of recurrence has been identified after 2 years of follow-up.

TEACHING POINTS

Fat necrosis, the great mimic, strikes again! In this case, a discrete new mass developed 3 years after breast conservation treatment, with marginal indistinctness on mammography and fine spiculation on ultrasound. Because of its small size, it was biopsied with 12-gauge, vacuum-assisted technique, to ensure adequate sampling. The lesion was seen at the time of biopsy to be largely excised. This case reminds us that image-guided biopsies can induce changes that may be visualized on subsequent follow-up exams, especially if there is a hematoma complicating the original procedure. Biopsies themselves can induce fat necrosis. Clips are variable in their appearances and conspicuity on follow-up imaging. Postoperative fluid collections generally contract and regress over time, but not inevitably. Some collections, like this 4-year-old example, become organized and chronic.

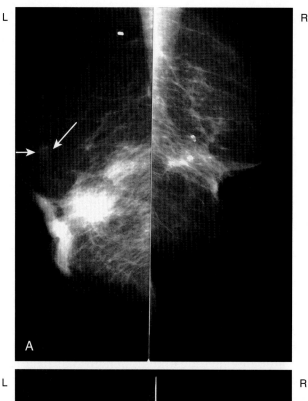

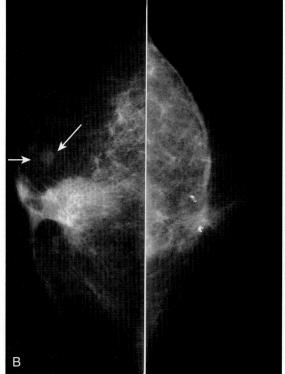

FIGURE 1.   MLO (**A**) and CC (**B**) mammograms show bilateral, central, postsurgical scarring. On the left, superomedial to the nipple, is seen an 8-mm mass, which was new compared with a mammogram 6 months before (*arrows*). Margins on spot compression are indistinct.

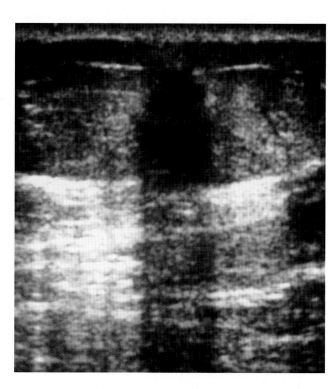

FIGURE 2.   Ultrasound of the corresponding mass shows highly suspicious features. The mass is very hypoechoic and shadows, and the margin is spiculated.

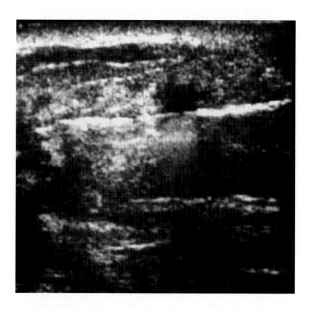

FIGURE 3.   Images obtained during a vacuum-assisted, 12-gauge core needle biopsy. The device is seen entering the field from the right and is positioned beneath the hypoechoic mass. Continuous sampling progresses upward through the mass, only a remnant of which was seen at the end of the procedure.

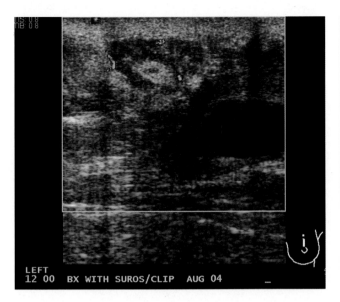

FIGURE 4. Follow-up ultrasound, 9 months later, of the site of the vacuum-assisted biopsy shows an echogenic clip surrounded by a hypoechoic rind of surrounding tissue reaction.

CASE 9

Fibrosis mimicking recurrence in implant-reconstructed breast cancer patient

A 54-year-old woman, treated 10 years earlier for left breast infiltrating ductal carcinoma (IDC), developed a palpable periareolar mass. She had bilateral subpectoral implants placed in the past year. Her original tumor was T1cN1M0, and was treated with partial mastectomy, radiation therapy, six cycles of Cytoxan, methotrexate, 5-fluorouracil (CMF) chemotherapy, and 5 years of tamoxifen.

Ultrasound of the palpable periareolar mass showed a very hypoechoic, taller-than-wide, irregularly marginated mass (Figure 1). This was biopsied with ultrasound guidance, with 14-gauge core needle biopsy technique.

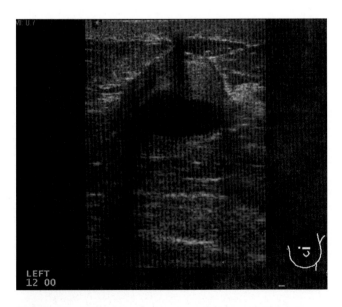

FIGURE 5. Image from the same ultrasound of the 4-year-old postoperative seroma in the same breast shows a complex fluid collection that is partly cystic and partly homogeneously echogenic.

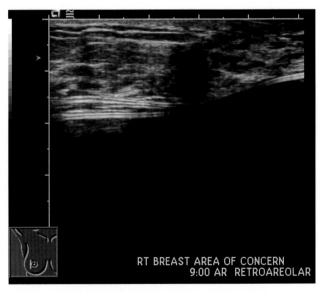

FIGURE 1. Ultrasound of the lateral retroareolar palpable lump shows suspicious sonographic features: extreme hypoechogenicity, taller-than-wide shape, irregular margins. The sonolucent implant is seen deep to the mass.

Pathology showed no carcinoma, with sclerosis, fibrosis, and foreign body giant cell reaction found.

TEACHING POINTS

This patient had implants placed in the prior year and had been treated with breast conservation for early-stage IDC 10 years before. The ultrasound appearance of this mass is highly suspicious and raised the specter of recurrent breast cancer in this patient. Fortunately, 14-gauge core needle biopsy confirmed a satisfactory alternate diagnosis. Fibrosis and foreign body giant cell reaction, presumably related to the patient's implant surgery, produced a mass that mimics recurrent breast cancer. See Case 7 in Chapter 6 for a very similar-appearing ultrasound mass, which did represent a recurrence.

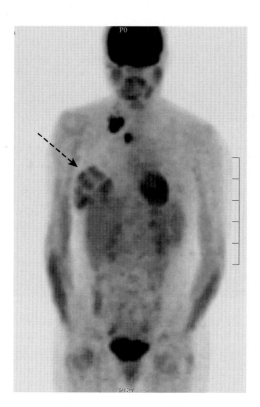

FIGURE 1. Anterior projection whole-body PET image shows diffuse tracer uptake within the right breast (*arrow*). Also seen is upper thoracic uptake corresponding to the known lymphoma, as well as normal activity within the heart and bladder.

CASE 10

Lactational asymmetry on PET

A 38-year-old woman with a recent diagnosis of lymphoma underwent a staging positron emission tomography (PET) scan. The patient was breast-feeding at the time. The PET scan demonstrated the known lymphoma within the upper thorax (Figure 1). In addition, diffuse uptake was seen involving the right breast. A subsequently performed breast MRI showed diffuse non-mass-like enhancement of the right breast, as well as breast edema (Figures 2 and 3). Upon questioning, it became apparent that the patient was breast-feeding only from the right breast, owing to difficulty on the left. The imaging findings of unilateral benign lactational change correlated with the history. No further breast workup or follow-up was required.

TEACHING POINTS

This case illustrates benign lactational breast changes, which should not be confused with a

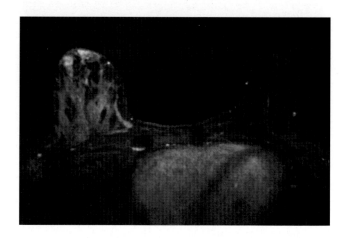

FIGURE 2. Postcontrast, subtracted, axial MRI of both breasts demonstrates diffuse non-mass-like enhancement of the right breast. No skin thickening or parenchymal distortion is seen.

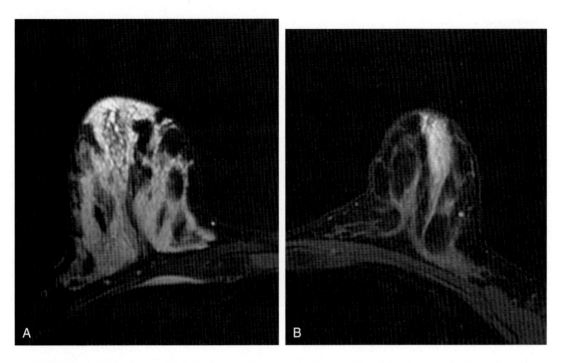

FIGURE 3. Right (**A**) and left (**B**) breast fat saturated T2-weighted MRIs show diffuse edema of the right breast.

malignant process. In this example, although there is diffuse uptake on the PET scan and enhancement on the MRI, the imaging features are consistent with a benign process, given the absence of mass effect, parenchymal distortion, or secondary signs of malignancy, such as skin thickening or adenopathy. In addition to lactational changes, infection and trauma may mimic malignancy. This case also emphasizes the importance of clinical history in establishing such alternative diagnoses.

CHAPTER 8

Identifying Bone Metastases

The most common site of distant metastasis from breast cancer is bone. In a study of almost 600 patients dying of breast cancer, Coleman and Rubens found that 69% had radiologic evidence of bone metastases before death.[1] These results antedated use of fluorodeoxyglucose (FDG) positron emission tomography (PET), suggesting the true incidence might be even higher. Bone metastases in breast cancer may be osteolytic, osteoblastic, or mixed blastic and lytic. This feature accounts for the variable sensitivity and specificity of different imaging modalities.[2] Of interest is that patients with blastic (versus osteolytic) bone metastases have been reported to have prolonged survival.[3]

The clinical presentation of bone metastases is most commonly pain in the axial skeleton. The most prevalent sites of bone metastases are spine, ribs, pelvis, skull, and femur. Prompt investigation of pain in weight-bearing bones is indicated to avoid pathologic fracture. Symptoms of back pain, concomitant with neurologic symptoms of cord compression, such as leg weakness, ascending numbness, or bowel and bladder symptoms, constitute a medical emergency to prevent permanent neurologic damage.

Other clues suggesting bone metastases include a rising alkaline phosphatase level, hypercalcemia, or, if tumor markers are being obtained, a rise in the carcinoembryonic antigen level or CA 27.29. It is not uncommon to find relatively asymptomatic bony metastases when obtaining staging studies in a patient with other sites of metastatic disease. When bone is the only site of metastatic disease, survival may be very prolonged, particularly in a postmenopausal woman with hormone receptor–positive disease.

Plain radiographs require 30% to 50% loss of bone mineral to visualize a metastasis.[4] Most breast cancer bone metastases demonstrate areas of lysis and sclerosis. Lesions can be permeative, moth-eaten, or geographic (Figure 1). Permeative and moth-eaten lesions predominate, whereas geographic lesions, exhibiting a sharp delineation between normal and abnormal bone, typically reflect a less aggressive metastasis.[5] Advantages of plain radiography include widespread availability, minimal imaging time, absence of patient preparation, favorable radiation dosimetry, and relatively low cost. Based on the higher sensitivity of nuclear medicine bone scintigraphy, as well as its ability to survey the whole body, plain radiographs are now typically used to add specificity or to clarify bone scan findings.

CT and MRI offer superb spatial resolution combined with excellent specificity. Nearly 50% of patients who are identified as having bony metastases on scintigraphy with negative plain radiographs will have detectable lesions on CT.[6] Additionally, CT and MRI may be quite helpful in determining the etiology of bone pain (e.g., concomitant fracture, arthritis, soft tissue pathology). These modalities are preferred to answer questions related to a specific area (e.g., CT for ribs, MRI for vertebral column) (Figure 2). However, the nuclear medicine bone scan remains the procedure of choice for whole-body screening.[7,8]

Bone scintigraphy has withstood the test of time and is very sensitive in identifying areas of osteoblastic change. Findings on scintiscan may antedate findings on plain radiographs by many months. The bone scan is widely available, requires minimal patient preparation (increased fluid intake is recommended), delivers low radiation, and is cost effective. Disadvantages include reduced sensitivity in the vertebral column (improved with the use of single-photon emission computed tomography, or SPECT), significantly reduced sensitivity for purely osteolytic lesions, and suboptimal specificity. Routine bone scanning in patients with early-stage breast cancer, in the absence of symptoms, is not recommended.[9]

Bone scanning can also be performed with the positron emitter ^{18}F sodium fluoride (NaF). Schirrmeister has published extensively on the use of ^{18}F sodium fluoride and has shown high sensitivity and specificity in multiple tumor types, including breast.[10–14] Compared with ^{99m}Tc-labeled polyphosphonates, ^{18}F sodium fluoride shows about twice the uptake as well as a significantly improved target-to-background ratio. Current PET and PET/CT scanners provide improved sensitivity, higher spatial resolution, and tomographic capability (Figures 3 and 4).

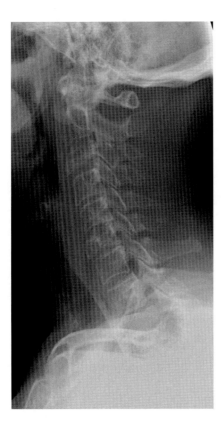

FIGURE 1. A 52-year-old woman with breast cancer metastatic to bone, identified 17 years after initial diagnosis of stage II disease, treated with mastectomy, chemotherapy, and tamoxifen. Lytic change is seen in C3 and C6, which show loss of height and indistinct cortices.

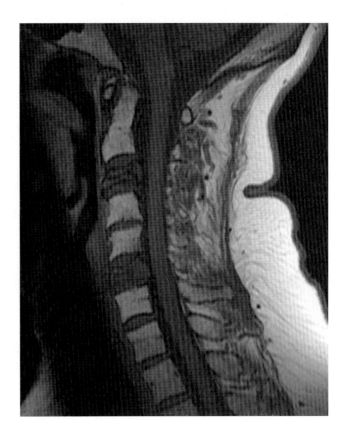

FIGURE 2. Same patient as in Figure 1. Sagittal T1-weighted, cervical spine MRI shows replacement of normal bright, fatty marrow signal in the C3 and C6 vertebral bodies, which show loss of height and end-plate invagination. The uniformly bright marrow signal elsewhere in the spine reflects prior radiation therapy.

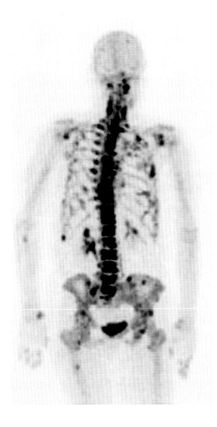

FIGURE 3. ^{18}F NaF bone scan volumetric image shows extensive bone metastases as nearly confluent intense uptake in the spine and tiny, scattered foci of activity in scapula, ribs, pelvis, and hips.

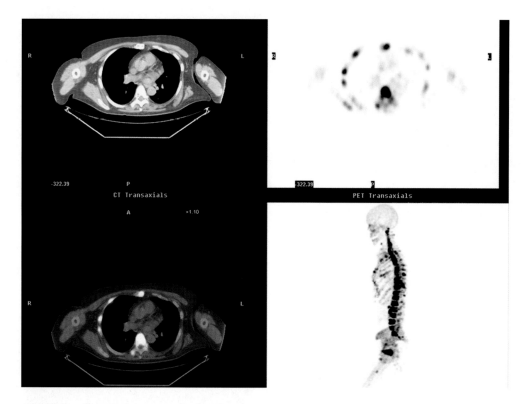

FIGURE 4. [18]F NaF bone scan PET/CT images of a patient with extensive breast cancer bone metastases provide whole-body, tomographic bone imaging with a high target-to-background ratio. Acquisition on a PET/CT unit allows precise anatomic localization and correlation with CT bone and soft tissue windows.

Uptake of NaF is not tumor specific. Therefore, both benign and malignant lesions will demonstrate NaF uptake. Current PET/CT scanners, with improved spatial resolution and precise anatomic localization of lesions, result in better differentiation of benign from malignant lesions.[14]

There does not appear to be enough scientific data or clinical experience to recommend the routine use of NaF bone scintigraphy over FDG PET or bone scintigraphy. NaF may be helpful in selected patients; however, FDG PET is an accepted modality for use as a whole-body screen, can reliably detect primary tumors, and allows accurate assessment of soft tissue metastases.[15–17]

[18]F fluorodeoxyglucose (FDG) is the current radiopharmaceutical of choice for PET imaging in cancer. FDG enters tumor cells via glucose transporter proteins on the cell membrane and, once intracellular, is trapped. Uptake of FDG in bone metastases is incompletely understood; however, it has been shown that uptake in osteolytic metastases may be up to 7 times higher than osteoblastic metastases.[18] Blastic metastases may

not be demonstrated on FDG PET (Figure 5). Most studies comparing bone scintigraphy and FDG PET suggest an advantage for FDG PET with respect to osteolytic metastases and specificity. Bone scintigraphy appears to be more sensitive for osteoblastic lesions, and the two studies are best viewed as complementary.

An important area of bone metastases is the spinal column. A patient's quality of life can be dramatically affected by metastases to the spine.[19] Available imaging modalities include plain radiography, MRI, and CT. PET/CT has gained popularity because of its ability to combine metabolic and anatomic data. Frontal, lateral, and dynamic plain films (e.g., flexion and extension views) are helpful in identifying instability. Neural compression is best evaluated with MRI. The presence and extent of metastases are well delineated by altered signal within bone. Bony anatomy is best defined by thin-section axial CT. Contrast enhancement is helpful in enhancing tumor visualization and more clearly defining neural compression.

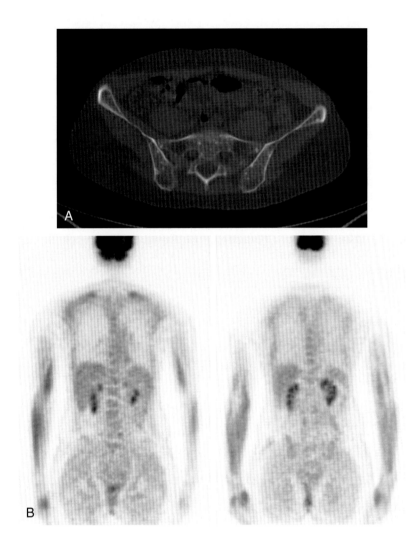

FIGURE 5. Pelvis CT bone window (**A**) and coronal FDG PET (**B**) images. It is possible for a patient to have extensive bone metastases and a negative PET scan. CT shows innumerable tiny sclerotic bone metastases, which are not apparent on PET. Presumably, this is because the lesions are blastic and tiny.

REFERENCES

1. Coleman RE, Reubens RO. The clinical course of bone metastases from breast cancer. *Br J Cancer* 1987; 55:61–66.
2. Even-Sapir E. Imaging of malignant bone involvement by morphologic, scintigraphic, and hybrid modalities. *J Nucl Med* 2005; 46:1356–1367.
3. Yamashita K, Koyama H, Inaji H. Prognostic significance of bone metastasis from breast cancer. *Clin Orthop* 1995; 312:89–94.
4. Edelstyn GA, Gillespie PJ, Grebell FS. The radiological demonstration of osseous metastases: experimental observations. *Clin Radiol* 1967; 18:158–162.
5. Wittig JC, Lamont JG. Bone metastases from breast cancer. In Roses DF (ed). Breast Cancer. Philadelphia, Elsevier Churchill Livingstone, 2005, pp 666–675.
6. Muindi J, Coombes RC, Golding S, et al. The role of computed tomography in the detection of bone metastases in breast cancer patients. *Br J Radiol* 1983; 56:233–239.
7. Hamaoka T, Madewell JE, Podoloff DA, et al. Bone Imaging in metastatic breast cancer. *J Clin Oncol* 2004; 22:2942–2953.
8. Love C, Din AS, Tomas MB, et al. Radionuclide bone imaging: an illustrative review. *RadioGraphics* 2003; 23:341–358.
9. Yeh KA, Fortunato L, Ridge JA, et al. Routine bone scanning in patients with T1 and T2 breast cancer: a waste of money. *Ann Surg Oncol* 1995; 2:319–324.
10. Schirrmeister H, Guhlmann CA, Elsner K, et al. Planar bone imaging vs 18 F-PET in patients with cancer of the prostate, thyroid and lung. *J Nucl Med* 1999; 40(10):1623–1629.
11. Schirrmeister H, Guhlmann CA, Kotzerke J, et al. Early detection and accurate description of extent of

metastatic bone disease in breast cancer with ^{18}F-fluoride ion and positron emission tomography. *J Clin Oncol* 1999; 17(8):2381–2389.

12. Schirrmeister H, Glatting G, Hetzel J, et al. Prospective evaluation of the clinical value of planar bone scans, SPECT and F-18 labeled NaF PET in newly diagnosed lung cancer. *J Nucl Med* 2001; 42(12): 1800–1804.

13. Schirrmeister H. Detection of bone metastases in breast cancer by positron emission tomography. *PET Clinics: Breast Cancer* 2006; 1(1):25–32.

14. Schirrmeister H, Diedrichs CG, Rentschler M, et al. Positron-emission tomography of the skeletal system using 18-F Na: the incidence, pattern of the findings and distribution of benign changes. *Fortschr Rontgenstr* 1998; 169(3):310–314 (in German).

15. Crippa F, Agresti R, Seregni E, et al. Prospective evaluation of fluorine–18-FDG PET in presurgical staging of the axilla in breast cancer. *J Nucl Med* 1998; 39(1):4–8.

16. Moon DH, Maddahi J, Silverman DHS, et al. Accuracy of whole body fluorinie-18 FDG PET for the detection of recurrent or metastatic breast carcinoma. *J Nucl Med* 1998; 39(3):431–435.

17. Even-Sapir E, Mester U, Flusser G, et al. Assessment of malignant skeletal disease: initial experience with ^{18}F-fluoride PET/CT and comparison between 18F-fluoride PET and 18F-fluoride PET/CT. *J Nucl Med* 2004; 45(2):272–278.

18. Cook GJ, Houston S, Rubens R, et al. Detection of bone metastases in breast cancer by 18 FDG PET: differing metabolic activity in osteoblastic and osteolytic lesions. *J Clin Oncol* 1998; 16(10):3375–3379.

19. Douglas AF, Cooper PR. Spinal column metastases from breast cancer. In Roses DF (ed). Breast Cancer. Philadelphia, Elsevier Churchill Livingstone, 2005, pp 644–652.

CASE 1

Stage IV presentation of breast cancer with bone metastases

A 60-year-old woman presented with a large, palpable right breast mass (same patient as in Case 19 in Chapter 4). Imaging workup, including mammography, ultrasound, breast MRI, and ultrasound-guided core needle biopsy and axillary lymph node aspiration, confirmed node-positive multifocal infiltrating ductal carcinoma (IDC). Based on physical examination, the patient was thought to have an advanced breast cancer, at least T3 by size, and she was started on neoadjuvant

chemotherapy while her staging workup was completed. The staging evaluation included a bone scan and positron emission tomography (PET)/CT. The bone scan, obtained before starting chemotherapy, showed several foci of increased activity, including in the left anterior third rib, one focus each in the cervical and thoracic spine, and a focus at the left upper sacroiliac joint region (Figure 1). A breast MRI, obtained a few days after the first round of chemotherapy, included a coronal short tau inversion recovery (STIR) series of the thorax, obtained with the body coil. This showed evidence of widespread bone metastases, with hyperintense foci in the right medial clavicle and in a lower thoracic vertebral body (Figure 2). A PET/CT scan was performed about 1 week after the first cycle of chemotherapy. In addition to showing hypermetabolism of the multifocal breast carcinoma, hypermetabolic foci were identified in multiple bony sites, including the right clavicular head, right upper cervical spine, two adjacent lower thoracic

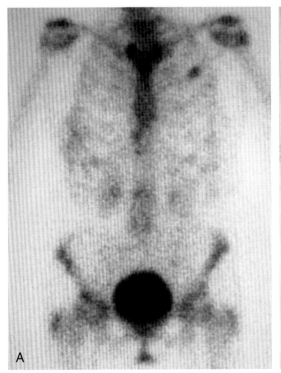
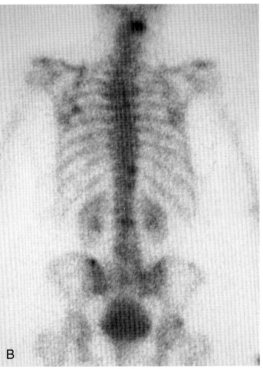

FIGURE 1. **A,** Anterior image from a prechemotherapy bone scan shows a focus of increased activity at the left anterior third rib level. The focus is less punctate than usually seen with trauma, although fracture is in the differential diagnosis. Note the slight asymmetry in sternoclavicular activity, with the right-sided activity slightly proximal to the joint compared with the left. **B,** Posterior view from the same prechemotherapy bone scan shows an intense focus of activity at the right upper cervical spine, with smaller foci of activity on the right at the lower thoracic spine level and a small focus at the left upper sacroiliac joint level. Degenerative changes, metastases, or some combination are in the scintigraphic differential diagnosis.

vertebrae, the left medial iliac crest, and a left anterior rib (Figure 3). These sites of abnormal activity overlapped in distribution with the abnormalities noted previously on limited chest MRI and the prechemotherapy bone scan. No definite correlates were found at these sites on CT. Thus,

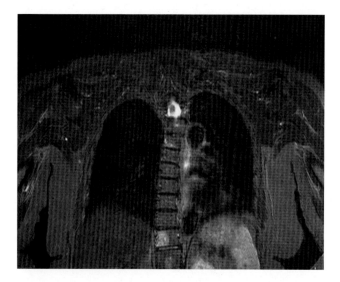

FIGURE 2. Coronal STIR image of the thorax, obtained with the body coil as part of the breast MRI, shows a hyperintense focus in a lower thoracic vertebral body. Similar findings were seen elsewhere, including the right clavicular head (not shown), suggesting bone metastases.

as the staging was completed in this patient, it became apparent that what was initially thought to be T3N1 disease (stage IIIA) was actually stage IV disease.

After one cycle of chemotherapy, CT scanning was repeated. The large breast mass and axillary adenopathy showed improvement, and new sclerosis was now evident at several levels in the spine (Figure 4).

Before undergoing repeat bone scanning and spine MRI, a second cycle of chemotherapy was given. The repeat bone scan, obtained 1 month after the prechemotherapy study, showed an increase in number of foci of increased activity (Figure 5). Several preexisting foci of activity appeared larger and more intensely active. MRI of the lumbar spine showed multiple areas of abnormal signal intensity, at levels corresponding to the prior bone and PET scans (Figure 6).

After completion of three cycles of neoadjuvant chemotherapy, the breast mass and axillary adenopathy had shrunk. Three months after diagnosis, the patient underwent bilateral mastectomies, right axillary dissection, left sentinel lymph node sampling, and removal of breast implants. The right mastectomy specimen contained a 3.5-cm IDC, with multiple satellite nodules and clear margins. Six of 16 axillary lymph nodes showed metastases.

Two weeks after surgery, CT-guided sampling of the sclerotic T11 lesion was performed and did not

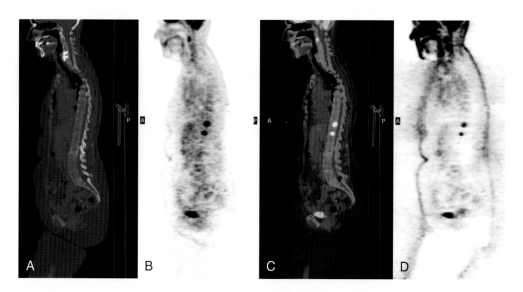

FIGURE 3. **A** to **D,** Sagittal images through the spine from PET/CT, performed 1 week after one round of chemotherapy. Two adjacent foci of hypermetabolism are seen in the lower thoracic spine, at T11 and T12. The corresponding CT bone window showed no definite lesions. A smaller hypermetabolic metastasis is seen in C2, above a prior surgical level.

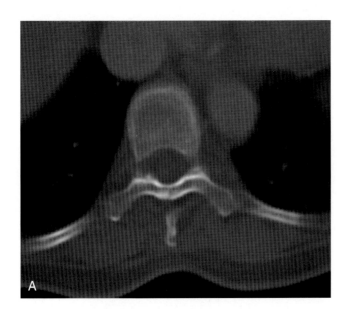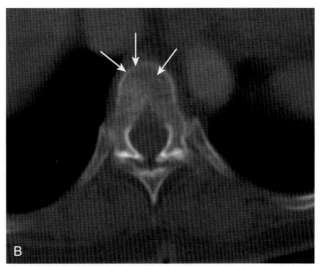

FIGURE 4. **A,** Detail of T11 vertebral body from staging CT, obtained before neoadjuvant chemotherapy. No definite osseous abnormality is seen to correlate with the hypermetabolism subsequently demonstrated at this level 1 week later on PET/CT. **B,** Detail of the same level, 3 weeks later, after one cycle of chemotherapy, shows new sclerosis (*arrows*), at the level where PET/CT had shown hypermetabolism.

confirm metastatic disease. The needle biopsy was repeated 2 months later, confirming metastasis. A nearly concurrent repeat PET/CT for restaging had normalized (Figure 7).

TEACHING POINTS

This case represents stage IV disease at presentation, with a locally advanced breast cancer, metastatic to bone. It provides an excellent take-off point for discussion of some of the imaging issues raised on initial identification of bone metastases, as well as the assessment of treatment responses.

Bone scanning is not routinely obtained in the initial staging of all newly diagnosed breast cancer patients, as it once was. The yield in early-stage disease is low. In general, bone scanning performed during initial staging is reserved for patients with stage III or greater disease, unless there is a symptom, physical examination finding, tumor marker, or other abnormal laboratory value to suggest advanced disease.

Bone metastases can have a variety of appearances on bone scintigraphy, from a solitary active lesion, to multiple focal areas of increased activity,

to diffuse involvement. Whether a bone metastasis is visualized on a bone scan depends on the size of the lesion, the location, and the type of bone reaction elicited. Because breast cancer metastases can be lytic, sclerotic, and frequently are mixed, a variety of manifestations are possible. Adding to the difficulty is the potential for conversion of successfully treated lytic metastases to blastic lesions. In general, bone scans most reliably depict osteoblastic metastases and can miss purely lytic disease. The converse is true of PET, which is highly sensitive for lytic bone lesions, but less sensitive for blastic metastases.

How then to resolve and explain the apparently conflicting imaging study results obtained in this patient?

The initial bone scan, obtained before starting chemotherapy, was abnormal, although not definitively diagnostic of bone involvement. Without imaging correlation, provided subsequently by a limited chest MRI, a number of the bone scan findings could have been accounted for by other explanations. The rib lesion, for example, could have been post-traumatic, and a possible trauma history was elicited from the patient. The activity is less punctate than generally seen with fractures, but a long segment of involvement, which would

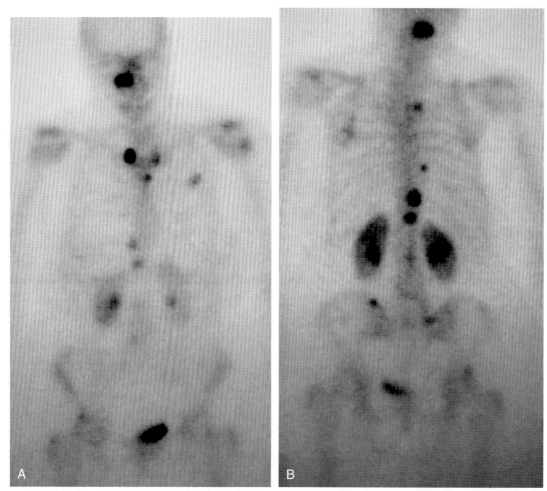

FIGURE 5. Repeat bone scan, 1 month after the prechemotherapy study, after two cycles of chemotherapy. **A,** Anterior planar view shows increased activity of the right clavicular head. The activity is now seen more clearly to be bone centered (versus joint centered). Intense shine-through activity of a larger right upper cervical spine lesion is seen, with less intense shine-through noted of adjacent right lower thoracic foci. The left anterior rib activity persists without clear change from before. **B,** Posterior planar bone scintigraphy shows more numerous and intense foci of activity compared with the prior study, including multiple spinal foci, correlating with hypermetabolism on PET/CT.

more compellingly suggest neoplasia, is not seen either. The patient had had prior cervical spine surgery, raising the possibility of accelerated degenerative change at an adjacent level. At the same time, the activity in both the cervical and thoracic levels is disturbingly focal and relatively intense. Degenerative findings frequently involve multiple adjacent levels and, unless actively degenerating, are often less intense in activity than the findings seen here.

The correlation provided subsequently by the limited chest MRI and PET/CT resolves the questions and provides compelling evidence of bony metastatic disease.

What is the significance of the apparent increase in disease seen on the second bone scan, performed 1 month later, after two cycles of chemotherapy? Does this mean the metastases are progressing? Not necessarily. In fact, the changes we see between these two bone scans are an excellent example of the flare phenomenon, whereby a patient responding to hormonal therapy or chemotherapy may actually appear worse on bone scanning. Increased activity of previously identified lesions and even new lesions may be seen (as in this case). Recall that it is the osteoblastic response to a bone abnormality (neoplastic, infectious, or traumatic) that we see as an increase in activity on a bone

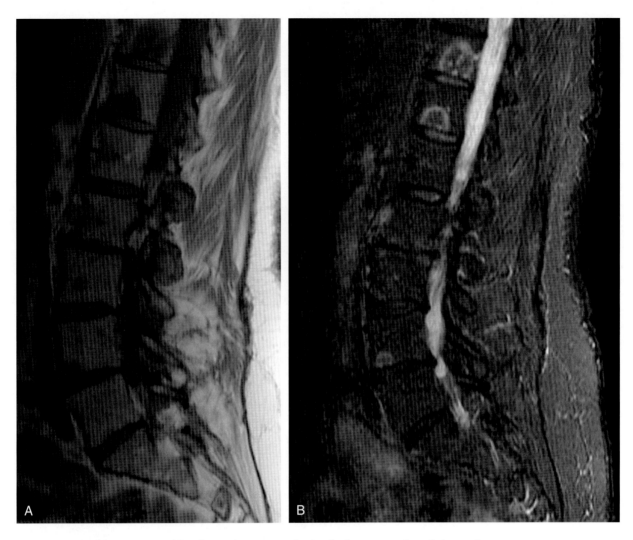

FIGURE 6. Sagittal lumbar spine MRIs, obtained after two cycles of chemotherapy. **A,** Sagittal, T1-weighted image shows hypointense foci of altered marrow signal, contrasting with the normal bright signal of fatty marrow. Lesions are seen at T11, T12, and the inferior-anterior L4 level. The larger lesions at T11 and T12 correlate with bone and PET scan findings. **B,** Sagittal STIR image through the same level shows corresponding peripheral hyperintensity of the metastases.

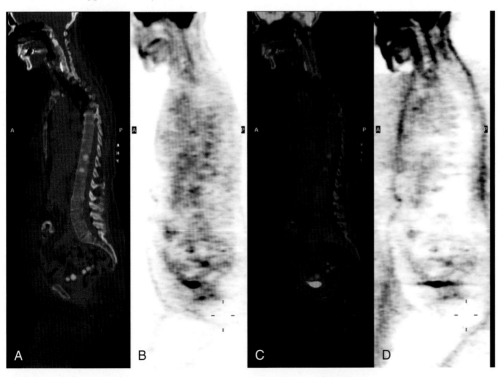

FIGURE 7. **A to D,** Sagittal images through the spine on follow-up PET/CT, 5 months after the initial staging PET/CT scan. The PET activity has resolved. The lesions can now be seen on the CT bone windows as sclerotic foci. The focus at T11 was biopsied 2 days before this study, confirming metastatic carcinoma.

scan. Metastases that are initially lytic may become sclerotic in response to treatment, and this is demonstrated in this case on the PET/CT. The hypermetabolic bone foci that were seen on the initial PET/CT were without a clear CT correlate (indicating they were lytic) but became sclerotic (within 3 weeks, after one cycle of chemotherapy!) and readily visible on the CT portion of the follow-up PET/CT, at which time the PET activity had resolved. This does not mean the patient is cured or that the disease is not active. This patient had biopsy confirmation of metastatic involvement of T11, concurrent with normalization of PET scan activity. This constellation of findings reflects the reality that initially lytic bone metastases, best seen on PET imaging, responded to treatment by developing sclerosis. In the process, the bone metastases became increasingly visible on CT and bone scan, and inactive on PET.

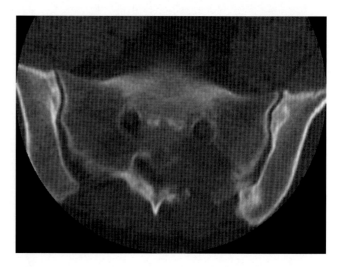

FIGURE 1.   Axial CT scan (bone window) through the sacrum shows lytic destruction of the left posterior sacrum, extending to the sacral foramina.

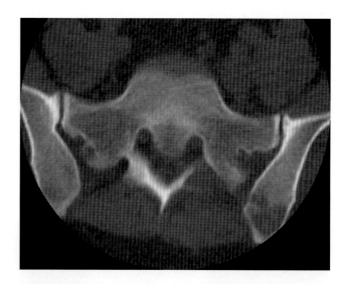

FIGURE 2.   More inferior axial CT image (bone window) through the sacroiliac (SI) joints shows another lytic lesion in the left medial ilium, adjacent to the SI joint.

CASE 2

Stage IV presentation with bone metastases (breast cancer presenting with back pain)

A 35-year-old obese woman presented with severe low back, knee, and hip pain and 5 days of intermittent fever up to 102 degrees. She was evaluated with abdominal, pelvic, and lumbar spine CT scans for suspicion of a spinal infection. These studies showed multiple lytic lesions in bone, including the L5 vertebral body, and left sacrum, ilium, and proximal femur (Figures 1, 2, 3, and 4). Bony metastatic disease was suspected, and a lung primary was sought with a chest CT. This showed a 2-cm spiculated right breast mass, suspicious for a breast cancer primary (Figure 5).

Bone scan showed corresponding, highly suspicious, multifocal findings suggesting bone metastases (Figure 6).

Breast imaging workup with diagnostic mammography, breast ultrasound, and ultrasound-guided core needle biopsy confirmed right breast cancer. The mammogram showed a dominant, central, 5-cm spiculated mass (Figure 7). Ultrasound showed a corresponding irregular hypoechoic mass in the retroareolar region, with a separate 1.7-cm suspicious shadowing focus in the upper outer quadrant (UOQ) (Figures 8 and 9). A suspicious axillary lymph node was also noted, with mild cortical mantle thickening (Figure 10).

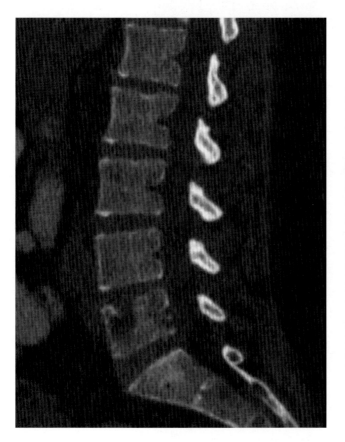

FIGURE 3. Sagittal lumbar spine reconstruction (bone window) shows another lytic lesion in L5, extending to the superior end plate.

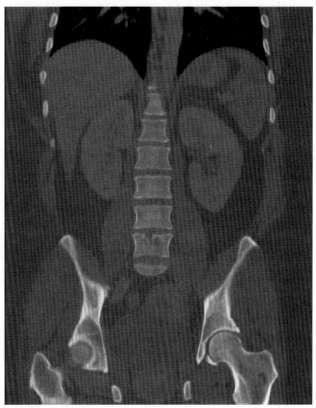

FIGURE 4. Coronal reconstruction (bone window) shows the lytic change in L5 and another small lytic lesion in the left intertrochanteric proximal femur.

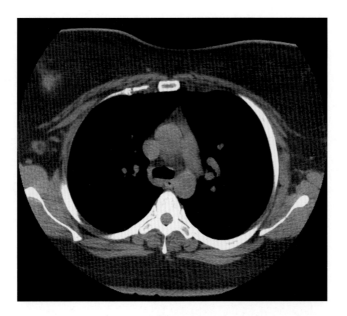

FIGURE 5. Axial unenhanced chest CT image shows a central right breast mass in largely fatty breasts.

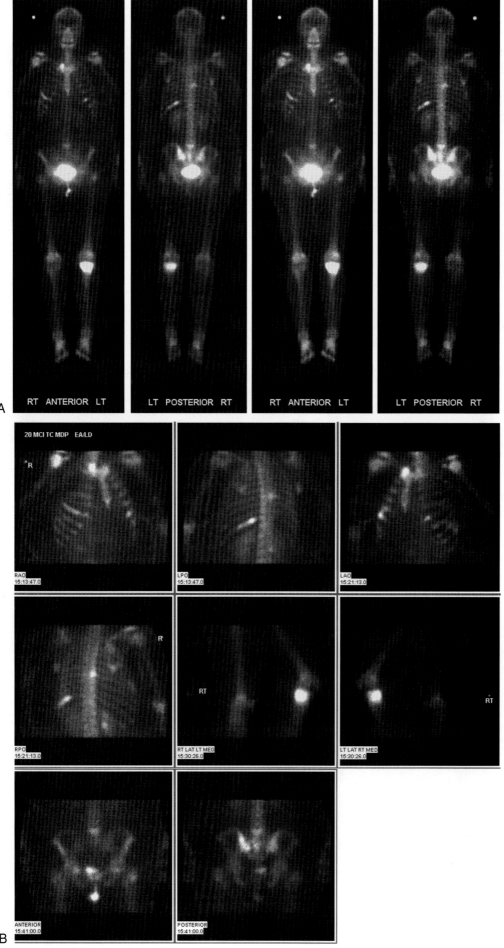

FIGURE 6. Bone scan images (**A,** anterior and posterior whole-body; **B,** spot views of the ribs [oblique], knees [lateral], and pelvis [anterior and posterior]) show multiple foci of abnormally increased activity in a highly suspicious pattern for bony metastatic disease. In addition to activity that corresponds to the known lytic foci in spine and pelvis on CT, sites are seen in the right clavicular head, ribs, and left proximal tibia, among others. The long segments of rib activity (left posterior, right anterior) are a pattern of activity that is highly suspect for neoplasia.

L

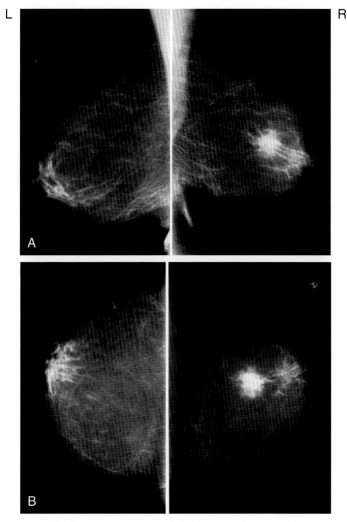

R

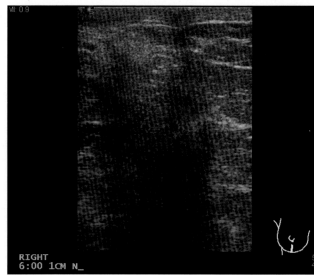

FIGURE 8.   Ultrasound of the right central breast shows a large area of ill-defined hypoechoic shadowing, which corresponds in location with the dominant mass on CT and mammography.

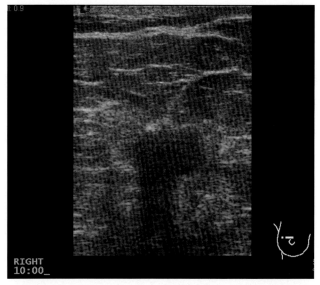

FIGURE 7.   MLO (**A**) and CC (**B**) mammograms show a dominant central, spiculated right breast mass behind the nipple, with stranding extending anteriorly toward the nipple. This mass corresponds to the mass identified on CT. The breasts are predominantly fatty.

FIGURE 9.   Ultrasound of the right UOQ shows a separate hypoechoic shadowing mass at 10 o'clock.

Histologic sampling of the breast masses confirmed infiltrating ductal carcinoma (IDC) from both sites, estrogen receptor and progesterone receptor positive, and *HER-2/neu* positive. Fine-needle aspiration of the axillary lymph node demonstrated metastatic carcinoma.

CT-guided sampling of a lucent sacral lesion showed metastatic adenocarcinoma, consistent with breast primary (Figure 11).

Palliative radiation therapy to the lumbar spine (L5 and sacroiliac region) and left knee were given for pain relief, and the patient was started on tamoxifen and zoledronic acid (Zometa). Repeat CT images, 7 months later, show

a variety of bone responses to these interventions (Figure 12).

TEACHING POINTS

This is a distinctly unusual presentation of breast cancer, with symptomatic bone metastases bringing this pre-screening-age patient with no notable

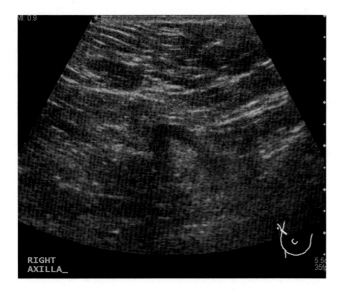

FIGURE 10. Right axillary ultrasound shows two lymph nodes with hypoechoic, thickened cortices. Fine-needle aspiration confirmed metastatic tumor.

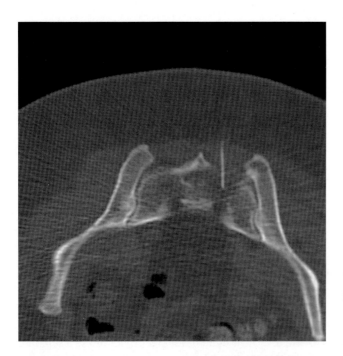

FIGURE 11. Sampling of the sacral lucent lesion was performed with CT guidance. Axial image with the patient in prone position shows the needle in the lesion. Histology confirmed metastatic adenocarcinoma, consistent with a breast primary.

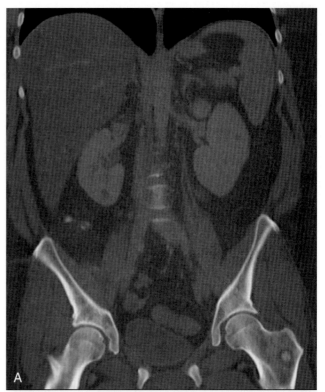

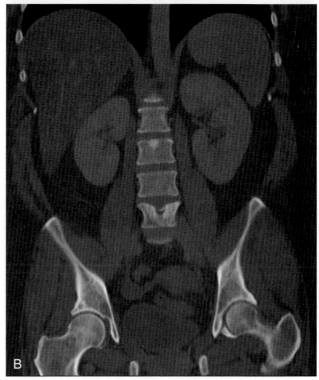

FIGURE 12. Coronal CT reconstructions (**A** anterior to **B**), 7 months after initial CT in Figure 4, after lumbar spine radiation, and treatment with tamoxifen and Zometa. In **A**, the left intertrochanteric metastasis has grown. It now displays a dominant central sclerotic component, with a lucent rim. In **B**, the lytic focus at the superior end plate of L5 remains visible, but now shows a thick surrounding blastic response. At the superior end plate of L3, a blastic lesion is now seen. This may reflect healing of a subradiographic lytic metastasis.

family history to attention. Less than 10% of breast cancer patients present with stage IV disease. This patient's primary tumor was also identified through an unusual route, being first seen on a chest CT. Breast cancers can certainly be picked up initially on chest CT, which usually is performed for other reasons. (See Case 15 in Chapter 1 for another example.) For this reason, CT interpreters should always scrutinize chest wall soft tissues and breasts as part of their routine search pattern.

The initial presentation of these bone metastases was lytic, manifested on CT as soft tissue replacement of bone. The lumbar spine was locally treated with radiation therapy for pain palliation. The follow-up study shows a new sclerotic metastasis at L3, which was not previously known. Sclerosis can be a manifestation of healing of a subradiographic lytic lesion. Sclerosis is now also seen surrounding the lytic end-plate change at L5. At the left hip level, the lytic lesion with central sclerosis grew between studies. On the later study, the lesion displays a larger and more sclerotic central component. Is this growth and progression of a mixed lytic and sclerotic metastasis, or growth despite a partial healing response manifested by the larger and more sclerotic central component? Unfortunately, this illustrates the difficulty of assessing by imaging the response of bone metastases to therapy.

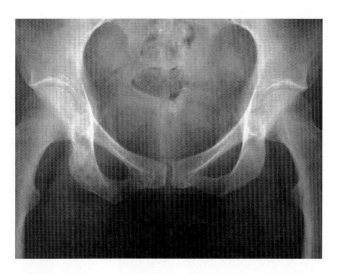

FIGURE 1. Anteroposterior view of the pelvis (cropped) shows expansion and abnormal bone mineral texture, with coarsened trabecula and mixed lucency and sclerosis, in the right ischium.

CASE 3

Relapse with bone metastases

A 36-year-old woman sought orthopedic advice for low back and right leg pain that developed while training for a half marathon. She had been treated 4 years before for an estrogen receptor and progesterone receptor positive, T1cN1b(4) infiltrating ductal carcinoma with breast conservation and axillary dissection, with 4 of 20 lymph nodes positive with microscopic extracapsular extension. Additional treatment was with chemotherapy (four cycles of doxorubicin [Adriamycin] plus cyclophosphamide [Cytoxan] [AC] and four cycles of paclitaxel [Taxol]); right breast, supraclavicular, and axillary radiation therapy; and tamoxifen.

A pelvis x-ray was abnormal, with a moth-eaten appearance of the right ischium (Figure 1). Subsequent evaluations with pelvis and lumbar spine MRI, body CT scans, positron emission tomography (PET), and bone scan suggested extensive bony metastases (Figures 2, 3, 4, and 5). A bone marrow aspirate confirmed metastatic breast cancer. The patient was placed on goserelin acetate (Zoladex),

zoledronic acid (Zometa), and anastrozole (Arimidex).

A year later, while on Zoladex, Zometa, and exemestane (Aromasin), the patient was restaged with PET/CT for symptoms of increased aching, weight loss, depressed appetite, and rising tumor markers. PET/CT showed new liver metastases. Chemotherapy was recommended, but declined. The patient was started on fulvestrant (Faslodex). Restaging after 2 months, at which time the patient had fatigue, shortness of breath, and rising tumor markers, showed progression of liver metastases as well as evidence of lung involvement (see Case 13 in Chapter 10). She died a month later, 15 months after bony metastases were detected.

TEACHING POINTS

This case illustrates well the hierarchy of bone imaging studies in terms of how completely they depict osseous metastases. Lowest on the totem pole are x-rays. Still useful to evaluate a site of focal symptoms or to further evaluate a focal bone scan abnormality, radiographs are known to be limited in depiction of bone metastases because up to 50% bone destruction must occur before radiographs will suggest an abnormality.

Higher in the hierarchy is bone scintigraphy. In most cancers, bone scans are 50% to 80% more sensitive than radiographs for detection of bone

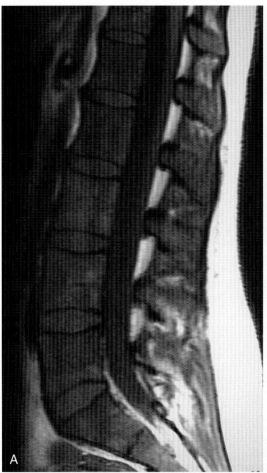

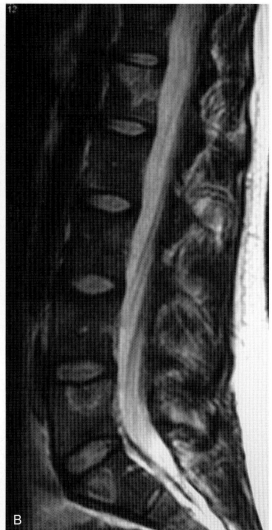

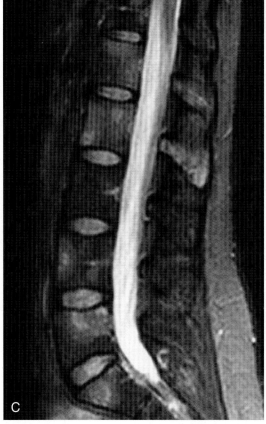

FIGURE 2. Sagittal MRIs of the lumbar spine show diffusely abnormal bone marrow signal. **A,** T1-weighted imaging shows complete loss of normal bright fatty marrow signal. **B,** T2-weighted, fat-saturated sequence shows heterogeneous patchy abnormal increased signal, involving portions of L1, L5, and S1 particularly. **C,** STIR sagittal view shows increased abnormal signal involving much of L1 and L2, and portions of L4, L5, and S1.

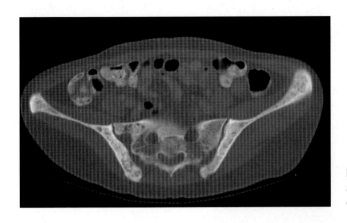

FIGURE 3. Axial pelvis CT image shows diffuse markedly abnormal bone mineral texture, with mixed lucency and osteosclerosis.

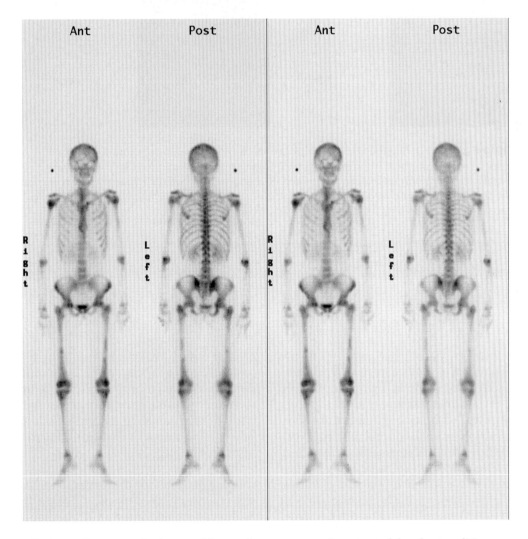

FIGURE 4. Bone scan is abnormal but under-represents the extent of the abnormalities apparent from MRI and CT. There are subtle abnormalities that correspond to known abnormalities (increased activity of the radiographically abnormal right ischium compared with the left), but overall the extent of disease suggested by bone scan is discrepant with other imaging studies. The most clear-cut evidence of bone metastases based on this study includes the patchy foci of increased activity in the shafts of both femurs and the increased activity in the right lower sternum. Activity is asymmetrically increased in the right proximal humerus, but also abnormal on the left. In fact, there is an overall "metabolic bone disease" pattern for much of the activity on this bone scan, with prominent periarticular activity of large joints.

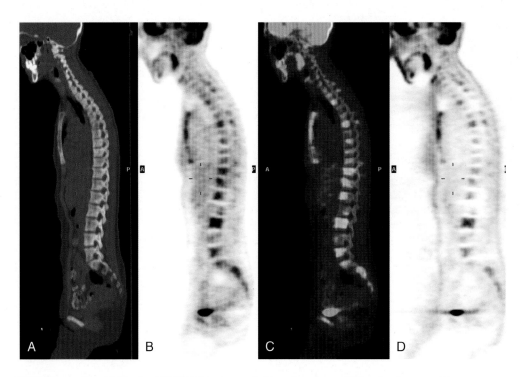

FIGURE 5. **A** to **D,** Sagittal PET/CT images of the spine show diffusely abnormal bone mineral texture on the CT portion (*left*), with some areas predominantly lytic and others mostly sclerotic. Diffuse, but markedly inhomogeneous increased PET scan activity is seen in the sternum and spine. In a general way, the sites of greatest PET scan activity appear to correlate with levels with more lytic than blastic change.

metastases. However, as in this case, there are instances in which bone scans can severely underestimate the extent of skeletal involvement (see also Case 5). A possible explanation is the very diffuse distribution, with such extensive involvement that there is essentially no normal intervening bone between lesions to increase the conspicuity of metastatic lesions. Such extensive bony metastases could result in a "superscan" pattern of diffuse increased skeletal activity, with high target-to–soft tissue ratio and minimal renal and bladder activity. In such scans, tracer uptake is so increased in the skeleton that less tracer is available to excrete through the urinary system. This bone scan does not demonstrate the classic features of a superscan, but shows some features in the spectrum of a superscan.

The sensitivity of bone scintigraphy can be improved with the addition of single-photon emission computed tomography (SPECT), especially in the spine. This is most applicable if there is a target area of symptoms or if planar bone scan suggests a localized abnormality, but is impractical and time-consuming for routine application. Improved performance of bone scintigraphy can also be achieved with performance of fluorine-18 bone scanning, but at higher cost of the radiopharmaceutical and in imaging time.

MRI is the most sensitive anatomic imaging modality overall for the detection of bone metastases, whether lytic or blastic. CT is the most sensitive radiographic modality. PET imaging is very sensitive, particularly for lytic disease, but may underestimate blastic bone disease. Because the converse is true for bone scans, PET and bone scintigraphy may be considered complementary for comprehensive evaluation of the skeleton for metastases, whether lytic or blastic. Particularly if the PET is a PET/CT, the combination of PET, CT, and bone scan information is a very comprehensive approach for the detection and characterization of osseous metastases.

CASE 4

Progression of bone metastases, epidural extension, radiation therapy effects

A 55-year-old woman with a remote history of treated breast cancer presented with breast recurrence and bone metastases. Her breast cancer history was 14 years earlier, a right T2N0 infiltrating ductal carcinoma (IDC), estrogen receptor and progesterone receptor positive, treated with lumpectomy and radiation. Tamoxifen had been declined. At this presentation with recurrent disease, her left breast showed firm hardening, partial nipple inversion, and peau d'orange. Core needle biopsy confirmed IDC. Increased right breast firmness and nipple retraction were also noted, as well as left supraclavicular fullness and nodularity. The patient noted right hip and back discomfort, and bone scan showed findings suspicious for bone metastases. Bone metastases were subsequently confirmed by lumbar spine MRI (Figures 1 and 2), and corresponding findings were noted on CT scans as well (Figure 3). The patient was placed on tamoxifen and monthly zoledronic acid (Zometa) after treatment with doxorubicin (Adriamycin) plus cyclophosphamide (Cytoxan) (AC) chemotherapy and monitored periodically with bone scans (Figures 4 and 5).

Over the subsequent years, the patient was maintained on multiple regimens, including letrozole (Femara) and pamidronate disodium (Aredia), and later Aredia and fulvestrant (Faslodex).

Four years after bone metastases were demonstrated, the patient was evaluated with PET, which showed multiple metabolically active bone lesions (Figures 6 and 7). At the time, the patient noted new left anterior thigh paresthesia, which progressed to excruciating. Lumbar spine MRI showed progression of bone metastases and new epidural disease at L2 (Figure 8). Radiation therapy was administered, with marked improvement in pain (Figure 9). The patient's therapy at this time included exemestane (Aromasin) and Aredia.

Nine months later, the patient developed pain above the radiated level, as well as hip pain, and was treated with samarium with a good clinical response.

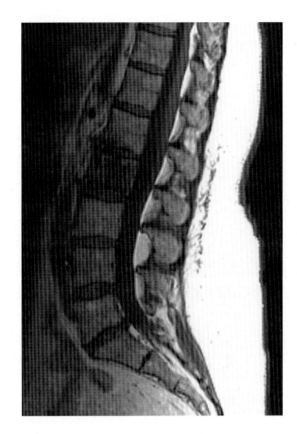

FIGURE 1. Sagittal, T1-weighted MRI of the lumbar spine, obtained 3 years after initial identification of bone metastases, shows replacement of the normal bright fatty marrow signal in the L2 vertebra, consistent with a metastasis.

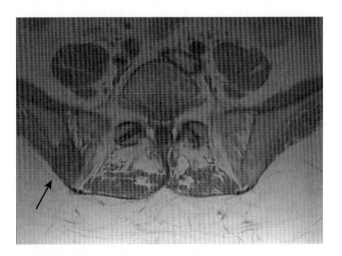

FIGURE 2. Axial T1-weighted image through the sacroiliac joints shows another focus of marrow hypointensity in the right posterior ilium (*arrow*).

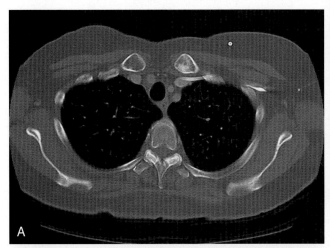

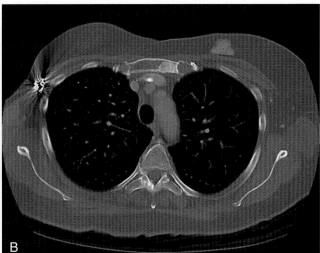

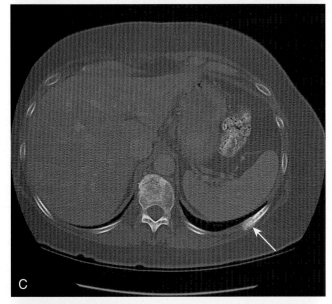

FIGURE 3. CT scans (bone windows) through the clavicular heads (**A**), the sternum (**B**), and the inferior thorax (**C**) show sclerotic metastases at the left medial clavicular head (**A**), left sternum (**B**), and in a lower thoracic vertebral centrum, as well as a left posterolateral rib (*arrow*) (**C**). A Porta-Cath is seen in left chest wall soft tissues, and there are axillary surgical clips on the right in **B**.

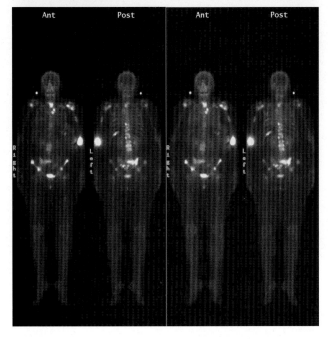

FIGURE 4. Anterior and posterior bone scan images show multiple abnormal foci of increased activity, including a long segment of left posterior lower rib activity. Multiple sites of abnormal activity are seen in the spine, sternal manubrium, left clavicular head, and in the pelvis, greatest at the right sacroiliac level. An "injectoma" is seen at the level of a left antecubital fossa injection site.

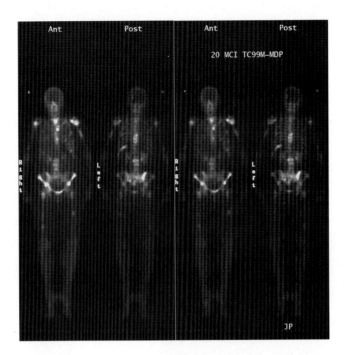

FIGURE 5.   Repeat bone scan, 10 months later, shows reduced activity at multiple adjacent thoracolumbar levels and the upper sacrum, which had been radiated. The patient had also been treated with samarium for bone pain. Findings at mid-thoracic, nonradiated levels are increased, and foci of increased activity are more evident in long bones of the extremities.

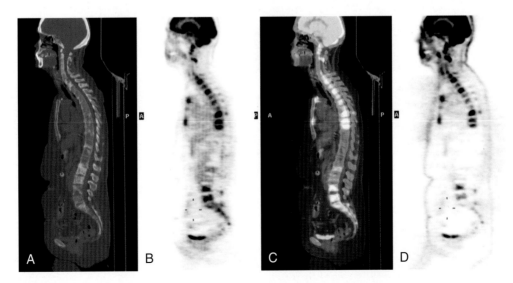

FIGURE 6.   Sagittal PET/CT scan shows intense, multilevel, increased activity in bone, seen here in spine and sternum. Adjacent thoracolumbar levels are photopenic, compatible with radiation therapy effect.

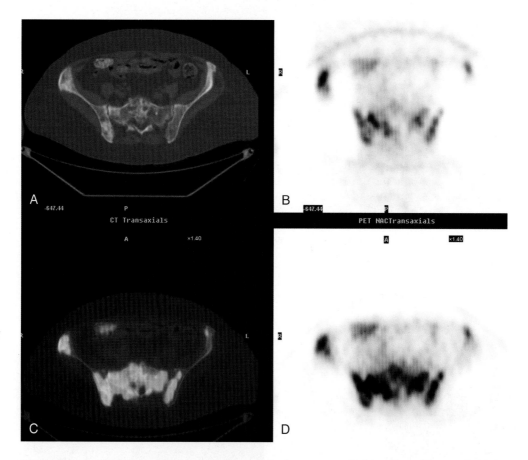

FIGURE 7. Axial PET/CT scan through the pelvis shows a mottled pattern of bone mineral density on CT, with lytic and sclerotic change and intense hypermetabolism at involved sites.

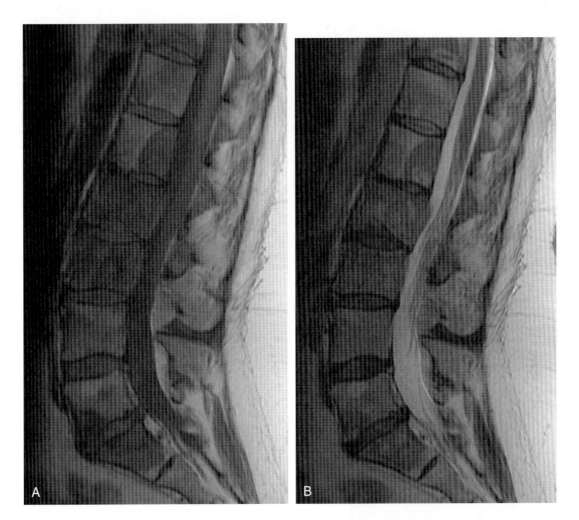

FIGURE 8.   Repeat lumbar spine MRI, 20 months later, shows progressive osseous metastatic disease, now with confluent involvement at L2 and L3, and patchy disease at other levels. The posterior cortex of the L2 vertebral centrum has been breached, with epidural extension. **A,** T1-weighted sagittal image. **B,** T2-weighted sagittal image.

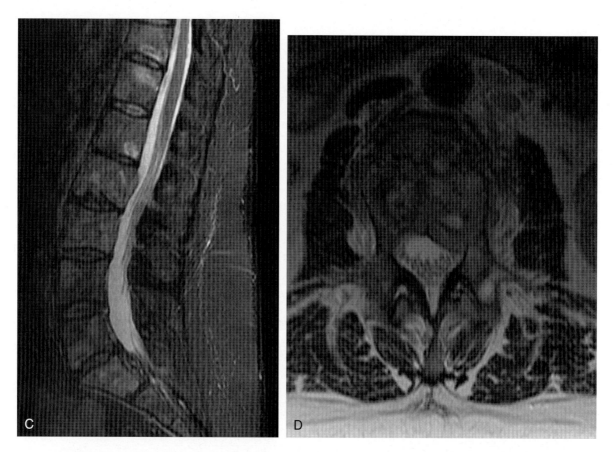

FIGURE 8, cont'd   C, STIR sagittal image. **D,** Axial T2-weighted slice through L2 shows epidural tumor in the left lateral recess and flattening of the adjacent thecal sac.

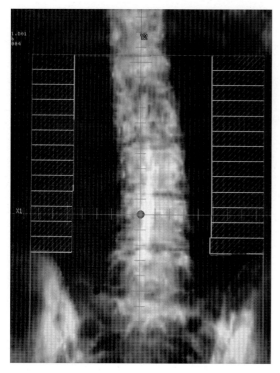

FIGURE 9.   Radiation therapy planning view of the lumbosacral spine shows the planned treatment field to encompass the entire lumbar spine, the sacrum, and sacroiliac regions.

Six months later, repeat spine MRI was obtained to evaluate new left leg sciatica. The patient noted increased fatigue, and her tumor markers were rising. Spine MRI showed progression of osseous metastases to near confluence (Figure 10). New epidural tumor was identified at the S1 level in the left lateral recess, explaining the patient's symptoms. Chemotherapy was restarted, with docetaxel (Taxotere).

TEACHING POINTS

This case demonstrates progressive bone metastases over a several year period and provides a take-off point for discussion of symptom management and radiation therapy effects on bone.

Bone scans are useful as whole-body skeletal maps reflecting the distribution, location, and activity of bone metastases. Although bone scans can underestimate purely lytic metastases, breast cancer metastases often have lytic and blastic components, with the associated bone turnover identifiable as increased activity on bone scintigraphy.

At this writing, reports of the use of whole-body MRI to identify bone metastases are appearing in the literature. Validation of this approach is ongoing, and in general today, MRI is used more selectively to image symptomatic regions or regions suspected based on other modalities to harbor metastatic

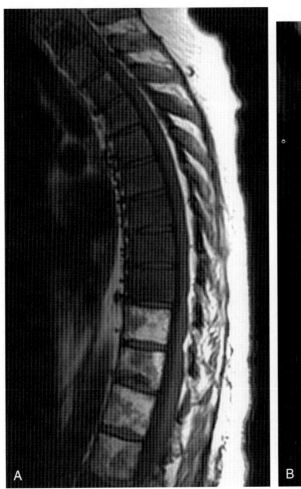
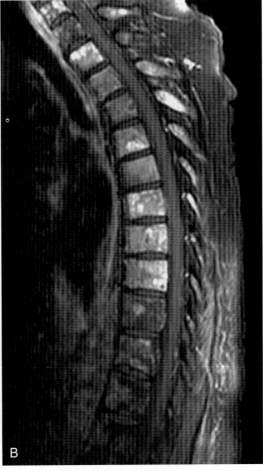

FIGURE 10.   Thoracic and lumbar spine MRI, obtained an additional 15 months later, after interval radiation therapy for the symptomatic L2 epidural disease, as well as administration of samarium for recurrent symptoms. Enhancing metastatic disease is now nearly confluent at upper thoracic and lower lumbar and sacral levels. Radiated levels are sharply delineated from untreated levels by the fatty signal of the marrow. Epidural tumor is now seen at the S1 level, accounting for the patient's new symptoms of left leg pain and numbness. **A,** Thoracic T1-weighted sagittal image. **B,** Thoracic enhanced, fat-saturated, T1-weighted sagittal image.

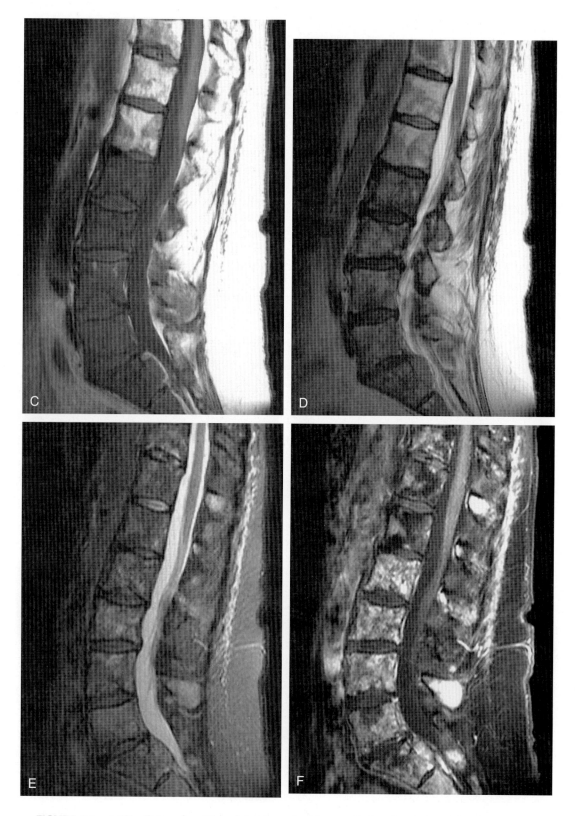

FIGURE 10, cont'd **C,** Lumbar T1-weighted, sagittal image. **D,** Lumbar T2-weighted, sagittal image. **E,** Lumbar sagittal STIR. **F,** Lumbar enhanced, fat-saturated, T1-weighted, sagittal image.

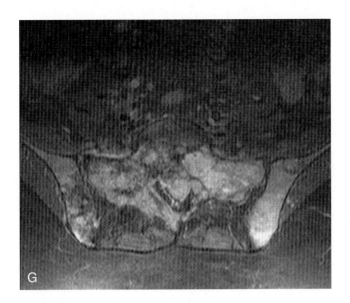

FIGURE 10, cont'd   G, Sacral enhanced, fat-saturated, T1 weighted axial image.

disease. Bone metastases are identified on MRI as areas of marrow replacement. T1-weighted sequences are sensitive for the detection of bone metastases because in adults, the normal marrow signal on T1-weighted sequences will be bright because of yellow (fatty) marrow. The signal intensity of metastases on T2-weighted sequences can help separate lytic from sclerotic lesions, with lytic metastases being relatively bright on T2 and STIR and sclerotic metastases hypointense on all sequences. Use of contrast enhancement, particularly with fat saturation, is useful to assess epidural tumor extension.

PET findings of bony breast cancer metastases can be complementary to bone scintigraphy. PET is sensitive to active bone metastases, particularly lytic disease, but may underestimate sclerotic bone metastases, which are identifiable on scintigraphy (see Case 10 in this chapter).

In this case, the patient had known bone metastases by scintigraphy for 3 years by the time of these imaging studies, which span 3 additional years. She had been on a variety of hormonal and chemotherapeutic regimens. Accordingly, some of the sclerotic lesions may reflect treatment effects as well as intrinsic characteristics of the lesions.

This case illustrates some of the neural complications of spinal metastatic disease. These findings may necessitate local therapies (radiation or surgery) to relieve pain and to prevent progression to loss of function.

Radiation therapy effects can be visualized on bone scan, PET scans, and MRI. The effect of radia-

tion is thought to be the result of small vessel insult. Radiated marrow becomes hypocellular, with fatty marrow replacing hematopoietic marrow. Because activity on bone scans results from delivery of the radiopharmaceutical and so is proportional to blood flow, the microvascular alterations induced by radiation may account for the photopenia seen on scintigraphy in radiated fields. Such changes have been reported to appear 4 to 6 months after treatment on scintigraphy.

The development of fatty marrow (manifest as increased signal on T1-weighted sequences) in radiated fields on MRI has been documented, in a prospective study by Yankelevitz and colleagues, to occur as early as 2 weeks after commencing therapy. The changes progress during treatment, with the greatest changes in the first 6 weeks.

SUGGESTED READINGS

Hattner RS, Hartmeyer J, Wara WM. Characterization of radiation-induced photopenic abnormalities on bone scans. *Radiology* 1982; 145:161–163.

Yankelevitz DF, Henschke CI, Knapp PH, et al. Effect of radiation therapy on thoracic and lumbar bone marrow: evaluation with MR imaging. *AJR Am J Roentgenol* 1991; 157:87–92.

CASE 5

Recurrence with bone metastases: Disease extent discordant between imaging and bone scan; pathologic fractures

A 65-year-old woman with a history of treated, early-stage breast cancer 1.5 years before, presented with progressive severe hip pain, to the point of being unable to walk. Her breast cancer was stage I, T1bN0, infiltrating ductal carcinoma, which was treated with lumpectomy and brachytherapy. The tumor was estrogen receptor and progesterone receptor negative, and *HER-2/neu* positive. The patient declined chemotherapy during initial treatment.

Her laboratory data were abnormal at the time of presentation with hip pain, with elevated alkaline phosphatase and CA27.29. The patient was admitted with suspicion of metastatic disease. The workup included a head CT; brain and spine MRI; chest, abdomen, and pelvis CT; and bone scan. Head CT and MRI showed intracranial metastases. CT showed suspicious findings for liver and lung metastases. Bone metastases were shown on spine MRI (Figure 1), as well as on CT (Figure 2). Bone scan was abnormal, most notably for rib, vertebral, and sacral fracture findings, but underrepresented the extent of diffuse osseous metastases (Figure 3).

TEACHING POINTS

The importance of imaging correlation when interpreting bone scans, PET scans, and other nuclear medicine studies cannot be overemphasized. Bone scans are highly variable in their depiction of metastases, depending on the size of the bone lesion, the location in the skeleton, and, importantly, the type of bone reaction incited (lytic, blastic, or mixed). There are patients with radiographic and imaging findings of extensive osseous metastases whose bone scans can appear deceptively benign. At first glance, the bone scan of this

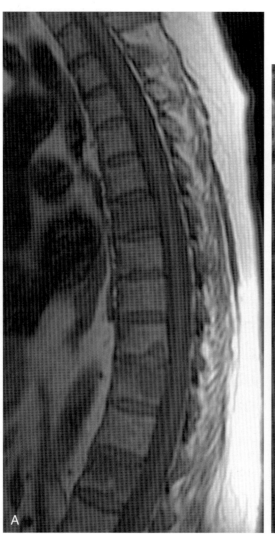 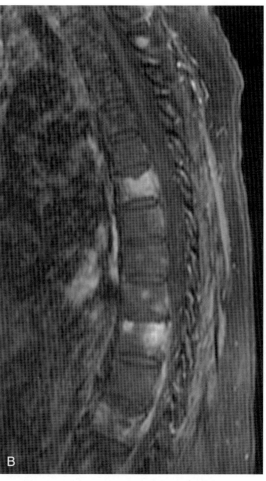

FIGURE 1.   Sagittal (**A**) T1-weighted and (**B**) fat-saturated, enhanced T1-weighted images through the thoracic spine show multiple foci of abnormal marrow signal and enhancement, consistent with metastases. There is also mild loss of height at the involved T12 level, suggesting pathologic fracture.

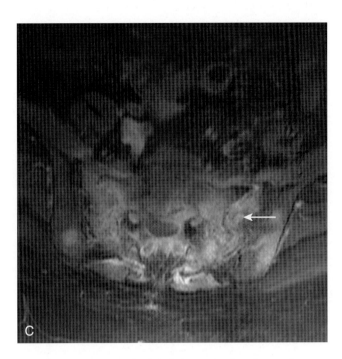

FIGURE 1, cont'd   C, Axial, fat-saturated, enhanced image through the sacrum shows diffuse, but heterogeneous enhancement of the sacrum and patchy enhancement of the adjacent ilia. A fracture line is visualized through the left sacral ala (*arrow*).

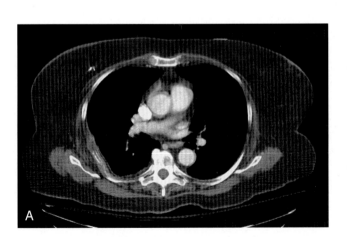
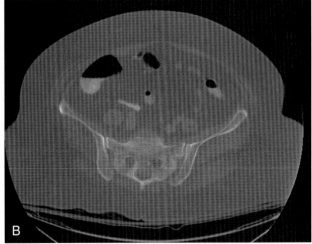

FIGURE 2.   Images from CT show (**A**) a destroyed, expanded, soft tissue replaced right posterior rib, and (**B**) a fracture line through the left sacral ala, with patchy lucency and sclerosis of the upper sacrum.

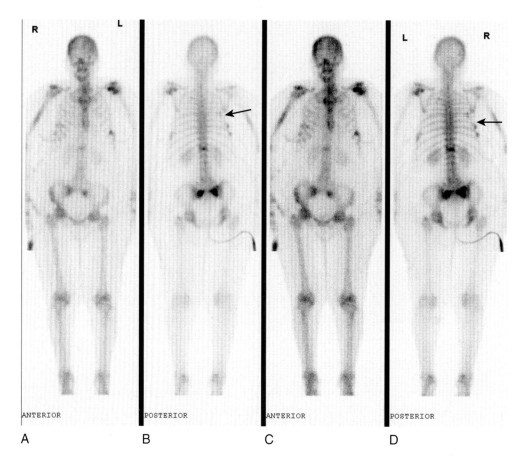

FIGURE 3. Anterior and posterior views from a whole-body bone scan are disconcertingly disproportionate in representing the findings of osseous metastases. Multiple abnormalities are noted, most of which represent fractures by correlation with CT and MRI. At many levels of known bony metastases, without pathologic fracture, the bone scan markedly under-represents the disease. The transverse band of activity at T12 corresponds to the partially replaced vertebral body with compression on MRI. The typical scintigraphic findings of sacral alar insufficiency fractures correlate with pathologic fractures on CT and MRI. Adjacent rib fractures are seen on the right, laterally (best seen on the posterior view). Just above this level, the lateral rib is absent, corresponding to the destroyed lytic rib metastasis and soft tissue mass seen on CT (*arrow*). Other levels of vertebral body involvement by MRI in the thoracic spine are not visualized on this bone scan. There are some findings, such as the long segment of increased activity in the right humerus, which do suggest bone metastases.

patient appears simply to be that of an elderly woman with typical scintigraphic findings of rib, vertebral compression, and sacral insufficiency fractures, with only subtle evidence on scintigraphy of metastatic disease as the etiology of the pathologic fractures. One of the most compelling findings on this bone scan for metastatic disease is the hardest to recognize: the cold lesion or absence of the destroyed right rib. With the roadmap provided by correlation with the CT, consequential oversights like this may be avoidable. At the same time, when presented with apparently discordant findings, the interpretation should reflect the fact that in individual patients, bone scintigraphy may not be the most accurate reflection of the full extent of osseous disease burden.

CASE 6

Diffuse bone metastases, underrepresented on bone scan

A 63-year-old woman was admitted from a rehabilitation center for evaluation of progressive anemia. She was recovering from an admission to another hospital for perforated ulcer, treated with gastrectomy. Her past medical history of right breast cancer was 7 years earlier, Stage 2, T1N2M0, treated with mastectomy, 6 months of adjuvant chemotherapy, and tamoxifen. A bone scan, performed for diffuse aches and bone pain, suggested metastatic disease as well as multiple fractures (Figure 1). Correlation with a concurrent body CT scan showed extensive bone mineral alterations of advanced and extensive osseous metastases, as well as multiple pathologic fractures (Figures 2 and 3). Metastatic adenocarcinoma, consistent with breast primary, was confirmed by CT-guided biopsy of a lytic focus in the left ilium (Figure 4).

TEACHING POINTS

Bone scans should never be interpreted in a clinical or imaging vacuum, as this case clearly illustrates. Correlation should always be made with any available radiographs, CT, or MRI. This CT scan demonstrates that the patient has very extensive and essentially confluent bony metastases, involving the entire skeleton, with virtually no normal intervening bone. The very confluence of this osseous disease presumably accounts for the surprising subtlety of the extensive metastases on scintigraphy. In the skull, with scattered, randomly distributed foci of increased activity, the diagnosis of metastatic disease is clearly suggested. Elsewhere, these extensive bony metastases are manifested predominantly by slight heterogeneity of activity. Other than the skull lesions, the bone scan is most remarkable for the multilevel fractures, which presumably are pathologic. In addition to the ribs, CT showed a right inferior pubic ramus fracture, which correlates with the discrete focus of increased activity on scintigraphy.

Considerations in choosing a site for biopsy of a suspected bone metastasis include ease and safety

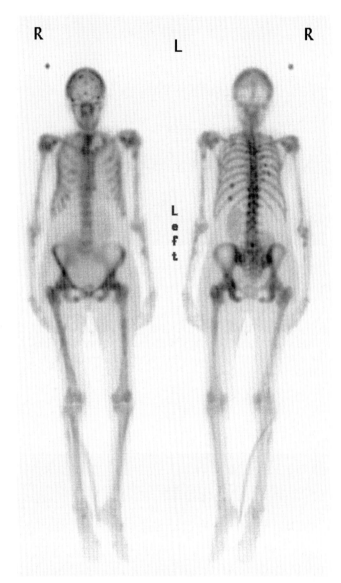

FIGURE 1. Anterior and posterior whole-body bone scan images show multiple foci of increased activity in the skull and posterior ribs. The foci in the skull are randomly distributed and highly suggestive of metastases. The posterior rib activity shows multiple adjacent foci bilaterally, in a pattern suggesting fractures. Note subtle heterogeneity of osseous activity elsewhere, best seen in the extremities, as in the left humerus (posterior view) and the femora (anterior view). The right kidney is ptotic. Increased soft tissue activity in the pelvis suggests malignant ascites. A small, focal area of increased uptake is seen in the right inferior pubic ramus.

of access (Can the patient lie prone? What structures might be injured?) and factors influencing the likelihood of obtaining adequate material (soft tissue replacing bone is easier to sample than bone forming tumor). In a case like this, in which there

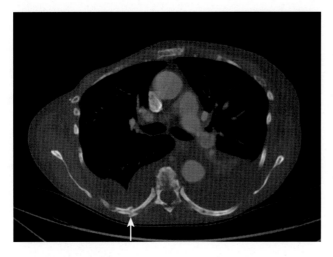

FIGURE 2. Bone windows from a concurrent body CT scan, at the level of the thorax, show a posterior rib fracture on the right (*arrow*). Additional fractures were seen at other levels (not shown). The bone mineral density is diffusely abnormal in the visualized sternum, spine, and ribs, indicating the rib fractures are most likely pathologic. There are moderate-sized bilateral pleural effusions as well.

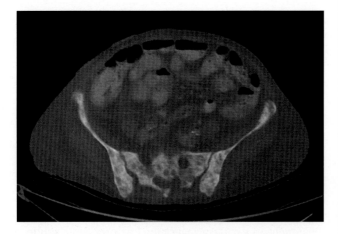

FIGURE 3. The diffuse nature of the abnormal bone texture is even more apparent on a slice through the sacrum. All of the bones show mottled, mixed sclerotic and lytic changes.

are diffuse changes, it makes sense to biopsy the pelvis, rather than risk a pneumothorax or neural injury sampling a rib or vertebral body. It is technically easier to obtain satisfactory material for analysis from a lytic bone metastasis than from sclerotic sites, when there is a choice.

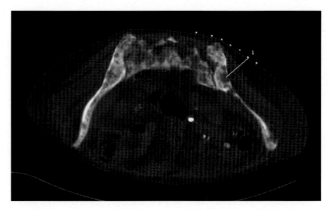

FIGURE 4. Image from CT-guided biopsy, showing the planned needle trajectory into a lytic focus in the left ilium.

CASE 7

Recurrence with mediastinal lymphadenopathy, vocal cord paralysis, and sclerotic bone metastases

A 59-year-old woman with a history of premenopausal breast cancer presented for medical oncologic evaluation for possible metastatic disease. Her breast cancer history was incomplete and obtained largely from the patient. It had been 10 years before, presenting as a large palpable left breast mass. She was treated with neoadjuvant chemotherapy with clinical response, followed by subsequent high-dose chemotherapy with stem cell rescue. A mastectomy and flap reconstruction was performed. The pathology specimen showed a 6-cm infiltrating lobular carcinoma (ILC). Six of 10 lymph nodes were involved. Chest wall radiation was performed. She declined recommended tamoxifen therapy.

A month before presentation, the patient developed left back pain, radiating laterally and to the front of the chest. A bone scan was abnormal at multiple levels, including T5, T11, the skull, and right humerus.

Oncologic evaluation included tumor markers, which were elevated (CEA and CA27.29). Positron emission tomography (PET) and CT imaging showed hypermetabolic mediastinal and hilar adenopathy and bone metastases (Figures 1, 2, 3, 4, 5,

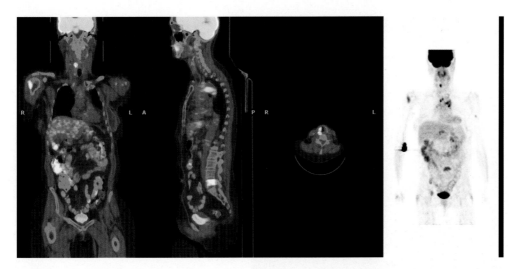

FIGURE 1. Three plane (*left to right:* coronal, sagittal, and axial), fused PET/CT with coronal projection volumetric image (*right*) shows multiple foci of hypermetabolism from soft tissue and bone metastases. Activity at the right proximal humeral (see coronal view) and L5 levels (seen on sagittal view) indicates bone metastases, whereas activity in the chest (seen on sagittal PET/CT and coronal projection image) shows aortopulmonary (AP) nodal disease, in a location to produce hoarseness. The coronal and axial views show asymmetry of vocal cord activity, with hypermetabolic muscular activity on the right at the level of the normally functioning cord, and absence on the left, paralyzed at the level of the left recurrent laryngeal nerve in the AP window.

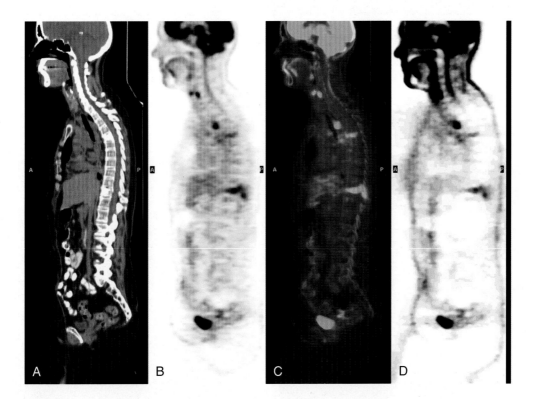

FIGURE 2. Sagittal PET/CT through the spine (*left to right:* CT, PET, fused PET/CT, non-attenuation-corrected PET) shows two foci of hypermetabolism in the thoracic spine, which on CT appear to be sclerotic. Anterior to the upper thoracic bone lesion is seen hypermetabolism in mediastinal nodes. Activity in the neck is vocal cord.

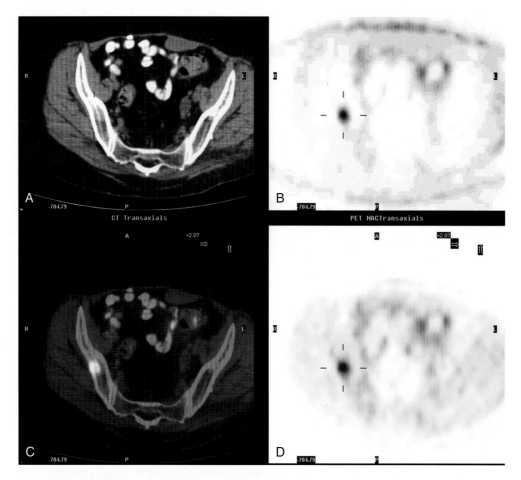

FIGURE 3.   Axial PET/CT images show a hypermetabolic metastatic focus in the right ilium.

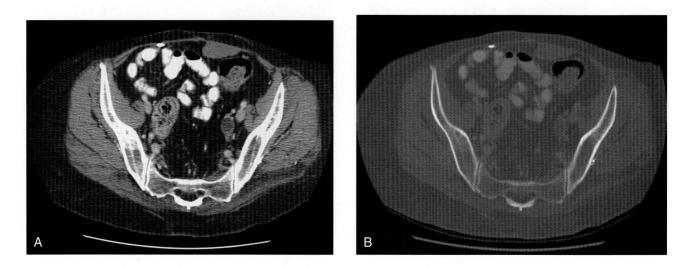

FIGURE 4.   CT images for correlation (**A,** soft tissue window; **B,** bone window). The blastic medullary bone change is visually much more apparent on soft tissue windows and comparatively subtle on the bone window.

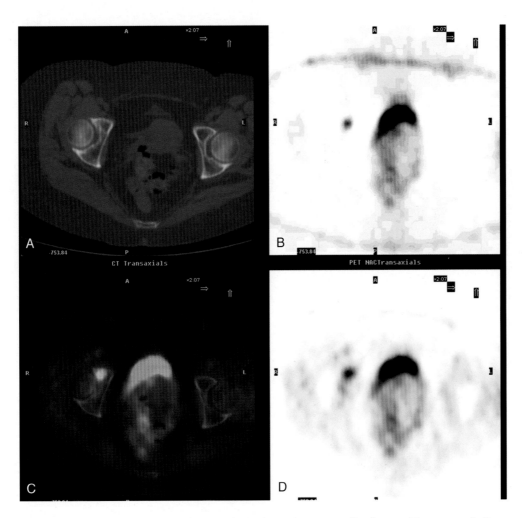

FIGURE 5. Axial PET/CT images through the hips show a smaller focus of hypermetabolism in another metastasis in the right anterior acetabulum.

and 6). The patient had been noted to be hoarse on physical examination, and PET showed asymmetrical muscular activity of the vocal cords. Metastases in the spine were further evaluated with MRI to assess epidural tumor extension (Figures 7, 8, 9, and 10).

A fine-needle aspiration was performed of a mediastinal lymph node, confirming metastatic disease, which was estrogen receptor and progesterone receptor positive and *HER-2/neu* negative. Radiation therapy was begun to the spine for palliation of pain.

TEACHING POINTS

Development of musculoskeletal symptoms is a clear clinical indication for restaging of a breast cancer patient. Systemic metastases occur most commonly to bone and are seen in up to one third of patients with recurrent disease. Traditionally, new focal pain would be evaluated with a radiograph of the joint or extremity, with the entire skeletal system surveyed with bone scintigraphy. Today, bone scanning is still indicated as a cost-effective

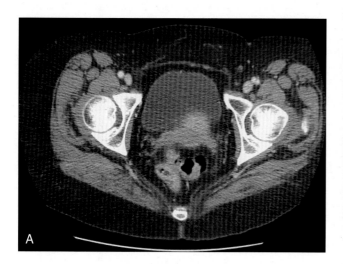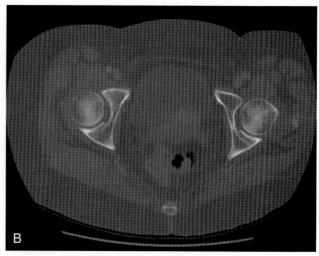

FIGURE 6. The corresponding CT images (**A,** soft tissue window; **B,** bone window) show subtle asymmetry, comparing the medullary density of one anterior acetabulum to the opposite side.

modality, which is particularly efficacious in identifying sclerotic metastases. If bone scanning does not provide an explanation for new symptoms, PET/CT may be indicated as the next imaging step for a highly sensitive comprehensive total-body evaluation for soft tissue and lytic bony metastases.

In this case, although bone scan showed evidence of bone metastases, PET/CT imaging showed soft tissue metastases to mediastinal lymph nodes. It also provided an explanation for the patient's hoarseness, showing PET-positive nodal disease in the aortopulmonary window and absence of vocal cord activity on the left. The CT component of the study provided an imaging correlate for the PET-positive bone metastases, showing some of the lesions to be blastic and others predominantly lytic. As demonstrated in this case, at times subtle blastic bony change can be easier to see on soft tissue windows than on bone windows, so assessment of the bones for metastases optimally should include review with more than one window setting.

This case also illustrates the limitations of CT for the evaluation of intraspinal and epidural disease. Although enhancing epidural soft tissue from the expanding bone metastasis is fairly clearly demonstrated in this case, identification of more subtle intraspinal extension is generally best undertaken with enhanced MRI.

It is highly desirable to obtain histologic confirmation when metastases from breast cancer are initially identified. In this case, mediastinal and bone metastases were identified essentially concurrently, and the question arises as to which lesion is preferable to sample. In this case, why biopsy the soft tissue disease in the mediastinum, when there are potentially less risky sites to sample in bone?

Multiple factors come into play when making this decision. Although it may be safer in terms of not entering a body cavity to sample an osseous site of suspected metastasis, it may be more difficult to obtain satisfactory material from bone than from soft tissue sites of disease. Not only does sufficient material need to be obtained to confidently diagnose malignancy if present, but estrogen receptor, progesterone receptor, and *HER-2/neu* information needs to be derived from the analysis if the lesion is metastatic breast cancer. At times, the receptor status of metastases can differ significantly from that of the original primary tumor, which has a major influence on treatment decisions.

Another factor to be considered is that thoracic disease could signify a new, potentially treatable, primary lung carcinoma, rather than metastatic disease from breast cancer. Such a distinction could be more difficult to make by analysis of a bone metastasis and is an argument for sampling of thoracic soft tissue disease.

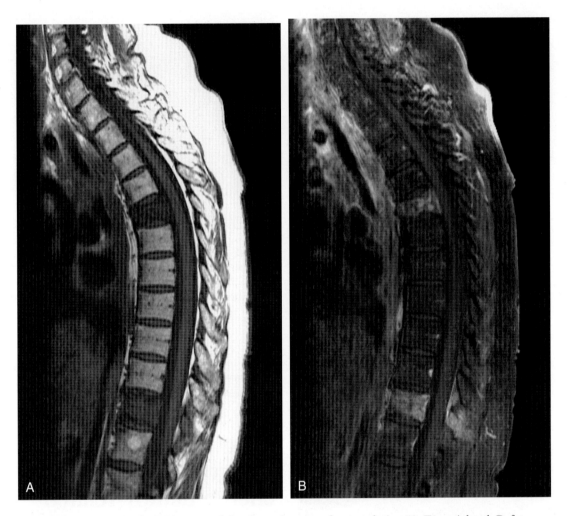

FIGURE 7. Sagittal MRI images of the thoracic spine, for correlation (**A,** T1-weighted; **B,** fat-saturated, enhanced, T1-weighted) show two thoracic metastases. **A,** On T1-weighted, unenhanced sequences, metastases show replacement of the normal bright fatty marrow of the vertebra with hypointense soft tissue intensity. The upper thoracic lesion shows evidence also of pathologic fracture, with loss of height. A small, hyperintense, fatty signal hemangioma is noted at the level below the lower thoracic metastasis. Increased soft tissue is seen in the visualized mediastinum anterior to the spine, corresponding to the nodal PET-positive disease. **B,** Fat-saturated, enhanced, T1-weighted image shows both vertebral lesions to be enhancing, as well as the mediastinal lymphadenopathy. Involvement of the lower thoracic posterior elements is easier to appreciate on this sequence. Enhancement is easier to visualize against a background of dark, suppressed fat signal. The hemangioma saturates, as would be expected on this sequence.

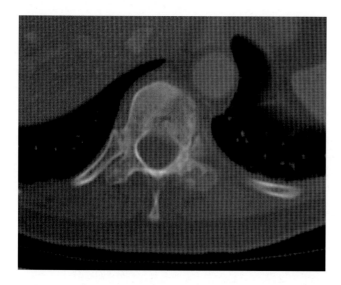

FIGURE 8. Axial CT images of T11 show lytic change of bone on the left, as well as the left transverse process. A subtle sclerotic margin is seen at the medial edge of the vertebral lysis.

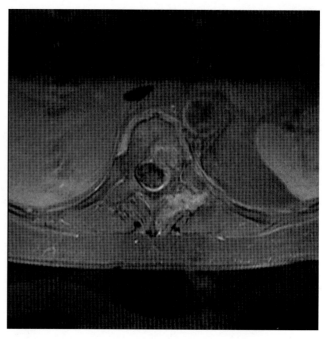

FIGURE 10. Corresponding axial fat-saturated, enhanced, T1-weighted image better shows the extent of enhancing tumor involvement of the left posterior elements, as well as the left anterolateral epidural tumor.

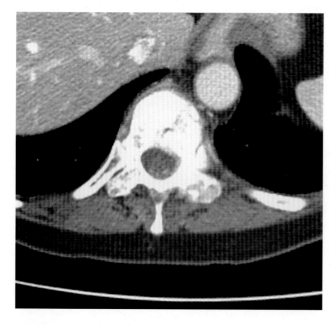

FIGURE 9. Enhanced soft tissue window from the same level shows an enhancing rim of soft tissue extending into the epidural space on the left anterolaterally.

CASE 8

Significance of solitary rib activity on bone scan; chemotherapy-related marrow activation changes on PET

A 39-year-old woman developed abdominal distention and increased fatigue a year after being treated for a high-risk breast cancer. This was an estrogen receptor– and progesterone receptor– positive, *HER-2/neu* positive, 2.7-cm infiltrating ductal carcinoma (IDC) with an extensive intraductal component of the right breast. Ten of 12 lymph nodes showed metastatic carcinoma, including a 3-cm lymph node with focal extracapsular extension. She was treated with a mastectomy, four cycles of doxorubicin and cyclophosphamide, followed by four cycles of paclitaxel, as well as chest wall, supraclavicular, and axillary radiation.

When the patient developed constitutional symptoms, she was restaged with CT scans, which showed extensive hepatic metastases. Chemotherapy with carboplatin, docetaxel (Taxotere), and trastuzumab (Herceptin) was initiated, with good response. Later the same year, brain metastases were identified, and treated with whole brain radiation therapy, with MRI resolution of lesions.

Evaluations for persistent right rib pain showed a fracture, seen on bone scan (Figures 1, 2, 3, and 4), CT (Figure 5), and PET scan. The patient had been coughing, and the activity seen on PET associated with the fracture was demonstrated subsequently to resolve on repeat PET.

PET scans obtained to monitor the patient's response to the chemotherapy given for liver metastases show typical findings of the frequently encountered treatment phenomenon of marrow activation (Figures 6 and 7).

TEACHING POINTS

A new, solitary bone scan finding in any patient with cancer poses a diagnostic dilemma. Unlike the more conclusive bone scan pattern of multifocal metastatic activity, such a bone scan result is often equivocal and will generally require correlation with imaging studies of the area with x-ray, CT, or MRI. Biopsy may ultimately be necessary to confirm or exclude metastatic bony disease. See a similar case, Case 9 in this chapter, for a discussion of bone scan rib findings.

In this case, in a patient with known liver and brain metastases, development of bone involvement would not be surprising.

How often is a solitary rib lesion on a bone scan in any cancer patient a metastasis? That depends on where the activity is located. Solitary spine foci are much more likely to be metastatic than a solitary rib focus: >40% versus <20%. This reflects the fact that vertebral bodies are highly vascularized and contain 75% of the body's red marrow.

This case also illustrates typical PET findings of marrow activation.

Granulocyte colony-stimulating factor (G-CSF) is frequently given in conjunction with myelosuppressive chemotherapy to stimulate neutrophil precursors in bone marrow. On PET imaging, a diffuse increase in marrow activity is seen, which resolves after cessation of therapy. Generally, the

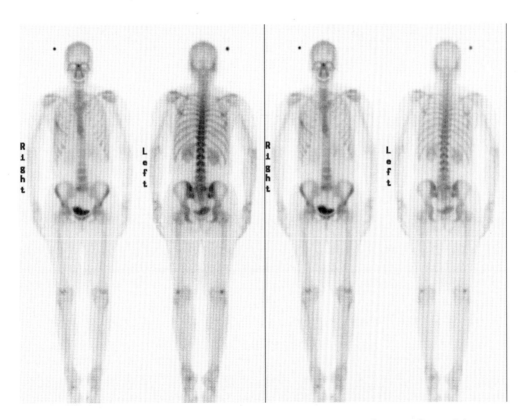

FIGURE 1. Anterior and posterior whole-body bone scan images show a solitary right anterolateral focus of increased activity.

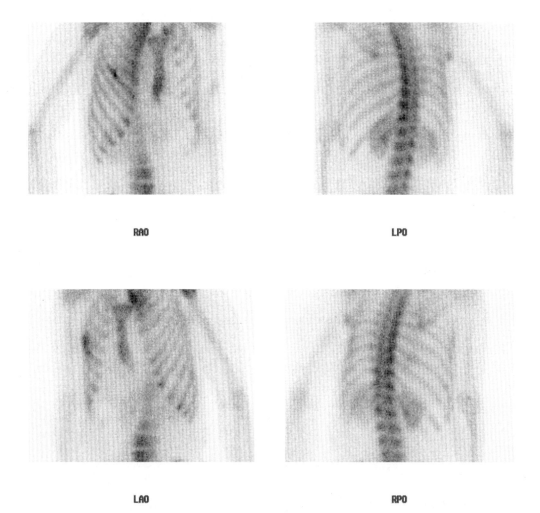

RAO

LPO

LAO

RPO

FIGURE 2. Oblique views of the ribs were obtained to better delineate the pattern of increased rib activity. No long segment involvement is seen to particularly suggest this is a metastatic lesion, but the activity is also less focal than seen in many rib fractures. Multifocal activity involving multiple adjacent ribs is a pattern of activity that would allow one to more confidently diagnose fractures.

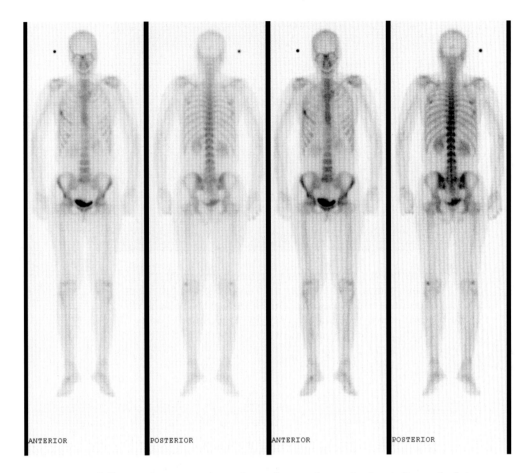

FIGURE 3.   A follow-up bone scan (anterior and posterior projections), 2 months later, shows persistent activity at the same level.

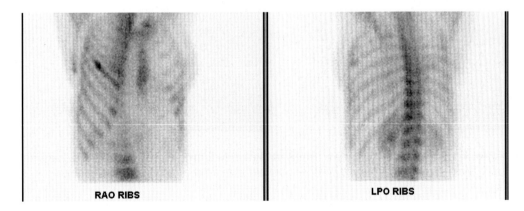

FIGURE 4.   Oblique rib views from this study show the activity to be focal and intense. This pattern of activity is more typical of a fracture.

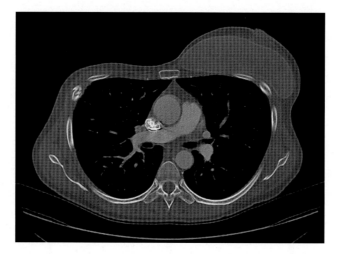

FIGURE 5.   Bone window from a concurrent chest CT scan shows a healing fracture. There is offset of the bone cortices, which may have contributed to the prolonged symptoms and bone scan activity. The patient is post–right mastectomy, and a left breast implant is noted.

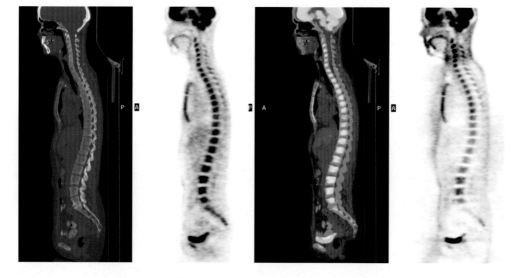

FIGURE 6.   Sagittal PET/CT images (*from left to right:* CT, attenuation-corrected PET, fused PET/CT, non-attenuation-corrected PET) obtained while the patient was undergoing chemotherapy for liver metastases show a uniform increase in marrow activity, new from a prior study. Note the ease of visualizing the sternum on the PET images, which generally is difficult to see. CT images show uniform bone mineral density, without evidence of diffuse osseous metastases.

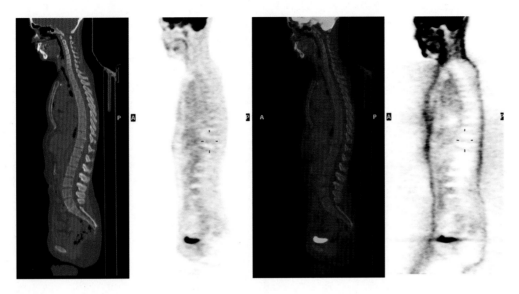

FIGURE 7. Comparable views from a repeat PET/CT, 2 months later, after cessation of chemotherapy, show resolution of the increased PET bone marrow activity. Bone mineral density on CT remains stable and normal.

increased marrow activity is diffuse and uniform. Rarely, this process may be less uniform and more difficult to differentiate from diffuse osseous metastases.

CASE 9

Significance of solitary rib activity on bone scan

A patient with a past history of left breast cancer presented with a complaint of left chest wall discomfort, with no known trauma. Her cancer had been diagnosed 5 years before, as an estrogen receptor–positive, *HER-2/neu* positive tumor, with one involved lymph node. She was treated with four cycles of doxorubicin (Adriamycin) plus cyclophosphamide (Cytoxan) (AC), four cycles of taxane, then tamoxifen for 3 years, followed by exemestane.

Tumor markers were negative. Bone scan showed a solitary focus of increased activity in the left eighth rib posteriorly (Figures 1 and 2). Rib x-rays suggested cortical loss of the corresponding rib. A positron emission tomography (PET)/CT scan showed a single site of modest increased metabolic activity at the same level (Figure 3). The corresponding CT identified an expansile focus at the level in question (Figure 4). This was biopsied under CT guidance, with specimens showing remodeling, with no evidence of malignancy. The patient's pain largely resolved over the next month. Repeat bone scan (Figures 5 and 6), 2 months later (4 months after the prior bone scan) showed the left rib activity to be resolving, but there was new right rib focal activity. The patient had recently fallen, resulting in recurrent left chest wall pain and new, more severe right chest wall pain. Her tumor markers remained normal throughout.

Another bone scan obtained 4 months later showed complete resolution of the original left rib focus, consistent with fracture healing, with persistence of the newer right rib fracture activity (Figures 7 and 8).

TEACHING POINTS

Chest wall pain occurring in a breast cancer patient may herald the development of recurrent or metastatic disease. Chest wall pain could be due to metastatic involvement of a rib, with or without pathologic fracture, or could be due to development of soft tissue recurrent disease, and must be differentiated from benign disease, such as rib fracture. If the symptoms seem likely to be due to a rib fracture (there is a history of trauma or coughing), and tumor markers are negative, bone scan is probably the most cost-effective means of assessing the rib cage. More sensitive to the presence of rib abnormalities than radiographs, the bone scan also provides a whole-body context against which to assess the significance of any identified rib activity.

If bone scan does show a rib focus of activity on the anterior or posterior whole-body views, oblique and lateral views of the thorax are often helpful to better visualize the scintigraphic morphology of the activity. The pattern of activity can be helpful in differentiating malignant involvement of a rib from trauma. Of course, fractures can be

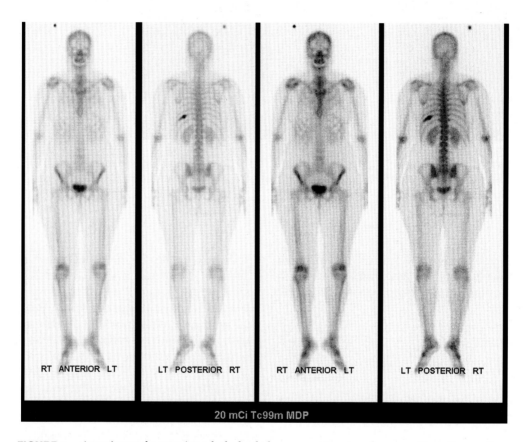

FIGURE 1. Anterior and posterior whole-body bone scan images show a solitary focus of increased activity in a left posterior rib. The most intense activity is focal, with less intense activity of the rib extending laterally. No additional foci of abnormal activity are seen.

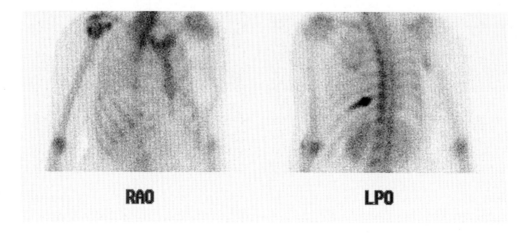

FIGURE 2. Oblique views of the thorax show the same pattern of activity.

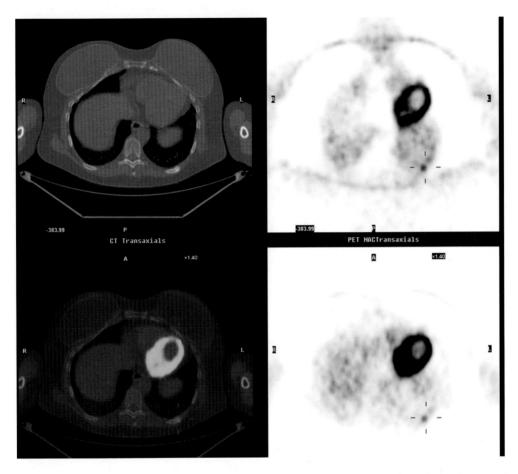

FIGURE 3.   Images from PET/CT (axial projection) show a solitary site of moderate increased metabolic activity at the same level, in a left posterior rib.

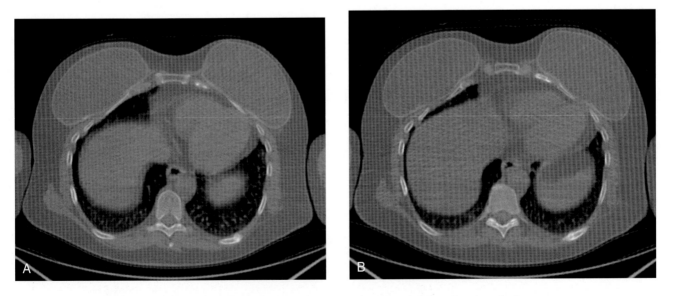

FIGURE 4.   Chest CT images (**A** and **B**) show hypertrophic callus at the site of a fracture, at the level in question on bone scan.

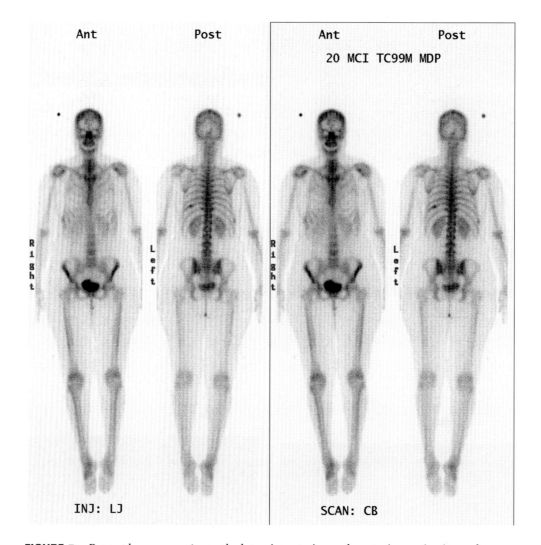

FIGURE 5. Repeat bone scan, 4 months later, in anterior and posterior projections, shows the left lower posterior rib activity to have diminished, consistent with fracture healing. A new focus of increased activity is suggested in a right lower lateral rib.

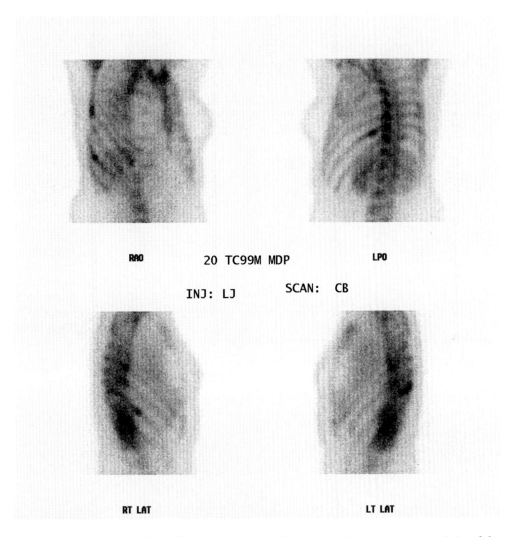

FIGURE 6. Oblique and lateral bone scan views of the thorax show regressing activity of the known left rib fracture and confirm relatively focal activity in a right lower lateral rib, suspected from the whole-body views.

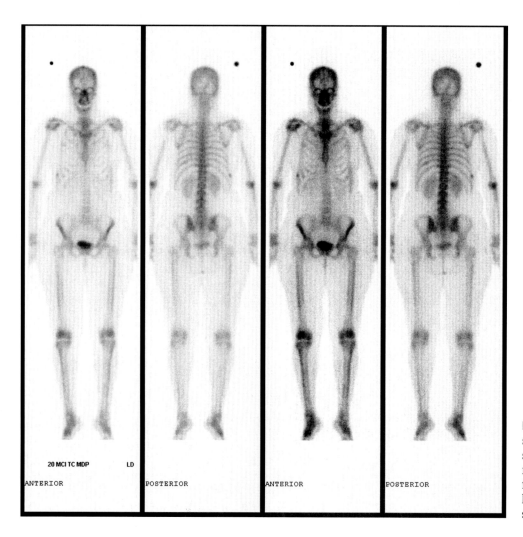

20 MCI TC MDP   LD

ANTERIOR   POSTERIOR   ANTERIOR   POSTERIOR

FIGURE 7. Repeat bone scan, 4 months later, shows complete resolution of the left rib fracture activity. The right lower lateral rib activity is still visualized.

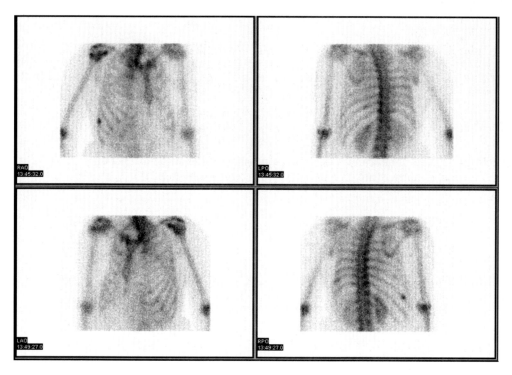

RAO
13:45:32.0

LPO
13:45:32.0

LAO
13:49:27.0

RPO
13:49:27.0

FIGURE 8. Oblique views of the thorax show persistent, very focal right lower lateral rib fracture activity.

pathologic, which adds to the difficulty. Views should be obtained to best visualize the pattern of activity, to determine whether the rib activity is solitary or multiple, and if multiple, whether it is scattered and randomly distributed or involving adjacent ribs. Multifocal involvement of adjacent ribs is a pattern strongly predictive of trauma as the etiology. This must be differentiated from longer segment involvement of adjacent ribs, which could signify chest wall invasion by neoplasia. If the activity is solitary, an assessment of the pattern of activity is helpful: Is the activity focal (punctate), which would favor fracture, or is there a longer segment of involvement, favoring tumor? This case illustrates that differentiation based on pattern of activity is not always possible. Fractures can have activity that is not typically focal.

If the rib activity is focal and rib fracture is suspected based on the pattern or the clinical history, and the patient's tumor markers are negative, the patient could be followed clinically and the bone scan repeated in 4 to 6 months for expected decline or resolution of fracture activity. If the activity or clinical history is not entirely typical, more workup can be considered, as in this case. High-resolution spiral CT images of the level in question will generally yield better and more useful detail of the bone than radiographs, and can be considered as a next step in further imaging. Alternatively, PET/CT can be considered for a more comprehensive whole-body survey for possible metastatic or recurrent disease. As in this case, recent fractures are metabolically active and will be visualized on PET/CT. The greatest utility of PET in such cases is in exclusion of disease elsewhere.

Increased uptake on a bone scan at the site of a fracture may persist for months, depending on the location. For ^{18}F fluorodeoxyglucose (FDG) PET, uptake has been reported in benign fractures for up to 8 weeks. In a retrospective study reported by Zhuang and colleagues, only 1 of 23 patients with a traumatic or surgical fracture showed FDG activity at the fracture site beyond 3 months. In this series, the one patient showing persistent FDG activity had complicating osteomyelitis.

SUGGESTED READINGS

Shon IH, Fogleman I. F-18 FDG positron emission tomography and benign fractures. *Clin Nucl Med* 2003; 28(3):171–175.

Zhuang H, Sam JW, Chacko TK, et al. Rapid normalization of osseous FDG uptake following traumatic or surgical fractures. *Eur J Nucl Med Mol Imaging* 2003; 30(8):1096–1103.

CASE 10

Solitary sclerotic rib metastasis (positive on bone scan, negative on PET)

A 57-year-old woman who had recently undergone bilateral mastectomies for newly diagnosed bilateral breast cancers was referred for medical oncology evaluation and therapy. Her breast cancer had been diagnosed the preceding month, when she presented with a palpable left-sided lump. The patient had never undergone mammographic screening.

On the left, her tumor stage was IIIA, T2N2, 3.2-cm infiltrating ductal carcinoma (IDC), with angiolymphatic invasion and negative margins. Eight of 16 lymph nodes were involved. The tumor was estrogen receptor and progesterone receptor positive and *HER-2/neu* positive.

Her right breast cancer was a T2NxM0, 2-cm IDC, estrogen receptor and progesterone receptor positive, and *HER-2/neu* negative, with negative margins and angiolymphatic invasion. One sentinel lymph node was involved.

The patient was staged with enhanced body CT scans, PET/CT, and bone scan. These evaluations showed a highly suspicious left anterior fourth rib focus of increased activity on bone scan (Figure 1), with subtle corresponding sclerosis at the same level on CT (Figure 2). There was no corresponding abnormal activity on PET. CT-guided biopsy showed metastatic adenocarcinoma, consistent with breast primary.

Because this seemed to be the only site of metastatic disease, aggressive chemotherapy was given, consisting of four cycles of doxorubicin (Adriamycin) and cyclophosphamide (Cytoxan) [AC], followed by 3 months of trastuzumab (Herceptin) and paclitaxel (Taxol). She then received Herceptin every 3 weeks for the remainder of the year, as well as anastrozole (Arimidex) and zoledronic acid (Zometa) every 6 months.

TEACHING POINTS

Systemic screening of this patient was indicated because of her high-risk tumor status (*HER-2/neu* positive and eight lymph nodes involved). The combination of studies obtained in this case to

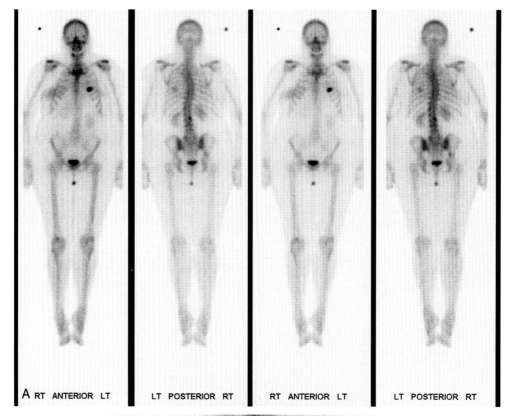

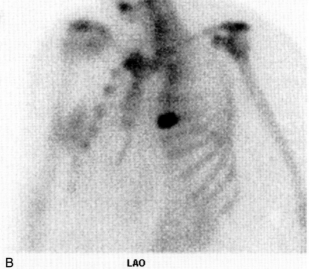

FIGURE 1. Whole-body bone scans (**A,** anterior and posterior whole-body views; **B,** oblique of the ribs) show a focus of intensely increased activity at the anterior left fourth rib level. Although the location brings trauma to mind, the activity is larger and less focal than generally seen with a rib fracture, especially when viewed in the left anterior oblique projection. The rib activity "shines through" on the posterior views. Increased chest wall soft tissue activity is seen, right greater than left, from recent mastectomies. Scoliosis is seen of the spine, but no other highly suspicious findings are noted (activity at L2 is indeterminate and seemed to correspond with degenerative spondylytic change on CT).

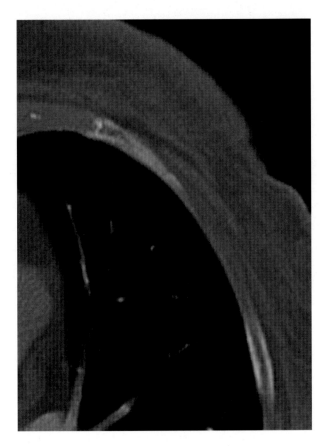

FIGURE 2. Detail views of the left anterior fourth rib from body CT scan show subtle blastic alteration of bone mineral density at the level in question, without expansion or fracture.

systemically stage this patient (PET/CT, enhanced body CT, and bone scan) is quite comprehensive, and arguably a very cost-effective combination. Even more cost-effective would be for the CT component of the PET/CT to be contrast enhanced, thereby eliminating one of the two CT scans obtained in the evaluation illustrated in this case. There are advantages and disadvantages to this approach.

This case illustrates well the complementary roles PET and bone scan play in the evaluation of breast cancer patients for osseous metastases. PET is a highly sensitive whole-body modality for the evaluation of soft tissue and visceral and lytic osseous metastases, but has known limitations in the demonstration of osteoblastic bone lesions. Conversely, bone scintigraphy is most reliable for identification of blastic bone metastases and may not show purely lytic lesions. As illustrated by this case, PET can miss osteosclerotic bone metastases that bone scan will find.

CASE 11

Assessing activity of sclerotic bone metastases

A 41-year-old woman with known sclerotic bone metastases taking letrozole (Femara) and monthly zoledronic acid (Zometa) developed generalized aches and pains, prompting imaging re-evaluation with bone scan, positron emission tomography (PET)/CT, and spine MRI. The patient had known sclerotic bone metastases for 3 years, which were inactive on prior bone and PET scans. Her initial diagnosis of breast cancer had been 7 years before at age 34, with T2N1M0, 3-cm, well-differentiated infiltrating ductal carcinoma. One of 11 lymph nodes was positive. She underwent right mastectomy with implant reconstruction, chemotherapy with four cycles each of doxorubicin (Adriamycin) plus cyclophosphamide (Cytoxan) (AC) and paclitaxel (Taxol), as well as chest wall and supraclavicular radiation.

When the development of symptoms prompted reimaging, a bone scan was obtained initially and showed new activity at T9 (Figures 1, 2, and 3), corresponding to a sclerotic metastasis known from CT (Figure 4). PET scan showed no associated hypermetabolism, and the size of the lesion on CT was unchanged. Spine MRI showed signal intensity characteristics of sclerosis at this and other levels. Subtle partial enhancement was noted of the T9 lesion, correlating with the new bone scan activity (Figure 5).

TEACHING POINTS

Assessing the activity of sclerotic metastases is difficult. Generally, radiography and CT are not particularly helpful. Only in the rare instance of development of a new superimposed soft tissue mass or lytic components might x-ray or CT suggest clear progression or activation of a blastic metastasis. Assessing degrees of sclerosis of blastic metastases, either qualitatively or quantitatively, is problematic. PET and PET/CT also are frequently limited in their utility for assessment of the activity of sclerotic bone metastases, with many such lesions not associated with increased activity on PET. Development of new activity on PET associated with a sclerotic bone metastasis is helpful

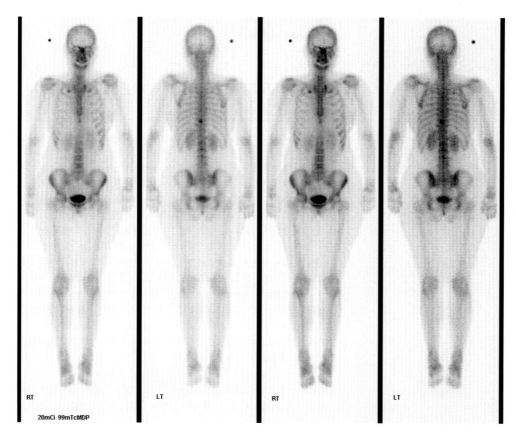

RT   LT   RT   LT

20mCi 99mTcMDP

FIGURE 1. Whole-body bone scan in anterior and posterior projections (right side marked at skull level) shows a new focus of increased activity at the T9 vertebral level. Based on these views, it is difficult to say whether the activity is in a spinous process or the vertebral centrum.

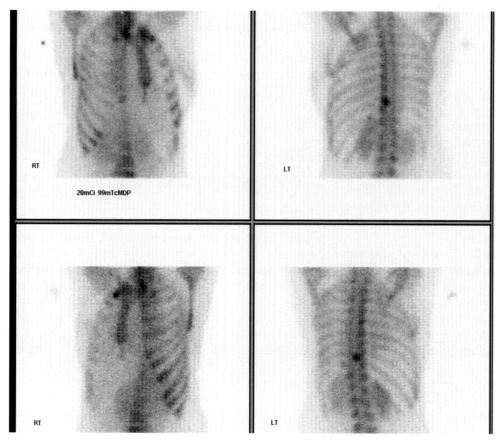

RT   LT

20mCi 99mTcMDP

RT   LT

FIGURE 2. Oblique views of the thoracic spine from the same bone scan localize the activity to the vertebral body.

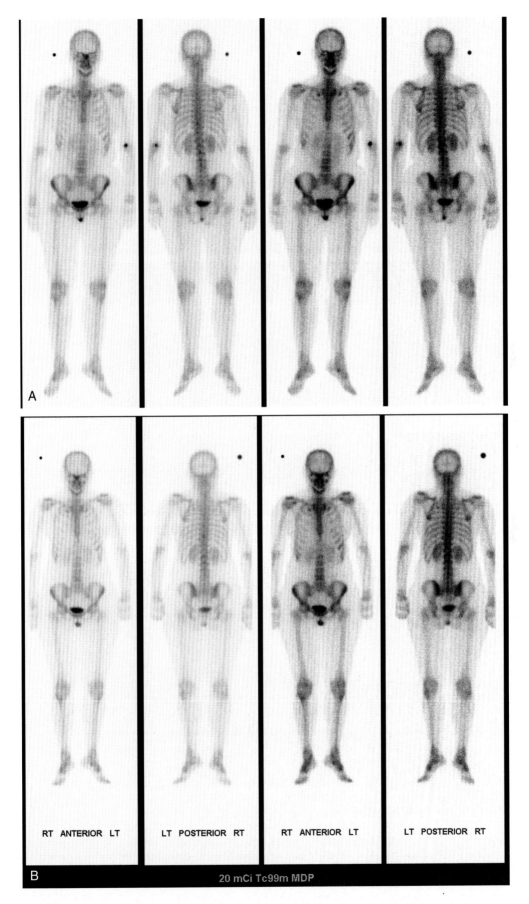

FIGURE 3.   Comparison whole-body bone scans for correlation, obtained 1 year (**A**) and 6 months (**B**) before. **A,** No abnormality is seen in the spine. **B,** No definite abnormality is seen. In retrospect, there may be very subtle change at the T9 level.

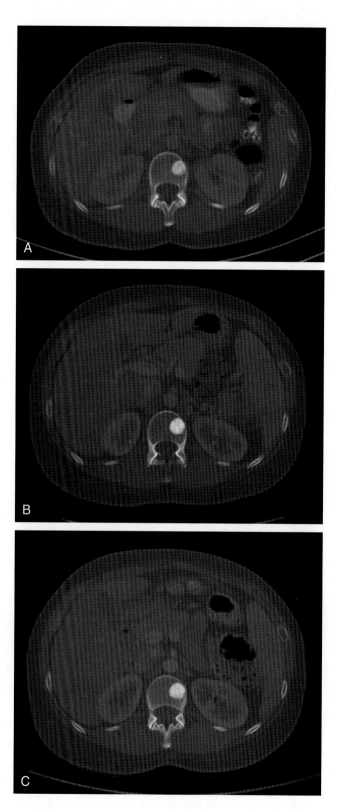

FIGURE 4. CT images for correlation (bone windows) from 3 years before (**A**), 1 year before (**B**), and concurrent with the bone scan in Figure 1 (**C**), show relatively stable findings of a sclerotic metastasis in the left side of the T9 vertebral body. No change in size is seen over this series of examinations. The lesion appears progressively more sclerotic, but the significance of this is uncertain.

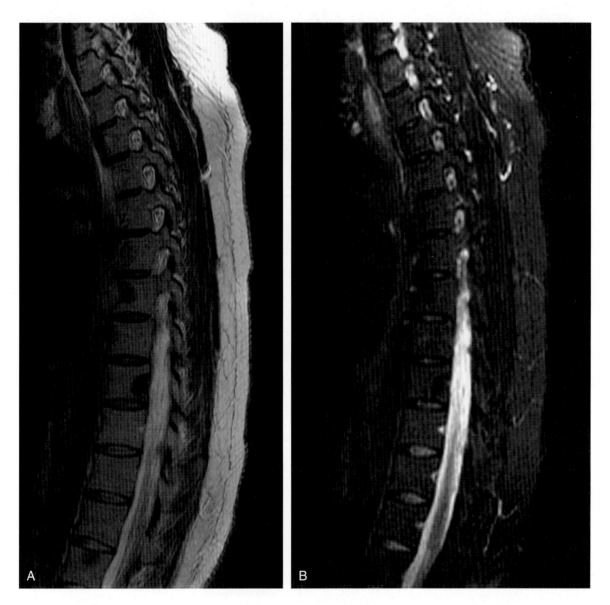

FIGURE 5.   Sagittal thoracic spine MRIs show foci of hypointensity on all sequences at T7, T9, and L1 (partially visualized). These signal intensity characteristics are consistent with sclerosis. Note subtle enhancement of the posteroinferior portion of the T9 lesion on **D**. This same component shows subtle higher signal on STIR than the rest of the sclerotic lesion. **A,** T2-weighted turbo spin echo (TSE). **B,** STIR.

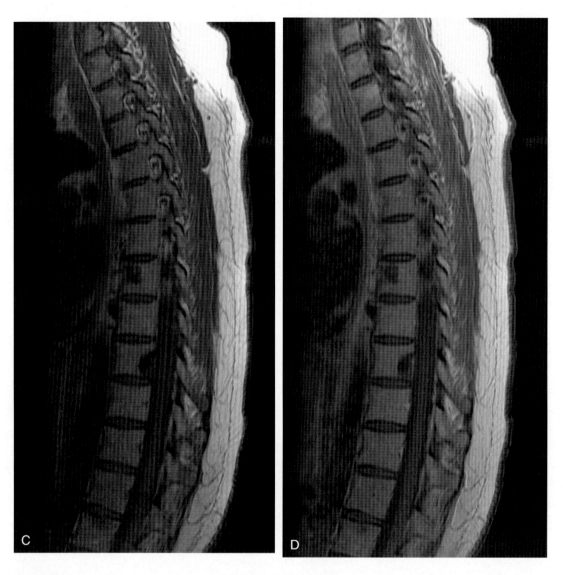

FIGURE 5, cont'd   C, T1-weighted image. **D,** Gadolinium-enhanced, T1-weighted image.

in suggesting disease reactivation (e.g., see Case 1 in Chapter 12). However, as this case illustrates, bone scan is very sensitive to changes in sclerotic metastases and may be the first or only modality to suggest disease reactivation. Typical imaging findings of sclerotic metastases are demonstrated by this case: focal increased activity on bone scan, increased bone density on CT, and hypointensity on all sequences on MRI. It is interesting to note the subtle enhancement seen on MRI at the level of the newly bone scan active T9 blastic metastasis. Other sclerotic bone metastases seen on the spine MRI of this patient did not show any enhancement and were scintigraphically inactive.

CASE 12

Diffuse bone metastases (superscan)

A 69-year-old woman with known extensive bony metastatic disease was evaluated with a bone scan (Figures 1, 2, and 3). Her bony metastatic disease had been diagnosed 6 years earlier, and she had undergone palliative radiation to the pelvis and

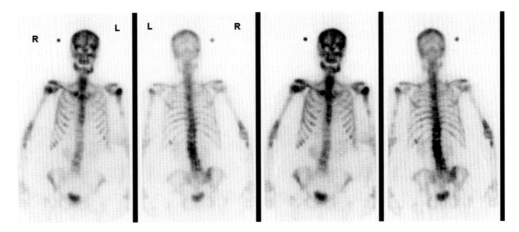

FIGURE 1. A diffuse, heterogeneous pattern of increased bone scan uptake is seen, with only faint renal activity. The pelvis and hips had been previously radiated, and a corresponding relative decrease in bone scan activity is seen. Activity in the sternum, spine, and skull is increased diffusely, with more patchy foci of activity in the humeri.

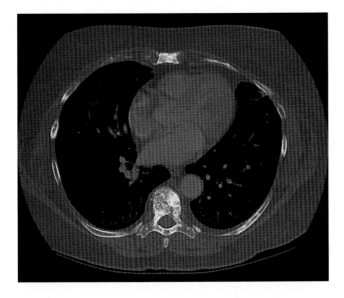

FIGURE 2. Correlation with a chest CT bone window shows patchy sclerotic bone metastases, seen here in the sternum, right lateral rib, left posterior rib, and vertebral body and posterior elements.

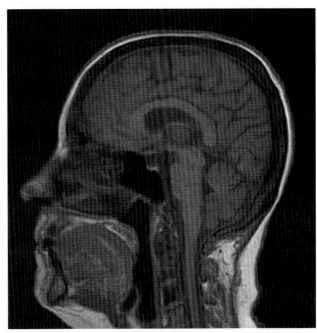

FIGURE 3. Correlation with a sagittal, T1-weighted brain MRI shows diffuse hypointensity of bone marrow signal throughout the calvarial and upper cervical spine, correlating with the CT findings of diffuse blastic metastases and the diffuse increased skull uptake on bone scan.

hips, as well as systemic treatment with samarium. Her original diagnosis of left breast cancer was 18 years earlier. This was a T1cN1M0, left, 1.9-cm infiltrating ductal carcinoma (IDC) with 1 of 20 lymph nodes involved. She had been treated with mastectomy and with breast and regional lymphatic radiation.

TEACHING POINTS

The term *superscan* can be applied to bone scans with markedly increased skeletal uptake, resulting in less tracer available for renal excretion and visualization. Conditions resulting in a high bone-to–soft tissue activity ratio, with faint or little renal activity, include extensive bone metastases and metabolic bone diseases. The primary tumors most likely to produce the superscan pattern are carcinomas of the breast, lung, and prostate. Metabolic bone diseases that can produce a similar superscan pattern include renal osteodystrophy, osteomalacia, hyperparathyroidism, myelofibrosis, and systemic mastocytosis. As in this example, the diagnosis of diffuse osseous metastases is suggested by inhomogeneity of the activity, and correlation with x-rays, CT, or MRI often enables ready confirmation.

CASE 13

Radiation therapy effects on bone

A 38-year-old woman with breast cancer metastatic to bone and bone marrow was followed with tumor markers, bone scans, CT, and positron emission tomography (PET). Her breast cancer had been diagnosed 4 years before when she presented with a palpable left breast lump, and underwent mastectomy. It was an estrogen receptor–positive, *HER-2/neu* negative, T3, infiltrating lobular carcinoma, with 12 involved axillary lymph nodes (largest, 2 cm, with extracapsular extension). At the time of initial diagnosis, the patient had low-grade fevers and myalgias. A bone scan suggested possible calvarial metastases. These were not confirmed on brain MRI, but the upper cervical spine marrow signal appeared abnormal. Cervical spine MRI showed diffusely abnormal marrow signal, suggesting diffuse metastases. A bone marrow biopsy showed more than 90% marrow space replacement with metastatic carcinoma.

The patient was treated with six cycles of doxorubicin (Adriamycin) and cyclophosphamide (Cytoxan) chemotherapy, and placed on tamoxifen. The following year, she underwent oophorectomy.

Three years after diagnosis of stage IV breast cancer, the patient developed low back pain, mild right leg weakness, and right lateral thigh numbness. Her tumor markers were rising. Lumbar spine MRI showed progressive metastatic disease, with new right L4-L5 epidural and neural foraminal involvement. Bone scan showed new L4 activity. Radiation therapy was given, including L3 to S2, and dexamethasone (Decadron) was started. The patient's symptoms resolved completely.

A bone scan obtained 14 months after radiation therapy showed photopenia in the radiated lumbosacral spine. New metastatic foci of increased activity were noted at the inferior tip of the right scapula and at the left proximal femoral level (Figure 1). The patient did have progressive left hip aching. Radiographs did not show a corresponding abnormality, but CT bone windows showed a corresponding sclerotic focus (Figure 2).

Radiation therapy was given to the left proximal femur, with complete relief of her pain. While on radiation therapy, the patient's regimen was changed from letrozole (Femara) to fulvestrant (Faslodex), while continuing on monthly zoledronic acid (Zometa). A repeat bone scan, 2 months after completion of hip radiation, showed resolution of the hip activity (Figure 3). Lumbar spine MRI was obtained for correlation and showed radiation therapy effects (Figure 4). Concurrent PET/CT and enhanced body CT scans, obtained to assess increased aches, rising tumor markers, and the response to Faslodex, showed new liver metastases (see Case 5 in Chapter 9 for liver imaging findings). Faslodex was discontinued and chemotherapy started with docetaxel (Taxotere) and capecitabine (Xeloda).

TEACHING POINTS

This patient had extensive bone marrow involvement detected at initial diagnosis. Bone imaging modalities, namely radiography, CT, MRI, and bone scan, have different capabilities in terms of their ability to demonstrate involvement of bone marrow compared with trabecular bone or cortical bone. This patient has diffuse, essentially confluent, spine metastases known from MRI. In this case, bone scan underestimates the full extent of her osseous metastatic tumor burden. Why?

Bone metastases are most commonly hematogenous. The vertebral venous plexus (Batson's plexus) is thought to be an important route for hematogenous dissemination of tumor cells to the spine, the most common site of osseous metastases. Within the medullary space of bones is the lacy reticular network of trabecular bone, with marrow cells and fat within the interstices. Early bone metastases are probably to marrow through hematogenous dissemination. With growth, destruction of trabecular bone results. Eventually, a lesion of

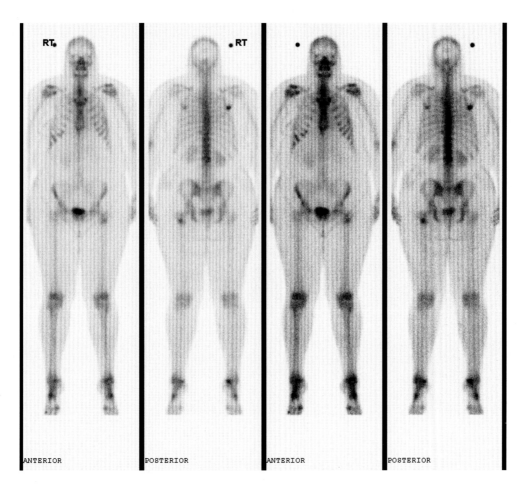

FIGURE 1. Bone scan, 14 months after L3-S2 radiation therapy for epidural disease, shows photopenia of the radiated lumbosacral spine, sharply demarcated from untreated levels above. Two new, presumably metastatic, sites of activity were seen compared with a prior study: right inferior scapular tip and the left proximal femur. Left anterior ribs are better seen than those on the right, owing to prior left mastectomy and the accompanying decreased soft tissue attenuation.

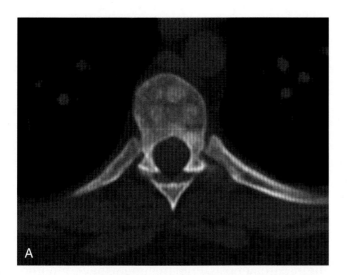

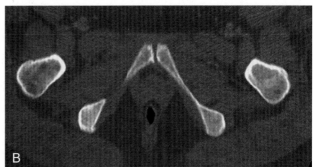

FIGURE 2. Bone window from body CT scans, for correlation with the concurrent bone scan. **A,** Lower thoracic spine: multiple sclerotic foci are seen on this single slice, belying the uniform activity of the thoracic spine on bone scintigraphy. **B,** Pelvis and hips: a mildly blastic focus is noted of the left proximal femur, corresponding to the bone scan.

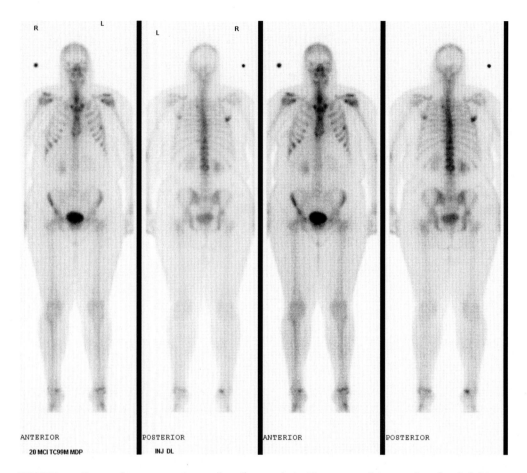

FIGURE 3. Repeat bone scan, 5 months after study in Figure 1 and 2 months after left hip radiation, shows resolution of the left proximal femoral uptake. The right inferior scapular focus is similar, but a new left anterolateral fifth rib focus of activity is seen.

sufficient size will involve and destroy the denser cortical bone. Cortical bone is so much denser than trabecular bone that even extensive trabecular destruction without cortical involvement is generally not visualized on radiographs, CT, and bone scan. With sufficient cortical bone destruction, abnormalities may then be identified by these modalities. It has been estimated that at least 50% of cortical bone destruction must occur before a lesion can be seen on radiographs. CT is far more sensitive to cortical bone involvement than radiography, but less reliable in depicting medullary space involvement than MRI. Bone scintigraphy is 50% to 80% more sensitive than radiographs in identifying bone metastases but is not as sensitive as MRI. MRI is the most sensitive imaging modality for detection of bone metastases.

Taoka and colleagues looked at the factors leading to different detection rates of vertebral metastases between MRI and bone scans and found

cortical involvement to be the key factor. They studied 74 patients with widely disseminated metastases. Vertebral body lesions found on MRI were analyzed for size and cortical involvement, as well as visibility on planar bone scans. Larger lesions and those involving cortex were more likely to be seen on scintigraphy. Intramedullary lesions found on MRI with no cortical involvement were not seen on bone scan, regardless of size.

Several explanations can be considered to explain the discrepancy between MRI and bone scan in this case example. One explanation is the dominance of marrow involvement as a feature of this patient's bone disease. The marrow involvement was essentially confluent in the spine from the initial diagnosis. Prior treatment may be another contributing factor. This patient had previously received both chemotherapy and hormonal therapy, and correlation with CT shows multiple sclerotic medullary foci in the thoracic spine, which appears

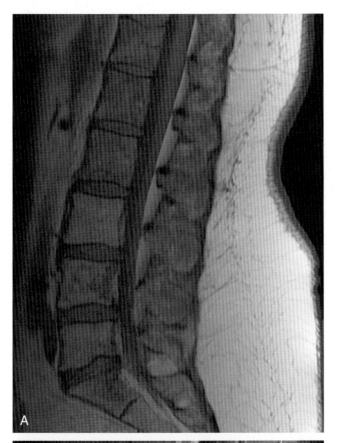

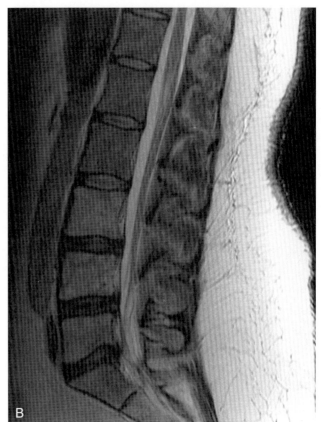

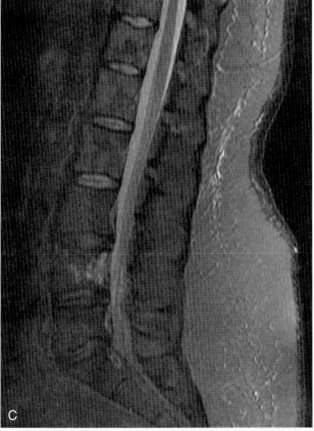

FIGURE 4. Sagittal lumbar spine MRIs, for correlation with bone scan, 10 months after lumbosacral radiation for epidural disease at L4. **A,** T1-weighted image. **B,** T2-weighted image. **C,** STIR. *(continued)*

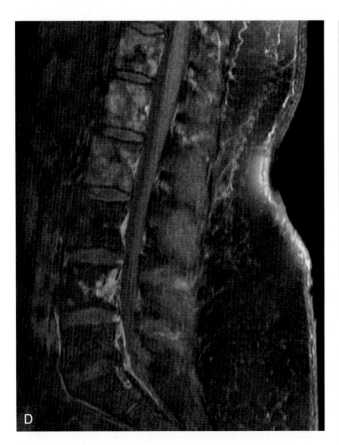

FIGURE 4, cont'd   D, Fat-saturated, enhanced, T1-weighted image. Diffuse marrow signal abnormalities and enhancement are seen at upper lumbar levels, with L3 and below generally better in appearance, with the exception of L4, where the most severe disease had been previously. There is conversion to fatty marrow at the radiated levels, L3 to the upper sacrum, with incomplete response at L4. Abnormal epidural enhancement is seen posterior to L5.

uniformly active on bone scan. Confluence may be another partial explanation—the uniform appearance of the thoracic spine activity on bone scan being a manifestation of superscan-like diffuse increased activity of extensive disease. We are able to appreciate it by its contrast with the radiation-induced photopenia in the lumbar spine.

This case does demonstrate that bone scans can still be useful to assess newly symptomatic areas and to gauge response to treatments, even if the full extent of bone metastases is not well represented.

SUGGESTED READING

Taoka T, Mayr NA, Lee HJ, et al. Factors influencing visualization of vertebral metastases on MR imaging versus bone scintigraphy. *AJR Am J Roentgenol* 2001; 176:1525–1530.

CASE 14

Extensive bone metastases; ^{18}F bone scan

A 93-year-old woman with known breast cancer metastases to bone (Figures 1 and 2) was evaluated with positron emission tomography (PET)/CT for rising carcinoembryonic antigen (CEA) level. She had been diagnosed with left breast cancer 3 years before, and had been treated with breast conservation surgery and radiation therapy. She had been taking tamoxifen, and was now taking anastrozole (Arimidex). She had no symptoms of bone pain.

PET/CT showed diffuse bone sclerosis, with no associated fluorodeoxyglucose (FDG) avidity (Figure 3). Mildly hypermetabolic mediastinal lymph nodes were seen. ^{18}F sodium fluoride bone scan showed intense uptake throughout the skeleton, which showed diffuse patchy sclerosis on CT (Figure 4).

TEACHING POINTS

This patient had progressive sclerotic bone metastases. Visually, these are easier to detect on the earlier bone scan, when they are patchy in distribution, than on the later superscan, when the metastases are more confluent. The faintness of the renal activity is a clue on the second bone scan to the diffuse extent of bone metastases. Comparing with the prior bone scan is a safeguard to correct interpretation of the later bone scan. The CT portion of the PET/CT scan obtained a few months later confirms that there is extensive blastic change of bone. The apparently discrepant bone uptake between FDG PET and bone scan is not surprising, with several potential explanations. Multiple studies have suggested that FDG PET is not as sensitive to detection of sclerotic metastases as lytic metastases. The converse is true of bone scans, in which purely lytic metastases may elude detection. In breast cancer, bone metastases can be purely lytic and predominantly blastic, can initially be lytic but respond to treatment by sclerosis, or can be intrinsically mixed, with elements of both lysis and sclerosis. This variety of possible manifestations suggests that for comprehensive imaging detection of breast cancer bone metastases, PET and bone scan are complementary.

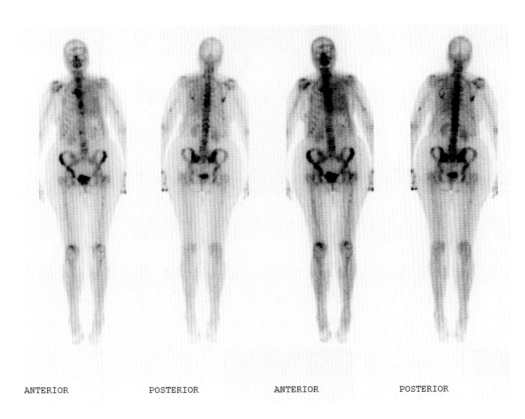

ANTERIOR   POSTERIOR   ANTERIOR   POSTERIOR

FIGURE 1. Abnormal whole-body bone scan shows multiple patchy regions of abnormal increased bone uptake in the spine, pelvis, sternum, and extremities (left mid-humerus, bilateral proximal femoral shafts).

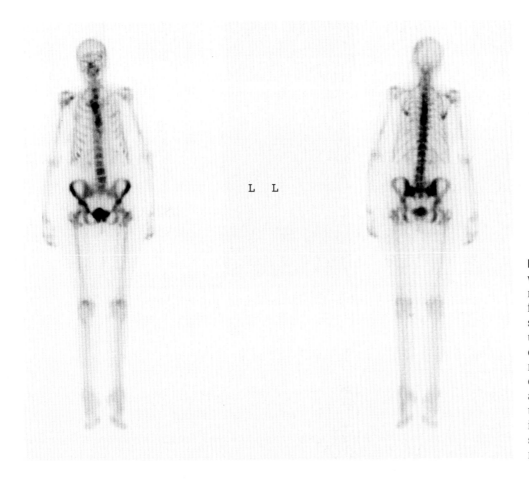

L L

FIGURE 2. Repeat whole-body bone scan, 6 months later, shows very faint renal activity. The spine and posterior pelvic uptake appears more diffuse and deceptively more uniform. Patchiness of the activity can still be appreciated, best seen in the sternum. The pattern is in the spectrum of a superscan of diffuse metastases.

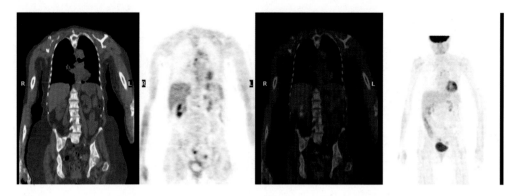

FIGURE 3.   Coronal PET/CT images, obtained to evaluate a rising CEA, show diffuse patchy sclerosis of bones, without accompanying FDG avidity. Small nodal foci of mild increased uptake are seen in the mediastinum.

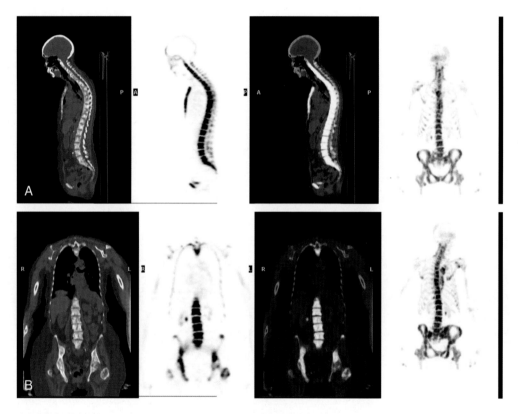

FIGURE 4. ^{18}F NaF bone scan images (**A,** sagittal; **B,** coronal; **C,** axial, through the pelvis) show diffuse patchy sclerosis of visualized bones, and intense diffuse accompanying ^{18}F bone uptake.

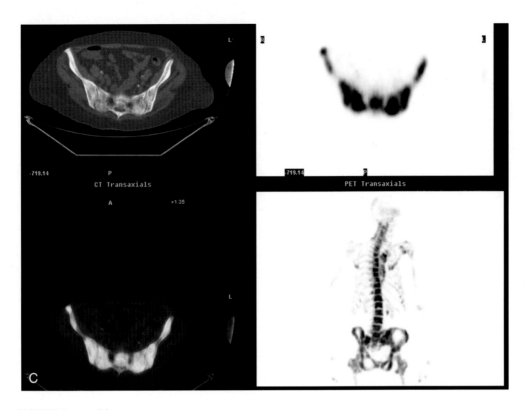

FIGURE 4, cont'd

Another possible explanation for inactivity of bone metastases on FDG PET is that the patient is being treated on an ongoing basis with Arimidex.

[18]F–sodium fluoride (NaF) PET is an alternative bone scanning modality. ^{18}F–sodium fluoride was first used as a bone scan agent in the 1960s with gamma cameras. Cyclotron production requirements for ^{18}F, the difficulty of gamma camera imaging of high-energy agents, and the development of ^{99m}Tc-polyphosphonate alternatives contributed to the decline of ^{18}F-NaF as a bone scanning agent, until re-emergence in the PET era. ^{18}F-NaF PET bone scans offer a number of advantages over bone scanning with ^{99m}Tc-polyphosphonates and gamma cameras. In particular, bone uptake of ^{18}F-NaF is 2 times greater than ^{99m}Tc-polyphosphonates, and blood clearance is faster, resulting in superior target-to-background ratio. As with conventional bone scan agents, uptake within metastases reflects regional blood flow and osteoblastic activity, with areas of increased bone turnover and remodeling seen as areas of increased uptake. The spatial resolution of ^{18}F-NaF PET is higher, and attenuation correction is superior. Osteolytic metastases, which may be overlooked on routine planar bone scans, may be depicted on ^{18}F-NaF PET scans as photopenic regions with a surrounding rim of increased activity, a pattern favoring neoplasia. Imaging can commence at 1 hour, an advantage over the 2- to 4-hour wait needed for routine bone scanning. Disadvantages are increased cost of the radiopharmaceutical and prolonged PET table time (in many practices, PET table time is at more of a premium than gamma camera time) of an hour or more.

Schirrmeister and colleagues prospectively evaluated the performance of ^{18}F-NaF PET compared with conventional planar bone scan in 34 breast cancer patients. ^{18}F-NaF PET outperformed bone scan on both a per-lesion and per-patient basis, detecting 64 metastases in 17 patients compared with 29 metastases in 11 patients with bone scan. Clinical management was changed in 4 patients (12%) and influenced in 6 patients (18%). In addition to a 2-times-higher sensitivity, there was a 2-times increase in detection of benign bone lesions, which are better visualized and anatomically localized because of the higher resolution and tomographic technique.

SUGGESTED READINGS

Even-Sapir E. Imaging of malignant bone involvement by morphologic, scintigraphic, and hybrid modalities. *J Nucl Med* 2005; 46(8):1356–1367.

Hall NC, Minerich SM. Focus: 18-F NaF for bone imaging. *White paper

Schirrmeister H, Guhlmann A, Kotzerke J, et al. Early detection and accurate description of extent of metastatic bone disease in breast cancer with fluoride ion and positron emission tomography. *J Clin Oncol* 1999; 17:2381–2389.

CHAPTER 9

Liver Metastases

LIVER IMAGING IN BREAST CANCER PATIENTS

The liver is the third most common site of breast carcinoma metastases, after bone and lung. Involvement of the liver at initial diagnosis is uncommon, with estimates ranging from 3% to 8%. However, autopsy series show liver involvement in up to 61% of breast cancer patients. Because two thirds of metastatic breast cancer (stage IV) patients will have involvement of the liver at some point in the course of their disease, it is a topic of considerable importance.

The yield of routine imaging for liver metastases in asymptomatic, early-stage breast cancer patients is very low. Accordingly, imaging evaluation of the liver for metastases is generally reserved for breast cancer patients with clinical indications, such as multiple hepatic enzyme elevations, elevation of serum alkaline phosphatase, hepatomegaly on physical examination, or symptoms such as right upper quadrant pain, jaundice, or weight loss. In addition, the use of imaging for systemic staging to exclude metastatic disease is indicated at initial diagnosis of locally advanced, high-risk breast carcinomas. The presence of hepatic metastases is an important prognostic factor, and liver imaging in breast cancer patients has generally focused on the presence or absence of metastases, rather than on planning for surgery or local ablative therapies. This is because few patients with breast liver metastases have solitary or localized liver disease that is suitable for ablative or surgical therapy. Liver metastases can respond well to systemic therapy, and decreased tumor burden correlates with improved survival. Imaging of the liver assumes an important role in the initial identification of liver metastases and in the follow-up and treatment assessment of patients with confirmed metastases.

MODALITY CHOICES AND TECHNIQUES

Options for imaging the liver include ultrasound, CT, MRI, and positron emission tomography (PET) or PET/CT.

Ultrasound

Of the available liver imaging modalities, ultrasound is overall the least widely applicable, in part because it is the most operator dependent. Its efficacy is also highly dependent on patient factors, including ability to suspend respiration, body habitus, and the presence of fatty infiltration, which hampers sonographic beam penetration and focal lesion detection. It is probably best reserved for select circumstances, such as pregnant patients, and in problem solving of difficult to characterize liver lesions identified on other modalities (e.g., CT). However, in this application, ultrasound is limited in utility for characterizing very small liver lesions (<0.5 cm).

Computed Tomography

CT is the most widely utilized modality for the detection and evaluation of breast cancer liver metastases, owing to its ready availability, speed, and lack of operator dependence. Disadvantages of CT include the necessity for intravenous contrast enhancement, with attendant risks for contrast reactions, allergies, and nephrotoxicity, as well as the ionizing radiation dose. Radiation exposure is becoming an increasing public health concern, particularly with multidetector CT enabling rapid, routine multiphasic imaging. Many cancer patients will require multiple CT scans over the course of their disease treatment, so prudence needs to be used when considering protocols for the imaging of these patients.

Options for CT imaging protocols for routine liver imaging of breast cancer patients include the following:

1. Triple-phase technique (noncontrast, followed by enhanced CT during hepatic arterial [HA] and portal venous [PV] phases of enhancement)
2. Dual-phase enhanced technique during HA and PV phases of enhancement
3. Without and with contrast enhancement (generally during the PV phase)
4. Enhanced (PV phase) alone

Generally, most metastases (any primary) are hypovascular and are best depicted on PV phase CT. Metastases that are considered hypervascular include renal cell carcinoma, carcinoid, neuroendocrine tumors, thyroid carcinoma, and melanoma and have been shown to be better seen on HA phase imaging. Breast carcinoma hepatic metastases can be hypervascular, but these represent a small minority of breast cancer liver metastases.

Triple-phase technique is desirable at initial imaging (referral for staging or clinical suspicion of liver metastases) to accurately characterize any lesions, benign or malignant, which may be encountered. However, follow-up of patients with known liver metastases with PV phase enhanced CT alone is generally sufficient and will avoid unnecessary radiation exposure. Support for this approach comes from work by Frederick and colleagues, who looked retrospectively at a series of 84 consecutive triple-phase CT scans in 80 women who were known or suspected to have breast cancer liver metastases.[1] They evaluated each phase independently for focal liver lesions and found that the PV phase outperformed noncontrast and HA phases for lesion detection and identified more malignant lesions than the other phases. Importantly, no CT interpretation was converted from negative to positive for the presence of liver lesions based on the addition of either noncontrast or HA phase images. The authors noted that noncontrast and HA phase imaging added additional information in some cases, but found it difficult to justify their routine use when the clinical question was the presence or absence of metastatic disease.

The same group subsequently published a larger, prospective study of liver metastases detection in 300 consecutive triple-phase helical CT examinations in breast cancer patients.[2] PV phase images were reviewed alone for the number and size of focal liver lesions. PV images were then reviewed in conjunction with noncontrast images, and again in conjunction with HA phase images. Little improvement in sensitivity for lesion detection was noted when comparing PV phase alone with PV phase in conjunction with noncontrast imaging (97% to 100%) or HA phase (96% to 98%), suggesting little additional benefit was derived from the addition of noncontrast or HA phases. Two to 4% of lesions were seen on HA phase imaging only. These represented either false-positive cases or were seen in conjunction with other metastases on the PV phase. The authors concluded that routine triple-phase imaging of breast cancer patients in whom liver metastases were suspected was not warranted, except at the time of initial examination when triple-phase technique is useful for characterizing focal lesions (e.g., cysts, hemangiomas, focal nodular hyperplasia) that may be encountered.

Magnetic Resonance Imaging

MRI is an excellent alternative for imaging of the liver, for initial evaluation for suspected metastases, characterization of lesions identified on other modalities, and follow-up of patients with known liver metastases. Advantages of MRI as a liver imaging modality include high intrinsic soft tissue contrast, higher sensitivity to contrast enhancement, lack of ionizing radiation, and better safety profiles of the gadolinium chelate contrast agents used in MRI compared with iodinated CT contrast agents. Reactions and allergies to gadolinium chelates are rare, and at standard doses, nephrotoxicity is generally not an issue.

Optimal liver imaging with MRI is performed on high-field strength magnets of 1 Tesla or greater, using phased array coils (for better signal-to-noise ratio than with body coil imaging), with breath-hold technique to minimize patient motion. Pulse sequences include T1-weighted gradient echo sequences (in and out of phase), fluid-sensitive sequences (short tau inversion recovery [STIR] and T2-weighted), and multiphasic fat-saturated, contrast-enhanced, T1-weighted sequences (either two- or three-dimensional gradient echo). With breath-hold technique, a complete evaluation of the liver, with and without contrast enhancement, including multiphasic dynamic enhanced technique, can be completed in 30 minutes.

Breath-hold, fat-saturated, gradient echo volumetric sequences can image the entire liver in thin slices (three-dimensional) in a reasonable breath hold, and can be repeated before and after contrast enhancement to obtain a dynamic assessment of the contrast enhancement pattern of any lesions that are identified. The sequence can be run repetitively to coincide with HA dominant, PV phase, and hepatic venous or interstitial phases of enhancement. The contrast agents are extracellular gadolinium chelates, which shorten T1 relaxation time, and are analogous in distribution to iodinated contrast agents used for enhancement in CT.

The HA dominant phase occurs 15 to 30 seconds after the bolus injection of contrast. During this phase, hypervascular lesions (lesions that enhance more than the liver parenchyma) are more readily visualized against a background of the minimally enhanced liver parenchyma. The hepatic arteries should be brilliantly enhanced during this phase, and the main portal veins show early enhancement as well, but the hepatic veins will not yet be enhanced.

The PV phase occurs 45 to 75 seconds after the start of bolus contrast injection, and during this phase, the liver parenchyma is maximally enhanced, as well as the portal and hepatic veins. This phase is optimal for depiction of most hypovascular liver lesions, including most metastases.

A delayed enhanced series, performed from 90 seconds to 5 minutes, depicts the hepatic venous or interstitial phase and is useful for characterization of lesions with persistent or late enhancement, such as cavernous hemangiomas and some cholangiocarcinomas.

Positron Emission Tomography

On PET, the normal liver generally displays a diffuse, low to medium level of activity. On attenuation-corrected images particularly, the liver activity often has a diffusely mottled appearance. Reconstruction artifacts contribute to this appearance and will be most apparent in larger patients. Non-attenuation-corrected images will show a gradient of activity (increased toward the liver periphery) but can be helpful to review in such patients. In general, the expected low level of activity of the normal liver provides an excellent backdrop for ready identification of hypermetabolic liver metastases. In the untreated patient, liver metastases as small as 1 cm can be identified. However, visualization of even considerably larger liver metastases may be less reliable when patients are receiving hormonal or chemotherapy.

FINDINGS OF LIVER METASTASES

Ultrasound

Liver metastases on ultrasound may manifest as solitary or multiple lesions, which most commonly are hypoechoic compared with the normal liver (Figure 1), or as diffuse inhomogeneity of the liver parenchyma (Figure 2).

Computed Tomography

On CT, breast cancer liver metastases typically are hypodense relative to normal liver on noncontrast series, may display rim enhancement or be hypervascular compared with the poorly enhanced liver on the hepatic arterial phase of enhancement, and on the portal venous phase, are hypodense relative to the enhancing liver (Figure 3).

Magnetic Resonance Imaging

On T1-weighted sequences, the liver normally is brighter than the spleen. Most liver lesions that are not of hepatocellular origin (including the most commonly encountered liver lesions, namely cysts, hemangiomas, and metastases), are hypointense compared with the liver parenchyma on T1-weighted sequences. Lesions that are of hepatocel-

lular origin (such as hepatocellular carcinoma, adenomas, and focal nodular hyperplasia) are often isointense or hyperintense to liver parenchyma on T1-weighted sequences. A variety of T1-weighted sequences are available, including conventional spin echo, turbo or fast spin echo (depending on the manufacturer), and gradient echo. Gradient echo T1-weighted sequences may be acquired with the echo time (TE) varied so that fat and water protons are in or out of phase. Such acquisitions are sensitive to the presence of microscopic fat and are very useful for identifying fatty infiltration, focal

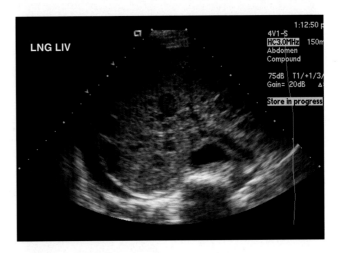

FIGURE 1. A 37-year-old woman with metastatic breast cancer to liver, thorax, and bone. Longitudinal ultrasound image of the liver shows multiple hypoechoic liver metastases scattered throughout the liver. There is a right pleural effusion as well.

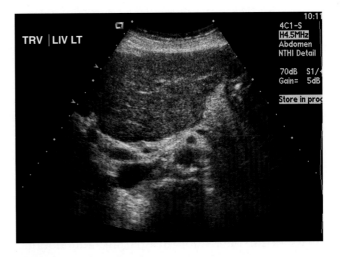

FIGURE 2. Another ultrasound manifestation of liver metastatic disease is diffuse inhomogeneity of the liver parenchyma, seen here in an 83-year-old woman who had known liver metastases for 3.5 years and had been treated with a variety of therapies. The liver contour is nodular, a recognized treatment effect, simulating cirrhosis.

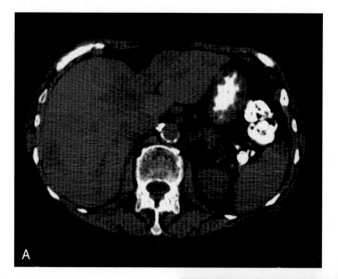

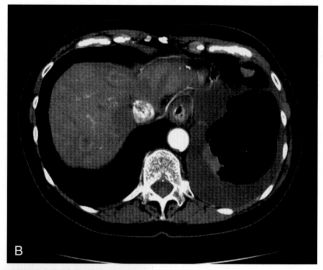

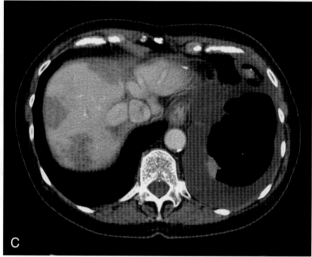

FIGURE 3.   CT images of liver metastases from an 83-year-old woman (same patient as in Figure 2) who developed a malignant pleural effusion and liver metastases 20 years after undergoing mastectomy for breast cancer. At the time of this study, the patient had known metastatic breast cancer for 3 years and had been relatively asymptomatic, first on letrozole (Femara) and then on fulvestrant (Faslodex), but progressive disease was suspected based on rising tumor markers. **A**, Unenhanced abdominal CT scan (acquired with arms at sides during tidal respiration for attenuation correction of PET) shows liver metastases as hypodense lesions compared with rest of the liver. **B**, Arterial phase enhanced CT scan shows three similar-appearing metastases, with thick peripheral enhancement and central hypodensity. The large hepatic veins are not enhanced during the HA phase of enhancement. **C**, PV phase enhanced CT image, same level, shows the lesions as larger hypodense regions, and an additional hypovascular metastasis is now seen in the peripheral right lobe, anterior segment, which was not previously seen on unenhanced or HA phase enhanced CT scans.

areas of fat deposition or sparing, and nodular forms of steatosis (Figures 4 and 5). On in-phase imaging, water and fat signal in the same voxel are additive, whereas on out-of-phase images, water and fat signal in the same voxel are opposed, leading to a loss of signal, which identifies fat-containing regions. The same principle is applied in the use of in-phase and out-of-phase imaging to confirm the identity of lipid-rich adrenal adenomas.

Fluid-sensitive sequences include T2-weighted and STIR sequences, which can be performed with or without fat saturation. Most liver lesions are hyperintense compared with liver parenchyma. The degree of hyperintensity is helpful in charac-

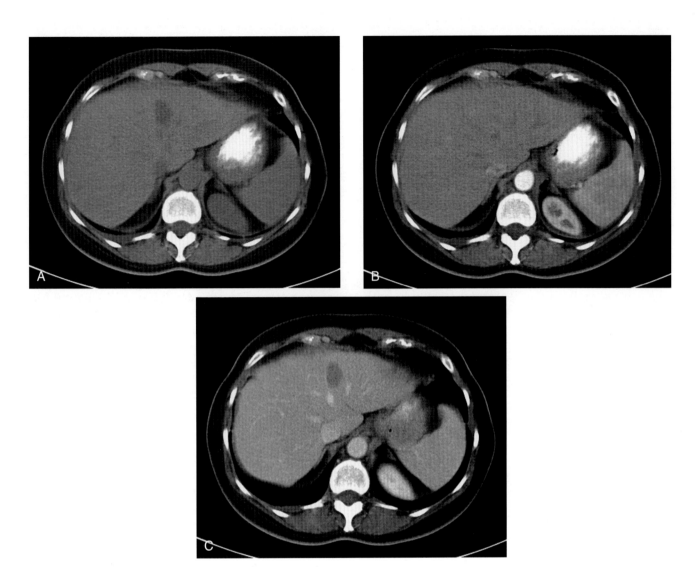

FIGURE 4. A 50-year-old woman with indeterminate hyperechoic liver lesions found on abdominal ultrasound, obtained to evaluate epigastric discomfort. **A**, Triple-phase abdominal CT was initially obtained to characterize the lesions. Noncontrast CT shows a hypodense lesion in the left lobe, one of four similar-appearing lesions. **B**, Arterial phase enhanced CT scan does not show the lesion to be hypervascular. It is not well seen on this phase of enhancement. **C**, PV phase enhanced CT scan shows the lesion to be hypodense compared with the enhancing liver. No peripheral nodular enhancement was seen to suggest a hemangioma.

terization of lesions, with cysts and hemangiomas more hyperintense and "fluid" in signal intensity than metastases and other more "solid" neoplasms. A good rule of thumb: the signal intensity of cysts and hemangiomas should be analogous to the cerebrospinal fluid (CSF) signal, whereas that of metastases and other neoplasms will approximate the signal intensity of the normal spleen.

Dynamic, enhanced imaging consists of repetitive performance of breath-hold, three-dimensional, fat-saturated, T1-weighted, gradient echo volumetric sequences, before, at 25 seconds, at 60 to 70 seconds, and at 2 or more minutes after bolus

administration of gadolinium chelate contrast media. The presence or absence of contrast enhancement and the pattern and timing of enhancement generally enable reliable differentiation of benign cysts and hemangiomas from metastases.[3]

As previously noted, breast cancer metastases have been variably considered in the literature to be hypervascular metastases. Danet and associates looked at a series of liver MRIs obtained on 165 consecutive patients with untreated liver metastases, from a variety of primary tumors, including 16 patients with breast cancer.[4] In this series, 69% of the breast cancer patients (11 of 16 patients) had metastases that were hypervascular, defined as enhancement greater than the liver on HA phase of enhancement, comparable to the pancreas. Smaller lesions (<1.5 cm) showed homogeneous hypervascular enhancement, whereas larger lesions (>3 cm) tended to show a peripheral ring of enhancement during the HA phase. In this series, 31% of the breast cancer patients (5 of 16) showed a hypovascular pattern of enhancement of liver metastases. Even for hypovascular metastases, the most common enhancement pattern seen during arterial dominant imaging was a faint peripheral ring of enhancement. The peripheral ring of enhancement was the most common enhancement pattern seen for all untreated metastases during arterial phase imaging in this series, and was seen in both hypervascular and hypovascular metastases and in 72% of the patients overall. This is considered a specific enhancement pattern for metastases. Incomplete central progression of enhancement was the most common pattern seen on delayed imaging in both hypervascular and hypovascular metastases, and was seen in 63% of the patients in this series of untreated metastases from a variety of primaries.

FREQUENCY OF LIVER INCIDENTALOMAS

On imaging of the liver for suspected metastases, a variety of benign "incidentalomas" will be encountered. These must be accurately characterized, reported, then dismissed. It is useful to gain perspective on the scope of this issue by reviewing series from the literature that address the incidence and significance of small focal liver incidentalomas. Depending on the series, small focal liver lesions have been variably defined as less than 10 or 15 mm. Jones and colleagues demonstrated that small focal liver lesions (<15 mm in this series) are common, found in 17% of 1454 consecutive outpatients undergoing contrast-enhanced abdominal CT over a 1-year period.[5] Eighty-two percent of the patients with small focal liver lesions had a malignancy history. Of these, lesions were found to be benign in 51%. This report found that in patients with no cancer history, small focal liver lesions are almost invariably benign.

Even in patients with a malignancy history, small focal liver lesions (<10 mm in the series of 2978 cancer patients undergoing CT over a 2-year period by Schwartz and associates) were benign 80% of the time.[6] In this series, focal liver lesions proved to be metastases in about 12% of patients overall and in 22% of patients when the malignancy history was breast cancer. However, this series did not include a control group of breast cancer patients without such lesions.

Krakora and colleagues evaluated the prognostic significance of the presence of small (<15 mm), hypoattenuating liver lesions on CT in breast cancer patients.[7] This was a retrospective review of 153 breast cancer patients who underwent serial abdominal CT, who did not have definite liver metastases at initial CT. Of these patients, 35% (54 of 153) had one or more small hypoattenuating liver lesions on initial CT. Twenty-eight percent (43 of 153) developed definite liver metastases on subsequent CT. These included 28% of patients (15 of 54) with hypoattenuating liver lesions on initial CT

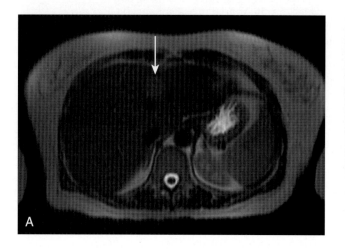
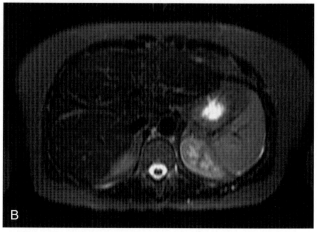

FIGURE 5. Abdominal MRI was then obtained to further assess the indeterminate liver lesions seen on CT in Figure 4. **A**, Axial half-Fourier acquisition single shot turbo spin echo (HASTE) (T2-weighted) shows the lesion to be brighter than the liver, similar to the spleen (*arrow*). **B**, Axial STIR does not clearly show the lesion.

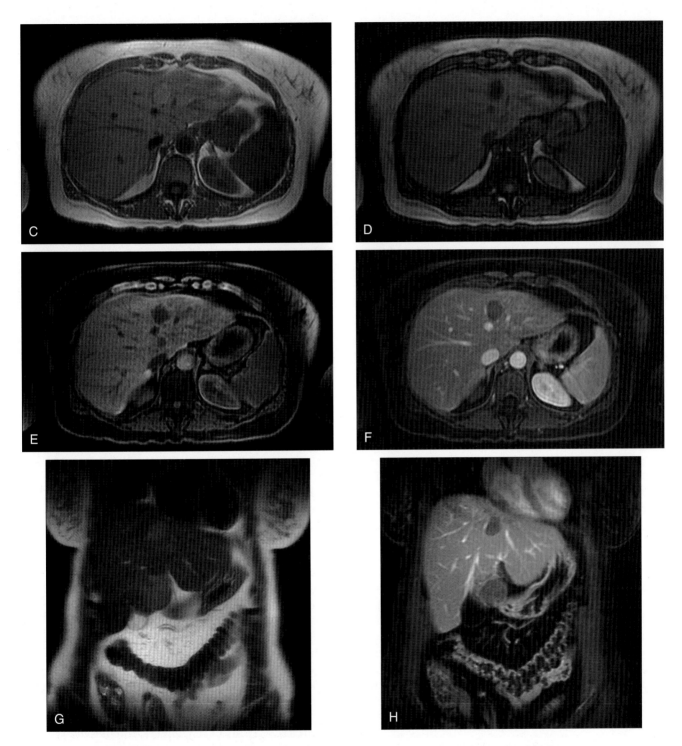

FIGURE 5, cont'd   **C,** In-phase, T1-weighted axial image shows the lesion to be slightly hyperintense compared with the rest of the liver. **D,** Out-of-phase, T1-weighted axial image shows the pivotal observation: there is a marked loss of signal of the lesion, indicating fat content. The other lesions behaved in a similar fashion. **E,** Axial fat-saturated, T1-weighted, gradient echo image before contrast administration shows the lesion as hypointense. **F,** PV phase, enhanced, fat-saturated, T1-weighted, gradient echo image shows the lesion as hypointense compared with the liver. No vascular displacement is evident. **G,** Coronal HASTE (T2-weighted) image shows two of the four similar-appearing lesions in the left lobe. **H,** Coronal fat-saturated, T1-weighted, gradient echo image of the same two lesions. Hyperechoic ultrasound lesions most commonly represent hemangiomas, but focal fat is also in the sonographic differential diagnosis. These lesions show none of the characteristic imaging features of hemangiomas on CT or MRI. The critical observation to make is the loss of signal of the lesions between in-phase and out-of-phase, T1-weighted, gradient echo imaging, confirming mass-like accumulations of focal fat. This was biopsy-confirmed macrovesicular steatosis.

and 28% (28 of 99) without such lesions. No association was demonstrated between the presence, size, or number of small hypodense liver lesions on initial CT and the subsequent development of liver metastases. The authors concluded that in breast cancer patients, the presence of small, hypoattenuating liver lesions on CT, without other evidence of hepatic metastases, was not associated with an increased risk for subsequently developing liver metastases.

Khalil and associates looked at the prevalence and significance of hepatic lesions considered to be too small to characterize (TSTC), which were identified on contrast-enhanced CT obtained in breast cancer patients.[8] At least one hepatic lesion considered TSTC (and no definite metastasis) was identified in 29% (277 of 941) of their patients. Subsequent imaging in 69% of patients (191 of 277) showed no change in 92% (175 of 191) or lesion nonvisualization in 4% (8 of 191). Interval enlargement of a lesion previously considered TSTC was noted in 6 of 191 patients (3%). Of these 6, 3 were metastatic breast cancer, 1 was metastatic pancreatic cancer, 1 was a growing cyst, and the final lesion was indeterminate. In this series, liver lesions that were initially TSTC were benign 93% to 97% of the time.

Similar series have looked at the incidence of benign liver incidentalomas detected on liver imaging by MRI in patients with breast cancer. An interesting series was reported by Noone and associates, who looked at 34 patients referred for liver MRI evaluation for suspected metastases at the time of initial breast cancer diagnosis.[9] The patients were referred for characterization of liver lesions noted on CT or ultrasound, or for liver function test abnormalities. A full third of the patients had benign lesions identified, including 11 (32%) with benign lesions only and an additional 2 patients with benign lesions coexisting with malignant lesions. The benign lesions were hemangiomas (7), cysts (5), adenomas (2), and one case each of focal fat deposition and focal fatty sparing. Three of 34 patients (9%) had multiple types of benign liver lesions.

In this series, liver neoplasia was identified in 62% of patients (21 of 34), of which 19 were breast cancer metastases, with one case each of metastatic carcinoid and hepatocellular carcinoma. There was one technically compromised false-negative case of sub-centimeter periportal biopsy-proven metastases, which was also false negative on ultrasound and CT. Overall results for the identification of malignant liver lesions were sensitivity of 95%, specificity of 100%, positive predictive value of 100%, and negative predictive value of 92%.

In this same series of 34 patients, only 2 (6%) patients had no focal liver lesions identified on MRI. Even allowing for the select nature of the study population, this result attests to the common occurrence of benign liver lesions when evaluating a population of breast cancer patients suspected of liver metastases.

Even when not directly evaluating the liver, it may be partially visualized during breast MRI (depending on the coil coverage). Accordingly, even the full-time breast imager needs to be familiar with focal liver lesions (Figure 6). In this setting, the imaging information will not be as complete as with a dedicated abdominal examination. It is important to have an understanding of when there is sufficient information to characterize a liver lesion or not. Similarly, not infrequently, focal liver lesions may have to be assessed based on a single phase of CT enhancement (usually portal venous), such as in metastases screening CT in patients with new diagnoses of locally advanced breast cancer (Figure 7).

Given the high likelihood of encountering liver incidentalomas in the imaging evaluation of breast cancer patients, a thorough review of their features is in order.

IMAGING FEATURES OF COMMONLY ENCOUNTERED BENIGN LIVER INCIDENTALOMAS

Cysts

Liver cysts are common, seen in 5% to 14% of the general population. They are thought to arise from bile duct epithelium. On ultrasound, cysts in the liver are anechoic, with sharp margins and enhanced through-transmission, analogous to breast cysts. On both CT and MRI, they are homogeneous, are near-water in density or signal intensity, have circumscribed margins and an imperceptible wall, and do not enhance (see Figures 6, 11B, and 11C). On CT, the density should be less than 20 HU, with the caveat that very small cysts may be volume-averaged with adjacent tissue and will have density greater than 20 HU. Readily visualizing a small, hypodense lesion on CT suggests it is cystic, because of the greater attenuation difference between a fluid density cyst and liver parenchyma than between a small metastasis and liver. On MRI, cyst signal intensity will approximate CSF on all sequences.

Rarely, cysts may be difficult to differentiate from cystic metastases. Identification of thick or

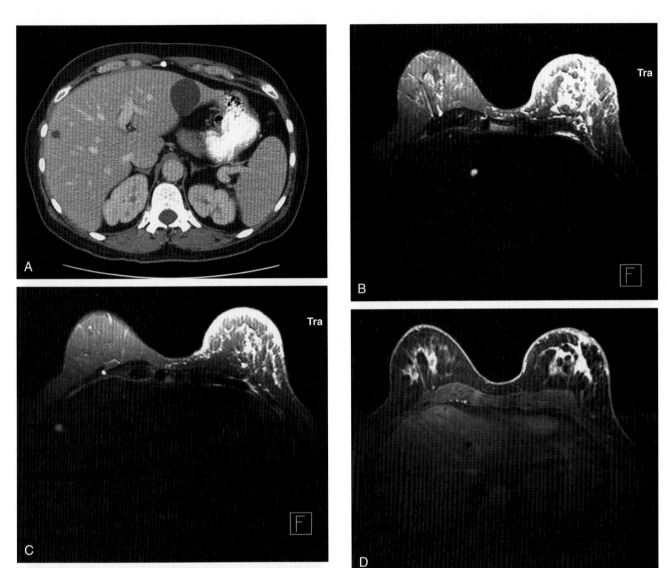

FIGURE 6. A 52-year-old woman with left breast inflammatory carcinoma, undergoing initial staging. **A**, PV phase, enhanced axial abdominal CT scan shows several sharply marginated, near water density, nonenhancing liver cysts. Additional cysts were noted on other slices. Lobular renal margins may be the residua of infection. **B** and **C**, Axial STIR images from staging breast MRI show diffuse skin thickening and edema of the left inflammatory carcinoma. In the liver, sharply marginated, hyperintense, fluid signal intensity, scattered lesions are seen in the liver. Based on this hyperintensity, a differential of small cysts or hemangiomas can be suggested. **D** and **E**, Fat-saturated, T1-weighted, gradient echo axial images through the same levels from the same study show no enhancement, confirming cysts.

irregular walls, internal septations, and any enhancement or density greater than 20 HU on CT usually allows cystic neoplasms to be distinguished from simple cysts.

Hemangiomas

Hemangiomas are the most commonly encountered benign liver tumor, seen in 7% of the normal adult population and 20% of autopsy specimens. Composed of communicating endothelium-lined vascular channels within a loose fibroblastic stroma, they are supplied by HA branches but have slow internal circulation. This structure is reflected in their characteristic enhancement pattern, with peripheral nodular or globular puddling enhancement, progressing centripetally to partially or completely fill in on delayed imaging. Larger lesions in particular may not fill in entirely, and complete fill-in is not necessary to confirm the diagnosis. The enhancement intensity should follow the aorta throughout all phases of imaging. Small hemangiomas may be completely opacified by the time of initial enhanced imaging, so-called flash filling. Hemangiomas are sharply marginated and may have internal septa that can be visualized, especially on MRI. On noncontrast CT, hemangiomas are hypodense to normal liver and isodense to the blood pool. On unenhanced MRI, hemangiomas are hypointense to liver on T1-weighted sequences and markedly hyperintense to liver (similar to CSF) on fluid-sensitive sequences (T2-weighted and STIR). On ultrasound, small hemangiomas are generally uniformly hyperechoic. Echogenicity of larger hemangiomas is more variable. For examples of the imaging features of hemangiomas, see Figures 7, 8, 12C and 12D, and Case 1 in this chapter.

Fatty Change of the Liver

Fatty infiltration of the liver can be diffuse, geographic, focal or multifocal, and nodular, termed *nodular steatosis*.[10] Fatty liver is commonly associated with alcoholic liver disease, metabolic syndrome (insulin resistance, obesity, and hyperlipidemia), viral infections or hepatitis, and drug exposure to steroids or prior chemotherapy. On ultrasound, fatty change is generally recognized by increased liver parenchymal echogenicity compared with normal renal cortex (Figure 9). The normal liver approximates or is minimally more echogenic than the normal kidney. The liver may be enlarged. With increasing degrees of fatty change, intrahepatic vessel visualization is hampered, as well as visualization of the diaphragm.

On CT, fatty change of the liver is recognized best on noncontrast images as reduced liver attenuation compared with the spleen (Figure 10). With marked degrees of fatty change, conspicuity of vessels and lesions is increased in comparison with the hypodense liver parenchyma, with the fatty change serving as a form of natural contrast. The liver density is normally 8 HU higher than the spleen. The diagnosis of fatty liver can be confirmed when the attenuation of the liver is at least 10 HU less than the spleen on unenhanced CT, or if the liver attenuation is less than 40 HU on enhanced CT.

Focal fat deposition is recognized as geographic or non-mass-like reduced attenuation and is commonly noted adjacent to the ligamentum teres (Figure 11A), as well as the porta hepatis and the gallbladder fossa. The location and appearance are usually sufficiently characteristic to enable recognition. Occasionally, focal fat deposition may be mass-like and will require further workup. If further characterization is needed, in-phase and out-of-phase T1-weighted, gradient echo MRI will show loss of signal in fat-containing regions on the out-of-phase images (see Figure 5).

CHARACTERIZING SMALL FOCAL LESIONS

Given that most routine liver imaging is with CT and that small, hypodense, difficult to characterize lesions will be regularly encountered, is there utility in additional imaging, with either ultrasound or MRI, to characterize indeterminate small lesions? We have seen that statistically, such too small to characterize (TSTC) lesions found on CT are most often benign.

Ultrasound is very operator dependent, and its sensitivity for identification of small liver lesions is greatly affected by a patient's body habitus. Eberhardt and colleagues looked retrospectively at the performance of sonography in evaluating small, indeterminate liver lesions found on CT in cancer patients.[11] In their series of 76 patients with 124 indeterminate, CT-identified, small (<1.5 cm) liver lesions, less than half (48%) of the lesions were found on ultrasound. The detection rate was influenced both by the size of the lesions and whether the sonographer was aware of the CT result and specifically sought an ultrasound correlate. Two thirds (66%) of lesions were found when the CT data were referenced, compared with only about one third (32%) when it was not. Lesion size was

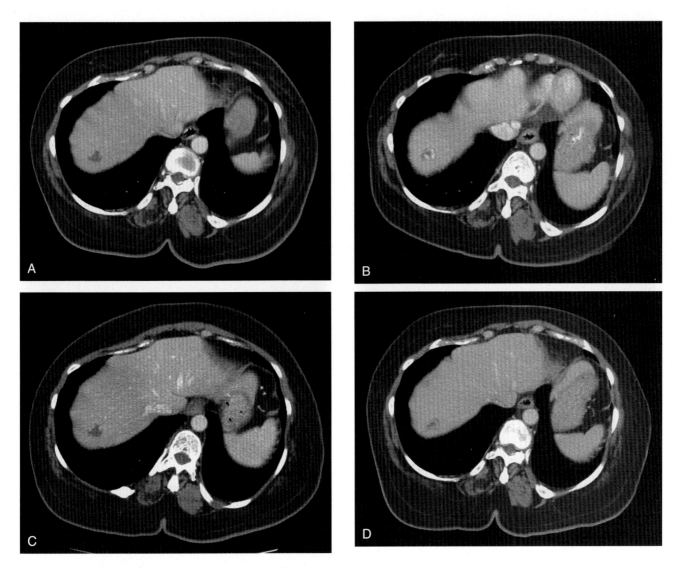

FIGURE 7. A 51-year-old woman with ulcerated, neglected, locally advanced, poorly differentiated infiltrating ductal carcinoma (IDC), presenting with lytic bone metastases (stage IV disease). Images from PV phase, enhanced abdominal CT images over a 1-year period show a variety of similar, overall stable appearances of a small incidental liver hemangioma, which was metabolically inactive on PET. **A**, Staging CT scan shows a hypodense lesion at the dome (posterior segment, right lobe), with nodular foci of enhancement on the periphery. **B**, Repeat PV phase enhanced CT scan, 3 months later, shows a similar appearance of nodular and globular peripheral enhancement of a small hemangioma at the dome. **C**, Repeat PV phase, enhanced CT scan, 2 months later, shows stable findings. **D**, PV phase, enhanced abdominal CT scan, 7 months later (1 year after study in **A**) shows no change.

the other major factor influencing detection, with 67% of lesions measuring 0.6 to 1.5 cm found, compared with 19% of lesions smaller than 0.5 cm. Patient body habitus was also a significant factor affecting lesion detection with ultrasound. The lesions ultrasound did find were successfully characterized in most cases (93%).

The authors concluded that ultrasound may be useful to characterize 0.6- to 1.5-cm indeterminate

liver lesions found on CT in cancer patients of average body habitus. The opposite conclusion could be drawn in reference to the same material: that ultrasound is too operator and patient body habitus dependent, as well as too limited for evaluation of very small (<0.5 cm) lesions to be routinely advocated to characterize small, indeterminate, CT-identified lesions, which are statistically highly likely to be benign (Figure 12).

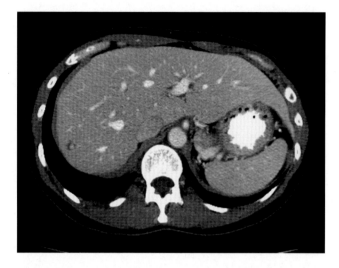

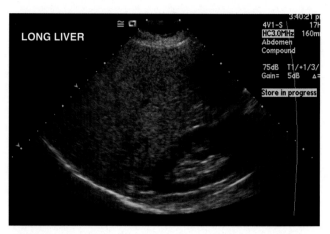

FIGURE 8. A 44-year-old woman with recurrent breast cancer, presenting 2 years after treatment of the primary with a malignant pleural effusion. Restaging CT shows in the abdomen a small hypodensity at the liver dome, with a nodular focus of associated enhancement, of similar density to other enhanced vessels. This focus was negative on PET and is compatible with a small hemangioma.

FIGURE 9. A 50-year-old woman with stage IV breast cancer metastatic to bone, diagnosed at presentation 2.5 years before, now has elevated liver function tests and rising tumor markers. The patient had been on exemestane (Aromasin) and zoledronic acid (Zometa) since her diagnosis, but had initiated chemotherapy recently and had undergone one cycle of capecitabine (Xeloda). Longitudinal abdominal ultrasound image shows diffuse hyperechogenicity of the liver, compared with the right kidney. There is loss of detail of intrahepatic vessels. Ultrasound findings are compatible with fatty change of the liver. This appeared to be new compared with CT performed 3 months before.

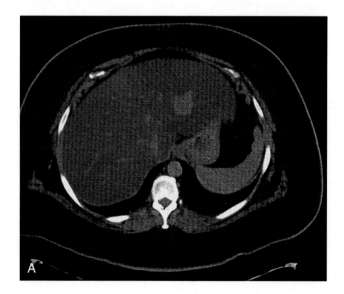

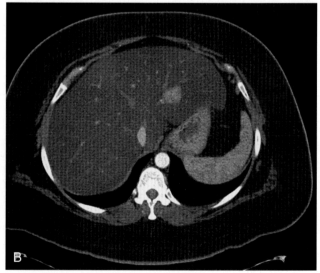

FIGURE 10. A 35-year-old woman with stage IV breast cancer (metastatic to bone) at presentation 7 months prior, treated with tamoxifen and Zometa until 1 month before, when chemotherapy with docetaxel (Taxotere) was begun and tamoxifen discontinued, for progression on bone scan of bone metastases. **A,** Unenhanced abdominal CT scan shows the liver to be markedly hypodense compared with the spleen. The liver fatty change serves as a natural contrast agent, delineating a new left lobe metastasis. **B,** HA phase, enhanced CT from the same study. Enhancement in the lesion is more difficult to discern visually.

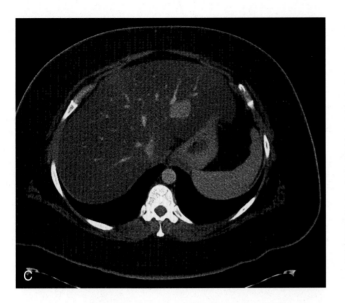

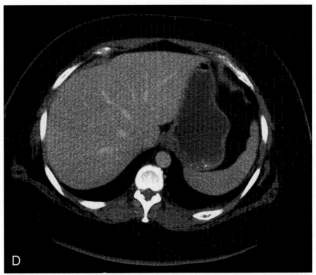

FIGURE 10, cont'd   C, PV phase, enhanced CT, from the same study, shows the same lesion. Enhancement is difficult to assess visually. Measurement of density confirms enhancement, increasing from 25 HU on the noncontrast study to 72 HU on this PV phase. **D**, Comparison study (PV phase, enhanced), 7 months earlier, at initial diagnosis of stage IV breast cancer, shows normal liver density.

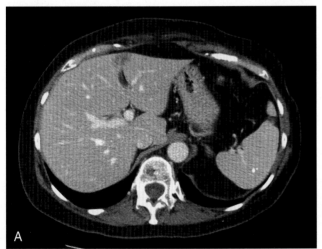

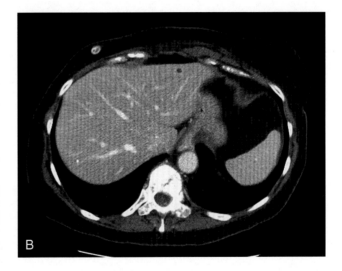

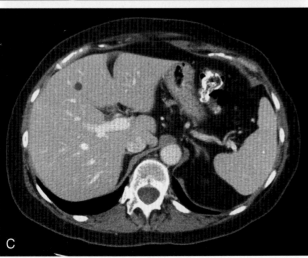

FIGURE 11.   Enhanced abdominal CT images from a 59-year-old woman with recurrent breast cancer, metastatic to mediastinal lymph nodes and bone. **A**, Localized region of hypodensity, consistent with focal fatty infiltration, is characteristic in location at the falciform ligament level. **B** and **C**, Additional sections from this patient show sub-centimeter, circumscribed, nonenhancing, near-water density cysts in the left lobe of the liver. Benign incidentalomas are not infrequently multiple, and multiple types of benign lesions can be seen in the same patient, as in this case.

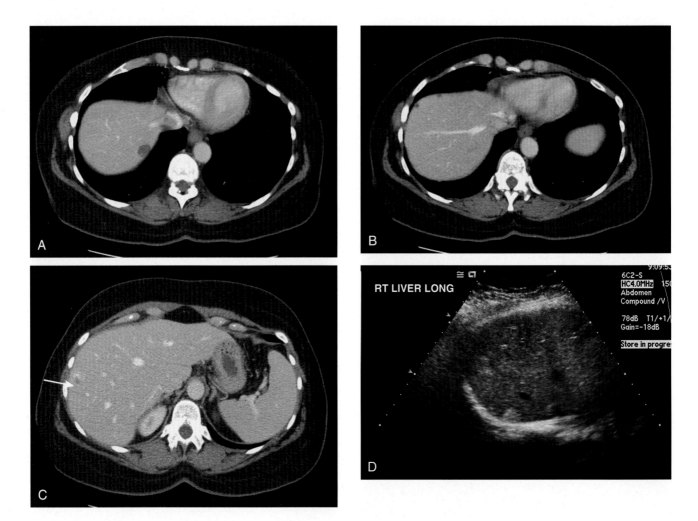

FIGURE 12. The difficulty of characterizing small, indeterminate liver lesions found on CT with ultrasound is demonstrated in this 49-year-old woman with newly diagnosed, node-positive (5 of 8, largest 1.9 cm, with extracapsular extension), 1.8-cm left breast IDC. Staging studies with PET and enhanced PV phase CT showed a variety of small, indeterminate, PET-negative liver lesions. Ultrasound or triple-phase CT was recommended for further characterization, and ultrasound was obtained. **A,** Enhanced abdominal CT, PV phase, at the dome of the liver, shows a sharply marginated, 1.5-cm, low-density (but not clearly fluid density by HU) lesion. No ultrasound correlate was identified, despite its size, probably because of its location. **B,** No ultrasound correlates were found for these two tiny lucencies at the liver dome, probably because of their small size and location at the dome. **C,** A vague hypodensity at the periphery of the right lobe of the liver appears to have a globule of associated peripheral enhancement (*arrow*), suggesting it may be a hemangioma. **D,** Ultrasound through the right lobe of the liver shows a corresponding, uniformly hyperechoic, peripheral lesion, compatible with a hemangioma.

Such a conclusion was drawn by Patterson and associates, who looked at evaluating small (TSTC) CT liver lesions in breast cancer patients with MRI.[12] Their study population consisted of 38 women with breast cancer who underwent abdominal MRI at or after initial diagnosis of breast cancer and who had at least one TSTC liver lesion previously identified on CT. In 11 patients (30%), indeterminate lesions on CT remained indeterminate on MRI. Follow-up imaging, biopsy, or both in 8 of

these 11 patients confirmed benignity of the indeterminate lesions. In 8 patients (21%), no lesion was confirmed on MRI at the site questioned on CT. Metastatic lesions were identified in 2 patients, and benign diagnoses were confirmed by MRI in 22. The authors concluded that only marginal benefit was derived from using MRI to characterize TSTC liver lesions found on CT in newly diagnosed breast cancer patients, if their initial CT did not show definite liver metastases. In this series, only

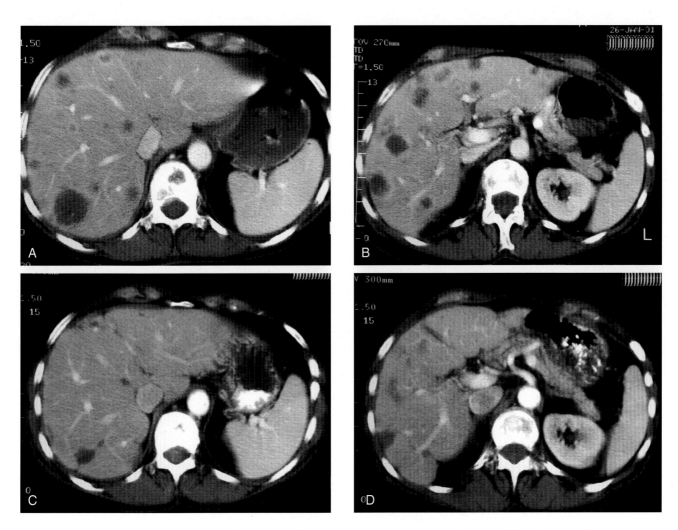

FIGURE 13. A 63-year-old woman with metastatic breast cancer to bone and liver. Liver metastases were biopsy proven, with three separate sites sampled. **A** and **B**, PV phase, enhanced abdominal CT images show multiple rim-enhancing necrotic metastases. **C** and **D**, PV phase, enhanced abdominal CT images, 1 year later, showing comparable levels. The patient had been receiving weekly chemotherapy. Liver metastases show marked improvement. Some lesions have resolved, whereas others have shrunk. Hypodense residual lesions, many with capsular contraction, remain where the larger metastases were and produce a pseudocirrhosis appearance of the liver. Concurrent PET scan showed extensive osseous metastases, but no foci of uptake in the liver.

about 5% of such TSTC lesions on CT proved on MRI to be metastases.

TREATMENT EFFECTS: IMAGING MANIFESTATIONS

A variety of morphologic changes can be seen in the liver after treatment with chemotherapy. These changes can be diffuse, such as fatty change (see Figure 10), or local changes may be seen at the site of treated liver metastases. Liver metastases may shrink, or largely resolve, in response to successful systemic therapy. A hypodense, scar-like residual may remain at the site of a treated lesion, and either growth or shrinkage of breast cancer metastases has been shown to induce changes in the overlying liver contour, resulting either from capsular retraction or nodular regeneration of uninvolved areas. The end result can on occasion mimic cirrhosis, with lobularity of the liver contour, atrophy of heavily involved lobes, enlargement of the caudate lobe, and even development of ascites on occasion (Figures 13 and 14). This appearance developing in response to chemotherapy for breast liver metastases has been termed *pseudocirrhosis* and is illustrated in Case 3 in this chapter.

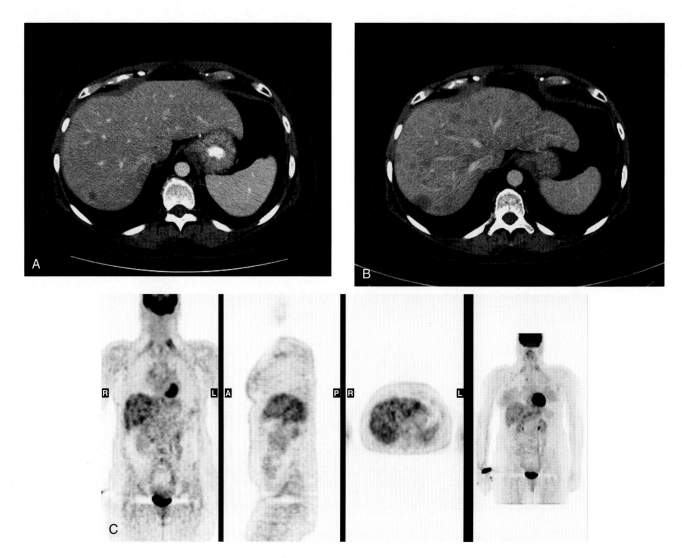

FIGURE 14.   A 50-year-old woman, treated the previous year with breast conservation for a high-risk left breast cancer, estrogen receptor positive, with angiolymphatic invasion and 10 of 11 lymph nodes involved. She had been treated with chemotherapy with doxorubicin (Adriamycin), cyclophosphamide (Cytoxan), and paclitaxel (Taxol), completed 3 months before, and started tamoxifen. Radiation therapy concluded 2 months before the patient presented with node-positive, inflammatory right breast cancer (IDC). There was no evidence of visceral metastatic disease by CT or PET, and the patient was treated with four cycles of chemotherapy using Taxotere and Xeloda. **A**, Restaging enhanced abdominal CT (PV phase) showed two new hypodense liver lesions. The larger of the two is shown, in the posterior segment of the right lobe, and measures 11 mm. PET/CT was negative at this time in the liver. **B**, Repeat CT scan, 3 months later, after two cycles of Taxol and bevacizumab (Avastin). The index lesion has grown, and there are multiple, additional, smaller, less well-defined hypovascular lesions seen throughout the liver. Note developing left lobe deformity, with surface nodularity due to capsular contraction. **C**, Concurrent PET scan shows multiple metabolically active liver metastases, new from a study 3 months prior.

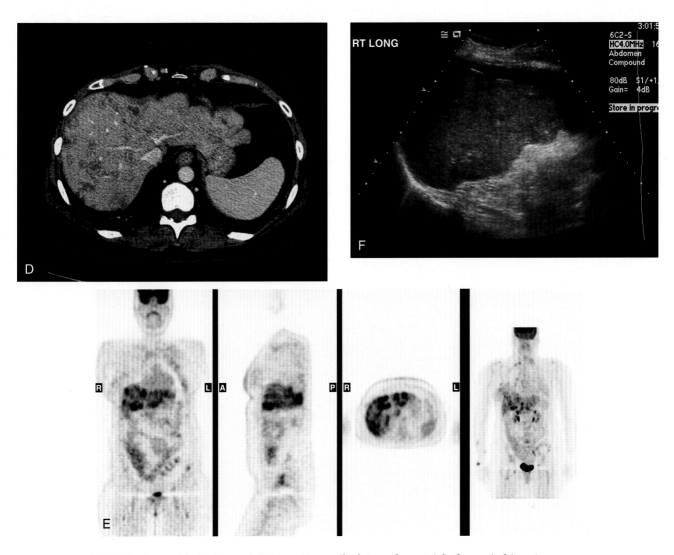

FIGURE 14, cont'd   **D**, Repeat CT scan, 3 months later, after a trial of gemcitabine. An increasingly nodular appearance of the left lobe is seen. The liver is diffusely heterogeneous, with multiple rim-enhancing metastases. **E**, Concurrent PET scan shows progressive bone, right chest wall soft tissue, and liver metastases. **F**, Abdominal ultrasound, later the same month as **D**, shows diffuse parenchymal heterogeneity and macronodular liver contour. Individual liver metastases are difficult to define. Ascites has developed, and the patient was now jaundiced.

Rarely, treated metastases may regress to leave cyst-like residuals (see Case 6 in this chapter).

REFERENCES

1. Frederick MG, Paulson EK, Nelson RC. Helical CT for detecting focal liver lesions in patients with breast carcinoma: comparison of noncontrast phase, hepatic arterial phase, and portal venous phase. *J Comput Assist Tomogr* 1997; 21:229–235.

2. Sheafor DH, Frederick MG, Paulson EK, et al. Comparison of unenhanced, hepatic arterial-dominant, and portal venous-dominant phase helical CT for the detection of liver metastases in women with breast carcinoma. *AJR Am J Roentgenol* 1999; 172:961–968.

3. Semelka RC (ed). Hepatic imaging. *Radiol Clin North Am* 2005; 43(5).

4. Danet I-M, Semelka RC, Leonardou P, et al. Spectrum of MRI appearances of untreated metastases of the liver. *AJR Am J Roentgenol* 2003; 181:809–817.

5. Jones EC, Chezmar JL, Nelson RC, et al. The frequency and significance of small hepatic lesions (<15 mm) detected by CT. *AJR Am J Roentgenol* 1992; 158:535–539.

6. Schwartz LH, Gandras EJ, Colangelo SM, et al. Prevalence and importance of small hepatic lesions

found at CT in patients with cancer. *Radiology* 1999; 210:71–74.

7. Krakora GA, Coakley FV, Williams G, et al. Small hypoattenuating hepatic lesions at contrast-enhanced CT: prognostic importance in patients with breast cancer. *Radiology* 2004; 233:667–673.

8. Khalil HI, Patterson SA, Panicek DM. Hepatic lesions deemed too small to characterize at CT: prevalence and importance in women with breast cancer. *Radiology* 2005; 235(3):872–878.

9. Noone TC, Semelka RC, Balci NC, et al. Common occurrence of benign liver lesions in patients with newly diagnosed breast cancer investigated by MRI for suspected liver metastases. *J Magn Reson Imaging*, 1999; 10(2):165–169.

10. Hamer OW, Aguirre DA, Casola G, et al. Fatty liver: imaging patterns and pitfalls. *RadioGraphics* 2006; 26:1637–1653.

11. Eberhardt SC, Choi PH, Bach AM, et al. Utility of sonography for small hepatic lesions found on computed tomography in patients with cancer. *J Ultrasound Med* 2003; 22:335–343.

12. Patterson SA, Khalil HI, Panicek DM. MRI evaluation of small hepatic lesions in women with breast cancer. *Am J Roentgenol* 2006; 187:307–312.

CASE 1

Workup of indeterminate liver lesion with MRI (hemangioma)

A 57-year-old woman with a remote history of treated breast cancer developed mild liver function test elevations while on statin therapy for elevated low-density lipoprotein cholesterol. Her breast cancer history was 17 years before at age 40 years, and was an early-stage, T1N0M0, 1.1-cm infiltrating ductal carcinoma, with negative lymph nodes and margins. She had been treated with lumpectomy, radiation therapy, and 5 years of tamoxifen. A triple-phase liver CT scan was obtained to further evaluate the liver. A hypovascular mass was identified, with rim enhancement, with subtle suggestion of rim nodularity (Figure 1). No delayed images were obtained. The findings were regarded as indeterminate and not diagnostic of a hemangioma. MRI was recommended for additional characterization, and confirmed signal intensity and enhancement characteristics of a hemangioma (Figures 2, 3, 4, 5, 6, 7, 8, 9, and 10).

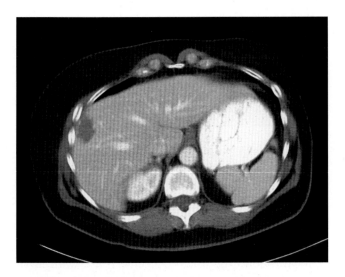

FIGURE 1. Enhanced abdominal CT image during the portal venous (PV) phase of imaging shows a lobular, hypovascular focal liver lesion in the periphery of the anterior segment right lobe. There is subtle rim enhancement, which is mildly nodular. No delayed images were obtained. Findings were regarded as indeterminate.

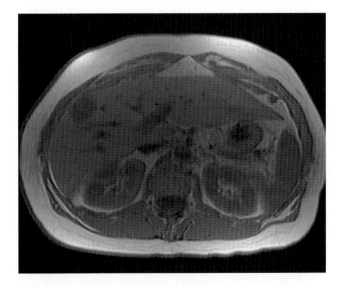

FIGURE 2. Axial T1-weighted MRI scan shows the lesion to have a lobular margin and to be hypointense to the liver parenchyma.

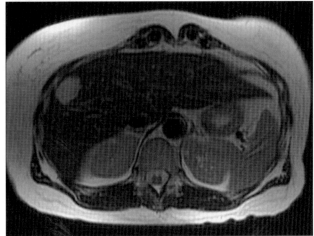

FIGURE 3. Axial T2-weighted MR image (HASTE) shows the lesion to be hyperintense, with thin septa within.

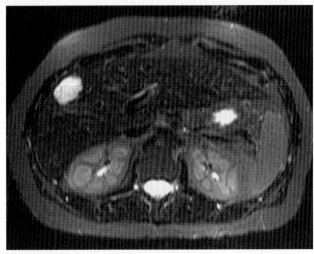

FIGURE 4. Axial STIR image of the lesion again shows a lobular contour, hyperintense signal, and internal septa.

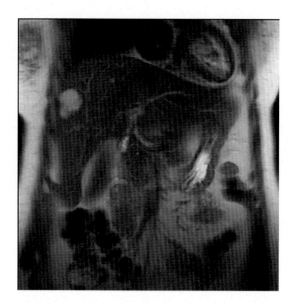

FIGURE 5. Coronal single-shot, T2-weighted, breath-hold image (HASTE) shows the lesion in question to be hyperintense, with faint internal septa. A second small, hyperintense lesion is seen in the left lobe medial segment, which proved to be a cyst.

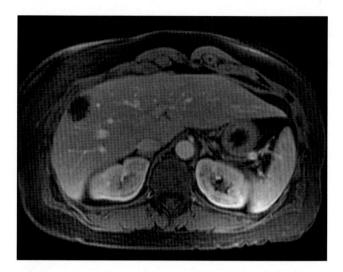

FIGURE 7. Fat-saturated, T1-weighted, three-dimensional, gradient echo, enhanced image obtained during the PV phase of enhancement shows progression of the nodular peripheral enhancement of the liver lesion. As expected during the PV phase of enhancement, there is maximal parenchymal enhancement of the liver, spleen, and kidneys compared with the HA phase.

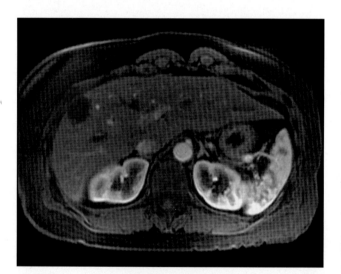

FIGURE 6. Fat-saturated, T1-weighted, three-dimensional, gradient echo, enhanced image obtained during the hepatic arterial (HA) phase of enhancement shows nodular peripheral enhancement of the lesion. As is normal for HA phase imaging, the hepatic veins and liver parenchyma are minimally enhanced, the kidneys are in the corticomedullary phase of enhancement, and there is heterogeneous enhancement of the spleen.

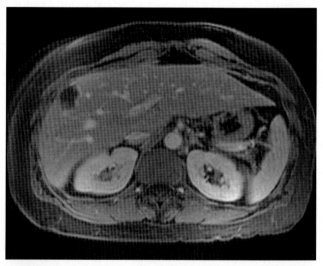

FIGURE 8. Repeat of the same sequence, about 2 minutes after injection of the gadolinium-based contrast agent, shows slow progression of the peripheral enhancement. The nodular enhancement seen earlier has coalesced to a thicker peripheral rim.

TEACHING POINTS

Imaging of the liver in patients with a history of breast cancer will frequently identify benign focal liver lesions, which will need to be accurately characterized in order to exclude liver metastatic disease. Most commonly encountered are liver cysts and hemangiomas. This case is an example of the most common benign liver tumor, the cavernous hemangioma, which can be seen in up to 7% of the normal adult population and in up to 20% of autopsy specimens. The lesion consists of interconnected, endothelium-lined, vascular channels within a loose fibroblastic stroma. Fed by branches of the hepatic artery, the lesion has slow internal

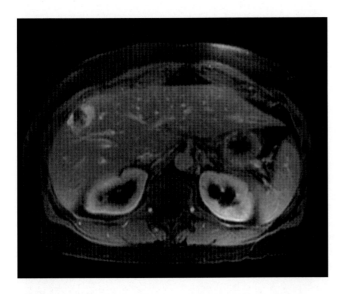

FIGURE 9. Repeat sequence, 5 minutes after injection, shows centripetal progression of the enhancement. The lesion is partly filled in.

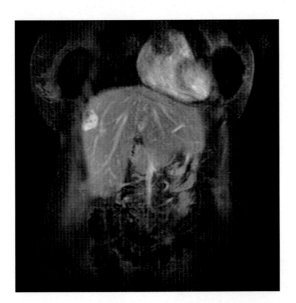

FIGURE 10. Coronal fat-saturated, enhanced, T1-weighted, gradient echo, three-dimensional image shows the lesion to be nearly completely filled in. Breast implants are noted.

circulation, leading to its characteristic enhancement pattern, which enables these lesions to be recognized and confidently characterized on CT and MRI. Early enhancement consists of peripheral puddling, with nodular or globular enhancement on the rim of the lesion. This progresses centripetally until most or all of the lesion is enhanced. On all phases of enhancement, the intensity of contrast enhancement should approximate that of the aorta. The lesions are sharply mar-

ginated. On MRI, the lesions are quite hyperintense or fluid in signal intensity on fluid-sensitive sequences, such as T2-weighted and STIR sequences, similar in intensity to cerebrospinal fluid. Internal septations can be seen, as in this case, and larger hemangiomas may not completely fill in. Small hemangiomas may completely fill in early in enhancement, termed *flash filling*.

CASE 2

Progression of liver metastases on CT and PET

A 37-year-old woman with extensive bony metastatic breast cancer known for 1 year developed increased aching, weight loss, depressed appetite, and rising tumor markers while on goserelin acetate (Zoladex), zoledronic acid (Zometa), and exemestane (Aromasin). Positron emission tomography (PET)/CT and enhanced body CT scans showed new liver metastases (Figures 1 and 2). Chemotherapy was recommended but declined by the patient. She was started on fulvestrant (Faslodex) and restaged 2 months later, at which time fatigue, shortness of breath, and rising tumor markers were

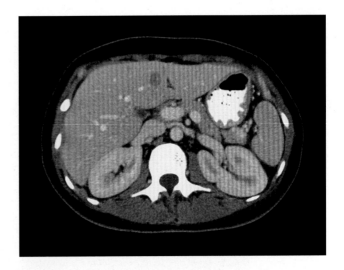

FIGURE 1. Contrast-enhanced abdominal CT scan, portal venous phase, showed multiple hypovascular new metastases in the liver, one of which is shown here, in the medial segment of the left lobe (segment IV).

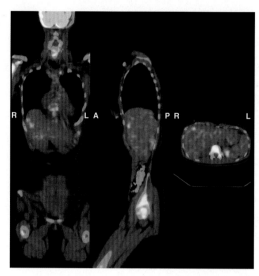
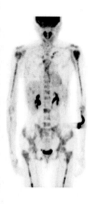

FIGURE 2. Representative concurrent PET/CT fused images (*left to right:* coronal, sagittal, axial, coronal projection volume image) shows hypermetabolic foci in the liver, corresponding to the CT findings. The coronal projection image on the right shows diffuse abnormal marrow hypermetabolism due to bone metastases, which is patchy and inhomogeneous. This is best seen in the spine and extremities. Although chemotherapy-related marrow activation could be considered in the scintigraphic differential of diffuse increased marrow activity, it could be dismissed in this case because the patient was not receiving chemotherapy and the activity was not uniform.

noted. Repeat PET/CT and enhanced body CT scans showed progression of liver metastases (Figures 3 and 4), as well as new lung involvement (see Case 13 in Chapter 10). One month later, the patient was admitted with mental confusion, thought to be hepatic encephalopathy due to the progressive and extensive liver metastases. Workup for alternative etiologies, including abdominal ultrasound and head CT, showed only the known disease, with no additional abnormality.

Her original tumor was diagnosed 5 years before and was an estrogen receptor– and progesterone

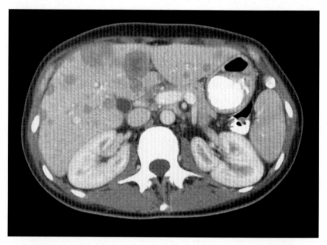

FIGURE 3. Repeat CT scan, 2 months later. Chemotherapy was declined by the patient, and 2 months of treatment with Faslodex was given instead. Marked progression of liver metastases is seen. The index left lobe lesion pictured in Figure 1 has grown, and innumerable additional metastases are seen.

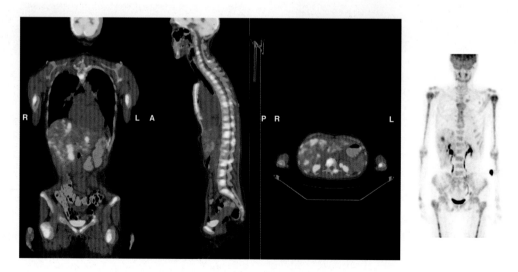

FIGURE 4. Repeat PET/CT, 2 months after study in Figure 2 and concurrent with CT in Figure 3. Fused PET/CT images show marked progression of liver metastases. Many more hypermetabolic liver foci are identifiable and correlate with the progressive CT findings.

receptor–positive, T1cN1b(4) infiltrating ductal carcinoma. It was treated with breast conservation and axillary dissection, with 4 of 20 lymph nodes positive. Additional treatment included chemotherapy (four cycles of doxorubicin [Adriamycin] plus cyclophosphamide [Cytoxan] [AC] and four of paclitaxel [Taxol]); right breast, supraclavicular, and axillary radiation therapy; and tamoxifen. One year before liver metastases were discovered, diffuse bone metastases were found when the patient sought orthopedic advice for low back and right leg pain. See Case 3 in Chapter 8 for discussion of the imaging manifestations of this patient's bone metastases.

TEACHING POINTS

This patient is typical in that liver metastases developed in the setting of widely metastatic disease, which in this case was in bone. More than half of patients with metastatic breast cancer develop liver metastases, which can be the cause of death in the 20% of patients who develop liver failure due to metastases. This patient's terminal presentation was notable for mental confusion, with multiple biochemical abnormalities, including elevated prothrombin time and liver function tests. Clinically, she was thought to have hepatic encephalopathy due to the extensive and progressive liver metastases. Workup for other etiologies did not yield an alternative explanation.

CASE 3

Pseudocirrhotic appearance of treated breast cancer liver metastases; mislocalization of right liver metastases into right lung base on PET/CT

A 39-year-old woman developed abdominal distention and increased fatigue a year after being treated for a high-risk breast cancer. This was a right breast estrogen receptor– and progesterone receptor–positive, *HER-2/neu*-positive, 2.7-cm

infiltrating ductal carcinoma with an extensive intraductal component. There were 10 of 12 lymph nodes with metastatic carcinoma, including a 3-cm lymph node with focal extracapsular extension. She was treated with a mastectomy, four cycles of doxorubicin and cyclophosphamide, followed by four cycles of paclitaxel, as well as chest wall, supraclavicular, and axillary radiation.

When the patient developed constitutional symptoms, she was restaged with CT scans, showing extensive hepatic metastases. Chemotherapy with carboplatin, docetaxel (Taxotere), and trastuzumab (Herceptin) was initiated, with good response. Follow-up surveillance CT scans showed resolution of the bulk of the liver metastases, with development of a progressively scarred liver, which has been termed *pseudocirrhosis*. Her disease status was periodically assessed while on vinorelbine tartrate (Navelbine) with enhanced abdominal CT scans and positron emission tomography (PET)/ CT (Figures 1, 2, 3, 4, and 5).

TEACHING POINTS

This patient had known, previously treated, extensive liver metastases, originally diagnosed 14 months before the earliest of these studies. She had had an excellent response to chemotherapy. Her particular healing response created pseudocirrhosis. These findings, described by Young and colleagues, included capsular surface retraction of the liver at the site of subjacent metastases, imparting a lobular contour to the liver, simulating cirrhosis. Volume loss in involved lobes was noted, with caudate lobe enlargement in the diffusely involved livers. In this series of 22 patients, pathologic correlation was available for 7 patients. All had residual tumor, and 6 of 7 showed nodular regenerative hyperplasia. No patients showed bridging portal fibrosis or pathologic evidence of true cirrhosis.

This case also illustrates a recognized misregistration artifact seen in PET/CT. In a series of 300 patients reported by Osman and colleagues, 2% of cases had mislocalization of liver dome lesions into the right lung base when CT was used for attenuation correction of PET. This occurs presumably because of respiratory variation between PET and CT. PET images, requiring several minutes of acquisition per position, are averaged over many respiratory cycles, as opposed to the more rapid CT acquisition. When such misregistration is suspected, review of the non-attenuation-corrected images (Figure 6) can be helpful in confirming this artifact.

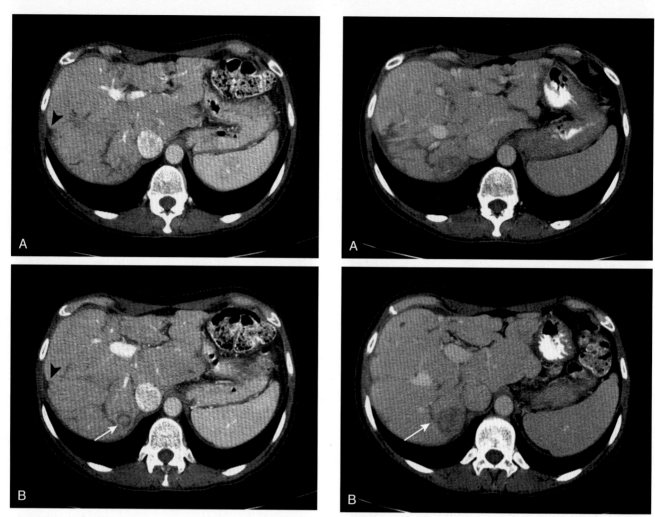

FIGURE 1. **A** and **B**, Portal venous (PV) phase enhanced images from abdominal CT scan show pseudocirrhosis treatment changes. The patient had previously been treated with chemotherapy for liver metastases. Linear, scar-like lucencies extend through the liver parenchyma, some extending to the liver surface where there is capsular retraction (*arrowheads*). A small, isodense residual lesion, outlined by surrounding lucency, is seen at the posterior right liver dome, best seen in **B** (*arrow*).

FIGURE 2. **A** and **B**, Repeat PV phase enhanced abdominal CT scan images at comparable levels, 3 months later, show interval growth of the hypodense liver metastasis in the posterior segment of the right lobe, adjacent to the inferior vena cava, best seen in **B** (*arrow*). The pseudocirrhosis changes impart a nodular contour to the liver surfaces.

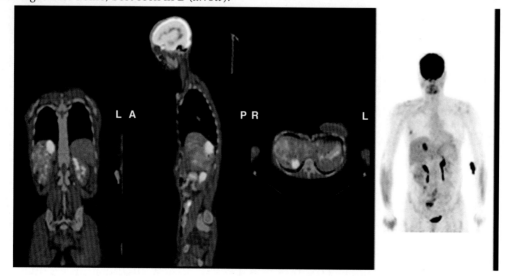

FIGURE 3. Fused PET/CT images (*left to right:* coronal, sagittal, axial, and coronal projection PET volume image), concurrent with CT scans in Figure 2, show the growing posterior segment right lobe liver metastasis at the dome to be intensely hypermetabolic. The coronal projection image shows a separate focus of activity in the right hemithorax, which proved to be a rib fracture. See Case 8 in Chapter 8 for a discussion of bone findings in this same patient.

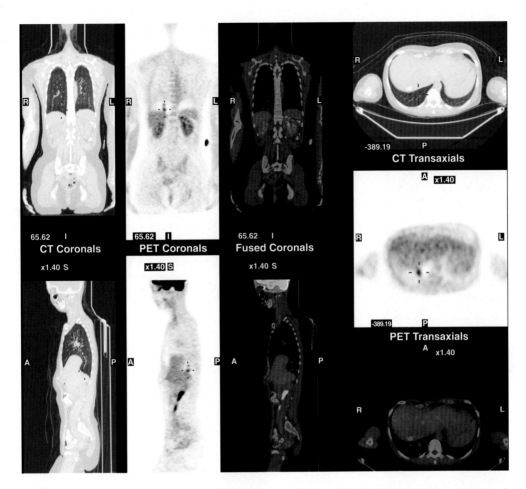

FIGURE 4. Repeat PET/CT scan, 6 months later, including CT with lung windows, PET, and fused PET/CT images, shows a small hypermetabolic focus (*cursors*), which projects in the right lung base. However, the lung windows show no corresponding abnormality. Note the abnormal step-off and abrupt change in contour of the right hemidiaphragm in the sagittal projection, a clue that respiratory variation produced this artifact.

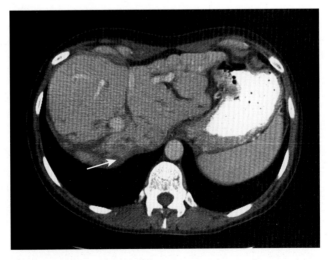

FIGURE 5. Concurrent enhanced chest and abdominal CT scans showed no lesion at the right lung base, but confirmed recurrent growth of the previously recognized waxing and waning metastasis in the posterior right liver dome (*arrow*). Pseudocirrhosis changes of the rest of the liver are again seen, with linear fibrosis in the right lobe, extending to the surface with capsular retraction, and macronodularity of the left lobe. The patient's therapy was changed from Navelbine to doxorubicin HCl (Doxil) in response.

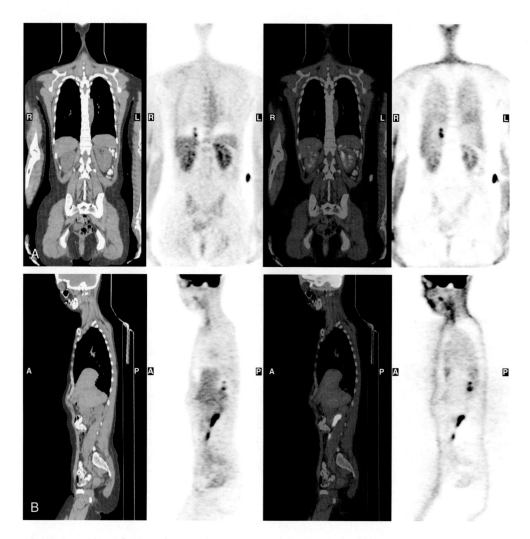

FIGURE 6. Coronal (**A**) and sagittal (**B**) PET/CT images (*from left to right:* CT, CT attenuation-corrected [AC] PET, fused PET/CT, non-attenuation-corrected [NAC] PET) allow comparison of the apparent position of the lesion between AC and NAC PET. On AC PET, the hypermetabolic bilobed lesion projects in an artifactual "clear zone" created by respiratory variation at the border between the lung base and liver dome, whereas on NAC PET, the lesion projects in the liver.

SUGGESTED READINGS

Osman MM, Cohade C, Nakamoto Y, et al. Mislocalization of lesions with PET/CT. *J Nucl Med* 2003; 44: 240–243.

Young ST, Paulson EK, Washington K, et al. CT of the liver in patients with metastatic breast carcinoma treated by chemotherapy: findings simulating cirrhosis. *AJR Am J Roentgenol* 1994; 163:1385–1388.

CASE 4

Progressive liver metastases on CT and PET

A 64-year-old woman, 3 years after right mastectomy, chest wall and supraclavicular radiation, and chemotherapy for breast cancer, was found to have an abnormally elevated tumor marker (CA 27.29). Her tumor was a 2.8-cm infiltrating ductal carcinoma, estrogen receptor and progesterone receptor positive, *HER-2/neu* positive, with 1 of 15 lymph nodes involved.

Evaluation with positron emission tomography (PET) and CT showed two liver metastases, one in each lobe, confirmed by biopsy of a left lobe lesion. The patient was evaluated for possible surgical or radiofrequency ablation therapy, but the presence of lesions in both lobes of the liver and lack of clinical data documenting benefit of resection in this setting resulted in the patient being treated instead with letrozole (Femara).

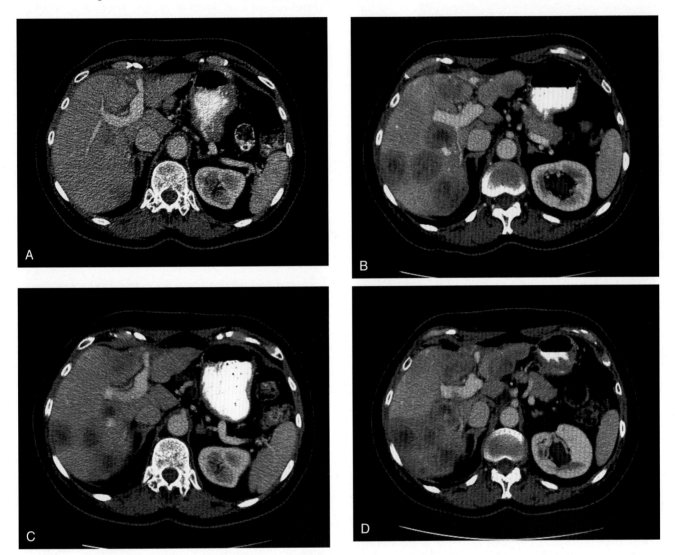

FIGURE 1. Enhanced abdominal CT images (displayed with liver windows, portal venous phase), obtained over a period of 14 months, showing a waxing and waning change in appearance of multiple metastatic breast cancer lesions, as this patient's therapy is adjusted. **A**, Vague, poorly defined hypodensities are seen in the liver. The corresponding PET scan showed five discrete foci of liver hypermetabolism. These findings were improved compared with 6 months before. **B**, Comparable repeat, enhanced abdominal CT at the same level, 5 months later, shows clear progression by CT. Five discrete individual liver metastases are now clearly defined, with low-density central necrosis and thick, enhancing tumor margins. The patient's therapy was changed from Herceptin and Navelbine to Xeloda. **C**, Repeat enhanced abdominal CT scan at the same level, 5 months later, shows the same number of liver metastases. Their size is similar, but there has been interval change in the appearance of the lesions, with less well-defined margins. **D**, Repeat enhanced abdominal CT scan at the same level, 4 months later (14 months after **A**) shows worsening. The metastases have grown, becoming nearly confluent in the posterior right lobe. Thick, enhancing tumor margins again show relatively well-defined edges. The patient's therapy was changed from Faslodex to Avastin and Taxol.

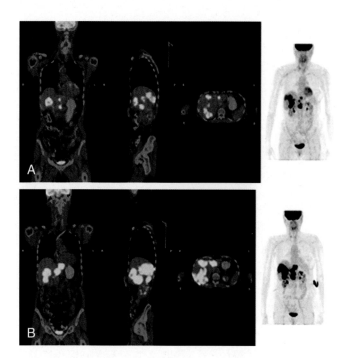

FIGURE 2. Three plane PET/CT fused images. **A**, This study is concurrent with Figure 1C. Multiple hypermetabolic liver lesions are seen, which were not clearly changed by PET compared with 5 months earlier. The patient had been on Xeloda during this time interval. On CT, the lesions were more ill-defined. **B**, Repeat study, 4 months later, concurrent with CT in Figure 1D. Clear progression of liver metastases is demonstrated by PET, correlating with the change in size and appearance of the liver lesions on CT. The patient's therapy was changed from Faslodex to Avastin and Taxol.

Periodic PET and CT evaluations were obtained over the next 3 years, to assess treatment responses, especially when tumor progression was suggested by rising tumor markers and liver function abnormalities (Figures 1 and 2). These showed a waxing and waning CT response of the liver metastases to adjustments in therapy, but there was an overall progression of her liver metastases. Her treatment regimen was adjusted numerous times, with multiple regimens utilized, including trastuzumab (Herceptin) and exemestane (Aromasin), Herceptin and vinorelbine tartrate (Navelbine), then capecitabine (Xeloda), followed by fulvestrant (Faslodex), and ultimately, bevacizumab (Avastin) and paclitaxel (Taxol). Over this time period, the patient remained relatively asymptomatic.

TEACHING POINTS

This patient was relatively asymptomatic while undergoing treatment for liver metastatic breast cancer. She was treated over a period of years with a variety of regimens, with initial responses, but ultimately progression. This was heralded by rising liver function tests and tumor markers, and confirmed by imaging with CT and PET scans. As shown here, sometimes the anatomic imaging responses to treatment can be ambiguous. These liver metastases seemed to wax and wane in conspicuity, becoming ill defined and less measurable when responding to treatment, and showing more aggressive characteristics when progressing. Supplementing the CT anatomic information with functional information from PET allows a higher confidence level in interpreting the significance of such changes in appearance.

CASE 5

Liver metastases arising in fatty liver, better seen on CT than PET

A 38-year-old woman with known metastatic breast cancer to bone on fulvestrant (Faslodex) was evaluated with PET and CT for increased aches and pains, and rising tumor markers.

Her breast cancer was diagnosed 3 years earlier when she presented with a left palpable estrogen receptor–positive, *HER-2/neu*-negative tumor and was treated with mastectomy. Bone metastases were identified at the time of her initial diagnosis, and the patient was treated with six cycles of doxorubicin (Adriamycin) and cyclophosphamide (Cytoxan) chemotherapy. She also received radiation therapy for lumbar spine epidural disease and a left proximal femoral metastasis.

PET/CT and contrast-enhanced body CT scans obtained to restage the patient showed new liver metastases. These were readily seen on CT as relatively hyperdense lesions against a background of a markedly fatty liver (Figure 1). The corresponding PET/CT scan, although abnormal and changed from a prior study, showed only subtle corresponding abnormalities, manifested as increased liver inhomogeneity (Figure 2).

The patient's therapy was changed to docetaxel (Taxotere) and capecitabine (Xeloda). She improved clinically and her tumor markers declined.

Repeat staging studies, 2 months later, confirmed the clinical and biochemical improvement (Figures 3 and 4).

TEACHING POINTS

This is an unusual case in which new liver metastases are more convincingly diagnosed on CT than from the PET scan. We are reminded of the complementary nature of anatomic (CT and MRI) and functional (PET) imaging. In this case, the extensive fatty change of the liver serves as an intrinsic contrast on CT, against which the new, solid, relatively hyperdense lesions are easily seen. We can speculate as to why these liver metastases are not more obvious on the PET study. Size likely is a contributing factor. The largest lesion by CT was 2 cm, but most of the lesions were on the order of 1 cm in diameter, about the lower limit to identify liver metastases on PET. Although the lower limit of

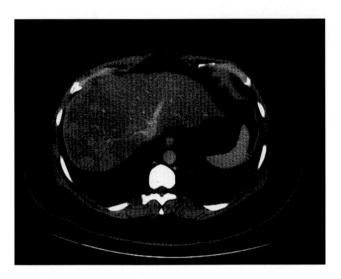

FIGURE 1. Contrast-enhanced abdominal CT scan (displayed with liver windows, portal venous enhancement) shows the liver to be fatty, with diffusely decreased density relative to spleen. Multiple, relatively hyperdense, focal liver lesions can be seen against this background in the right lobe of the liver.

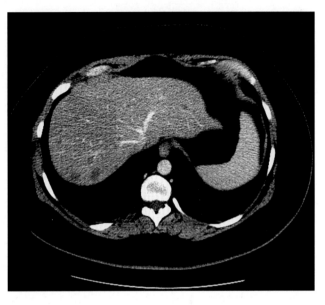

FIGURE 3. Repeat contrast-enhanced abdominal CT scan (displayed with liver windows, portal venous enhancement) shows the focal liver lesions to be hypodense relative to liver parenchyma, which does not appear as fatty as before.

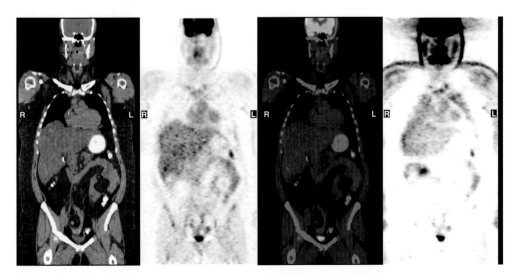

FIGURE 2. Concurrent coronal PET/CT scan shows subtle corresponding findings, with heterogeneity of the liver activity.

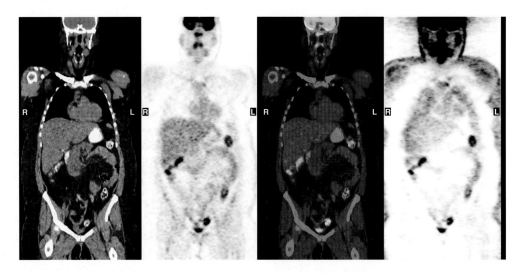

FIGURE 4. Repeat coronal PET/CT scan, concurrent with CT in Figure 3, shows improved homogeneity of liver activity compared with the prior study. The patient's symptoms had improved, and her previously rising tumor markers had stabilized.

resolution for PET scanners today is about 6 mm, what can be seen at this size depends on the intrinsic metabolic activity of the particular tumor and its location. The liver itself has a standardized uptake value (SUV) of about 2.5, so a small metastasis within it has to be that much more metabolically active to be visualized.

Another potential contributing factor is that this patient was on long-standing treatment for breast cancer bone metastases and was on Faslodex at the time of imaging. Her liver metastases may have been partially treated by this agent.

CASE 6

Evolution of liver metastases with treatment to cyst-like residuals

A 61-year-old woman with known, long-standing metastatic breast cancer to bone and skin developed fatigue and rising tumor markers, which was assessed with enhanced body CT scans and PET/CT. Her original breast cancer was 20 years earlier, a right, T2N0, infiltrating ductal carcinoma (IDC), estrogen receptor and progesterone receptor positive, which was treated with lumpectomy and radiation. Tamoxifen had been declined. Metastatic

disease was detected 14 years after the original diagnosis (6 years before the current evaluations) with new left breast biopsy-confirmed IDC, as well as clinically apparent left supraclavicular adenopathy and bone scan evidence of osseous metastases. The patient received chemotherapy (doxorubicin [Adriamycin] and cyclophosphamide [Cytoxan]) (AC) and was subsequently managed over a period of years with a variety of regimens, including tamoxifen and monthly zoledronic acid (Zometa), letrozole (Femara) and pamidronate disodium (Aredia), and later Aredia and fulvestrant (Faslodex).

By the time liver metastases were identified, the patient had progressive bone metastases for 6 years. In addition to the systemic therapies, she had been treated with radiation to the lumbar spine for painful epidural disease and with samarium for recurrent back pain. See Case 4 in Chapter 8 for a discussion of imaging manifestations of this patient's bone metastases and neural consequences.

Enhanced CT scan of the abdomen showed new, peripherally enhancing, centrally necrotic liver masses, with typical CT findings of liver metastases (Figures 1 and 2). After treatment with chemotherapy (docetaxel [Taxotere]), an interesting evolution in appearance of the liver lesions was seen on CT (Figures 3, 4, and 5).

TEACHING POINTS

Ideally, treated metastases would respond unambiguously, with complete resolution. In reality, responding liver metastases can show a host of

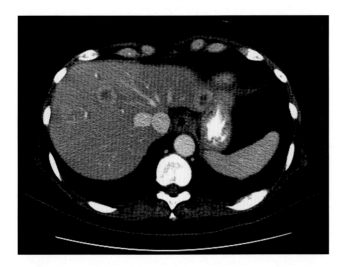

FIGURE 1. Enhanced axial CT image through the liver (portal venous [PV] phase, displayed with a liver window) shows two similar-appearing new metastatic lesions, one in the right lobe, anterior segment (segment 8) and one in the left lobe, lateral segment (segment 2). Both show typical CT features of metastases, with central hypodensity reflecting necrosis, as well as thick, peripheral rims of enhancing tumor.

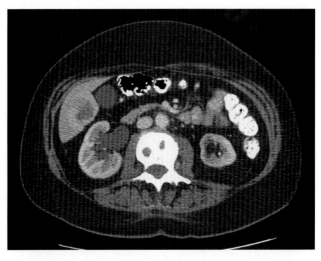

FIGURE 2. In the posterior segment of the right lobe inferiorly (segment 6), a larger lesion with necrosis is seen. Only this lesion showed increased metabolic activity on a concurrent PET scan.

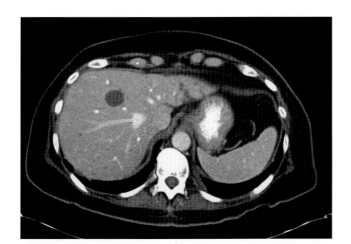

FIGURE 3. Repeat enhanced, PV phase abdominal CT, 3 months later, after treatment with Taxotere chemotherapy, shows the index lesion in segment 8 to have changed in appearance (compare with Figure 1). It now appears cystic, although careful inspection shows a thin, enhancing rim. Irregular, linear hypodensity is now seen at the level of the previously seen lesion in the lateral segment of left lobe (segment 2). Tiny hypodensities are also suggested in the posterior right lobe.

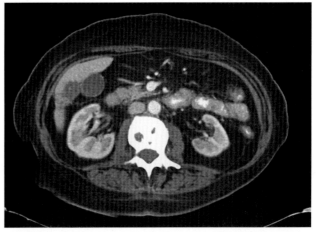

FIGURE 4. Three-month follow-up enhanced, PV phase abdominal CT scan through the lesion in segment 6 (compare with Figure 2) shows a hypodense residual, with resolution of the associated enhancement. Note development of capsular contraction at this level.

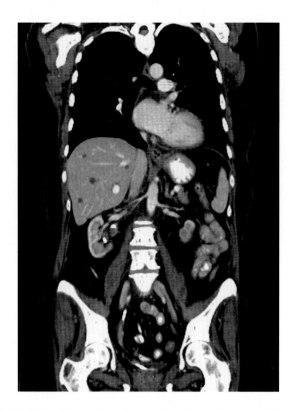

FIGURE 5. Coronal reconstruction from the same CT scan shows scattered small lucencies throughout the liver. Their appearance resembles cysts, but the patient was known from earlier studies not to have liver cysts. These developed after treatment of fairly typical-appearing liver metastases. These represent a relatively unusual response to treatment.

responses, ranging from complete resolution to shrinkage in size to morphologic alterations, generally with a decrease in size. Not only can treated liver metastases change in appearance but also treatment can induce changes in the liver. Capsular contraction, such as seen at the level of the largest metastasis in this case, is a frequently observed finding. The pretreatment appearance of these metastases is typical, with central necrosis and peripheral enhancement of the viable rim. A variety of post-treatment appearances are demonstrated here. The largest lesion in the inferior right lobe is smaller, with retraction of the adjacent capsule. Other lesions show a pseudocystic appearance. A larger lesion in the anterior right lobe in Figure 3 resembles a cyst at first glance. However, the presence of any enhancement, such as this thin, enhancing rim, differentiates it from a cyst.

CHAPTER 10

Thoracic Metastases, Mimics, and Treatment Effects

Most breast cancer patients with intrathoracic metastases are asymptomatic, the exception being those with significant pleural effusions. Therefore, unless pleural, parenchymal, or nodal metastases are demonstrated at initial staging, thoracic metastases are most commonly found at the time of follow-up imaging. A significant number are found on chest x-rays done for other reasons. Isolated involvement of the lung or pleural space occurs in 15% to 25% of women with metastatic breast cancer.[1]

Pulmonary metastases are typically peripheral,[2] and, if large enough, may be discovered on preoperative chest radiographs. Because of its low cost, chest radiography may be a reasonable choice as a baseline study or in follow-up; however, the extremely low yield, false-positive results, inferior sensitivity compared with CT, and lack of data supporting an outcome benefit limit routine use in follow-up.

CT is the preferred modality for investigation of thoracic metastases. CT has proven efficacy for detecting local, regional, and distant disease. Normal-sized internal mammary nodes are not visualized on CT, so a patient in whom CT identifies a node or nodes larger than 6 mm is at risk for malignant involvement.[3] Because of the recognized problem of relying on size only to diagnose disease, positron emission tomography (PET)/CT is presently considered the modality of choice for assessing internal mammary nodes (Figure 1). In women who die from disseminated breast cancer, intrathoracic nodal metastases may occur in more than 70% of patients.[4] As with internal mammary nodes, using size as the major criterion for disease identification reduces both sensitivity and specificity. Magnetic resonance imaging (MRI) can detect most lesions larger than 5 mm, does not expose the patient to ionizing radiation, and has acceptable imaging times; however, it is generally viewed as complementary to CT, rather than as a replacement for CT (Figure 2).[5–9] Cardiac and respiratory motion, reduced sensitivity for lesions smaller than 5 mm (compared with CT), calcified metastases, and suboptimal ability to assess lymphangitic spread are recognized limitations of MRI in the thorax.[10]

PET using fluorodeoxyglucose (FDG), an analogue of glucose, has assumed a primary role as a whole-body survey examination in many types of cancer, including breast. PET, and more recently PET/CT, excels at identifying the metabolic status of intrathoracic nodes, including internal mammary nodes, and solitary pulmonary nodules. Metabolic changes, resulting in pathologic or increased uptake on PET scan, can occur months before changes in size or shape. Additionally, it is now well recognized that lymph nodes larger than 10 mm may be benign or reactive, and lymph nodes smaller than 10 mm may represent metastases. With one important caveat, PET does not rely on the size of a lymph node or nodule to characterize it as benign or malignant. The caveat relates to the sensitivity of the PET/CT system based on lesion size. Presently, most scanners in clinical practice are able to reliably identify hypermetabolic foci down to about 8 mm. The addition of CT capability in PET/CT combination units will in many cases further improve sensitivity by allowing relatively precise image registration. The ability to confirm hypermetabolic activity in very small lesions may complicate reliance on the standardized uptake value (SUV). This calculated value is a measure of radioactivity in a lesion divided by the average value of radioactivity in the body, corrected for body weight. Many centers use a cut-off value of 2 to 2.5 or higher to indicate malignancy, with values less than 2 as evidence for benignity. The SUV is dependent on a multitude of factors, including serum glucose at the time of FDG injection, time between injection and imaging, and lesion size. Many investigators believe that any uptake above background in small (i.e., 5 to 7 mm) lesions should be regarded as suspicious for malignancy.

In one series of 73 patients who underwent FDG PET and CT for recurrent or metastatic disease, PET proved more sensitive (85% versus 50%) and specific (90% versus 83%) than CT. Also, PET uptake in mediastinal and internal mammary nodes was 2 times more prevalent than enlarged nodes on CT.[11]

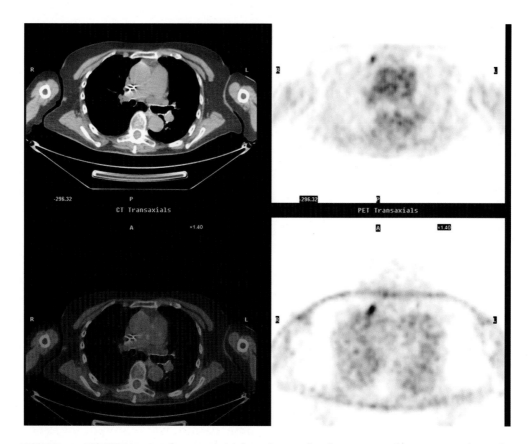

FIGURE 1. PET/CT images from an initial staging study of a 77-year-old woman with newly identified locally advanced infiltrating ductal carcinoma (IDC). Internal mammary nodal involvement is seen on the right. Normal internal mammary lymph nodes are not usually visualized on chest CT. This enlarged node, measuring 8 mm, is readily seen on CT and is hypermetabolic on PET. Although not biopsy proven, these imaging features are strong presumptive evidence of internal mammary nodal involvement. Seven of 12 axillary nodes were involved with tumor at surgery.

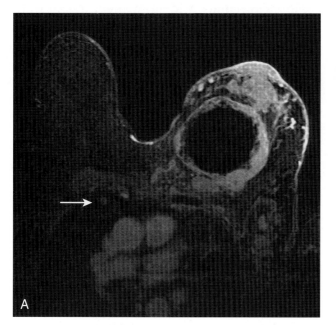

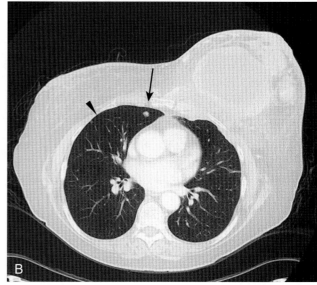

FIGURE 2. **A,** Breast MRI of a neglected, locally advanced left breast cancer with chest wall, skin, and nipple involvement shows a lung nodule on the right, suggesting possible stage IV disease (*arrow*). **B,** Chest CT confirmed a lung nodule, with an additional tiny subpleural nodule seen on this slice as well (*arrowhead*).

FDG PET has been shown to be significantly more accurate in staging the mediastinum in patients with non–small cell lung cancer, using histology as the gold standard.[12–13] Extrapolation of these data to patients with breast cancer may be problematic. It has been recognized that certain subtypes of breast cancer (e.g., invasive lobular, tubular, carcinoma in situ) show relatively low FDG uptake, resulting in reduced sensitivity compared with infiltrating ductal carcinoma (IDC) primary tumors.[14–15] Theoretically, patients whose initial staging FDG PET is negative in these tumor subtypes (especially if the primary has not been excised) may demonstrate reduced sensitivity for detection of metastases, including within the chest, on restaging studies.

Pleural involvement may be suspected based on clinical signs on physical examination or symptoms (e.g., cough, shortness of breath, pleuritic-type chest pain, orthopnea), the discovery of a pleural effusion on plain radiography or CT, or the identification of pleural abnormalities on CT or FDG PET (Figure 3). Pleural effusion is often unilateral and on the same side as the breast primary.[16] The effusion can be confirmed by chest radiography, CT, or even ultrasound. Thoracentesis may be performed for both diagnostic and therapeutic purposes. If the result is nondiagnostic, or negative with a strong clinical suspicion of malignancy, consideration may be given to FDG PET imaging (preferably, PET/CT).

FDG PET commonly identifies more pleural involvement than other imaging modalities and may be especially helpful in delineating the caudal extent of disease. The effusion itself tends to be only mildly positive on PET or frankly negative, presumably owing to the paucity of malignant cells relative to the volume of the effusion.

Many special circumstances exist with respect to the thoracic manifestations of breast cancer, reviewed in depth by Jung and associates.[17] One important consideration is radiation therapy–related complications. Radiation pneumonitis typically occurs within 3 months of radiation therapy

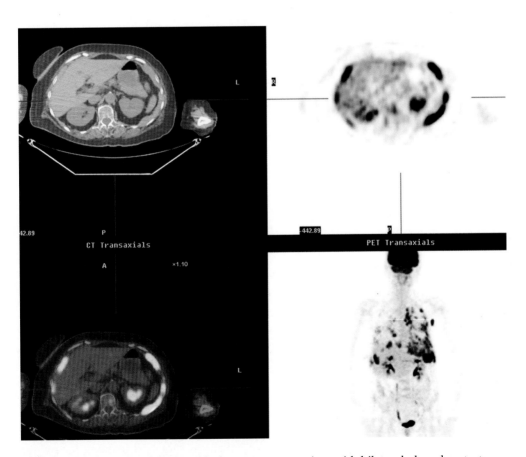

FIGURE 3. PET/CT axial images of a breast cancer patient with bilateral pleural metastases, more extensive on the left than the right. The pleural spaces extend far inferiorly, so that hypermetabolic pleural metastases appear to project in the periphery of the abdomen, overlapping the liver and spleen. The coronal projection image also shows a large, hypermetabolic left axillary lymph node.

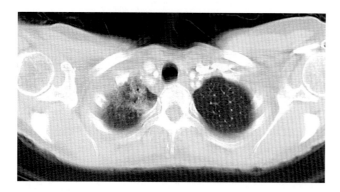

FIGURE 4. Axial lung window chest CT image from a 56-year-old woman, 4 years after treatment for a high-risk IDC involving 19 of 26 lymph nodes with lumpectomy, axillary dissection, systemic chemotherapy, and radiation to the breast, axillary, and supraclavicular nodal basins, shows asymmetrical right apical radiation fibrosis. This was stable on imaging, corresponded to the radiation field, and showed stable, low-level activity on FDG PET.

and progresses from diffuse haziness to coalescence of areas of consolidation to fibrous changes on chest x-ray or CT. Findings in the irradiated field may persist for months to years (Figure 4). Although PET/CT has demonstrated efficacy in separating scar from active tumor in many malignancies, its use following radiation therapy in the irradiated field may be problematic for months to 1 year or more. The heightened metabolic activity of activated monocytes at sites of radiation pneumonitis can last for a variable period of time, especially in the lung and with head and neck tumors. A negative FDG PET study at a site of postirradiation change on chest x-ray or CT is reassuring; however, a positive study must be interpreted with caution and reassessed or further investigated before initiation of additional tumor-targeted therapy.

The development of a solitary pulmonary nodule in patients who have been treated for breast cancer should not be assumed to be a breast recurrence without histologic proof. About half of these patients will have lung cancer, and a small percentage of cases will be benign.[18] These patients are excellent candidates for PET/CT. Hypermetabolic uptake in the nodule directs the patient to tissue sampling (sometimes obviated by the finding of widespread metastases). Absent FDG uptake, as well as an otherwise negative study, may allow watchful waiting with short-term CT follow-up (e.g., 3 to 6 months). Recall the limitations of PET with respect to histology and lesion size.

Lymphangitic metastases are extremely common in women who die from breast cancer.[19] CT is the imaging modality of choice for the identification of

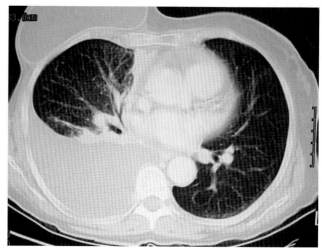

FIGURE 5. Axial lung window chest CT image from a 63-year-old woman with bone, thoracic, and brain metastases shows a large right pleural effusion. The lung parenchyma, particularly on the right, shows bronchovascular thickening and a finely nodular appearance of the interstitium, highly suggestive of lymphangitic tumor spread.

this process, which is most often bilateral (Figure 5). Findings include irregular thickening of the interlobar septa and peribronchovascular sheaths as well as thickening of the structures in the central regions of the secondary pulmonary lobules.[20]

REFERENCES

1. Patanaphan V, Salazar OM, Ricco R. Breast cancer: metastatic patterns and their prognosis. *South Med J* 1998; 81 (9):1109–1112.
2. Shaw JP, Glassman LR. Thoracic metastases from breast cancer. In Breast Cancer. Philadelphia, Elsevier Churchill Livingston, 2005, pp 661–666.
3. Meyer JE, Munzenrider JE. Computed tomographic demonstration of internal mammary lymph-node metastases in patients with locally recurrent breast carcinoma. *Radiology* 1981; 139:661–663 (A).
4. Thomas JM, Redding WH, Sloane JP. The spread of breast cancer: importance of intrathoracic lymphatic route and its relevance to treatment. *Br J Cancer* 1979; 40:540–547.
5. Feierstein IM, Jicha DL, Pass HL, et al. Pulmonary metastases: MR imaging with surgical correlation—a prospective study. *Radiology* 1992; 181:123–129.
6. Müller NL, Gamsu G, Webb WR. Pulmonary nodules: detection using magnetic resonance and computed tomography. *Radiology* 1985; 155:687–690.
7. Panicek DM. MR imaging for pulmonary metastases? *Radiology* 1992; 182:10–11.
8. Webb WR, Sustman HD. MR imaging of thoracic disease: clinical uses. *Radiology* 1992; 182:621–630.
9. Ohno Y, Sugimura K, Hatabu H. MR imaging of lung cancer. *Eur J Radiol* 2002; 44(3):172–181.

10. Vogt FM, Herborn CU, Hunold P, et al. HASTE MRI versus chest radiography in the detection of pulmonary nodules: comparison with MDCT. *AJR Am J Roentgenol* 2004; 183:71–78.

11. Eubank WB, Mankoff DA, Takasugi J, et al. [18]Fluorodeoxyglucose positron emission tomography to detect mediastinal or internal mammary metastases in breast cancer. *J Clin Oncol* 2001; 19:3516–3523.

12. Vansteenkiste JF, Stroobants SG, De Leyn PR, et al. Lymph node staging in non-small-cell lung cancer with FDG-PET scan: a prospective study on 690 lymph node stations from 68 patients. *J Clin Oncol* 1998; 16(6):2142–2149.

13. Scott WJ, Gobar LS, Terry JD, et al. Mediastinal lymph node staging of non-small-cell lung cancer: a prospective comparison of computer tomography and positron emission tomography. *J Thorac Cardiovasc Surg* 1996; 111(3):642–648.

14. Crippa F, Seregni E, Agresti R, et al. Association between [^{18}F]-fluorodeoxyglucose uptake and postoperative histology, hormone receptor status, thymidine labeling index and p53 in primary breast cancer: a preliminary observation. *Eur J Nucl Med* 1998; 25:1429–1434.

15. Avril N, Menzel M, Dose J, et al. Glucose metabolism of breast cancer assessed by ^{18}F-FDG PET: histologic and immunohistochemical tissue analysis. *J Nucl Med* 2001; 42:9–16.

16. Connolly JE, Jr, Erasmus JJ, Patz EF, Jr. Thoracic manifestations of breast carcinoma: metastatic disease and complications of treatment. *Clin Radiol* 1999; 54:487–494.

17. Jung JI, Kim HH, Park SH, et al. Thoracic manifestations of breast cancer and its therapy. *RadioGraphics* 2004; 24:1269–1285.

18. Casey JJ, Stempel BG, Scanlon EF, et al. The solitary pulmonary nodule in the patient with breast cancer. *Surgery* 1984; 96:801–805.

19. Kreisman H, Wolkove N, Finkelstein HS, et al. Breast cancer and thoracic metastases: review of 119 patients. *Thorax* 1983; 38:175–179.

20. Webb WR, Müller NL, Naidich NP, High-Resolution CT of the Lung, 3rd ed. Philadelphia, Lippincott Williams & Wilkins, 2001.

Solitary pulmonary nodule in the breast cancer patient: Primary lung cancer versus breast cancer metastasis

An 80-year-old woman with emphysema was found to have a left upper lobe (LUL) mass on chest x-ray. This was confirmed on chest CT, which also showed a similar-appearing, suspicious right lower lobe (RLL) lesion (Figure 1). Fine-needle aspiration (FNA) of the LUL lesion was consistent with a non–small cell lung carcinoma. The patient's past medical history was significant for prior left mastectomy for breast cancer nearly 20 years earlier. Lymph nodes were reportedly negative, and the patient did not undergo additional therapy at that time. She also had a significant past smoking history, on the order of 1.5 packs per day.

The PET scan showed both the LUL and RLL lesions to be hypermetabolic (Figure 2). Based on the information available, this result seemed most consistent with synchronous lung cancers. However, subsequent immunocytochemical stains performed on the material obtained from FNA suggested the cause to be metastatic breast carcinoma.

TEACHING POINTS

This is not an uncommon clinical scenario. Identification of solitary pulmonary nodules in patients with a history of breast cancer represents new diagnoses of lung cancer rather than metastatic breast cancer in about 50% of cases. Differentiation between these two diagnoses generally cannot be reliably made on morphologic grounds, as seen in this case, and requires histologic sampling. The distinction between primary lung adenocarcinoma (60% to 70% of lung cancers) and metastatic adenocarcinoma of breast is particularly difficult. Differentiation generally comes down to immunohistochemical stains.

In the rare patient who has a true solitary pulmonary breast cancer metastasis, there are data to suggest survival benefit from metastasectomy. However, consideration of surgical treatment requires careful imaging exclusion of other metastases. Today, such an evaluation should include bone scan; enhanced chest, abdomen, and pelvis CT scans; and positron emission tomography (PET) scan.

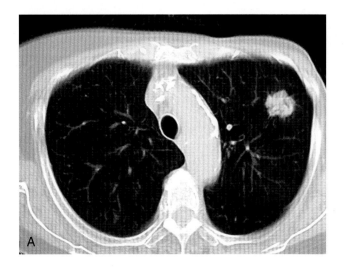 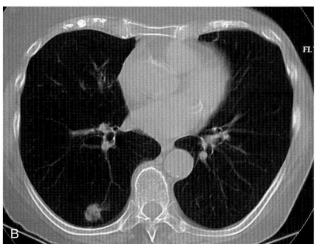

FIGURE 1. Two chest CT sections show similar-appearing lung masses, one in the anterior segment of the LUL (**A**), and the other in the superior segment of the RLL (**B**). Both display suspicious morphology, with irregular spiculated margins, suggesting primary bronchogenic cancers in appearance.

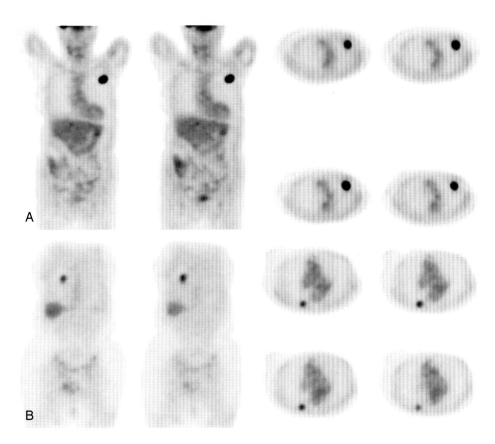

FIGURE 2. **A** and **B**, PET shows both lesions to be hypermetabolic, consistent with malignancy at both sites.

CASE 2

Lung metastases, progression to pleural metastases

A 56-year-old woman with biopsy-proven lung metastases, taking exemestane (Aromasin), was restaged after transferring her care. She was 8 years post diagnosis of a palpable node-negative, 3.5-cm left breast cancer, estrogen receptor positive, *HER-2/neu* negative. She had been treated with lumpectomy, radiation, and chemotherapy (four cycles of doxorubicin [Adriamycin] plus cyclophosphamide [Cytoxan] (AC)), but no hormone therapy.

Four years after her initial diagnosis, a chest x-ray showed lung nodules. Malignancy was confirmed with fine-needle aspiration. She was started on tamoxifen. Subsequent progression prompted a change in therapy to Aromasin.

At the time of restaging, the patient was essentially asymptomatic. Chest CT and positron emission tomography (PET) showed four lung nodules on CT, three of which were hypermetabolic on PET (a 3 × 7-mm nodule was probably too small) (Figures 1, 2, 3, 4, and 5).

Seven months later, follow-up CT scans showed new right pleural and mediastinal disease, confirmed as fluorodeoxyglucose avid on PET (Figures 6 and 7). The patient was not particularly symptomatic, and was reluctant to have chemotherapy. She began a trial of androgenic hormone therapy (Halotestin).

When she was re-evaluated 3 months later, she noted right posterior chest pain and dry cough. Imaging showed further progression. She was restaged in conjunction with the entrance requirements of a chemotherapy clinical trial. These studies showed progression of right pleural metastases and new liver metastases (Figure 8).

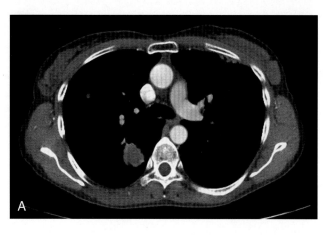
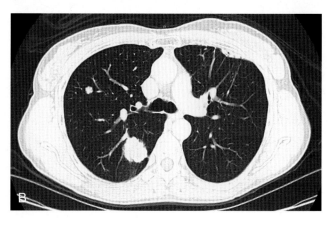

FIGURE 1. Contrast-enhanced chest CT (**A**, soft tissue window; **B**, lung window) images show two right lung nodules. The superior segment right lower lobe lesion measures 3 cm, whereas the right upper lobe lesion measures 1 cm. Fibrosis of the left anterior subpleural lung is from prior radiation therapy for breast cancer.

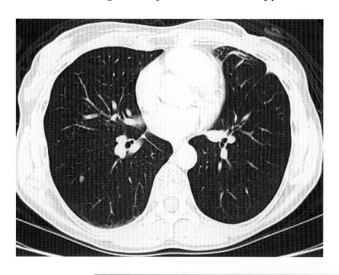

FIGURE 2. Lung window through the lower lobes shows a 3 × 7-mm nodule in the right lower lobe, which showed no correlate on PET, probably because of its size.

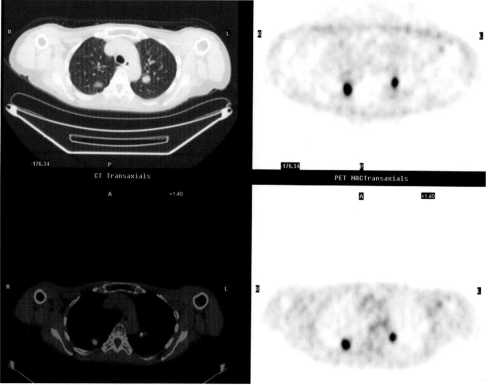

FIGURE 3. Axial PET/CT images show two hypermetabolic lung metastases.

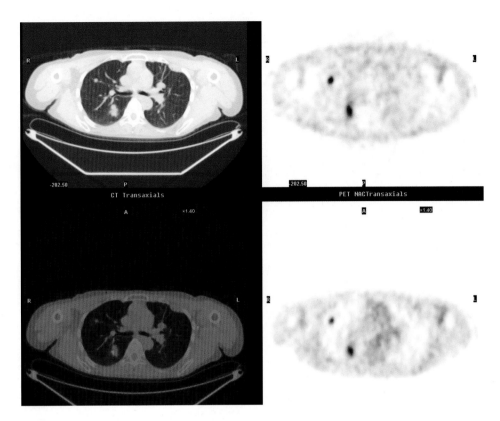

FIGURE 4.   A more inferior PET/CT image shows hypermetabolism in the two right lung lesions depicted in Figure 1.

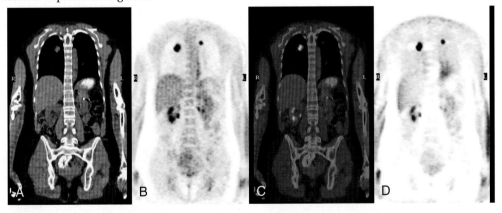

FIGURE 5.   **A** to **D**, Coronal PET/CT images show uptake in bilateral upper lobe metastases.

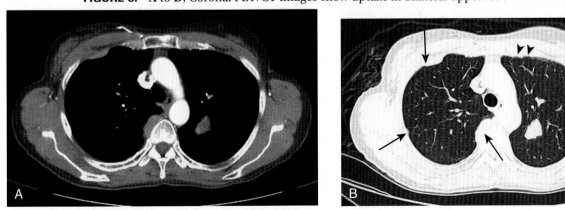

FIGURE 6.   Repeat chest CT, 7 months later. **A**, New, plaque-like right pleural soft tissue masses are now seen, in addition to the known left upper lobe (LUL) metastasis. **B**, Lung window from the same level as in **A** shows the LUL metastasis, left anterior subpleural radiation therapy change (*arrowheads*), and right pleural metastases (*arrows*).

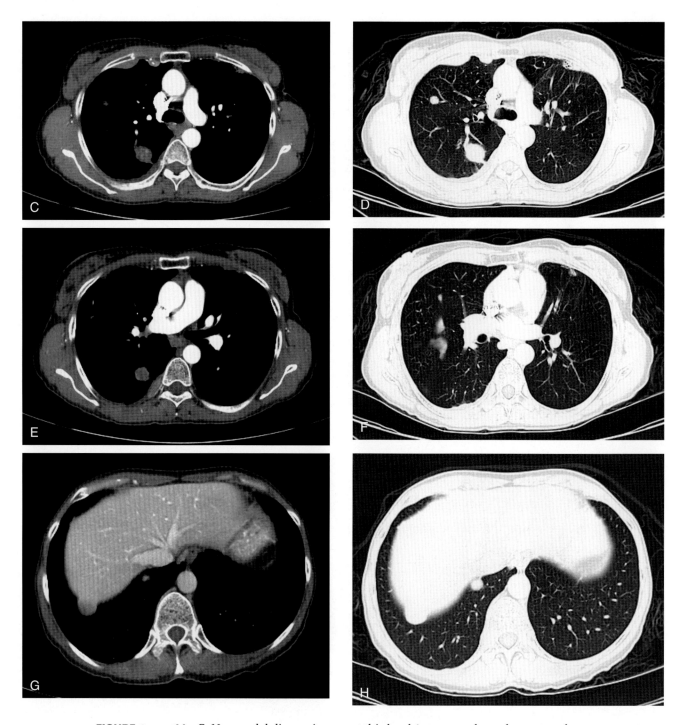

FIGURE 6, cont'd **C**, New nodal disease is seen at this level (azygoesophageal recess and right internal mammary), in addition to new right pleural metastases and the preexisting right lung nodules. A new pleural effusion is also noted. **D**, Lung window from the same level as **C**. **E**, A right paraspinal pleural based mass is outlined by pleural effusion at this level. **F**, Pleural metastases are seen in major and minor fissures on the right on this slice. **G**, Pleural metastases stud the right diaphragmatic pleura. **H**, Lung window from the same level as **G**.

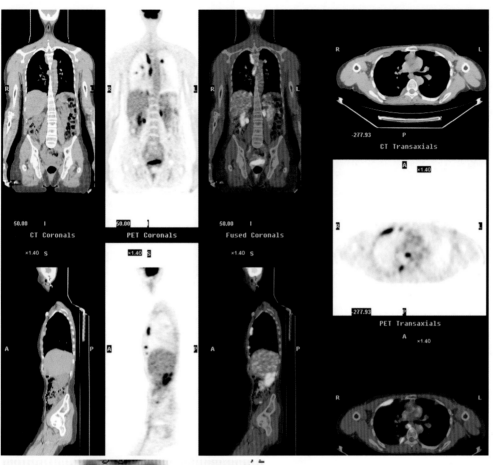

FIGURE 7. Concurrent PET/CT, 7 months after PET scan in Figures 3 to 5, shows new peripheral linear and nodular right hemithoracic hypermetabolism, which corresponds to the new pleural masses on CT and represents pleural metastases.

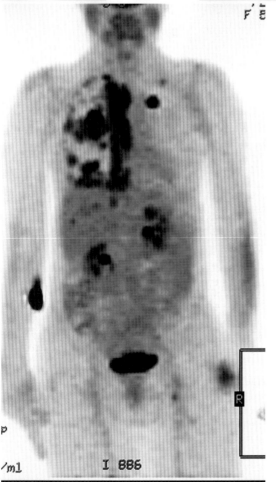

FIGURE 8. Coronal volumetric projection image, 5 months later, documents disease progression. The right hemithorax is encased in hypermetabolic tumor. Small metabolically active foci now are seen in the liver as well.

TEACHING POINTS

Malignant pleural effusions developing in breast cancer patients occur more frequently on the side ipsilateral to the breast cancer. This is thought to be lymphatic in etiology, due to transthoracic lymphatic communications, such as between internal mammary and mediastinal lymph nodes. Malignant pleural effusions can also result from hematogenous spread. Malignant pleural effusions developing contralateral to breast cancer may be more likely hematogenous in origin than ipsilateral pleural recurrences. In this case, this patient had known pulmonary metastases for more than 4 years, with little symptomatology on a variety of hormonal regimens, before progressing rapidly to pleural metastases and malignant effusion contralateral to her breast cancer.

This case reminds us of the resolution limits of whole-body PET scanners. With current technology, the lower limit of whole-body PET resolution is about 6 mm. Accordingly, it is not surprising that the smallest lung nodule found in this patient (3 × 7 mm) was not visualized on PET.

CASE 3

Chest wall, pleural, and thoracic nodal recurrence

A 55-year-old woman noted a palpable abnormality in her right breast, which had been treated for breast cancer 8 years before with lumpectomy, axillary lymph node dissection, radiation, and chemotherapy. Physical examination showed an obvious nodular skin recurrence. Her prior tumor was a poorly differentiated, 6.5-cm primary, estrogen receptor and progesterone receptor negative, HER-2/neu negative, with negative lymph nodes.

Mammography confirmed a corresponding 2.5-cm spiculated mass with suspicious pleomorphic microcalcifications, new from a prior study 4 years earlier. Palpation-guided fine-needle aspiration (FNA) was positive for malignant cells, and a concurrent skin punch biopsy showed adenocarcinoma involving the dermis, estrogen receptor

negative, progesterone receptor weakly positive, and HER-2/neu negative.

Initial evaluations suggested local recurrence only, and mastectomy was planned. However, her CA-125 was noted to be elevated, leading to restaging with positron emission tomography (PET)/CT, diagnostic enhanced body CT scans, and bone scan. PET and CT findings suggested thoracic recurrence (Figures 1, 2, 3, 4, and 5). CT scans showed a moderate-sized right pleural effusion with modest associated metabolic activity on PET. A 1-cm nodule in the right major fissure was metabolically active, as was a left hilar lymph node. The known right breast local recurrence was intensely hypermetabolic and could be faintly visualized as soft tissue activity on bone scan (Figure 6).

Based on the PET and CT findings, CT-guided thoracentesis and FNA of the right pleural nodule were performed. Both confirmed metastatic breast cancer by morphology and immunohistochemistry. Thyroid transcription factor-1 was noted to be

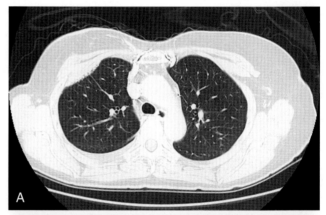
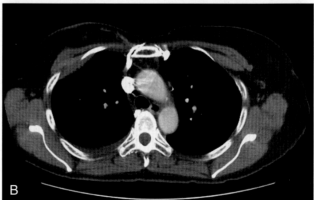

FIGURE 1.   Enhanced chest CT images (**A**, lung window; **B**, soft tissue window) show a right pleural effusion. Right anterolateral subpleural lung consolidation is seen, in a characteristic distribution for radiation fibrosis. Note the straight linear edge of the lung changes. Right breast skin thickening is also seen on this slice.

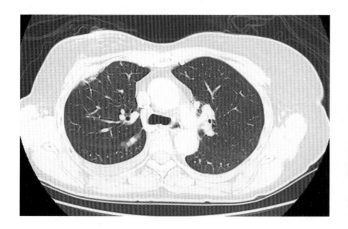

FIGURE 2. A more inferior lung window section, at the level of the aortopulmonary window, again shows right anterolateral subpleural radiation fibrosis changes and a right pleural effusion. Nodules up to 1 cm are seen in the right major fissure, suggesting that the etiology of the pleural fluid is neoplastic.

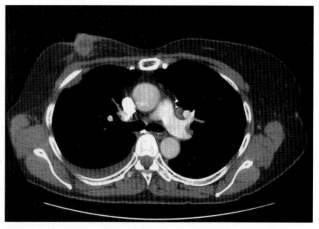

FIGURE 3. A more inferior slice, soft tissue window, shows a right breast mass, extending to the skin, which is locally thickened. A left hilar lymph node seen at this level was metabolically active on PET.

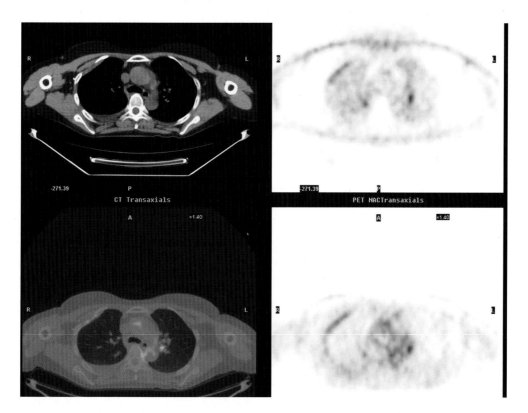

FIGURE 4. Axial PET/CT images, corresponding in level to Figure 2, show the right pleural nodules to be metabolically active. The associated activity is better seen on the NAC image (*upper right*) than on the AC image (*lower right*). A linear band of right anterolateral subpleural activity corresponds with the radiation fibrosis changes on CT, and was 8 years old. Activity corresponding with the left hilar lymph node is also seen. Note also subtle increased dependent activity in the right hemothorax compared with the left, seen on fused PET/CT (*lower left*) and AC PET (*lower right*), correlating with the pleural effusion. This, coupled with the pleural nodularity and activity, suggests a malignant etiology of the effusion, which was subsequently confirmed histologically.

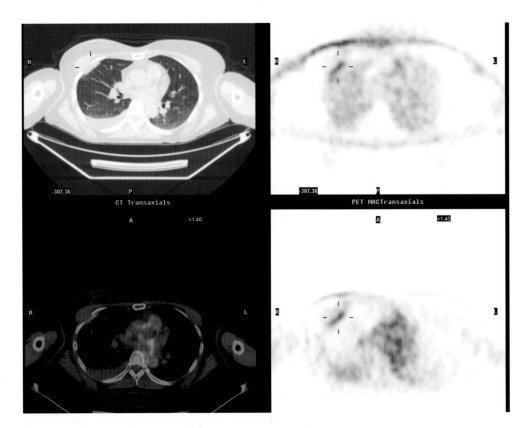

FIGURE 5. A more inferior axial PET/CT section shows similar findings, with subtle increased activity associated with the dependently layering right pleural effusion. Right subpleural anterolateral radiation fibrosis changes and activity is denoted by cursors.

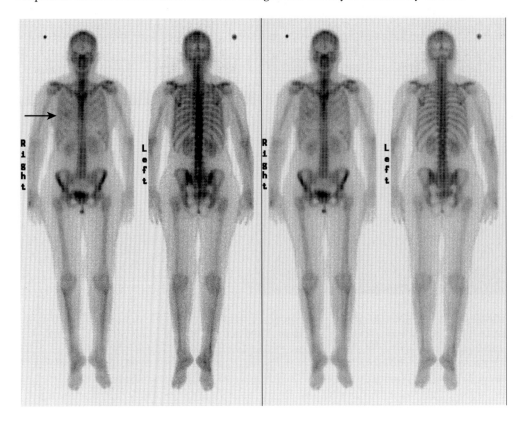

FIGURE 6. Anterior and posterior whole-body bone scan images showed no evidence of bony metastases, but subtle soft tissue activity can be seen in the right breast recurrence (*arrow*).

negative, largely eliminating lung cancer from the differential.

The patient's management was changed to chemotherapy, and the planned mastectomy was canceled. On paclitaxel (Taxol) and bevacizumab (Avastin), the patient demonstrated a good clinical and imaging response. The local recurrence, which had been symptomatic with fungation, healed well and largely resolved, and the PET scan activity regressed as well.

TEACHING POINTS

Pleural metastases are commonly manifested by the development of pleural fluid, which most often occurs on the same side as the primary breast carcinoma. The route of spread is thought to be lymphatic rather than hematogenous, which would be expected to be bilateral. This propensity for same-side laterality of pleural metastases is demonstrated in this case. The findings can range from effusion alone to fluid with variable degrees of pleural thickening and enhancement. This can be fairly smooth, as in this case, or frankly nodular and mass-like (see Case 5). Activity of pleural effusions on bone scans (see Case 4) and PET scans suggests a malignant etiology. In this case, both the pleural fluid and the nodules in the major fissure showed metabolic activity on PET, a constellation of findings strongly suggesting a malignant etiology, which was subsequently confirmed histologically.

Note that the PET scan findings are relatively subtle on the attenuation-corrected (AC) images, and are better seen on non-attenuation-corrected (NAC) images. This reminds us of the utility of reviewing the NAC data set, especially if no abnormalities are seen or to increase one's confidence level in subtle abnormalities suspected from the AC images.

The bone scan in this patient does not show soft tissue activity within the right hemithorax to correspond with this proven malignant pleural effusion. It does show subtle soft tissue uptake of the radiopharmaceutical in the right breast dominant mass recurrence.

This patient's radiation fibrosis changes show associated metabolic activity on PET 8 years after treatment. Radiation-induced lung fibrosis PET activity can persist indefinitely.

CASE 4

Pleural recurrence; bone scan and CT findings

A 57-year-old woman was found on preoperative evaluation for symptomatic mitral regurgitation to have a large right pleural effusion on chest x-ray. The patient noted concurrent right-sided chest tightness. Her history of breast cancer was 10 years before, stage II on the right, and was treated with mastectomy, postoperative radiation therapy, and chemotherapy. Three lymph nodes showed metastatic disease.

Diagnostic thoracentesis showed malignant cells consistent with breast primary, which were estrogen receptor and progesterone receptor positive. The patient was placed on anastrozole (Arimidex) after restaging studies showed no evidence of other disease (Figures 1 and 2).

TEACHING POINTS

This case illustrates many typical features of metastatic breast cancer in the pleura. As in this patient, metastases may develop years after the initial breast cancer diagnosis. The patient can be relatively asymptomatic, and the diagnosis may be made inadvertently during evaluation for other problems. Recurrences to pleura most commonly are to the same side as the original breast cancer. This is thought to be due to pleural interconnections through the internal mammary and intrathoracic lymph nodes.

Causes of asymmetrical nuclear medicine activity of the hemithoraces in breast cancer patients include prior surgery or radiation, presence of implants, and chest wall and pleural metastases. Knowledge of the prior clinical history is essential to assess the significance of asymmetry. Patients who have undergone mastectomy without reconstruction have less breast soft tissue to attenuate bone scan activity and consequently may show better visualization of rib activity on anterior views on the mastectomy side. Patients who have been treated with mastectomy and implant reconstruction may show decreased rib activity due to attenuation on the treated side. Radiation to the breast or chest wall may result in discernible photopenia of ribs on the treated side. In general, these treatment-induced changes are better visualized on

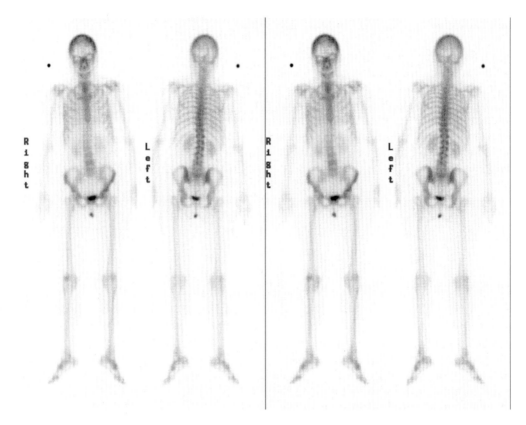

FIGURE 1.   Anterior and posterior whole-body bone scan images show subtle increased soft tissue activity of the right hemithorax compared with the left. This is a scintigraphic correlate for a malignant pleural effusion. No bone scan evidence of bony metastases is seen.

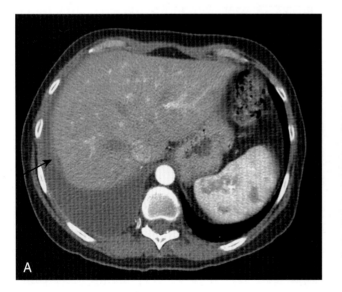
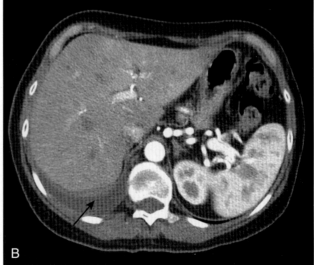

FIGURE 2.   Enhanced CT scans (hepatic arterial phase of enhancement) through the lower thorax and upper abdomen (**A**, above; **B**, below) show intense arterial enhancement in the aorta, heterogeneous splenic enhancement, and no enhancement of hepatic veins. A moderate-sized right pleural effusion is seen. Smooth thickening and enhancement of the right pleura is outlined by the fluid and is compatible with pleural metastases (*arrows*).

anterior views. Asymmetrical soft tissue activity such as seen here, visualized both anteriorly and posteriorly, suggests the possibility of tumor-related soft tissue activity. Most commonly, findings such as these are seen in the setting of a malignant pleural effusion, although such findings could be produced by extensive chest wall soft tissue recurrence.

CT findings of pleural recurrences range from effusion alone, to variable degrees of pleural enhancement and thickening (smooth or otherwise), to frank nodularity (see Case 5). The presence of pleural fluid serves as a natural contrast agent to allow interpreters to better visualize the pleura itself, which normally is thin to nearly imperceptible. Ready visualization of a thickened pleura in the presence of pleural fluid, in a patient with a cancer history, should heighten suspicion for a possible malignant etiology.

CASE 5

Pleural and chest wall recurrence

A 44-year-old woman with a history of breast cancer developed shortness of breath, and a chest radiograph showed a large right pleural effusion (Figure 1). The patient was 2 years post–right mastectomy and flap reconstruction for a node-negative, estrogen receptor–positive, progesterone receptor–negative, 1.5-cm infiltrating ductal carcinoma. The patient had declined chemotherapy and hormonal therapy.

Cytology of the serosanguineous thoracentesis aspirate confirmed carcinoma, consistent with breast primary. Workup with positron emission tomography (PET)/CT (Figures 2, 3 and 5) and enhanced body CT scans (Figures 4 and 6) showed findings of a malignant right pleural effusion, with abnormal right hemithoracic pleural thickening, nodularity, and enhancement, with a corresponding pleural rind of hypermetabolism on PET. Right anterior chest wall involvement was demonstrated, with hypermetabolism in asymmetrical soft tissue masses (Figures 2–6).

The patient was begun on chemotherapy with doxorubicin (Adriamycin) and docetaxel

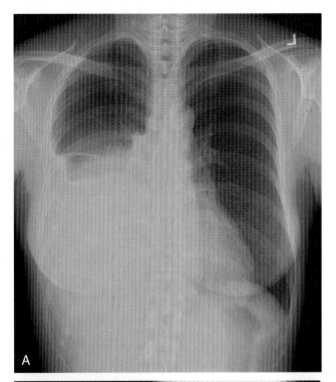

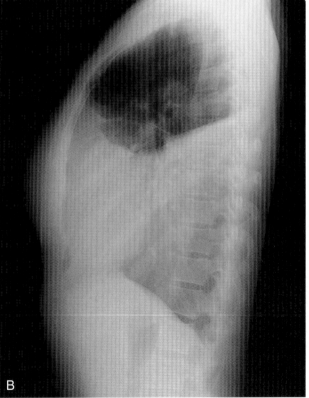

FIGURE 1. Posteroanterior (**A**) and lateral (**B**) chest x-rays obtained at presentation for shortness of breath show a large right pleural effusion, filling two thirds of the right hemithorax.

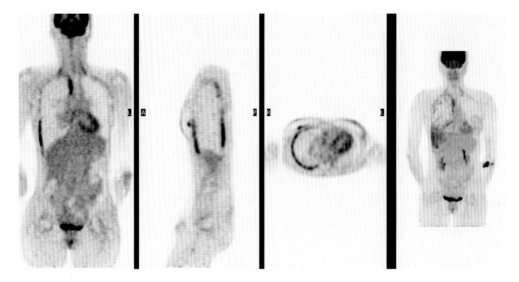

FIGURE 2.   PET scan images (*from left to right:* coronal, sagittal, axial, and coronal projection volume image) show intense linear hypermetabolism surrounding the right lung. This hypermetabolic pleural rind is a characteristic PET appearance of pleural metastases. The sagittal and axial images also show a separate focus of nodular hypermetabolism in the right chest wall soft tissues. The coronal projection image shows hypermetabolism in inferior pleural reflections overlapping the liver.

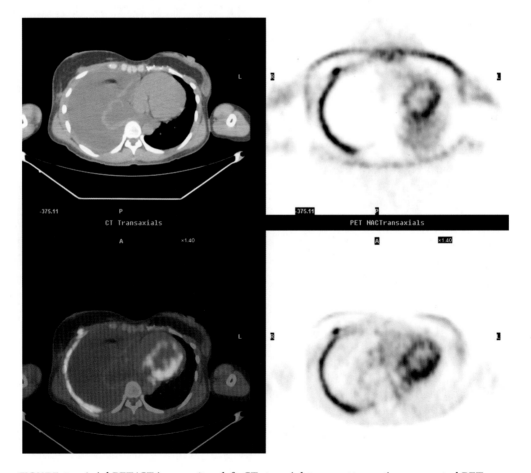

FIGURE 3.   Axial PET/CT images (*top left*, CT; *top right*, non-attenuation-corrected PET; *bottom left*, fused PET/CT; *bottom right*, attenuation-corrected PET) show the linear rind of metastatic pleural hypermetabolism, with a hypermetabolic soft tissue density nodule anteriorly in the right chest wall.

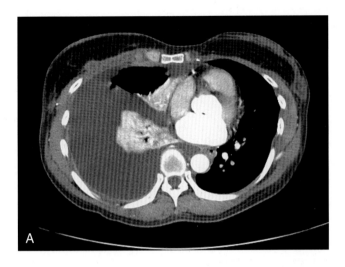 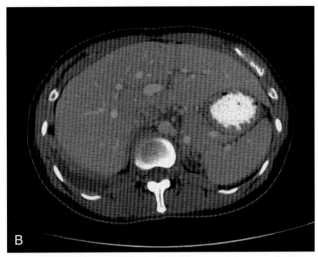

FIGURE 4. Contrast-enhanced CT images show corresponding findings. **A,** The large right pleural effusion is accompanied by a thickened, enhancing pleural rind. The right lower lobe is compressed and atelectatic because of the effusion. The reconstructed right neo-breast appears largely fatty, in contrast to the left breast. An enhancing nodule is seen at the anterior aspect of the asymmetrically thickened right anterior chest wall. This nodule corresponds with the focal anterior chest wall hypermetabolism on PET. **B,** Inferiorly, the thickened, enhancing pleura overlying the liver is more frankly nodular with metastatic tumor masses.

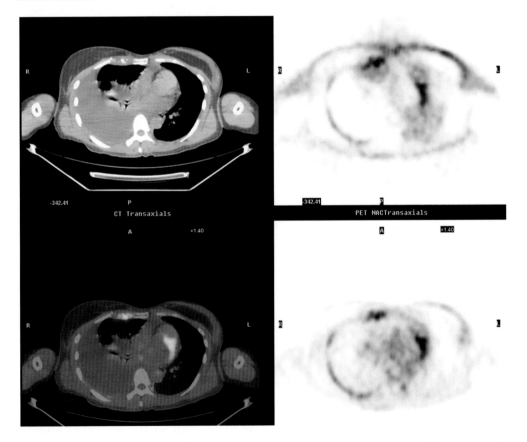

FIGURE 5. Axial PET/CT (*top left,* CT; *top right,* non-attenuation-corrected PET; *bottom left,* fused PET/CT; *bottom right,* attenuation-corrected PET) through the heart, with metabolically active left ventricular myocardium, shows the large malignant right pleural effusion with hypermetabolic pleural tumor rind. In addition, hypermetabolic soft tissue tumor thickening with destruction of costal cartilage is seen at the right parasternal level.

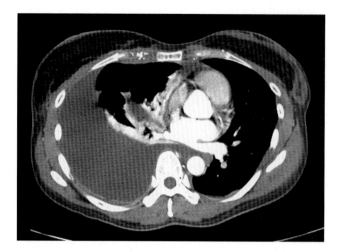

FIGURE 6. Corresponding enhanced chest CT level shows the large right malignant pleural effusion, enhancing pleural rind, atelectatic right lung base, and right parasternal soft tissue tumor expansion of the chest wall. Disorganized mineralization within the soft tissue presumably reflects costal cartilage replacement and destruction.

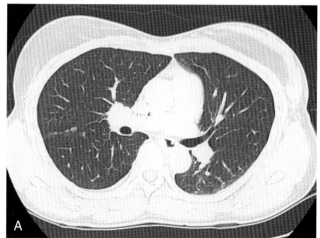

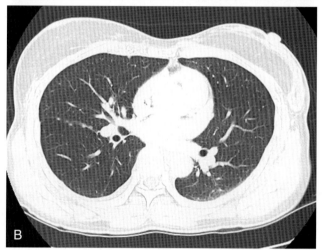

FIGURE 7. Chest CT images (lung windows, **A** and **B**) of repeat chest CT, 2 months later, after three cycles of chemotherapy, show improvement, with resolution of the right pleural effusion. Residual nodularity of the pleura is best seen along the major fissure, but also noted as subtle nodularity of pleural surfaces and tiny pleural-based nodules. Dependent density is noted on the left.

(Taxotere), as well as zoledronic acid (Zometa). Two months later, after three chemotherapy cycles, the chest CT was repeated to assess the response (Figures 7 and 8). In addition to resolution of the right pleural effusion, reduced pleural tumor burden was present, with tiny residual nodules where there previously had been bulky disease. In addition, small occasional sclerotic bone foci were now identified, thought to represent healing, formerly lytic bone metastases, previously unrecognized. These findings were stable and unchanged at repeat CT imaging 1 month later, after completion of chemotherapy, at which time the PET scan had normalized. The patient was then begun on tamoxifen.

TEACHING POINTS

Breast cancer is the most common cause of a malignant pleural effusion in women. Development of a pleural effusion in a patient with a history of breast cancer should be viewed as malignant until proved otherwise. The diagnosis is most easily established by thoracentesis with cytologic evaluation of the pleural fluid, with a diagnostic yield of 60% to 70%. More technically difficult and invasive options of percutaneous or thoracoscopic pleural biopsy may be required to make the diagnosis if pleural fluid cytology is inconclusive.

As this case illustrates, some patients respond well to chemotherapy. As in all of imaging, knowledge of the clinical history and familiarity with the prior imaging studies is critical to the accurate interpretation of follow-up examinations. Correlation of the follow-up CT with the prior study enables the correct conclusions to be drawn, namely that the patient is responding well to chemotherapy, with the pleural effusion resolved and the bulky pleural nodules reduced to tiny pleural-based residuals. This excellent response was subsequently confirmed by a repeat PET scan, which showed complete resolution of the hypermetabolic pleural rind. Interpreting the follow-up study without considering the prior studies could lead to serious misinterpretation, such as that the nodules are new parenchymal disease, which could suggest the patient is not responding and mislead the oncolo-

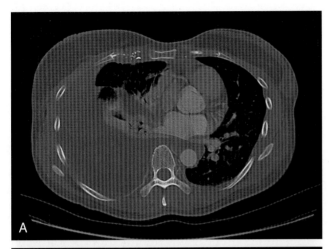

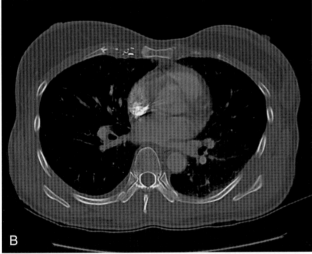

FIGURE 8. Bone windows from the two chest CT studies (**A**, initial; **B**, 2 months later, after three chemotherapy cycles) show conversion of lytic bone metastases to sclerotic, consistent with a healing response to treatment. Lytic change of the right anterior sternum on the initial study shows new sclerosis on the follow-up study. The right anterior chest wall soft tissue mass is diminished after therapy.

gist into considering an alternative chemotherapeutic course. Critical observations on the way to the correct interpretation of the follow-up study are that all of the tiny nodules are along pleural surfaces. Of course, comparison with the preceding study showing bulky pleural nodular disease, aids in the correct assessment.

This case also serves to remind us of important anatomic relationships. Disease overlying the surface of the liver may be below the diaphragm and may represent serosal implants on the liver surface or peritoneal implants. This disease overlying the liver (see coronal projection image from the PET, Figure 2, far right; and abdominal CT image, Figure 4B) is above the diaphragm, in the pleural space, which PET reminds us extends far inferiorly to overlap the liver.

Finally, this case demonstrates an interesting manifestation of clinically unrecognized and asymptomatic bone metastases. The follow-up study, after initiation of chemotherapy, showed several tiny new osseous sclerotic foci in the spine. No corresponding abnormality could be seen, even in retrospect, at some of these levels on the prior study. This response is illustrated in the right side of the sternum (see Figure 8). Lytic change can be seen on the initial study in the right sternum, where sclerosis develops on the follow-up study after chemotherapy. Presumably, these lytic, small bone metastases (too small to be seen on PET and mostly subradiographic on pretreatment CT) developed sclerosis as a healing response to chemotherapy.

CASE 6

CT and PET findings of talc pleurodesis for malignant pleural effusion

A 36-year-old woman was diagnosed with metastatic carcinoma to bone and the left hemithorax 4 years after mastectomy for a 1-cm left breast infiltrating lobular carcinoma. Her breast cancer was stage II, T1N1Mx, and was estrogen receptor positive and *HER-2/neu* 3+ positive. The patient had declined adjuvant therapy.

A left-sided pleural effusion was initially identified when the patient was evaluated for a cough 4 years after surgical treatment for breast cancer. An abnormality at T10 was noted during the same period, and biopsy confirmed metastatic breast cancer. The patient underwent thoracenteses twice of 1.5 liters of fluid, with negative cytologies. Ultimately, for management of the recurrent effusion, the patient underwent left hemithoracic thoracoscopy and thoracotomy, with drainage of the left pleural effusion, visceral and parietal pleurectomy, decortication of the left lung, and mechanical and talc pleurodesis. A pericardial effusion was also drained and a pericardial window created. Cytologies of both the pericardial and pleural fluid were positive for carcinoma, consistent with breast primary. Biopsies of the pleura, diaphragm, and pericardium confirmed metastatic carcinoma, consistent with metastatic lobular carcinoma. Evaluation of the visceral pleural specimens noted carcinoma extending into the subpleural alveolar septa.

The patient was begun on chemotherapy. Positron emission tomography (PET)/CT scans 1 and 3 months after the left pleurodesis showed similar findings, with left linear pleural space hypermetabolism (Figure 1), corresponding to the distribution of hyperdense talc on CT (Figures 2 and 3).

TEACHING POINTS

Talc pleurodesis is a known cause of prolonged pleural hypermetabolism on PET, and so effectively mimics pleural metastatic activity, particularly in patients thus treated for malignant pleural effusions. Pleurodesis is used to treat recurrent pleural effusions, and talc is one of the most effective agents used. Talc incites an intense granulomatous pleural inflammatory response, and expected post-treatment CT findings include pleural thickening and nodularity. These changes and residual loculated pleural effusion are difficult to differentiate from pleural metastases. Talc accumulations on CT resemble pleural calcifications and plaques. In case reports in the literature, PET activity corresponding to pleural deposition of talc has been seen years after pleurodesis.

In this case, the distribution of the PET activity corresponds precisely to the location of talc seen on CT. No pleural activity had been visualized in this patient when imaged with PET before pleurodesis, at a time when the patient was repeatedly undergoing large-volume thoracenteses, with negative cytologies.

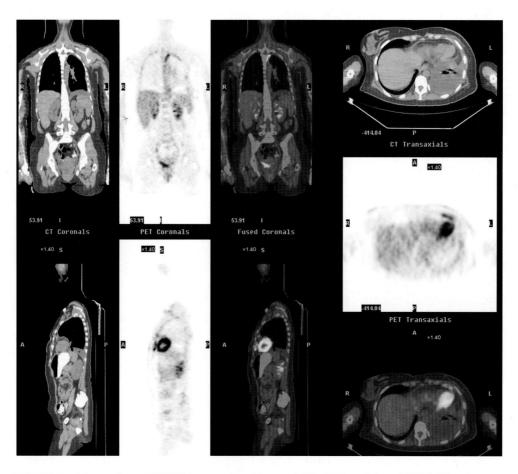

FIGURE 1. Three plane PET/CT images (unenhanced CT, PET, and fused PET/CT) show linear hypermetabolism in the left pleural space. On coronal slices, this is well seen at the left lung apex. Sagittal and axial images show linear hypermetabolism in the left anterior pleural reflection, anterior to the heart.

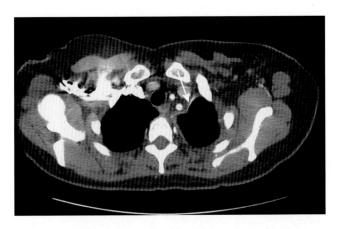

FIGURE 2. Contrast-enhanced chest CT slice through the lung apices shows linear hyperdensity along the left lateral aspect of the mediastinum (*arrow*).

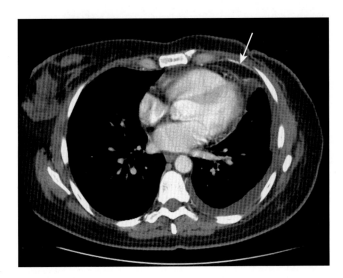

FIGURE 3. A slice from the same contrast-enhanced chest CT, through the heart, shows residual loculated pleural fluid. Anterior to the apex of the heart, linear hyperdensity can be seen along the pleural lining, consistent with talc (*arrow*).

SUGGESTED READINGS

Asad S, Aquino SL, Piyavisetpat N, et al. False-positive FDG positron emission tomography uptake in non-malignant chest abnormalities. *AJR Am J Roentgenol* 2004; 182(4):983–989.

Kwek BH, Aquino SL, Fischman AJ. Fluorodeoxyglucose positron emission tomography and CT after talc pleurodesis. *Chest* 2004; 125:2356–2360.

Murray JG, Erasmus JJ, Bahtiarian EA, et al. Talc pleurodesis simulating pleural metastases on F18 FDG PET imaging. *AJR Am J Roentgenol* 1997; 168:359–360.

CASE 7

Infraclavicular and mediastinal nodal recurrence presenting with brachial plexopathy symptoms

A 38-year-old woman elected to undergo prophylactic left mastectomy and bilateral transverse rectus abdominis musculocutaneous (TRAM) flap reconstruction 10 months after finishing radiation therapy for a right stage II, T2N1, 3-cm infiltrating ductal carcinoma, estrogen receptor and progesterone receptor negative and *HER-2/neu* negative, with 3 of 22 involved axillary lymph nodes. She had been treated with right mastectomy with clear margins, chemotherapy with four cycles each of doxorubicin (Adriamycin) and cyclophosphamide (Cytoxan) (AC) and paclitaxel (Taxol), and right chest wall, supraclavicular, and posterior axillary boost radiation therapy (see Case 18 in Chapter 3 for the presenting imaging features and staging of this patient).

Her initial staging workup had identified elevated tumor markers (CEA and CA 27.29). A PET/CT scan and enhanced diagnostic chest, abdomen, and pelvic CT scans were obtained and showed intense hypermetabolism in the known breast cancer and in a right axillary lymph node. Increased metabolic activity was also seen in a 5-mm right interpectoral (Rotter's) lymph node.

The patient had undergone genetic testing subsequent to her diagnosis and treatment, and proved to be *BRCA-1* positive. Her family history was of premenopausal breast cancer in a maternal aunt. She decided to undergo hysterectomy and oophorectomy, which was performed at the same time as prophylactic left mastectomy and bilateral TRAM flap reconstruction. Her left breast mastectomy specimen was benign.

The patient's postoperative course was complicated by development of abdominal wound infection, requiring débridement twice of infected, necrotic tissue and intravenous antibiotic therapy. She also required anticoagulation for pulmonary embolism. (See Case 3 in Chapter 6 for imaging features of a complicated TRAM flap donor site.)

During the patient's recovery from these procedures, she began to complain of right upper arm and shoulder pain. A lump developed under her

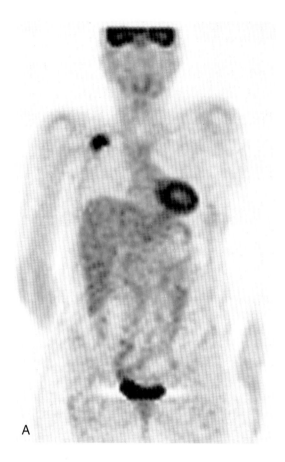

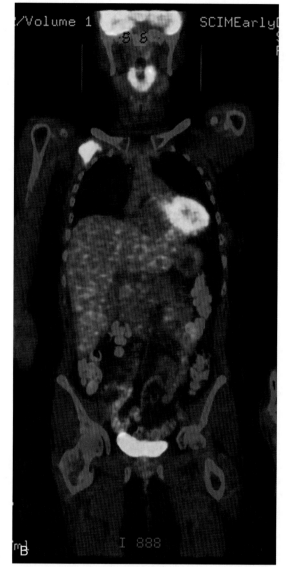

FIGURE 1. Coronal PET (**A**) and fused PET/CT (**B**) images show intense hypermetabolism at the right infraclavicular level.

right clavicle. She was imaged with enhanced body CT and PET/CT, which showed hypermetabolic nodal masses in the right paratracheal mediastinum and in the right infraclavicular region (Figures 1, 2, 3, and 4). These findings represented changes from prior studies, indicative of recurrent disease. Ultrasound of the right infraclavicular region identified a corresponding nodal mass (Figure 5), which was sampled with fine-needle aspiration technique, and confirmed recurrent adenocarcinoma, consistent with breast primary. To better define the extent of disease in light of the patient's symptoms of right shoulder pain, a brachial plexus MRI was obtained (Figures 6, 7, 8, 9, 10, and 11).

TEACHING POINTS

The anatomy of the brachial plexus is challenging to learn. Much of the confusion arises from the multiplicity of components. A simplified approach is suggested for the imager (adapted from Castillo), concentrating on landmarks for identification of the trunks and cords.

The brachial plexus is formed from the anterior rami of C5 through T1 in most people. The anterior rami reside just beyond the neural foramen. They form the trunks, which course between the anterior and middle scalene muscles (Figure 12), above the subclavian artery. The interscalene fat pad is an

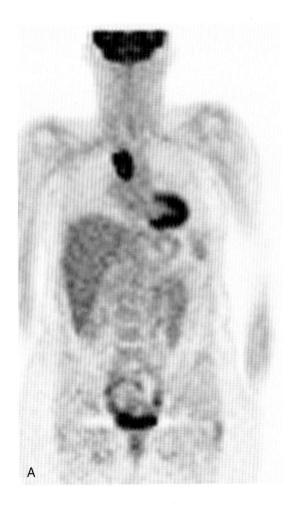

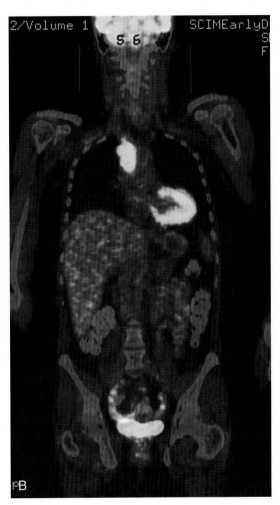

FIGURE 2. Coronal PET (**A**) and fused PET/CT (**B**) images show a second site of intense hypermetabolism, localizing to the right paratracheal mediastinal level.

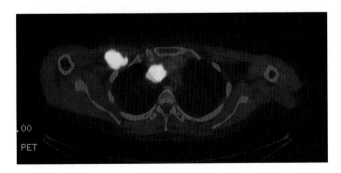

FIGURE 3. Axial fused PET/CT image shows the two sites of hypermetabolic uptake, one at the right infraclavicular level and the other at the right paratracheal mediastinum.

important anatomic landmark to evaluate for symmetry or effacement on coronal sequences because tumors or other processes at this level will impinge on brachial plexus trunks (Figure 13). These trunks ramify to form divisions posterior to the clavicle, which run in the supraclavicular triangle above the subclavian artery. These divisions ramify again to form cords inferior to the clavicle. These cords are the infraclavicular component of the brachial plexus with which we are most concerned in breast cancer patients. (Remember: Cords are the brachial plexus component behind the clavicle.) Although breast cancer metastases can arise anywhere along the course of the brachial plexus, the critical area is in the retroclavicular region around the cords of the brachial plexus. At this level, the cords are in close proximity to the axillary artery and vein (as the subclavian artery and vein are known lateral to the first rib).

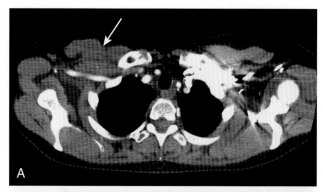

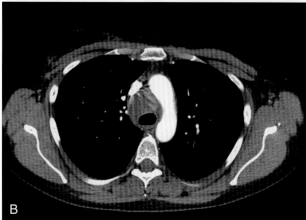

FIGURE 4. Contrast-enhanced chest CT images for correlation (**A** above **B**). **A**, A rounded, soft tissue mass (*arrow*) imparts increased bulk to the right retropectoral region. **B**, An enlarged right paratracheal nodal mass corresponds to the PET.

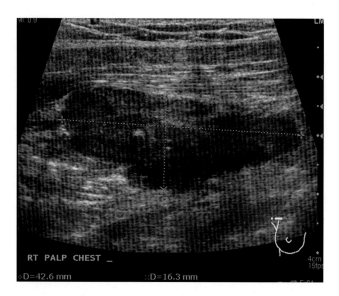

FIGURE 5. Ultrasound of the right infraclavicular fullness shows a lobular nodal mass. Ultrasound-guided fine-needle aspiration confirmed metastatic adenocarcinoma.

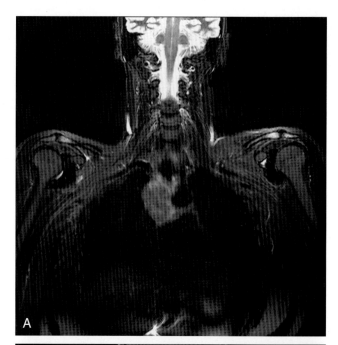

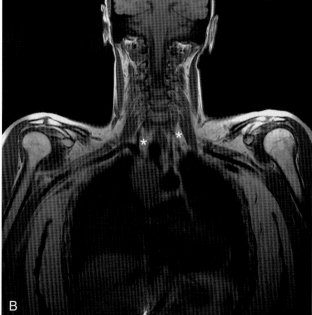

FIGURE 6. Coronal short tau inversion recovery (STIR) (**A**) and T1-weighted (**B**) brachial plexus MRIs at the same level show the bulky right paratracheal nodal mass. Portions of the subclavian arteries are seen on these sections, accompanied by cords of the brachial plexus. Note on the T1-weighted image the symmetry of the interscalene fat triangles, through which trunks of the brachial plexus pass (*asterisks*).

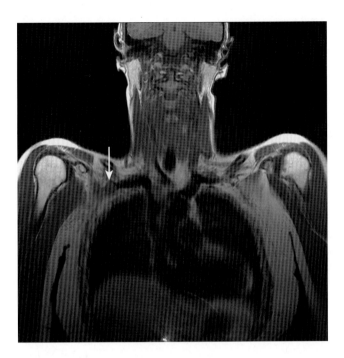

FIGURE 7. A more anterior coronal T1-weighted image shows the subclavian veins. A nodule is seen at the level of the right subclavian vein (*arrow*).

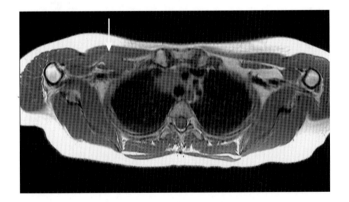

FIGURE 8. Axial T1-weighted image through the infraclavicular region and superior mediastinum. The top of the bulky right paratracheal nodal mass is seen. An oval mass is seen deep to the right pectoralis major muscle on the right (*arrow*), which posteriorly displaces the right pectoralis minor muscle. The normal appearances of the pectoralis major and minor are well depicted on the left.

Patients like this, with axillary nodal disease, are at a known 10% to 20% risk for recurrence at the apical axillary nodal level (axillary level III). Lymph node dissections target lymph nodes at axillary level I (lateral to pectoralis minor muscle) and level II (under the pectoralis minor muscle) and generally do not extend to encompass apical axillary

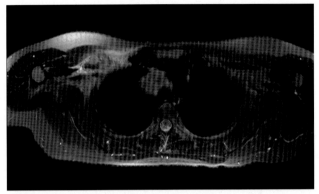

FIGURE 9. Fat-saturated, T2-weighted image, at a comparable level to Figure 7, shows hyperintensity of both the right paratracheal nodal mass and the interpectoral (Rotter's) nodal mass. The medial aspects of both the right pectoralis major and minor muscles are also increased in signal intensity.

nodes (level III), which lie in an infraclavicular site superior to the medial border of the pectoralis muscle. These apical axillary nodes are in continuity with supraclavicular nodes and are clustered around the axillary vessels in proximity to the cords of the brachial plexus.

This patient was known to be high risk. In addition to axillary disease, she had a PET-positive interpectoral (Rotter's) node identified at presentation. This is not a nodal site typically addressed surgically. She received aggressive systemic therapy and underwent chest wall radiation after mastectomy.

Development of symptoms (shoulder pain) is cause for concern and appropriately should lead to further investigation for possible recurrence. In this case, the clinical picture was clouded by the imaging evaluations addressing the abdominal wall and pulmonary embolism complications of this patient's TRAM flap surgery. CT scans were being obtained to assess these acute problems. The interpectoral nodal mass responsible for this patient's symptoms was poorly depicted on CT. This is not surprising, given the limitations of soft tissue contrast inherent in CT. These same findings are dramatically more conspicuous with either functional imaging (PET) or better soft tissue contrast (MRI).

As depicted by this case presentation, the combination of PET or PET/CT and brachial plexus MRI is optimal for comprehensive imaging evaluation of the breast cancer patient manifesting symptoms of a possible brachial plexopathy.

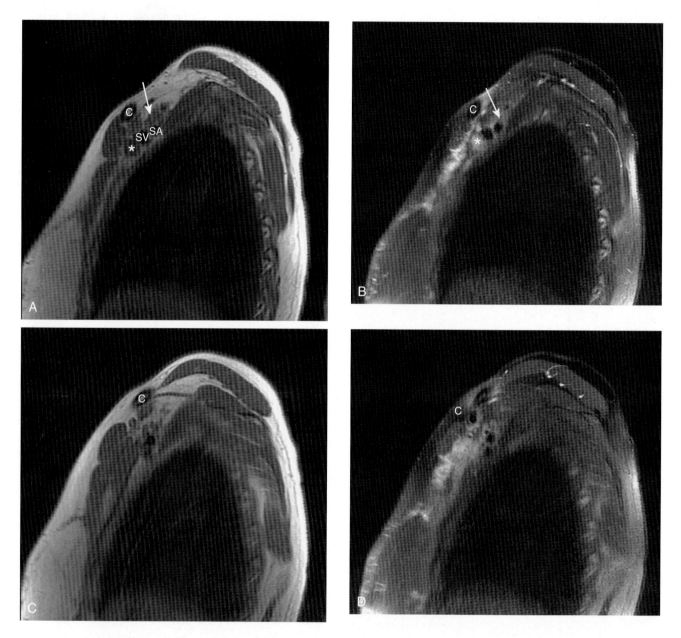

FIGURE 10. Sagittal MRIs of the retroclavicular components of the brachial plexus (at the level of the subclavian artery and vein, and brachial plexus cords). **A**, T1-weighted sagittal image. **B**, Matching fat-saturated, T2-weighted, sagittal image. **C**, T1-weighted, sagittal image, lateral to **A** and **B**. **D**, Matching fat-saturated, T2-weighted, sagittal image, lateral to **A** and **B**. Subclavian artery (SA) is above subclavian vein (SV). SV is anterior to the artery. In **A** and **B**, a nodule abuts the SV (*asterisk*). The fat around the artery is occupied by abnormal soft tissue (*arrow*), effacing cords of the brachial plexus. Further laterally (**C** and **D**), abnormal infiltration of the pectoralis muscle is seen anterior to the vessels (clavicle, C).

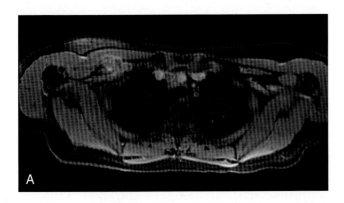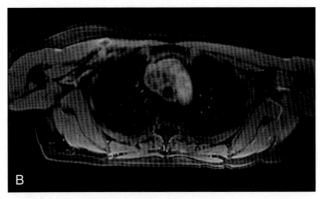

FIGURE 11.   Axial fat-saturated, enhanced, T1-weighted, breath-hold, gradient echo images (**A** above **B**). **A**, Peripheral enhancement of a multilobular, necrotic mass is seen in the right chest wall. The epicenter is interpectoral at the Rotter's node level. This mass extends anteriorly into the posterior pectoralis major muscle and infiltrates the pectoralis minor muscle. **B**, A more inferior section, showing pectoralis major and interpectoral components, with a similar enhanced appearance of the right paratracheal nodal mass.

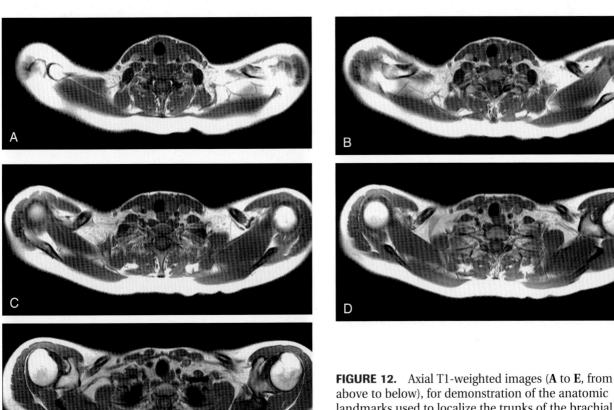

FIGURE 12.   Axial T1-weighted images (**A** to **E**, from above to below), for demonstration of the anatomic landmarks used to localize the trunks of the brachial plexus. The trunks course between the anterior (colored *yellow*) and middle (*pink*) scalene muscles. The trunks are best visualized in **C**. No evidence of pathology is seen at these levels.

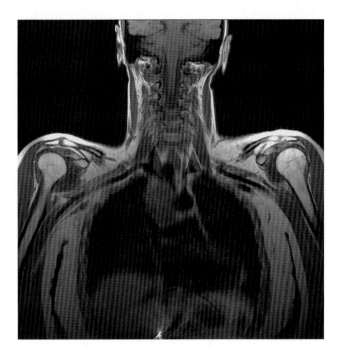

FIGURE 13. Coronal T1-weighted image, demonstrating the landmarks used to localize the position of the trunks of the brachial plexus. The anterior scalene muscles have been colored *yellow*, and the interscalene fat pads *orange*. Asymmetry of or effacement of an interscalene fat pad is an important clue to possible infiltration of the brachial plexus at the trunk level (not present here). The bulky right paratracheal nodal mass is seen.

SUGGESTED READINGS

Castillo M. Imaging the anatomy of the brachial plexus: review and self-assessment module. *AJR Am J Roentgenol* 2005; 185:S196–S204.

Hathaway PB, Mankoff DA, Maravilla KR, et al. Value of combined FDG PET and MR imaging in the evaluation of suspected recurrent local-regional breast cancer: preliminary experience. *Radiology* 1999; 210:807–814.

Qayyum A, MacVicar AD, Padhani AR, et al. Symptomatic brachial plexopathy following treatment for breast cancer: utility of MR imaging with surface-coil techniques. *Radiology* 2000; 214:837–842.

CASE 8

Brachial plexus involvement

A 64-year-old woman with stage IV breast cancer metastatic to bone developed pain in the left occip-

ital region and numbness of the left shoulder. She had been diagnosed with infiltrating ductal carcinoma the previous year, with biopsy-confirmed bone metastases identified at the same time. She had previously been treated palliatively with radiation for right shoulder and left hip pain.

At the time of evaluation of the mild brachial plexopathy symptoms, a palpable left supraclavicular nodal mass was noted on physical examination. Fine-needle aspiration confirmed metastatic adenocarcinoma. CT and MRI of the brachial plexus confirmed stippled, nodular infiltration of the left supraclavicular triangle (Figures 1, 2, 3, 4, and 5). After progression on a trial of an experimental chemotherapeutic agent, the supraclavicular region was radiated. The supraclavicular mass decreased in size and became more mobile, and the patient's shoulder paresthesias improved.

The left neck progressive disease had developed on hormonal therapy, and so chemotherapy was begun. Later the same year, the patient developed intractable nausea, vomiting, abdominal pain, and abnormal liver function tests. Abdominal ultrasound confirmed liver metastases. The patient elected hospice care.

TEACHING POINTS

This patient had mild symptoms of an early left brachial plexopathy and developed a palpable supraclavicular node to suggest the etiology and location of the causative disease. From an anatomic perspective, MRI is the imaging modality

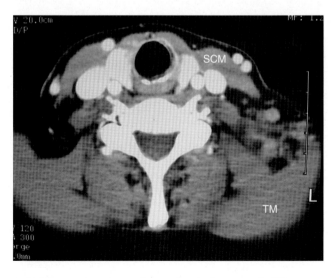

FIGURE 1. Contrast-enhanced soft tissue neck CT scan shows small nodules and stippled soft tissue densities effacing fat in the left supraclavicular region. SCM, sternocleidomastoid muscle; TM, trapezius muscle.

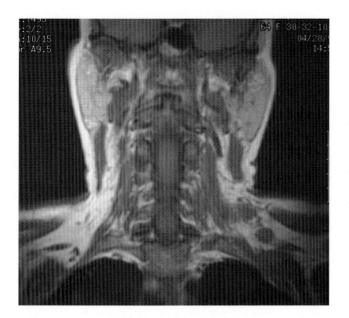

FIGURE 2. T1-weighted coronal MRI shows left supraclavicular abnormalities. In addition to a round lymph node, there is ill-defined soft tissue infiltration effacing fat.

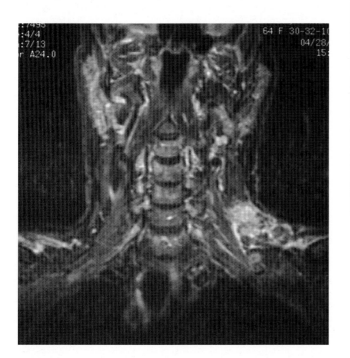

FIGURE 3. Coronal STIR image shows hyperintense mass lesions at the left supraclavicular level.

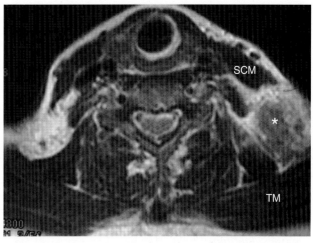

FIGURE 4. Axial T2-weighted MRI through the supraclavicular regions shows relatively bright signal of the left soft tissue infiltrative process (*asterisk*). SCM, sternocleidomastoid muscle; TM, trapezius muscle.

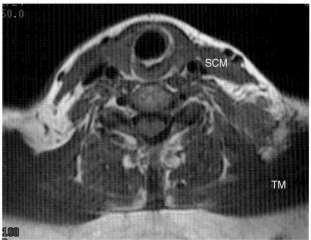

FIGURE 5. Corresponding axial T1-weighted MRI through the same level shows the left-sided soft tissue process to abut the muscles, with loss of the intervening fat plane. SCM, sternocleidomastoid muscle; TM, trapezius muscle.

with the best combination of soft tissue contrast and resolution for delineation of the location, size, and distribution of disease recurrence affecting the brachial plexus. If the findings were more subtle, positron emission tomography (PET) could be a valuable adjunct to image the region functionally, especially if the area had been previously surgically altered or radiated, which would make anatomic evaluation more difficult. The bulk of this recurrent disease is in the supraclavicular triangle, delineated by the sternocleidomastoid (SCM) muscle anteriorly and the trapezius muscle (TM) posteriorly. The brachial plexus divisions pass through the supraclavicular triangle above the subclavian artery, before ramifying behind the clavicle to form cords, which constitute the infraclavicular components of the brachial plexus, en route to the axilla. For a case of infraclavicular brachial plexus recurrence, see Case 7 in this chapter.

SUGGESTED READINGS

Castagno AA, Shuman WP. MR imaging in clinically suspected brachial plexus tumor. *AJR Am J Roentgenol* 1987; 149:1219–1222.

Castillo M. Imaging the anatomy of the brachial plexus: review and self-assessment module. *AJR Am J Roentgenol* 2005; 185:S196–S204.

Hathaway PB, Mankoff DA, Maravilla KR, et al. Value of combined FDG PET and MR imaging in the evaluation of suspected recurrent local-regional breast cancer: preliminary experience. *Radiology* 1999; 210: 807–814.

Qayyum A, MacVicar AD, Padhani AR, et al. Symptomatic brachial plexopathy following treatment for breast cancer: utility of MR imaging with surface-coil techniques. *Radiology* 2000; 214:837–842.

Wittenberg KH, Adkins MC. MR imaging of nontraumatic brachial plexopathies: frequency and spectrum of findings. *RadioGraphics* 2000; 20:1023–1032.

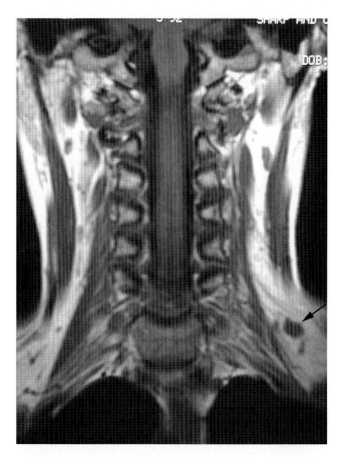

FIGURE 1. T1-weighted coronal MR image shows only a normal (1 cm) size left supraclavicular lymph node (*arrow*) and was the only MR finding relevant to the persistent palpable abnormality in this region.

CASE 9

Nodal recurrence to mediastinum and supraclavicular regions

A 43-year-old woman with recurrent breast cancer was evaluated with positron emission tomography (PET) for a persistent palpable left supraclavicular abnormality 1 year after finishing chemotherapy for left neck nodal disease.

The patient was first diagnosed with a 1-cm left breast infiltrating ductal carcinoma at age 32 and treated with mastectomy. Fifteen lymph nodes were negative. Two and a half years before PET scanning, left neck nodal recurrence was found and treated with 6 months of chemotherapy. Six months later, she again developed a recurrent left neck lump and was treated with an additional eight cycles of chemotherapy, which finished 1 year before. At the time of PET evaluation, she had a persistent hard, fixed, palpable left supraclavicular nodule. MRI showed only a normal-sized (1 cm) left supraclavicular lymph node at that level (Figure 1).

PET scan confirmed a small left supraclavicular hypermetabolic nodule at the level in question

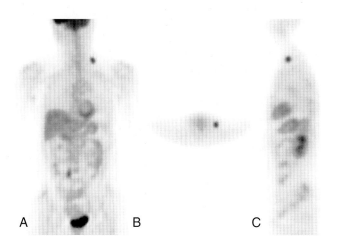

FIGURE 2. PET scan images show a small hypermetabolic nodule of activity at the left supraclavicular level, corresponding precisely to the normal size lymph node in question on MRI. This was subsequently excised and proven to be metastatic breast cancer. Coronal (**A**), transaxial (**B**), and sagittal (**C**) views are depicted.

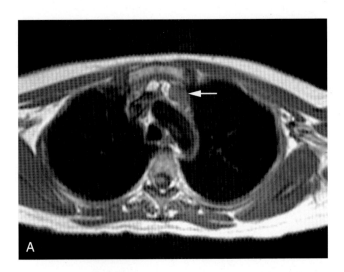 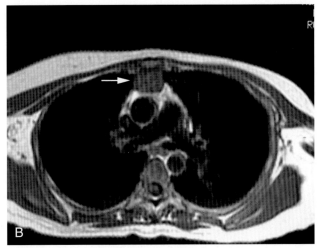

FIGURE 3. **A** and **B**, T1-weighted axial MR images through the superior mediastinum show two prevascular soft tissue masses (*arrows*).

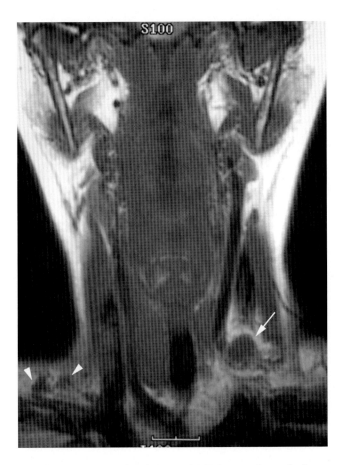

FIGURE 4. T1-weighted coronal MR image through the anterior neck shows a round, new left supraclavicular nodule (*arrow*). Smaller soft tissue nodules are noted in the right supraclavicular fat (*arrowheads*).

(Figure 2). A trial of hormonal therapy yielded no clinical response, so 3 months later, the node was surgically excised and proved to be metastatic breast cancer. She was restarted on chemotherapy and had completed four cycles when she was re-evaluated with neck and chest MRI and PET scan. Unfortunately, these studies showed interval progression, with new prevascular mediastinal and bilateral neck and supraclavicular foci of activity on PET, which correlated with MRI masses (Figures 3, 4, 5, and 6).

TEACHING POINTS

At the time of this patient's initial PET scan, she had had a protracted course with left neck recurrent disease and was left with a palpably suspicious hard and fixed left neck lump. The corresponding MRI showed only a normal-sized lymph node. This discordance was bridged with the addition of PET imaging, which showed this node to be intensely hypermetabolic. Metastatic breast cancer was subsequently confirmed at this site by surgical excision. PET also confirmed the progressive findings demonstrated subsequently on imaging follow-up.

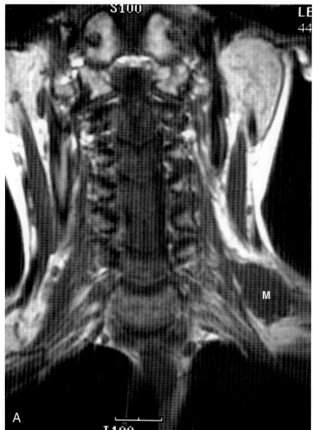

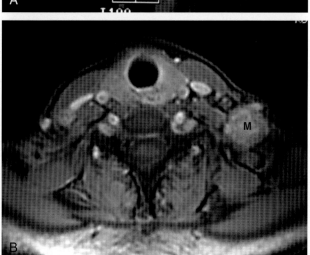

FIGURE 5. T1-weighted coronal (**A**) and enhanced, fat-saturated fast multiplanar spoiled gradient recalled (FMPSPGR) (gradient echo) (**B**) axial sequences show a new, lobular mass (M) in the left posterior triangle.

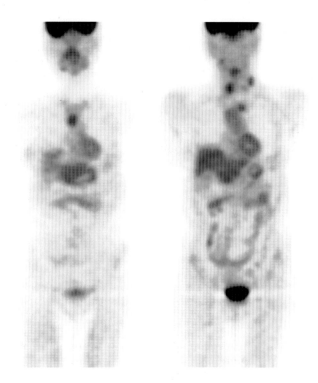

FIGURE 6. Corresponding coronal PET scan images shows some of the multiple new foci of activity in the anterior mediastinum and neck, corresponding to the MRI findings.

CASE 10

PET-positive thoracic nodal recurrence mimic due to silicone implant leak

A 63-year-old woman with a remote history of treated breast cancer presented from an outside facility for medical oncology follow-up. Her breast cancer was on the left 17 years before, a 5-cm infiltrating lobular carcinoma with 10 of 14 lymph nodes involved. She was treated with a modified radical mastectomy and subsequently underwent a prophylactic right mastectomy. Additional therapy was six cycles of chemotherapy Cytoxan, Adriamycin, 5-fluorouracil (CAF) and radiation to the chest wall and peripheral lymphatics. The patient had been on tamoxifen about 10 years. Breast reconstruction with implants was revised 4 years before the current presentation, and the replacement implants were removed 2 years before.

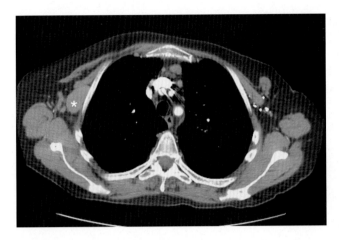

FIGURE 1. Enhanced chest CT image through the great vessel origins shows left axillary surgical clips. In the right axilla is a markedly enlarged lymph node (3.7 × 2.4 cm) (*asterisk*). Enlarged lymph nodes are also seen in the prevascular mediastinum.

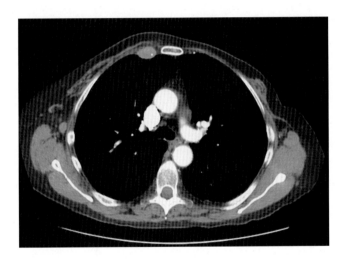

FIGURE 2. A more inferior enhanced chest CT image shows an enlarged right internal mammary lymph node containing a small focus of calcium.

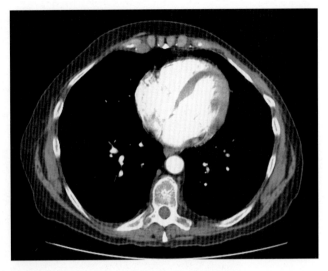

FIGURE 3. Another, more inferior enhanced chest CT image shows a second enlarged right internal mammary lymph node, also containing a small focus of calcium.

Physical examination identified a 2-cm right axillary lymph node. Positron emission tomography (PET)/CT and contrast-enhanced CT scans showed multiple abnormally enlarged and metabolically active lymph nodes in the right axilla, prevascular mediastinum, and right internal mammary regions (Figures 1, 2, 3, 4, 5, and 6). Correlation with right axillary sonography showed characteristic findings suggesting silicone as the etiology, rather than nodal recurrent disease (Figure 7).

TEACHING POINTS

Not all increased metabolic activity in regional lymphatics of treated breast cancer patients repre-

sents recurrent tumor. Like Case 16 in Chapter 6, iatrogenic etiologies of lymphadenopathy can simulate recurrent disease and should be considered when there is a prior history of reconstruction, implant rupture, or other viable alternative explanation. As in this case, it may take another modality or even tissue sampling to completely characterize such abnormalities.

In this case, the patient was known to have had ruptured silicone implants replaced previously. The CT and PET scan findings are nonspecific, and by themselves, would not allow exclusion of recurrent disease. However, correlation with the characteristic ultrasound findings is reassuring and provides a reasonable, benign alternative etiology.

Unlike metastatic tumor cells, which lodge preferentially in the subcapsular and cortical sinusoids of lymph nodes, foreign material such as silicone tends to accumulate in medullary sinusoids. There is a range of appearances on ultrasound of lymph nodes containing silicone, depending on the amount of material accumulated. Hardest to recognize are lesser degrees of involvement, with ill-defined shadowing arising from the mediastinum (illustrated to variable degrees by Figures 7A and 7B). With progressive accumulation of silicone in the medullary sinuses, the hilus becomes increasingly hyperechoic and may shadow, as in Figure 7A. Most characteristic is the snowstorm appearance of lymph nodes so silicone laden that even the cortex is hyperechoic and not readily differentiated from the medulla, with dirty shadowing emanating from the whole of the extensively involved lymph node, as in Figure 7C.

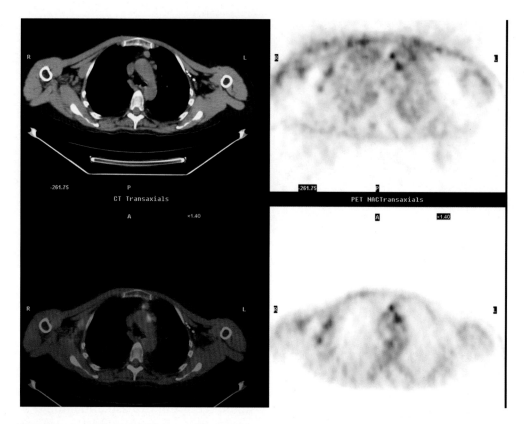

FIGURE 4. Axial PET/CT images show modest increased metabolic activity of the enlarged prevascular and right axillary lymph nodes.

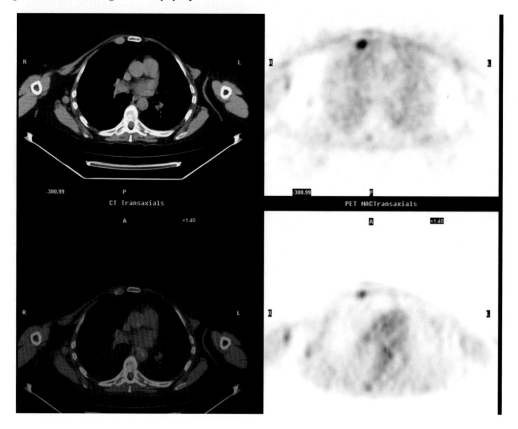

FIGURE 5. Axial PET/CT images show moderate increased metabolic activity of one of the enlarged right internal mammary lymph nodes.

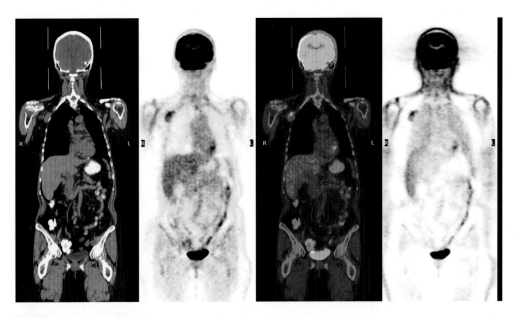

FIGURE 6. Coronal PET/CT scans show the right axillary nodal hypermetabolism (*from left to right*): CT, attenuation corrected PET, fused PET/CT, and non-attenuation corrected PET.

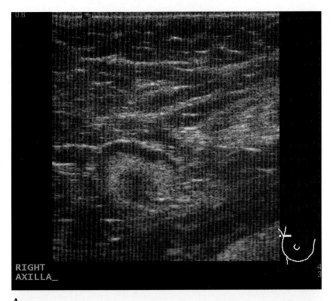

A

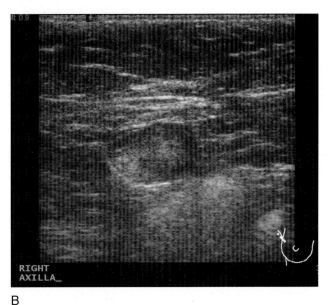

B

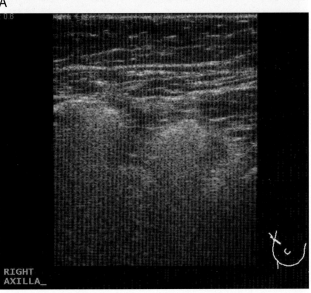

C

FIGURE 7. Three views of right axillary lymph nodes by ultrasound. **A**, This lymph node shows a smooth hypoechoic cortex of normal thickness. The medulla is abnormally hyperechoic with dirty shadowing beyond. **B**, A second abnormal axillary lymph node shows a similar appearance. Hyperechogenicity with dirty shadowing is seen deep to this, representing a completely replaced silicone-laden lymph node. **C**, Adjacent silicone snowstorms in additional silicone-laden axillary lymph nodes.

CASE 11

Unusual pattern of chest wall recurrence (intercostal muscle infiltration)

A 47-year-old woman with previously treated recurrent left breast lobular cancer presented with dimpling and a tender palpable lump at the superior aspect of her left breast implant. She also complained of chronic left chest wall pain, between the reconstructed breast and the axilla, in a region of dense fixation.

She had originally been diagnosed with left breast lobular cancer at age 37, presenting as a pea-size palpable lump. Her tumor was 2 cm, a T2N0M0 lesion, estrogen receptor and progesterone receptor positive, *HER-2/neu* negative, and was treated with mastectomy. The margins were close, and she underwent chest wall and supraclavicular radiation as well as six cycles of Cytoxan, methotrexate, 5-fluorouracil (CMF) chemotherapy.

Subsequently, she was on tamoxifen for 3 years, before developing a left axillary recurrence. This was excised, confirming metastatic breast cancer, and treated with left axillary radiation. Additional staging workup showed ovarian cysts. Bilateral oophorectomy was negative for malignancy, and the patient was placed on anastrozole (Arimidex).

Seven years later, the patient presented with small palpable subcutaneous nodules and chronic left chest wall pain. Ultrasound showed hypoechoic subcutaneous nodules (Figure 1). An ultrasound-guided biopsy confirmed recurrent infiltrating lobular carcinoma (ILC), estrogen receptor positive, progesterone receptor negative, infiltrating skeletal muscle and adipose tissue.

Restaging with positron emission tomography (PET) and CT showed multiple small hypermetabolic subcutaneous nodules as well as hypermetabolism lateral to the implant in the region of dense fixation and along an intercostal space in the left chest wall (Figures 2, 3, 4, 5, 6, and 7).

The patient was referred to surgery for consideration of chest wall excision and reconstruction. CT-guided biopsy of the hypermetabolic intercostal space obtained skeletal muscle, heavily infiltrated by adenocarcinoma with breast morphology, estrogen receptor positive and progesterone receptor negative.

TEACHING POINTS

An unusual pattern of chest wall recurrence is illustrated by this case. The curvilinear, obliquely oriented activity was confounding to sort out. Based on its appearance on the PET volumetric image and sagittal projections, the course of the activity suggests it is in an involved rib. In fact, it had previously been suggested clinically that perhaps the patient's chronic chest wall pain was due to radionecrosis of a rib. However, this was never substantiated. A bone scan 8 months before was negative, review of the CT bone windows showed no rib

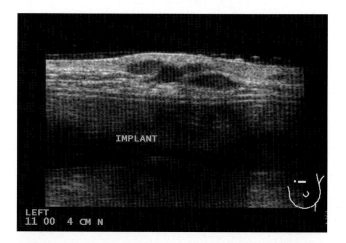

FIGURE 1. Ultrasound of the palpable lump at the superior margin of a left breast implant shows a lobular hypoechoic nodule superficial to the anechoic implant below. Ultrasound-guided biopsy confirmed recurrent ILC.

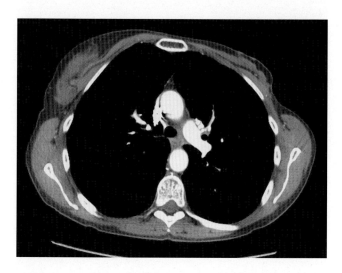

FIGURE 2. Enhanced chest CT image shows tiny left chest wall skin nodules. These were metabolically active on PET.

abnormality, and the activity seemed to localize to an intercostal space and not to a rib. Although there was some asymmetry in the CT appearance of the chest wall musculature, there did not appear to be any focal correlate in the intercostal space implicated on PET. Because respiratory motion can significantly affect localization of PET abnormalities, this was carefully scrutinized. The registration between the CT and PET data appeared perfect.

After much discussion among the consultants (the patient was being considered for surgery, with chest wall reconstruction), it was elected to pursue the intercostal abnormality despite the lack of a focal CT correlate. Using landmarks, the interspace was identified, and biopsy confirmed recurrent breast carcinoma.

With the second positive biopsy confirming the PET impression of much more extensive chest wall

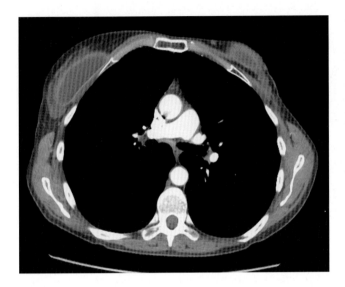

FIGURE 3. A more inferior section from the same chest CT shows a larger subcutaneous soft tissue nodule medial to the left breast implant. This was also metabolically active on PET. Soft tissue seen lateral to the left breast implant was intensely hypermetabolic on PET.

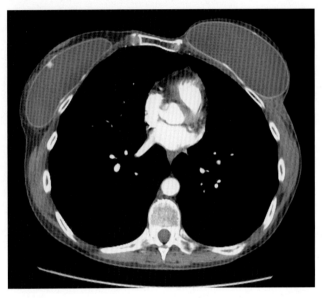

FIGURE 4. A more inferior slice through the saline implants (implant valves can be visualized on this slice) shows asymmetrical soft tissue lateral to the left breast implant.

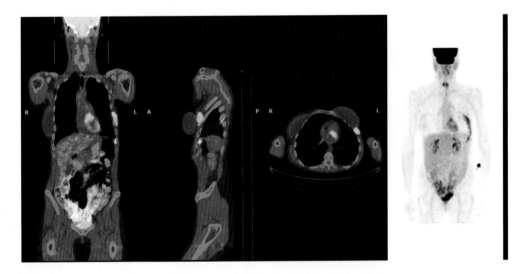

FIGURE 5. Three plane fused PET/CT images show multiple foci of intense hypermetabolism in the left chest wall. The coronal projection volumetric image (*right*) displays a curvilinear shape, following the oblique orientation of a rib. Intense hypermetabolism lateral to the implant (best seen on the axial section) corresponds with the asymmetrical soft tissue lateral to the left breast implant shown in Figure 4.

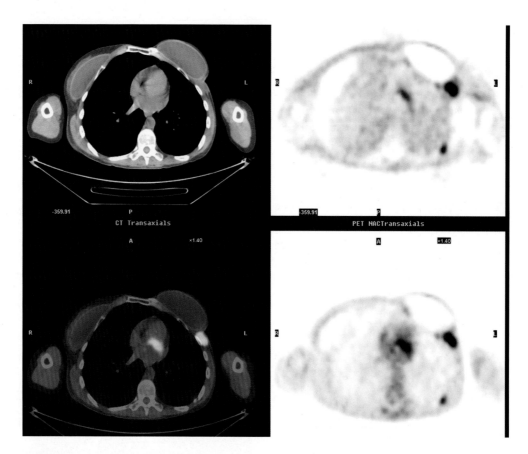

FIGURE 6. Axial PET/CT images showing the intense hypermetabolism lateral to the left breast implant. Note a second, separate focus in the left posterolateral chest wall, localizing to an intercostal space. Normal variant myocardial activity is also seen here.

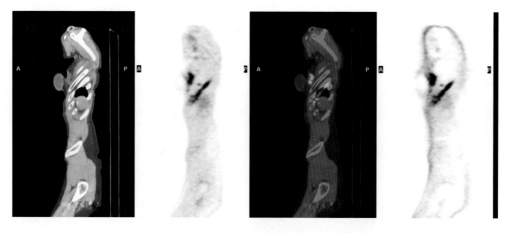

FIGURE 7. Sagittal PET/CT images show intense, curvilinear, obliquely oriented activity, separate from hypermetabolism on the lateral margin of the implant.

involvement than suspected previously, it became clear that surgery was unlikely to render this patient disease free. She was started on fulvestrant (Faslodex), a direct estrogen receptor blocker.

This case illustrates how helpful PET data can be in clarifying the significance of indeterminate or ambiguous CT findings. The relatively poor soft tissue contrast of CT is also demonstrated by these findings, with areas of tumor activity on PET showing the same soft tissue density on CT as other apparently uninvolved and inactive chest wall muscles.

Drug reaction (pulmonary toxicity) due to chemotherapy

A 42-year-old woman was found to have lung and nodal breast cancer metastases after evaluation with positron emission tomography (PET) and CT for rising tumor markers. Her diagnosis of breast cancer was 4 years before, and was stage IIB, T2N1. She underwent bilateral mastectomy and received adjuvant CMF chemotherapy and tamoxifen. Her prior medical history was notable for treatment of Hodgkin's lymphoma at age 17 with radiation and chemotherapy.

The diagnosis of recurrent breast cancer was made by biopsy of a lung nodule, confirming malignant adenocarcinoma, consistent with breast primary. The patient was begun on a regimen of docetaxel (Taxotere) and gemcitabine (Gemzar).

A chest CT obtained just before cycle seven of chemotherapy showed that the index lung metastases were responding (Figures 1 and 2). However, new, vague, bilateral ground-glass lung opacities were noted. A drug reaction was suggested as the etiology. The patient complained of fatigue but was otherwise asymptomatic. Her tumor markers had normalized.

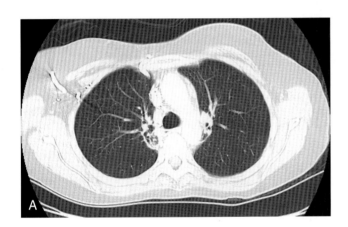
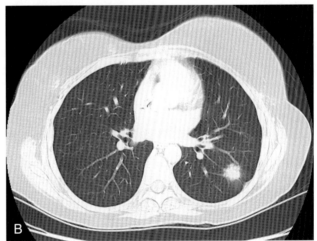

FIGURE 1. **A**, CT scan through the superior mediastinum shows paramediastinal fibrosis from prior radiation for Hodgkin's lymphoma. The lungs at this level are clear. **B**, CT scan through the lower lobes shows a spiculated left lower lobe (LLL) metastasis, with localized pleural thickening.

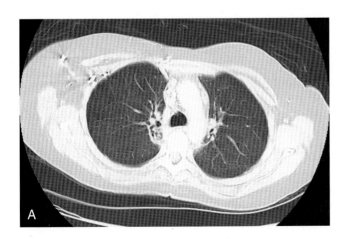
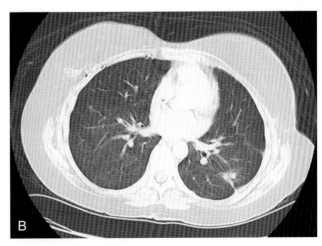

FIGURE 2. **A** and **B**, Three months later, through comparable levels, CT scan shows new, vague increase in lung opacity diffusely. Subtle new intralobular septal thickening is present. The LLL metastasis shows marked diminution in size and volume.

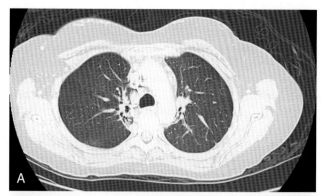

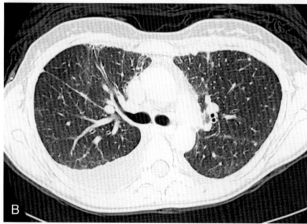

FIGURE 3.   **A** and **B**, Six months since the CT in Figure 1, and after chemotherapy was discontinued 3 months, CT scan shows that the diffuse lung changes have resolved. The index LLL lung metastasis has grown.

direct pulmonary toxicity and indirectly through inflammation and hypersensitivity reactions. Imaging findings are best demonstrated on high-resolution CT and reflect chronic pneumonitis and fibrosis. CT manifestations of pulmonary toxicity may include fibrosis, air space consolidation, ground-glass opacities, and air trapping due to obliterative bronchiolitis. A retrospective review of the high-resolution CT findings of drug-induced pneumonitis found the most common manifestation of chemotherapy-induced reactions were diffuse or multifocal ground-glass opacities with intralobular interstitial thickening, which this case illustrates (albeit a subtle example). Drug reactions are generally diagnoses of exclusion, requiring correlation of the time course of drug administration to the development of imaging findings and symptoms to suggest the diagnosis.

SUGGESTED READINGS

Akira M, Ishikawa H, Yamamoto S. Drug-induced pneumonitis: thin-section CT findings in 60 patients. *Radiology* 2002; 224:852–860.

Camus PH, Foucher P, Bonniaud PH, Ask K. Drug-induced infiltrative lung disease. *Eur Respir J* 2001; 18:93S–100.

Padley SP, Adler B, Hansell DM, et al. High-resolution computed tomography of drug-induced lung disease. *Clin Radiol* 1992; 46(4):232–236.

Four months later, the patient noted increasing dyspnea with exertion. Her chemotherapy was interrupted and consultation with chest medicine obtained. Additional symptoms of intermittent cough and low-grade fever were noted by this time. Pulmonary function tests were abnormal, with evidence of moderate restriction and low diffusing capacity, suggesting interstitial lung disease. Bronchoscopy was performed to exclude an infectious etiology. All cultures were negative. On a chemotherapy holiday, the patient's symptoms improved dramatically, and the ground-glass infiltrates seen on chest CT resolved (Figure 3). Repeat pulmonary function tests 3 months later showed improvement.

TEACHING POINTS

Numerous chemotherapeutic agents are implicated in toxic pulmonary side effects, both through

CASE 13

Lymphangitic tumor

A 37-year-old woman with extensive bony metastatic breast cancer known for 1 year developed increased aching, weight loss, depressed appetite, and rising tumor markers while on goserelin acetate (Zoladex), zoledronic acid (Zometa), and exemestane (Aromasin). Positron emission tomography (PET)/CT and enhanced body CT scans showed new liver metastases (see Case 2 in Chapter 9). Chemotherapy was recommended but declined. She was started on fulvestrant (Faslodex) and restaged after 2 months, at which time fatigue, shortness of breath, and rising tumor markers were noted. Repeat PET/CT and enhanced body CT scans showed progression of liver metas-

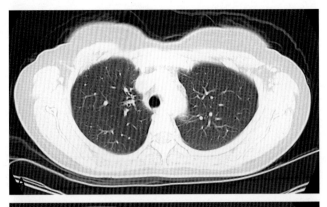

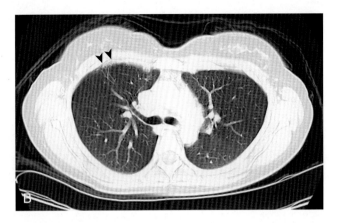

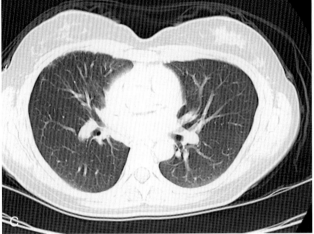

FIGURE 1. Baseline chest CT images, 7 months before identification of liver metastases. **A**, Axial slice through the upper lobes. **B**, Through the mid-thorax, at the level of the carina. **C**, Through the lower lobes. These images show linear, right anterior, subpleural, parenchymal consolidation (*arrowheads*), in a distribution compatible with radiation fibrosis from radiation therapy 4 years earlier.

tases, new pleural and pericardial effusions as well as pulmonary metastases, and evidence of lymphangitic spread (Figures 1, 2, 3, 4, 5). One month later, the patient was admitted with confusion, thought to be hepatic encephalopathy due to the extensive liver metastases. She died soon thereafter.

Her original tumor had been treated 5 years earlier and was an estrogen receptor– and progesterone receptor–positive, T1cN1b(4) infiltrating ductal carcinoma. She was treated with breast conservation and axillary dissection, with 4 of 20 lymph nodes positive and showing microscopic extracapsular extension. Additional treatment was with chemotherapy (four cycles of doxorubicin [Adriamycin] and cyclophosphamide [Cytoxan] [AC] and four of paclitaxel [Taxol]); right breast, supraclavicular, and axillary radiation therapy; and tamoxifen. Four years after the original breast cancer diagnosis and 1 year before detection of liver metastases, diffuse bone metastases were found. See Case 3 in Chapter 8 for discussion of the imaging manifestations of this patient's bone metastases.

TEACHING POINTS

Lymphangitic, pleural, and pericardial metastases appear to be related phenomena in women with metastatic breast cancer. The major intrathoracic lymphatic vessels are in centriacinar bronchovascular bundles, interlobular septa, and subpleural regions of the lungs. Development of malignant pleural effusions in breast cancer patients has been observed to occur most commonly unilaterally and ipsilateral to the side of the primary. The theory is that tumor spread is through lymphatics, namely the ipsilateral internal mammary, with secondary involvement of the lung, pleura, and pericardium.

Autopsy series of women who die of metastatic breast cancer show that 83% had lymphangitic tumor. This is less frequently appreciated by imaging than the prevalence suggested by autopsy data. The pathologic hallmark is tumor thrombi in lymphatic vessels of bronchovascular bundles, interlobular septa, and pleura, with localized foci of subpleural tumor. Pleural effusions are seen in patients with extensive disease.

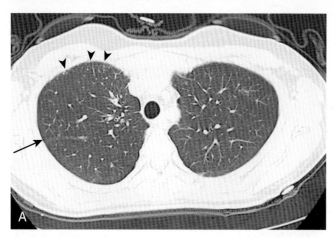

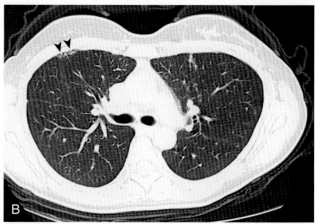

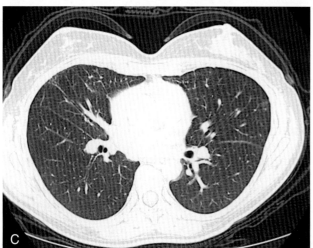

FIGURE 2. Comparable levels on repeat chest CT, 7 months later. The patient was being evaluated for aching, weight loss, depressed appetite, and rising tumor markers. She had diffuse bone metastases identified 1 year earlier, and liver metastases were identified at this time. **A,** Axial slice through the upper lobes. **B,** Through the mid-thorax, at the level of the carina. **C,** Through the lower lobes. No pleural fluid is identified. The radiation therapy changes in the right anterior subpleural lung were again noted. No other lung parenchymal abnormalities were identified. In retrospect, very subtle ominous changes may be appreciated. The major fissure can now be visualized on these slices, and displays very subtle new nodular thickening (*arrow*). New subpleural interlobular pleural thickening is suggested as well, best seen on the right anteriorly in **A,** at the level of the prior radiation therapy change (*arrowheads*). Subtle nodular bronchovascular thickening is also suggested in right middle and lower bronchi visualized in **C.**

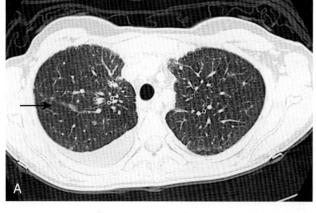

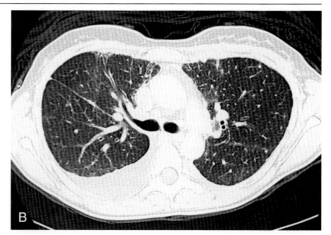

FIGURE 3. Comparable sections on a third chest CT, 2 months later. Liver metastases were identified on the prior study. The patient had declined recommended chemotherapy and at this point had undergone 2 months of therapy with fulvestrant (Faslodex). Progressive fatigue, shortness of breath, and rising tumor markers were noted at this time. **A,** Axial slice through the upper lobes. **B,** Through the mid-thorax, at the level of the carina. **C,** Through the lower lobes. Pleural effusions have developed bilaterally, right greater than left. Nodular thickening of the right major fissure is more apparent (*arrow*). Parenchymal findings of lymphangitic tumor are now readily apparent, especially anteriorly, right greater than left, with subpleural interlobular septal thickening and occasional tiny subpleural nodules. Bronchovascular thickening and nodularity is notable on the right centrally (**A**) and in the anterior right upper lobe (**B**).

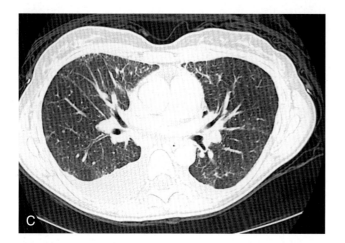

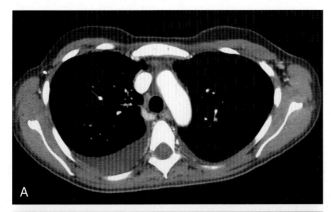

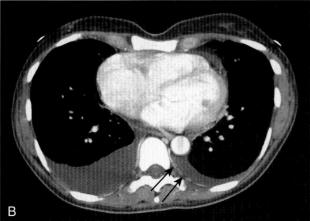

FIGURE 4. Contrast-enhanced chest CT images (**A** and **B**, soft tissue window) from the final CT (same study as Figure 3) show bilateral pleural effusions, right greater than left. The pleura is enhancing, smoothly in some places and nodularly in others (as seen here best on the left, *arrows*), suggesting malignant effusions. A small new pericardial effusion is also partially visualized here.

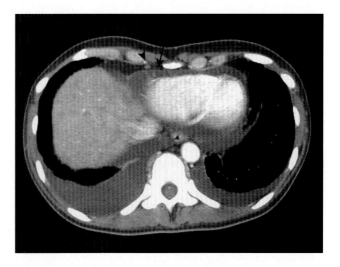

FIGURE 5. A contrast-enhanced image from the same chest CT shows the pericardium distended by a moderate-sized effusion. The enhancing pericardium is visualized, evidence that this is a malignant effusion. A right pericardial lymph node is seen (*arrowhead*), and there is an enhancing soft tissue nodule within the pericardial fluid (*arrow*). The liver is heterogeneous. Liver metastases were better demonstrated on other slices (not shown). Malignant pleural effusions with enhancement of the pleura are again seen.

The diagnosis is suggested by high-resolution CT showing reticular or reticulonodular interstitial markings, irregular and nodular thickening of interlobular septa (Kerley B lines), and uneven thickening of bronchovascular bundles, especially with a beaded or nodular appearance. CT underestimates the extent of subpleural tumor compared with pathology.

Bilateral lymphangitic disease is generally seen with most malignancies; however, unilaterality is more common in breast cancer. Additional findings that may be seen on CT in patients with lymphangitic tumor are hilar and mediastinal lymphadenopathy and pleural effusion and thickening (all of which were seen in this patient).

SUGGESTED READINGS

Connolly JE Jr, Erasmus JJ, Patz EF Jr, et al. Thoracic manifestations of breast carcinoma: metastatic disease and complications of treatment. *Clin Radiol* 1999; 54:487–494.

Thomas JM, Redding WH, Sloane JP. The spread of breast cancer: importance of the intrathoracic lymphatic route and its relevance to treatment. *Br J Cancer* 1979; 40:540–547.

CASE 14

Lymphangitic tumor

A 55-year-old woman with stage III breast cancer diagnosed 3 years before was noted to have rising tumor markers (CA 27.29), while finishing a delayed year of trastuzumab (Herceptin) therapy. She had been treated at another facility for a 4.5-cm, estrogen receptor– and progesterone receptor–negative, *HER-2/neu* positive, infiltrating ductal carcinoma, with mastectomy, chemotherapy (four cycles of doxorubicin [Adriamycin] plus cyclophosphamide [Cytoxan] [AC] and four cycles of docetaxel [Taxotere]), and radiation. Ten of 12 lymph nodes were involved. The patient presented for medical oncology second opinion 9 months after finishing primary treatment and began a year's therapy with trastuzumab (Herceptin).

The patient's rising tumor markers prompted a restaging workup with CT and positron emission tomography (PET). Tiny (2 to 3 mm) micronodules were noted in the right upper lobe (RUL) on chest CT. The PET scan was negative. She was evaluated by pulmonary medicine. A short interval follow-up was recommended because the patient was essentially asymptomatic, other than left knee pain.

A repeat chest CT 4 months later showed increased interstitial lung changes, and the specter of lymphangitic tumor was raised (Figures 1 and 2). Repeat PET scan showed new abnormalities, with bilateral suprahilar hypermetabolic uptake, as well as new mild, generalized, increased upper lobe activity, corresponding to the new parenchymal findings (Figure 3).

Bronchoscopy showed a normal tracheobronchial tree. RUL lavage and transbronchial biopsy confirmed metastatic breast cancer, estrogen receptor and progesterone receptor negative. Bone scan, obtained to evaluate complaints of left knee pain, showed findings suggesting hypertrophic osteoarthropathy as a possible etiology for the pain (Figure 4).

TEACHING POINTS

This patient's tumor markers began rising during the last few months of a year of Herceptin therapy. Workup showed only minimal RUL peripheral micronodularity (Figure 2B) and PET was negative. Repeat chest CT and PET, 4 months later and 2 months after completing Herceptin, show dramatic interval change, suggesting lymphangitic tumor spread. Metastatic breast cancer was confirmed by bronchoscopic biopsy, directed to the RUL, where the most extensive findings were seen.

Hypertrophic osteoarthropathy may cause bone pain and arthralgias due to periostitis. This is manifested scintigraphically by increased long bone

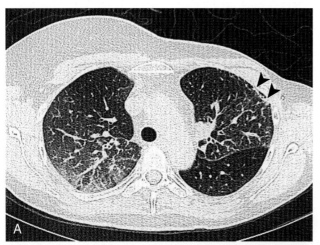

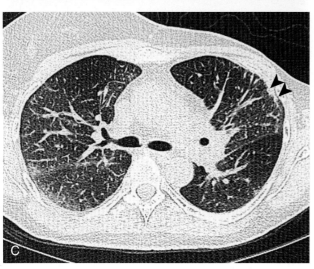

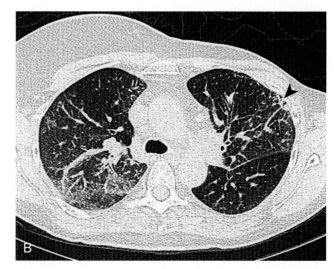

FIGURE 1. Chest CT images (**A** to **C**, from above to below) show increased parenchymal ground-glass opacity, with thickening of peripheral interlobular septa. These findings are most evident in the posterior RUL, with similar but lesser changes in the superior segment right lower lobe and posterior left upper lobe. Note subtle nodularity of prominent bronchovascular structures in the RUL. Anterolateral subpleural lung changes on the left are consistent with radiation fibrosis (*arrowheads*). Note prior left mastectomy.

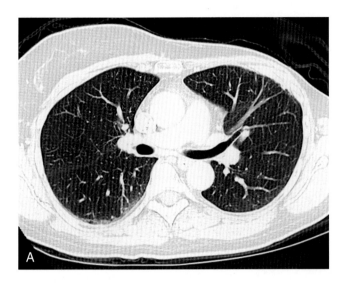
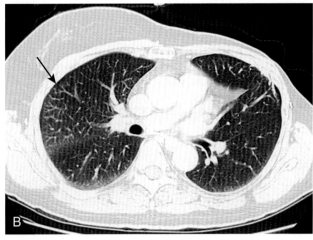

FIGURE 2. Prior chest CT images, for comparison, 15 months (**A**) and 4 months (**B**) before. Note new prominence of RUL peripheral interstitial markings and interlobular septa. Tiny peripheral RUL subpleural micronodules are now suggested (*arrow*).

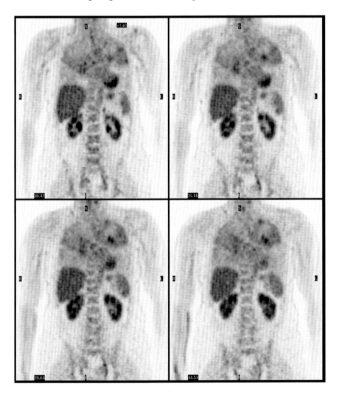

FIGURE 3. Coronal PET images show new bilateral perihilar hypermetabolism, with lower-level, generalized, mild increased activity of both upper lobes.

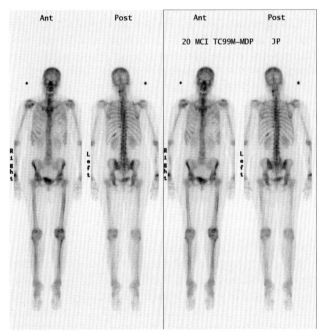

FIGURE 4. Bone scan images show a long segment of mild increased uptake at the left 11th rib level posteriorly, a pattern suspicious for metastasis. Left neck degenerative activity is similar to the PET scan findings at this level. Cortex of the left femur is unusually well seen. Given the lung findings, this could be a subtle case of hypertrophic osteoarthropathy.

SUGGESTED READING

Munk PL, Muller NL, Miller RR, et al. Pulmonary lymphangitic carcinomatosis: CT and pathologic findings. *Radiology* 1988; 166:705–709.

cortical activity, most often recognized in the lower extremities, which can be seen before clinical symptoms develop. It is seen with a variety of thoracic conditions, both malignant and benign. Lung cancer is the most common association, but thoracic metastases are one of the less often seen causes.

CHAPTER 11

Breast Cancer Metastases to the Neural Axis

Breast cancer is the second most common primary tumor to metastasize to the central nervous system (CNS), after lung cancer.[1,2,3] Breast cancer metastases to the neural axis typically occur late in the disease, with lung, liver, or bone metastases preceding the diagnosis of CNS metastases. The median interval between the diagnosis of breast cancer and brain metastases is 34 months. The historical 1-year survival rate after diagnosis of brain metastases is 20%.[3]

CNS metastases can be a challenging management issue. Brain metastases are often more debilitating and more rapidly fatal if untreated than metastases to other organ systems.

Based on data from the 1960s and 1970s, the incidence of clinically apparent brain metastases in women with stage IV breast cancer is 10% to 16%. However, autopsy data show the incidence to be greater and has been reported to be as high as 30%.[1]

Younger patients are at higher risk for CNS metastases. In an autopsy series of 1044 breast cancer patients, the median age of patients with CNS metastases was 5 years younger than patients without CNS metastases.[1]

Studies suggest a relationship between hormone receptor status and the incidence of CNS metastases.[1,3,4] A study of 217 breast cancer patients found a difference in the rate of brain metastases between estrogen receptor–negative and –positive tumors (10% versus 4%). In a multivariate model, *HER-2/neu* overexpression was the strongest predictor of CNS relapse, with a 10-fold increase in the incidence of brain metastases (4.3% versus 0.4%). However, it is unclear whether *HER-2/neu* positive patients are actually at higher risk for CNS metastases or whether the natural history of their disease is affected by more effective systemic disease control with trastuzumab (Herceptin). *HER-2* amplification occurs in 25% to 30% of breast cancers and correlates with decreased disease-free and overall survival rates. Treatment with Herceptin improves systemic disease control and overall survival of *HER-2/neu* positive patients with metastatic breast cancer. However, it does not cross the blood-brain barrier. The theory is that the natural history of the disease may be changed as a result of improved extra-CNS systemic disease control from Herceptin therapy, resulting in an increase in the incidence of CNS metastases. Circumstantial evidence for this includes the statistic that the incidence of CNS metastases in stage IV breast cancer patients who are treated with Herceptin is higher than historical norms, and ranges from 28% to 43%.

DISTRIBUTION OF CRANIAL METASTASES

Brain metastases result from hematogenous spread. Their predilection for the gray-white matter junction is thought to result from decreased vessel caliber at this level acting as a trap for embolized clumps of tumor cells. Similarly, there is a predilection of metastases to occur at intracranial vascular watershed levels. The distribution of metastases within brain compartments is roughly proportionate to the blood supply, with about 80% occurring in the cerebrum, 15% in the cerebellum, and 5% in the brainstem. Metastases occur most commonly at the junction of gray and white matter in the cerebral hemispheres, followed by deep gray matter (basal ganglia, thalami), intraventricular (choroid plexus), and cerebellum.[3,6]

CNS metastases can be categorized as intra-axial, extra-axial, or cerebrospinal fluid (CSF) dissemination. Breast cancer more commonly involves multiple compartments (parenchyma, meninges, bone) than other tumors. It is the solid tumor most commonly associated with leptomeningeal involvement, although this is considerably less common than parenchymal metastases, occurring in 5% to 16% of patients at autopsy.[1] Breast cancer also metastasizes to the eye at a higher rate than other tumors. A small percentage of breast cancer metastases target the meninges or the skull diploic space. Growth of such lesions may be intracranial and can compress the brain surface, whereas metastases to the skull base dura or bone can exert mass effect on the brainstem or cranial nerves.

The most common imaging manifestation of intracranial metastatic disease is multiple intra-axial brain masses.[6] These vary in size, shape, and enhancement patterns; the amount of associated edema can range from negligible to intense. Lesions can be solid and enhance uniformly (Figure 1), or can be cystic (Figure 2) or necrotic, with peripheral rim enhancement. Rim enhancement can be thin, thick, uniform, or irregular (Figure 3). Identifying single or multiple intracranial mass lesions in a breast cancer patient is highly suspicious for intra-cranial metastases, although it has mimics with other diagnoses, including other neoplasms (metastases from other primaries, brain primary neoplasia, and CNS lymphoma), demyelinating disorders such as multiple sclerosis, multifocal infectious or granulomatous processes, and multi-focal ischemic or vasculitic lesions.[6]

Extra-axial mass lesions may be formed by metastases to the skull or dura. Dural-based meta-static masses can be nodular and mass-like (Figure 4) or elongated and plaque-like (Figure 5). The underlying cerebral cortex may be compressed and edema incited in the underlying parenchyma. Mor-phologically, dural-based metastases may mimic meningiomas, or subdural collections.[6]

Leptomeningeal tumor consists at pathologic studies of sheet-like growth of tumor on the brain, spinal cord, or nerve root surfaces. Three mecha-nisms are postulated for CSF dissemination of tumors.[3] Tumor cells may rupture out of the sub-arachnoid space or pial vessels. Growing metasta-ses in the brain cortex or pia may contact and be bathed by CSF, and thereby shed cells into it. Alter-natively, hematogenous metastases to the choroid plexus may seed the CSF. Lobular carcinoma has been noted in clinical and autopsy series to be more likely to manifest as leptomeningeal tumor

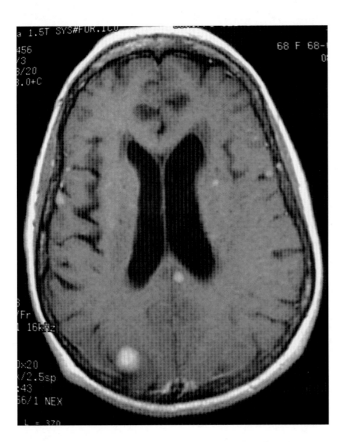

FIGURE 1. Enhanced T1-weighted axial MRI from a 68-year-old woman with metastatic breast cancer shows multiple, scattered, rounded, uniformly enhancing masses. Most are peripheral in location, near the brain surface.

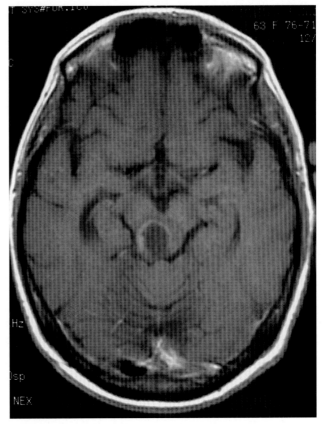

FIGURE 2. Enhanced T1-weighted axial MRI from a 63-year-old woman with metastatic breast involvement shows a cystic midbrain lesion with an enhancing rim of variable thickness. The patient presented with new onset of ataxia. Brain metastases were identified 3 years after diagnosis of breast cancer and 1 year after development of thoracic and bone recurrent disease.

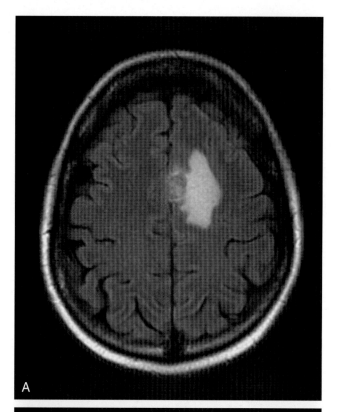

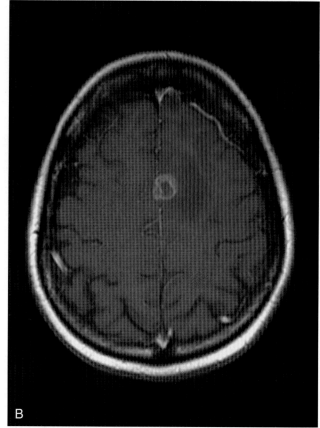

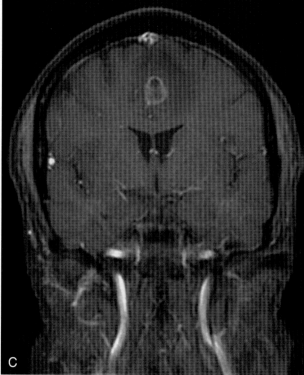

FIGURE 3. A 52-year-old woman with metastatic breast cancer to pleura and peritoneum, who developed numbness of the lips and slurred speech. Her original diagnosis of infiltrating ductal carcinoma was 14 years before, with axillary recurrence at 5 years. Brain MRIs (**A,** axial fluid attenuated inversion recovery (FLAIR); **B,** enhanced T1-weighted axial; **C,** coronal, fat-saturated enhanced T1-weighted) show a single brain metastasis to the left paramedian frontal lobe, adjacent to the falx. On FLAIR, the lesion itself is isointense to mildly hyperintense to brain parenchyma, but is outlined by the associated edema. Contrast-enhanced sequences show thick and irregular peripheral enhancement, which suggests central necrosis.

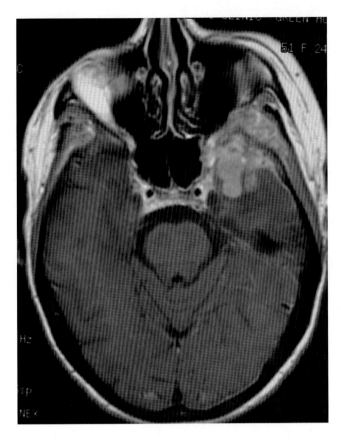

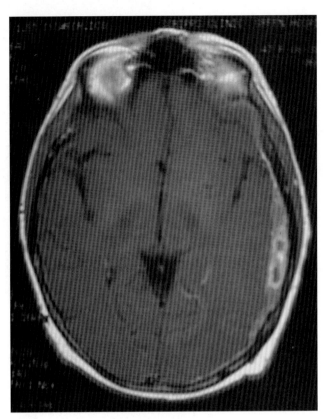

FIGURE 4. Enhanced axial T1-weighted MRI of a 51-year-old woman with metastatic breast cancer shows an enhancing, lobular, dural- and bone-based mass centered on the left sphenoid wing. The component extending into the left middle cranial fossa mimics a meningioma, being dural based and extra-axial, with well-defined margins and an enhancing dural tail. The underlying brain is compressed and edematous. Enhancing tumor also replaces the sphenoid wing bones, and on other levels, extended into the left orbit (not shown). See additional images from the same patient in Case 6 in this chapter.

FIGURE 5. A 47-year-old woman with new-onset expressive aphasia and prior gamma knife therapy 7 months before for right posterior parietal metastasis. Enhanced axial T1-weighted MRI shows a localized region of plaque-like metastatic dural enhancement over the left cerebrum. Additional images on this case can be seen in Case 7 in this chapter.

than ductal carcinoma. The diagnosis can be suggested by characteristic imaging findings on gadolinium-enhanced MRI or can be established by CSF cytology. The imaging hallmarks are enhancement of the leptomeninges (pia and arachnoid) on the brain or cord surface, which can be confluent and sheet-like or nodular, with extension into sulci or along cranial nerves or around the cauda equina (Figure 6).

DETECTION OF CNS METASTASES BY IMAGING

Gadolinium-chelate contrast-enhanced MRI is acknowledged to be the most sensitive imaging modality for the diagnosis of neural axis metasta-

ses.[7,8] Enhanced MRI is superior to enhanced CT for both brain parenchymal and brain and spine leptomeningeal disease due to its higher soft tissue contrast, higher sensitivity to contrast enhancement, direct multiplanar capability, and lack of artifacts related to bone. It particularly excels in demonstration of lesions in the posterior fossa and brainstem, where beam-hardening artifacts can be problematic on CT. MRI is also superior to CT in identifying multiple lesions, which is helpful in the differential diagnosis.[6]

The role of brain PET is limited in evaluating for metastases. Although brain metastases can be seen occasionally on whole-body PET scans (see Case 4 in this chapter), the sensitivity of PET for detection of brain metastases is inferior to MRI and is size dependent. The likelihood of detecting a 1-cm lesion with PET is reported to be about 40%. On a retrospective evaluation of whole-body PET performance in identifying brain metastases, Rohren and colleagues found that PET detected only 61% of lesions found by MRI.[5]

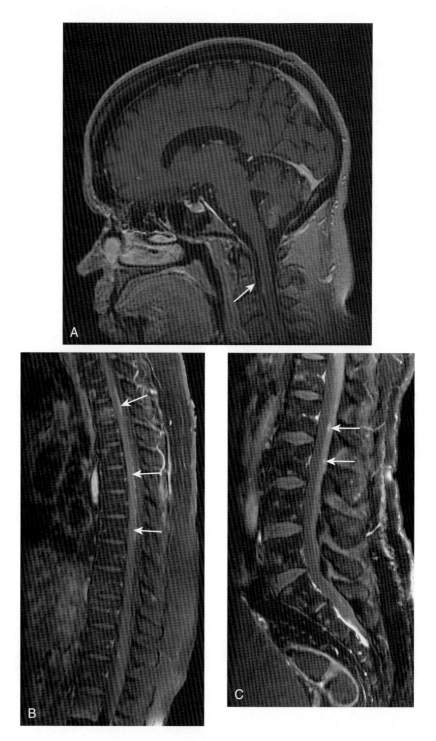

FIGURE 6. A 51-year-old woman with metastatic breast cancer to liver, bone, and brain, imaged for progressive symptoms, with new perineal numbness, worsening weakness, and urinary incontinence. Based on prior evaluations for headache, the patient was known to have predominantly infratentorial brain parenchymal metastases, diagnosed 5 months before and treated with whole-brain radiation. Her original diagnosis of breast cancer was 9 years before, treated with mastectomy, radiation, and chemotherapy. She had been known to have liver metastases for 6 years and bone involvement for 2 years at the time of identification of brain metastases. **A,** Sagittal, enhanced (double-dose technique), high-resolution, T1-weighted, gradient echo image shows an enhancing inferior vermis metastasis. In the upper cervical spine included here, linear surface enhancement is seen on the cord (*arrow*). **B,** Fat-saturated, enhanced, T1-weighted sagittal view of the thoracic spine shows evidence of known spine and liver metastases. The cord surface also shows linear surface enhancement, compatible with leptomeningeal tumor (*arrows*). **C,** Fat-saturated, enhanced, T1-weighted sagittal view of the lumbar spine also shows foci of linear enhancement of cauda equina roots (*arrows*).

INDICATIONS FOR IMAGING

CNS metastases may be heralded clinically by focal neurologic symptoms, seizure activity, or symptoms reflecting increased intracranial pressure, such as headache, nausea, vomiting, and mental status changes.[1,3] Focal neurologic symptoms may result from tumor-induced chemical changes causing neuron dysfunction and swelling, or from mass effect from compression of normal tissue. Tumor-induced electrical dysfunction can lead to seizure activity. Increased intracranial pressure may result from obstructive hydrocephalus, such as from mass effect from a parenchymal metastasis to the posterior fossa, or from communicating hydrocephalus due to leptomeningeal metastases.

The most common presenting symptom for brain parenchymal metastases is headache, followed by mental status changes and cognitive disturbances. Less common manifestations of CNS metastases include visual and sensory disturbances, focal weakness, seizure, ataxia, and nausea and vomiting. Leptomeningeal disease more often presents with nonlocalizing symptoms of headache or neck or back pain, although cranial neuropathies may result.

TREATMENT OPTIONS

After corticosteroid treatment for edema, therapeutic choices for brain metastases include whole-brain radiation therapy (WBRT), neurosurgery, stereotactic radiosurgery (SRS), and chemotherapy.[1,2,3] If there are multiple metastases, WBRT has been shown to improve survival and quality of life compared with corticosteroids alone. Median survival is 4 to 5 months. Most patients (75% to 85%) will have improvement of symptoms, with best palliation achieved of seizures and headache. Imaging responses to effective radiation therapy range from complete resolution to shrinkage in size of lesions, to decreased number of identifiable lesions, to alterations of morphology, with improved mass effect and associated edema (Figure 7).

A single metastasis to the brain can be treated either neurosurgically or with SRS. The major advantage of neurosurgery is immediate relief of mass effect from debulking. The decision making is highly dependent on the lesion location.

Surgery can be beneficial to treat a solitary brain metastasis if the breast cancer history is remote (e.g., there is a long tumor-free interval between diagnosis and development of brain metastasis), and there is no other evidence of metastases. Survival is improved in patients undergoing surgery and WBRT for solitary brain metastasis than for those treated with radiation alone. Average survival after resection of a solitary brain metastasis and WBRT is about 1 year.

Selected patients with brain metastases from a variety of primary types (single lesions, better performance status, controlled extra-CNS disease) have better outcomes with surgery than with WBRT. Postoperative external-beam radiation is usually given after gross total tumor excision to treat microscopic residual disease. The addition of WBRT does not appear to confer a survival advantage, although there is improved local control with lower rates of relapse. The major risk of WBRT is progressive dementia.

Single or few metastases can also be treated noninvasively with SRS. Decision making is based on the size and location of the lesion. Ideal lesions for SRS are less than 3 cm in diameter. Stereotactic radiosurgery involves many radiation beams intersecting at a point, resulting in the delivery of a high additive lethal dose to a target tumor, while largely sparing the surrounding brain. Typically, SRS is given as a single, outpatient treatment. Gamma knife is one form of SRS. Contraindications are tumors of large size (>3 cm) and those with significant edema because the treatment can be expected to incite further edema. It is an option to consider for surgically inaccessible metastases (e.g., the brainstem) and can be used to treat multiple tumors.

These treatment options can also be combined. There is evidence that administration of WBRT after SRS reduces the risk for CNS relapse.

There appears to be no clear survival advantage between surgery and SRS in appropriately selected patients. Either treatment confers a survival advantage over WBRT alone.

Chemotherapy plays a lesser role in treatment of breast cancer brain metastases. Most agents used do not cross an intact blood-brain barrier; however, the blood-brain barrier may be dysfunctional with brain metastases, and responses have been reported with agents that do not cross the intact barrier.

Because CSF metastatic disease most commonly manifests as hydrocephalus, and less commonly with carcinomatous meningitis, treatment is directed toward relief of hydrocephalus with shunting, and intrathecal chemotherapy may be considered, administered either by lumbar punctures or Ommaya reservoir.

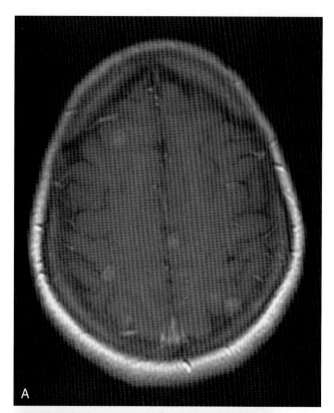

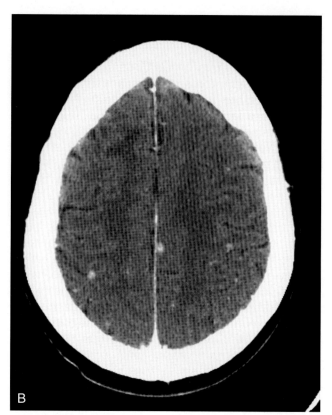

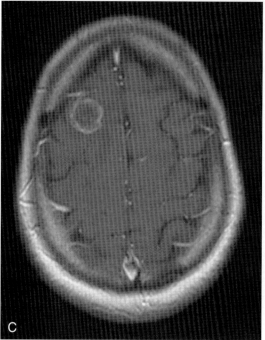

FIGURE 7. A 43-year-old woman with metastatic breast cancer to bone developed headaches. Her breast cancer had been diagnosed 3 years before, and bone metastases were identified 8 months before evaluation for headache. Whole-brain radiation was given for palliation, with improvement in the patient's symptoms. **A,** Axial, enhanced, T1-weighted brain MRI at a supratentorial level shows multiple scattered, uniformly enhancing, round newly diagnosed metastases at the gray-white matter junction. **B,** Enhanced head CT, 4 months later, after whole-brain radiation, shows tiny scattered, smaller residual enhancing metastases, which have shrunk in response to radiation therapy. **C,** Seven months later, the patient presented with a new seizure. Repeat brain MRI showed progressive disease, with interval growth of several lesions and increased associated edema. A right frontal lesion has grown, and now displays ring enhancement.

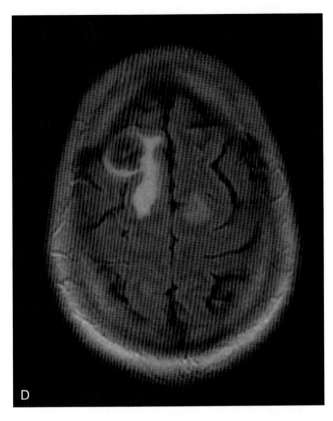
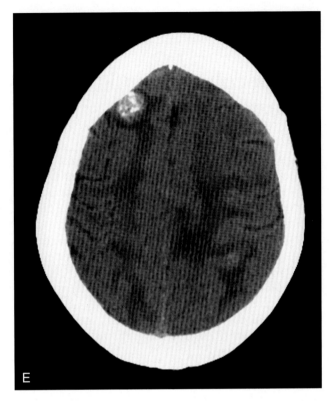

FIGURE 7, cont'd D, Axial FLAIR of the same lesion shows the associated edema, as well as edema associated with a left paramedian frontal lesion. **E,** Unenhanced head CT scan, 2 months later, after gamma knife therapy of the same lesion. Calcification is now seen of the treated lesion.

SPINAL METASTASES

Metastases that compress the spinal cord most commonly present with pain at that level. With increased compression, symptoms progress to numbness below that level and eventually to difficulty ambulating. If untreated, there can be progression to paralysis. Bowel and bladder dysfunction may occur late.

Metastases to the cauda equina produce back pain and, variably, radicular symptoms.[9]

REFERENCES

1. Lin NU, Bellon JR, Winer EP. CNS metastases in breast cancer. *J Clin Oncol* 2004; 22:3608–3617.
2. Chang EL, Lo S. Diagnosis and management of central nervous system metastases from breast cancer. *Oncologist* 2003; 8:398–410.
3. Parker EC, Kelly PJ. Brain metastases from breast cancer. In Roses DF (ed): Breast Cancer. Philadelphia, Elsevier Churchill Livingstone, 2005, pp. 633–643.
4. Bendell JC, Domchek SM, Burstein HJ, et al. Central nervous system metastases in women who receive trastuzumab-based therapy for metastatic breast carcinoma. *Cancer* 2003; 97(12):2972–2977.
5. Rohren EM, Provenzale JM, Barboriak DP, et al. Screening for cerebral metastases with FDG PET in patients undergoing whole-body staging of non–central nervous system malignancy. *Radiology* 2003; 226: 181–187.
6. Yock DH. Magnetic Resonance Imaging of CNS Disease: A Teaching File. St. Louis, Mosby, 2002, pp. 2–19, 101, 439.
7. Sze G, Milano E, Johnson C, et al. Detection of brain metastases: comparison of contrast-enhanced MR with unenhanced MR and enhanced CT. *AJNR Am J Neuroradiol* 1990; 11:785.
8. Davis PC, Hudgins PA, Peterman SB, et al. Diagnosis of cerebral metastases: double-dose delayed CT vs contrast-enhanced MR imaging. *AJNR Am J Neuroradiol* 1991; 12:293.
9. Douglas AF, Cooper PR. Spinal column metastases from breast cancer. In Roses DF (ed): Breast Cancer. Philadelphia, Elsevier Churchill Livingstone, 2005, pp. 644–652.

CASE 1

Multilocular thalamic cystic metastasis

A 43-year-old woman with metastatic breast cancer to the thorax developed nausea, one episode of vomiting, progressive headache, confusion, and speech difficulty.

Her diagnosis of stage T2N1 breast cancer was 5 years before, a 4.5-cm poorly differentiated adeno-carcinoma, with one positive lymph node. She underwent bilateral mastectomy and received adjuvant Cytoxan, methotrexate, 5-fluorouracil (CMF) chemotherapy and tamoxifen. Her prior medical history was notable for treatment of Hodgkin's lymphoma at age 17 with radiation and chemotherapy.

Lung and nodal breast cancer metastases had been identified the year before with PET and CT evaluation for rising tumor markers. The diagnosis of recurrent breast cancer was confirmed by a lung nodule biopsy, which showed malignant adenocarcinoma, consistent with breast primary. The patient was begun on a regimen of docetaxel (Taxotere) and Gemzar. This was eventually discontinued because of pulmonary toxicity (see Case 12 in Chapter 10) and disease progression. The patient's regimen was changed to capecitabine (Xeloda) for six cycles, with a good initial response, but subsequent regrowth.

When the patient developed symptoms of headache, nausea, and mental status changes, a non-contrast head CT scan was obtained (Figure 1). The head CT identified a lesion and suggested that secondary hydrocephalus was developing. Unenhanced head CT excluded a hemorrhage. Brain MRI was obtained next, which better showed the internal structure of the mass, which was solitary (Figure 2).

The patient was evaluated by neurosurgery and radiation oncology. She was started on dexamethasone (Decadron) and elected to undergo whole-brain radiation therapy (WBRT). Her symptoms improved.

TEACHING POINTS

This patient was treated for Hodgkin's disease with radiation as an adolescent, a demographic at

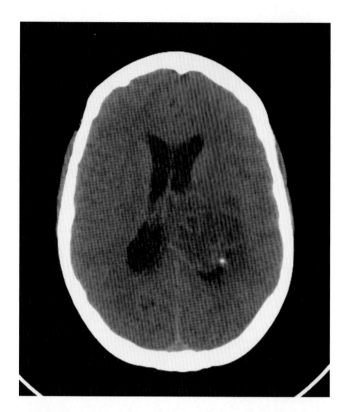

FIGURE 1. Noncontrast head CT scan shows a large mass lesion centered in the left thalamus. A portion of the mass has a multilocular, cystic appearance. The lateral ventricles appear prominent, suggesting developing hydrocephalus.

known higher risk for development of breast cancer. As is usual with breast cancer CNS metastases, which typically occur late, this patient already had known extracranial metastases in the thorax at the time she presented with this presumed solitary brain metastasis.

Brain metastases may be cystic or solid. Larger lesions in particular can have associated cystic or necrotic regions. The surrounding rim of enhancing tumor can be fairly smooth and thin, irregularly thickened, or both, as seen here. Based on imaging features alone, the differential diagnosis of a neoplasm with this appearance would include a primary malignant glioma. The clinical context and presence of additional lesions in the case of metastases generally allow differentiation.

Although hematogenous brain metastases classically favor a peripheral distribution, often at the gray-white matter junction, brain metastases not uncommonly occur in deeper locations, frequently the periventricular regions. Masses such as this, occurring adjacent to ventricles, can be difficult to distinguish from masses within ventricles. MRI is very helpful in this distinction, because of its multiplanar capability and better soft tissue contrast.

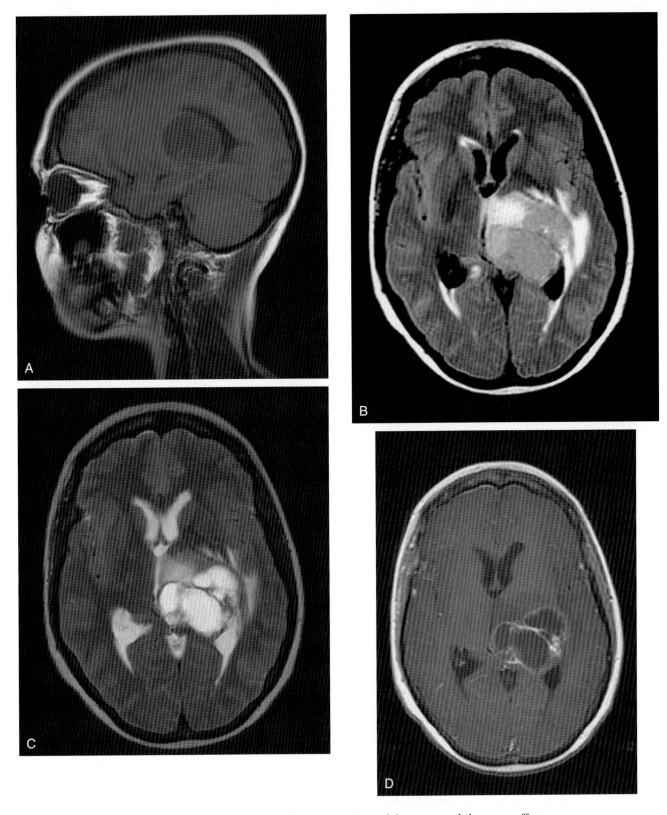

FIGURE 2. Brain MRIs better show the composition of the mass and the mass effect upon adjacent structures. **A,** T1-weighted sagittal image shows no hyperintense components to suggest hemorrhage. **B,** Axial FLAIR. **C,** Axial T2-weighted image. **D,** Contrast-enhanced axial T1-weighted image. *(Continued)*

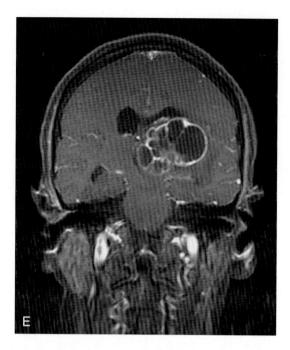

FIGURE 2, cont'd **E,** Contrast-enhanced, fat-saturated, coronal T1-weighted image. FLAIR and T2-weighted sequences show the cyst-like components of the mass to differ in fluid signal intensity from cerebrospinal fluid (CSF). Edema is seen anterior and lateral to the mass. The third ventricle is deviated to the right. Periventricular edema at the lateral ventricular margins, well seen on FLAIR, is compatible with transependymal migration of CSF, and suggests developing hydrocephalus. Enhanced T1-weighted sequences show rim enhancement of the cystic locules. The mass pushes up on and distorts the trigone of the lateral ventricle, as well as deviating the third ventricle to the right.

The higher sensitivity of MRI is also useful in the evaluation of suspected metastases by identification or exclusion of additional lesions.

Solitary brain metastases may be considered for local therapy with surgery or stereotactic radiosurgery (SRS). The available data suggest prolonged survival of suitable candidates with local therapy than patients treated with whole brain radiation therapy (WBRT) alone. The location and size of a metastasis and the control status of extra-CNS disease are factors considered in decision making. The best candidates for local therapy are those with limited disease in an accessible location who have well-controlled systemic disease. Of note, the limited data available come from series that include brain metastases from a variety of primary sources.

In this case, the lesion size (4.7 cm) would generally preclude consideration of SRS, which is usually reserved for lesions smaller than 3 cm. Surgery enables immediate decompression of large, symp-tomatic metastases, while establishing a histologic diagnosis.

Treatment with WBRT confers a survival advantage over treatment with corticosteroids alone, with a median survival of 4 to 6 months. Most patients (75% to 85%) can expect improvement or stabilization of their neurologic symptoms with WBRT. Administration of WBRT also decreases the incidence of subsequent CNS relapse.

CASE 2

Brain metastases mimicking multiple sclerosis

A 60-year-old woman with metastatic breast cancer to the left orbit, lungs, and bones was evaluated with brain CT for intractable nausea. Her breast cancer had been diagnosed 3 years before as a stage I infiltrative ductal carcinoma of the right breast, estrogen receptor and progesterone receptor positive, *HER-2/neu* positive, with five negative lymph nodes. She was treated with lumpectomy and radiation. She received no adjuvant therapy except for 1 month of tamoxifen, which was discontinued because of intolerance.

Metastatic breast cancer, estrogen receptor positive, progesterone receptor negative, *HER-2/neu* negative, was identified 2 years later, as a left axillary lump. Later the same year, metastatic orbital and lung involvement was identified. The lung disease was biopsy proven, with a left lower lobe wedge excision showing metastatic carcinoma to pleura and lung with lymphovascular invasion.

The patient was treated with radiation to the orbit, and systemic chemotherapy with trastuzumab (Herceptin) and capecitabine (Xeloda), without response.

At the time of evaluation for intractable nausea and dry heaves, additional symptoms of dysphagia, coughing, anorexia, and weight loss were noted. Head CT, with and without contrast enhancement, showed small, enhancing periventricular white matter lesions, and a sclerotic clivus lesion (Figures 1, 2, and 3). MRI showed comparable findings (Figures 4, 5, 6, and 7).

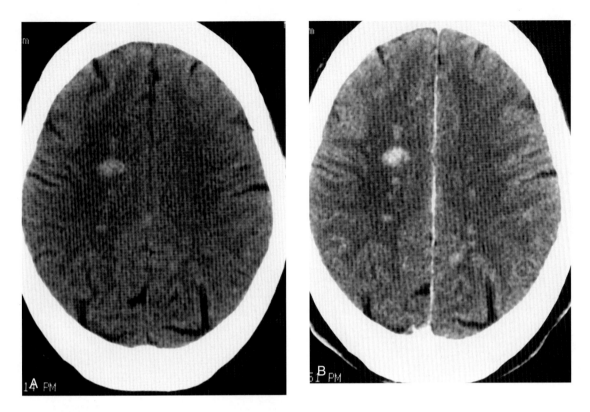

FIGURE 1. Unenhanced (**A**) and enhanced (**B**) head CT images obtained at the centrum semiovale level show multiple white matter lesions. On unenhanced imaging, the visualized lesions are hyperdense. The lesions enhance, and more are seen with contrast administration.

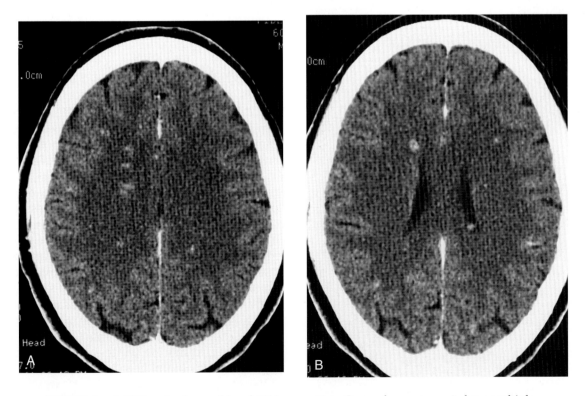

FIGURE 2. Additional enhanced head CT images (**A** to **C,** see also next page) show multiple, small, white matter, enhancing lesions in a periventricular distribution.   (*Continued*)

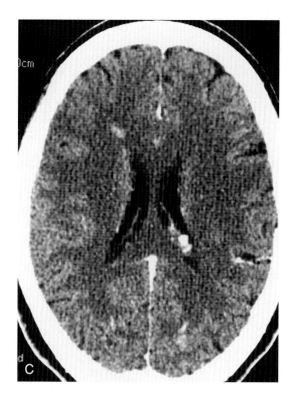

FIGURE 2, cont'd

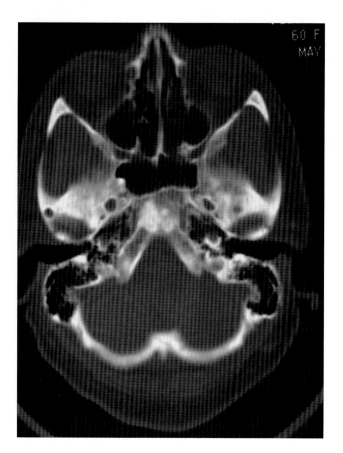

FIGURE 3. Head CT bone window through the skull base shows a sclerotic bone lesion in the clivus.

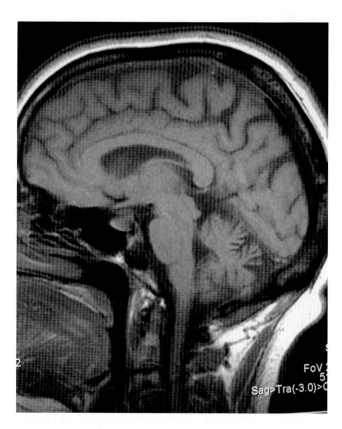

FIGURE 4. Sagittal T1-weighted image through the midline of the brain shows hypointensity of the calvarial and upper cervical spine bone marrow. A hypointense lesion is seen in the clivus, with some preservation of fatty marrow signal surrounding the hypointense lesion.

TEACHING POINTS

The differential diagnosis of multiple enhancing intracranial lesions is long and includes neoplasms (metastases and primary CNS lymphoma), demyelinating processes (e.g., multiple sclerosis and acute disseminated encephalomyelitis), infection (e.g., cysticercosis, tuberculosis, histoplasmosis, toxoplasmosis), granulomatous processes (e.g., sarcoid), ischemia, and vasculitis. These multiple intracranial lesions represent a relatively unusual presentation of brain metastases, with morphology and distribution mimicking multiple sclerosis plaques. The features suggesting this include the relatively uniform size of the lesions, lack of significant associated edema, and the central periventricular distribution, rather than the more typical peripheral gray matter–white matter junction location favored by many hematogenous metastases.

In this case, a repeat study obtained 11 days later showed worsening, with edema now associated with left cerebellar lesions.

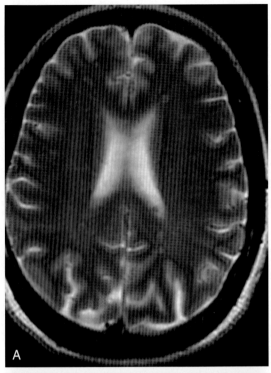

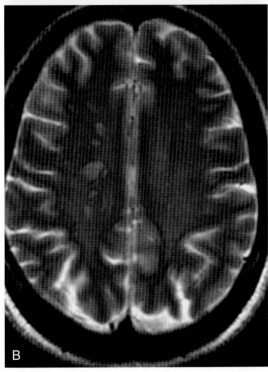

FIGURE 5.   Axial T2-weighted images (**A,** through the ventricles; **B,** through the centrum semiovale) show multiple foci of white matter hyperintensity, many in the periventricular regions. No associated edema is seen. Some of lesions are elliptical in shape.

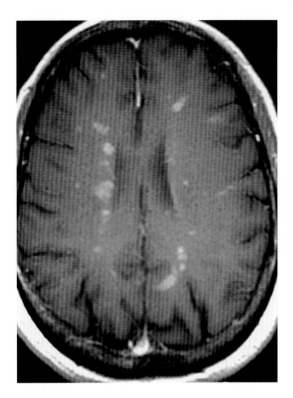

FIGURE 6.   Enhanced T1-weighted axial series shows that most of the white matter lesions enhance. The predominant periventricular distribution is well seen here, with some of the linear and elliptical-shaped lesions oriented perpendicular to the long axis of the lateral ventricles.

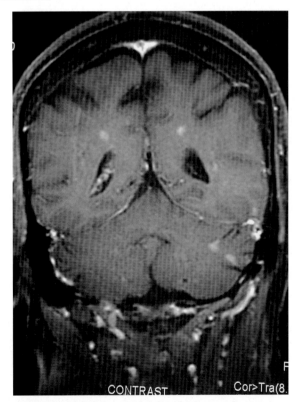

FIGURE 7.   Fat-saturated coronal, T1-weighted, enhanced image shows additional small, enhancing lesions in the subcortical left cerebellum.

Brain metastases mimicking multiple sclerosis

A 38-year-old woman treated for breast cancer 2 years earlier developed episodes of visual disturbance, with scintillating scotomas. Enhanced brain MRI was abnormal, with multiple enhancing elliptical white matter lesions, without edema (Figures 1 and 2). A differential diagnosis of brain metastases versus demyelinating process (multiple sclerosis) was considered.

The patient's breast cancer was a stage II, T2N0, estrogen receptor– and progesterone receptor–positive, *HER-2/neu* positive, 2.5-cm left breast high-grade infiltrating ductal carcinoma with extensive ductal carcinoma in situ, which was treated with lumpectomy, chemotherapy (four cycles of doxorubicin [Adriamycin] and cyclophosphamide [Cytoxan]), and radiation. Zero of 6 lymph nodes were involved. At the time of evaluation for the visual disturbance, the patient had recently been diagnosed with liver, mediastinal, and bone metastases and was being treated for these with vinorelbine (Navelbine) and trastuzumab (Herceptin). A symptomatic left hip metastasis was prophylactically treated with an intramedullary femoral nail. Tissue from this procedure confirmed breast metastasis.

Repeat brain MRI 2 months later showed more numerous and larger enhancing brain lesions, with a more typical appearance for metastases than on the prior study (Figure 3).

A cervical and thoracic spine MRI was obtained at the time of the initial brain MRI to evaluate complaints of back pain. Spine MRI showed metastatic involvement of T4 (Figure 4), and the patient underwent T3-T5 radiation for palliation of symptoms.

TEACHING POINTS

Intracranial lesions in patients with cancer histories most often represent brain metastases, although not invariably. The differential diagnosis includes primary brain neoplasia, infection, inflammation, infarction, and as raised in this case, demyelinating processes. In a randomized trial reported by Patchell and colleagues of 54 patients who underwent

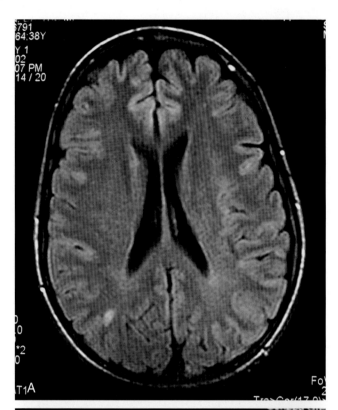

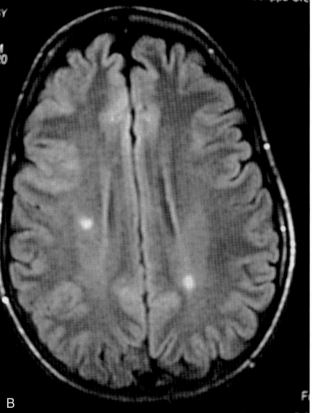

FIGURE 1. Axial FLAIR images through the ventricles (**A**) and centrum semiovale (**B**) show scattered, small, round to elliptical foci of white matter hyperintensity, without associated edema or mass effect.

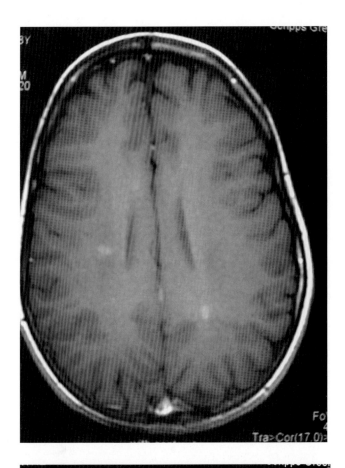

FIGURE 2.   Enhanced axial T1-weighted sequence, at the same level as Figure 1B, shows enhancement of the lesions.

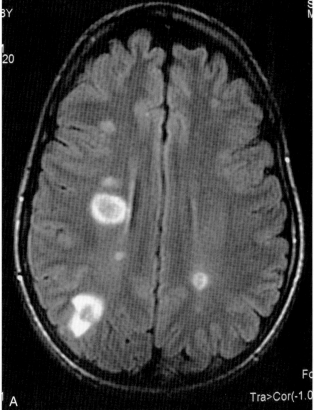

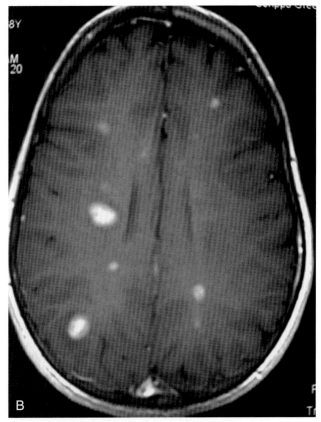

FIGURE 3.   Repeat brain MRI, 2 months later, at levels corresponding to Figures 1B and 2 (**A,** axial FLAIR; **B**, enhanced axial T1-weighted) shows the lesions to be larger, with collars of perilesional edema demonstrated on FLAIR. Multiple similar appearing new enhancing lesions are seen in addition.

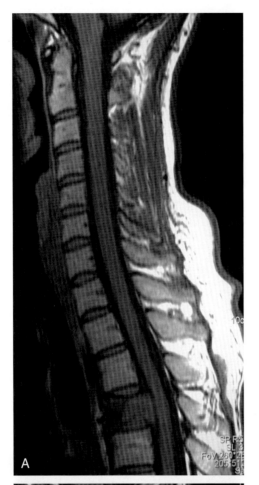

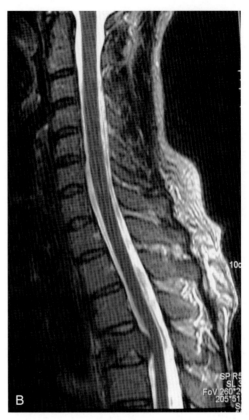

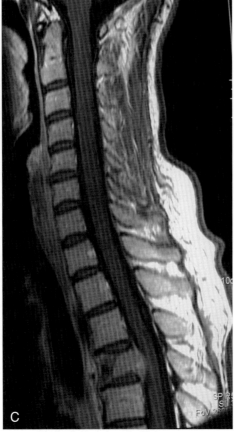

FIGURE 4. Sagittal spine MRIs through the cervical and upper thoracic spine (**A,** T1-weighted, sagittal; **B,** T2-weighted sagittal; **C,** enhanced T1-weighted sagittal) show abnormal signal intensity at T4. This is most conspicuous on unenhanced T1-weighted imaging as loss of the normal bright fatty marrow signal. Expansion of the replaced vertebral body into the anterior epidural space is well seen on all sequences. Delineation of the mass effect and ventral impression on the cord are aided by use of T2-weighted imaging, in which CSF fluid signal is bright. Dural tails of enhancement associated with the bony and epidural metastasis are depicted on the enhanced T1-weighted sequence.

either surgery and radiation therapy compared with radiation therapy after needle biopsy for treatment of single brain metastases from a variety of primaries, 11% were found to have an alternative diagnosis on pathology.

Atypical imaging presentations may require biopsy or follow-up imaging to differentiate metastatic disease from other possibilities. This case initially was a surprisingly good imaging mimic for multiple sclerosis, with the lesions small and discrete, many being elliptical in shape, located in the deep white matter and lacking associated edema. The repeat study shows more typical metastatic findings, with the larger lesions now seen on FLAIR as isointense to parenchyma, with collars of perilesional edema. The interval growth and increase in number also are strong presumptive evidence of progressive metastatic disease.

The bone metastasis depicted here at T4 shows typical imaging features (see Figure 4). The bone lesion conspicuity, based on replacement of the normal fatty marrow signal, is greatest on T1-weighted images. Bone lesion conspicuity is comparatively poor with T2-weighting where the lesion is essentially isointense to other vertebral levels. The expansion of the replaced body into the epidural space and mass effect on the cord are well depicted against the bright cerebrospinal fluid (CSF) signal afforded by T2-weighted technique. Contrast enhancement also decreases the conspicuity of the bony lesion, although depiction of the epidural extent, associated dural enhancement, and mass effect on the cord are improved.

MRI protocols for evaluation of the spine need to be designed to detect most significant pathology. Bone metastases can generally be identified without contrast enhancement, and as demonstrated in this case, contrast enhancement can actually decrease the conspicuity of bone lesions. Protocols generally include a T1-weighted sequence and a fluid-sensitive sequence, either T2-weighted or short tau inversion recovery (STIR) sequence. Contrast enhancement, although not essential for the diagnosis of bone metastases, is necessary for complete evaluation of the spinal contents. This can be obtained with a fat-saturated, T1-weighted sequence to compensate for the decreased conspicuity of enhancing bone metastases.

SUGGESTED READING

Patchell RA, Tibbs PA, Walsh JW, et al. A randomized trial of surgery in the treatment of single metastases to the brain. *N Engl J Med* 1990; 322:494–500.

CASE 4

Brain metastases identified on PET in an asymptomatic metastatic breast cancer patient

A 52-year-old woman on chemotherapy for metastatic breast cancer to bone was being followed with positron emission tomography (PET)/CT (Figure 1). Although she was asymptomatic from a neurologic standpoint, PET suggested new brain metastases (Figures 2 and 3). These were confirmed on enhanced brain MRI, which showed multiple additional lesions (Figures 4, 5, 6, 7, 8, 9, and 10).

The patient initially presented 16 months before with a greater than 1 year history of a central, firm, and retracted left breast mass involving the nipple, with fungation and drainage. The patient had not sought medical attention. Evaluations at presentation confirmed a locally advanced, poorly differentiated infiltrating ductal carcinoma, estrogen receptor and progesterone receptor positive, and *HER-2/neu* positive, involving axillary lymph nodes and metastatic to bone (see Case 1 in Chapter 12).

The patient received chemotherapy for locally advanced and metastatic breast cancer. The patient had an excellent clinical response to chemotherapy (six cycles of trastuzumab [Herceptin], docetaxel [Taxotere], and carboplatin), with improved bone pain and partial regression of the breast mass. PET scan hypermetabolism at both the breast and bony levels dramatically improved. She was then maintained on a regimen of Herceptin, zoledronic acid (Zometa), and letrozole (Femara) with continued clinical response. About 1 year after presentation, her tumor markers began to rise, and reimaging with CT and PET showed tumor progression. PET hypermetabolism in the index breast mass and in bone metastases, which had markedly regressed with chemotherapy, showed recurrent increased metabolic activity. The patient's therapy was changed to vinorelbine (Navelbine) and Herceptin. The efficacy of this therapy was being assessed with PET/CT at the time the unsuspected brain metastases were noted.

Palliative whole-brain radiation therapy was performed (Figure 11). The Navelbine was discon-

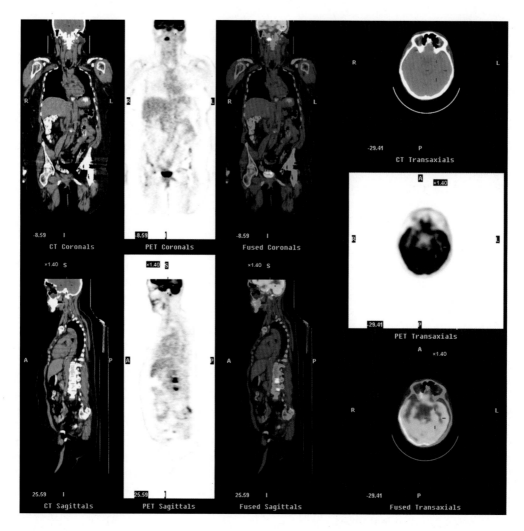

FIGURE 1.   Images from three-plane PET/CT show multiple foci of hypermetabolism localizing to bone, demonstrated here in the upper cervical spine, at adjacent lumbar spine levels and in the pelvis. The intensity is adjusted for optimal display of the PET scan data in the body, so the brain is intensely hypermetabolic at this setting. The location of one of the two identified brain lesions is marked here with *cursors*, but no lesion is visualized with the brain activity displayed at this threshold.

tinued, and Herceptin was held because of decline in left ventricular ejection fraction.

TEACHING POINTS

Brain metastases generally are heralded by the development of symptoms, leading to further imaging, usually with enhanced brain MRI. This case is unusual in that brain metastases were first identified on whole-body PET in a neurologically asymptomatic breast cancer patient being treated for bone metastases. Visualization of brain metastases on a whole-body PET scan depends on the lesions being of sufficient size and hypermetabo-

lism to be seen against the background of normal brain activity. As demonstrated in this case, this depends on the interpreter adjusting the intensity of brain to a much lower level than would be used for evaluating the rest of the scan. Although the yield is low, this case illustrates the utility of routinely including in one's search pattern a review of the brain with the intensity threshold adjusted to a level at which one can "see through" the brain background activity. In this case, the patient presumably would have become symptomatic with growth of the lesions. This allowed early intervention.

How frequently are brain metastases identified on whole-body PET? The answer is: not often enough to justify inclusion of the brain in whole-body fluorodeoxyglucose (FDG) PET studies performed for

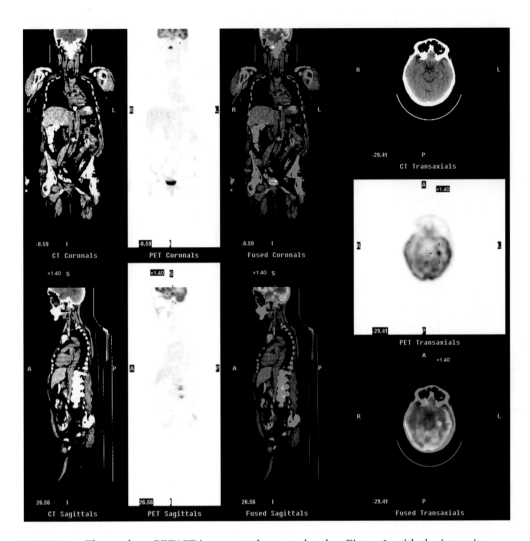

FIGURE 2. Three-plane PET/CT images at the same level as Figure 1, with the intensity "dialed down" to better visualize the brain parenchyma. The bone metastases are less well seen, but a small hypermetabolic metastasis can now be seen in the left temporal lobe of the brain (*cursors*).

staging purposes. Most of the information in the literature is derived from studies of lung cancer staging, but the same principles and limitations should apply to detection of breast cancer brain metastases. In general, even dedicated brain PET is not sensitive enough to be relied on over CT or MRI. A retrospective study of PET compared with enhanced brain MRI by Rohren and associates showed PET to identify only 61% of the metastases seen on MRI. The sensitivity of FDG PET for detecting brain metastases in this study was 75%, with specificity of 83%. Lesion size is a major factor in the ability of brain PET to depict metastases. The likelihood of detecting a 1-cm metastasis has been estimated to be 40%.

Although not biopsy-proven, the diagnosis is quite certain in this case. Multiplicity is a hallmark of metastases, and as demonstrated here, metasta-ses can vary significantly in size, appearance, and presence or absence of associated edema. It is no surprise that many more lesions were seen on MRI than were suggested on PET. It is interesting to correlate the number, size, and appearance of brain metastases seen on PET versus MRI. The metastases seen on PET scan were the largest of the lesions confirmed on MRI. "Solidity" of a lesion also contributes to conspicuity on PET. The rim-enhancing, cystic metastasis seen only on brain MRI at the right temporal lobe level is similar in overall size to the more uniformly enhancing and solid metastasis at the left temporal level, which could be seen on both PET and MRI. This result is not surprising because the right temporal cystic lesion is less cellular, and would be expected to be less metabolically active than the more solid left temporal metastasis.

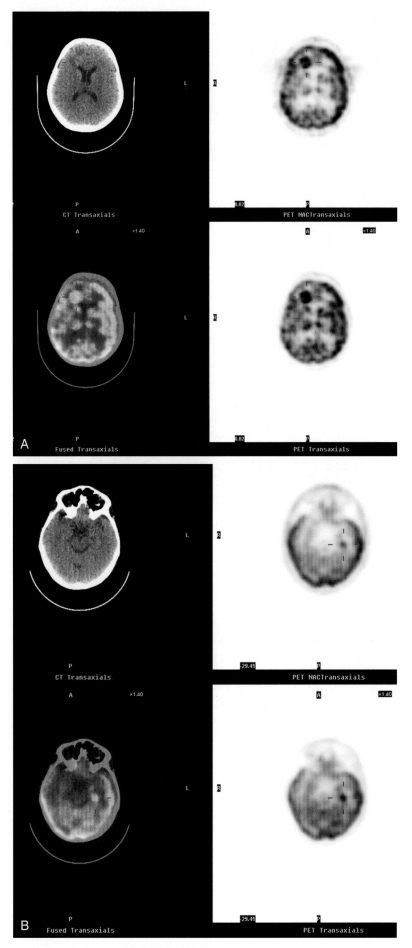

FIGURE 3. Axial PET/CT images (**A,** through the lateral ventricles; **B,** through the temporal and occipital lobes) show two hypermetabolic foci (the larger in the right frontal lobe, and a smaller lesion in the left temporal lobe). The clinical setting and multiplicity are strong presumptive evidence of brain metastases.

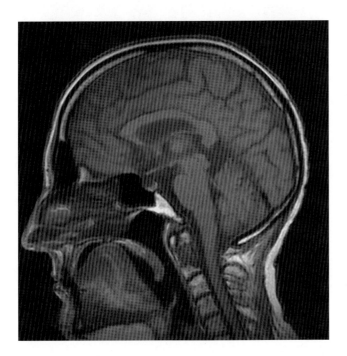

FIGURE 4. Sagittal T1-weighted midline brain MR image shows replacement of normal fatty marrow signal at the C2 level, correlating with known PET-positive disease.

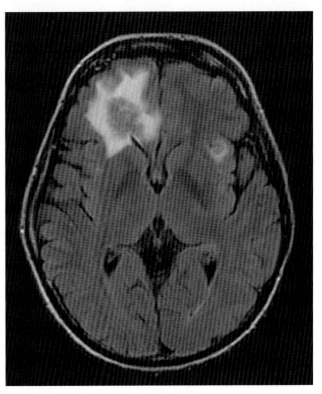

FIGURE 6. Axial FLAIR brain MRI at the same level as Figure 5, showing both isointense frontal lobe lesions to be surrounded by high signal vasogenic edema.

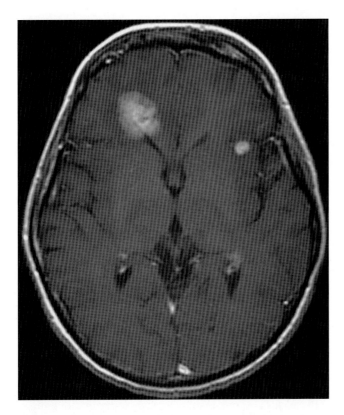

FIGURE 5. Axial enhanced, T1-weighted brain MRI shows two enhancing frontal lobe lesions. The larger of the two abuts the right frontal horn and corresponds to one of the two lesions first seen on PET imaging (see Figure 3A).

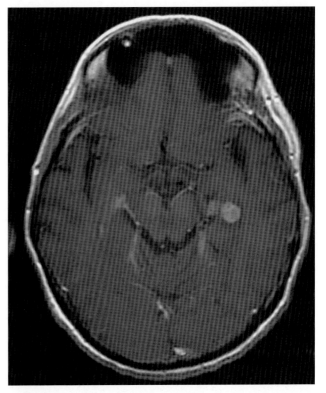

FIGURE 7. Axial enhanced, T1-weighted image through the temporal lobes shows a small, uniformly enhancing metastasis at the left temporal lobe level, representing the other lesion identified on PET (see Figures 2 and 3B).

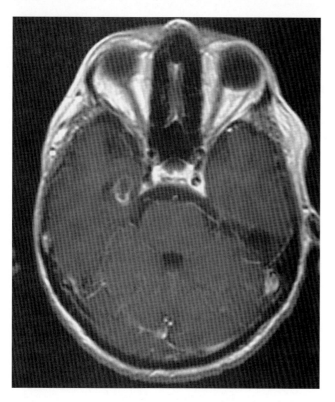

FIGURE 8. An enhanced T1-weighted image, through the orbits and inferior temporal lobes, shows a right temporal lobe ring-enhancing metastasis, which was not seen on PET.

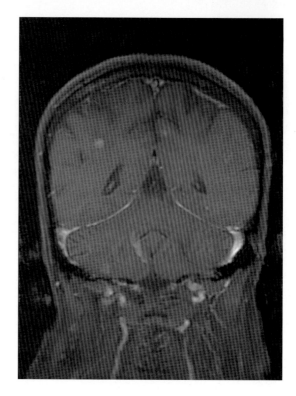

FIGURE 10. A more posterior, enhanced, fat-saturated, T1-weighted coronal image shows three additional small, enhancing metastases. One is on the right, superolateral to the ventricle, with another on the left, adjacent to the falx, and the third at the inferior right cerebellar level.

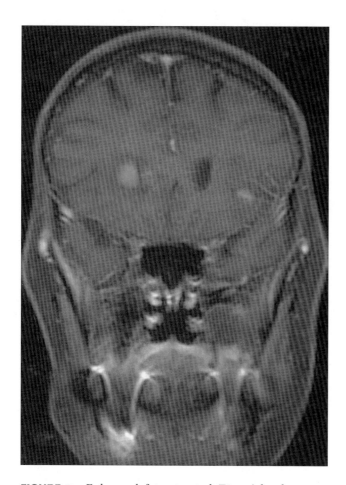

FIGURE 9. Enhanced, fat-saturated, T1-weighted coronal view through the frontal lobes shows the same two metastases seen in Figures 5 and 6.

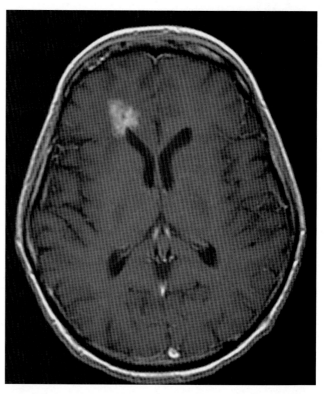

FIGURE 11. Three months later, repeat enhanced brain MRI (axial T1) shows response to whole-brain radiation. The largest lesion, at the right frontal level, is shown and has decreased in size. The additional smaller lesions had also improved, manifested as decreased size and intensity of enhancement, with resolution of the associated edema (not shown).

SUGGESTED READING

Rohren EM, Provenzale JM, Barboriak DP, et al. Screening for cerebral metastases with FDG PET in patients undergoing whole-body staging of non–central nervous system malignancy. *Radiology* 2003; 226: 181–187.

CASE 5

Unusual miliary pattern of brain metastases

A 57-year-old woman with locally recurrent and metastatic breast cancer to the pleura developed new symptoms of flashing visual disturbance, progressive lower extremity weakness, low back pain, nausea, occasional vomiting, and difficulty with balance.

Her original breast cancer was treated 9 years before with lumpectomy, axillary lymph node dissection, radiation, and chemotherapy. Her tumor was a poorly differentiated, 6.5-cm primary, estrogen receptor and progesterone receptor negative, *HER-2/neu* negative, with negative lymph nodes. She had a biopsy-proven local recurrence identified 1 year before, as well as biopsy-proven right pleural metastases. She had been treated with chemotherapy, with paclitaxel (Taxol) and bevacizumab (Avastin), with response clinically and by imaging.

Brain MRI obtained to evaluate the new neurologic symptoms showed an unusual pattern of metastases, with innumerable, tiny, miliary, enhancing nodules, concentrated in the cerebellum and scattered supratentorially (Figures 1, 2, 3, and 4). The patient was treated with whole-brain radiation therapy for palliation of symptoms.

TEACHING POINTS

This is an unusual pattern of brain metastases, with innumerable tiny, enhancing foci without much associated edema. The scattered supratentorial distribution of lesions, favoring the gray matter–white matter junction, is fairly typical, but the disproportionate concentration of lesions in the

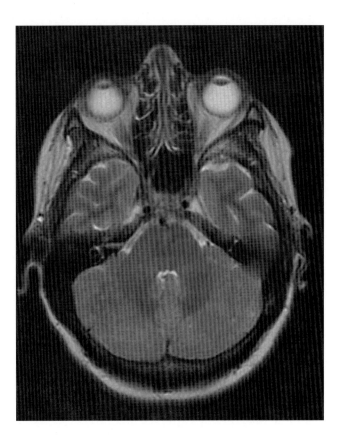

FIGURE 1. Axial T2-weighted brain MRI shows subtle diffuse cerebellar parenchymal heterogeneity.

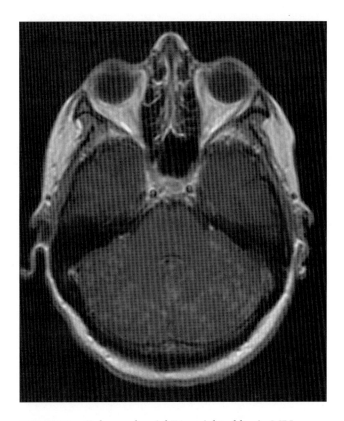

FIGURE 2. Enhanced, axial T1-weighted brain MRI shows innumerable, tiny, cerebellar foci of enhancement.

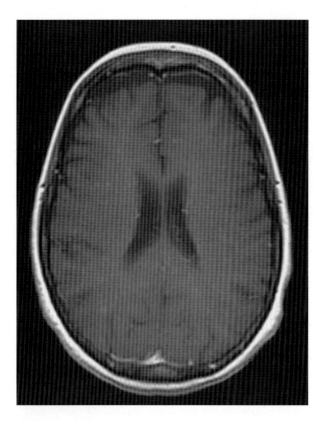

FIGURE 3. Enhanced, axial T1-weighted brain MRI through the lateral ventricles shows scattered, tiny enhancing parenchymal foci.

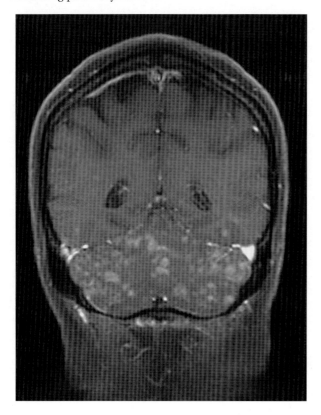

FIGURE 4. Fat-saturated, enhanced, coronal T1-weighted brain MRI shows the nearly confluent cerebellar enhancing metastases and comparatively rare, scattered, supratentorial metastases at the gray matter–white matter junction.

cerebellum is distinctly unusual. The near confluency of the cerebellar lesions suggests leptomeningeal metastases as a possibility, although these lesions are more nodular than the typical appearance of leptomeningeal metastases.

CASE 6

Dural-based sphenoid wing metastasis with orbital extension

A 50-year-old woman with metastatic breast cancer to liver and bone developed lethargy and hallucinations while on medications for intractable pain. Her right breast infiltrating ductal carcinoma with 27 involved lymph nodes had been diagnosed 5 years earlier. She was treated with partial mastectomy, radiation, and chemotherapy.

Bone and liver metastases were detected 4 years after initial diagnosis and treatment for breast cancer. Severe intractable bone pain led to prophylactic pinning of the left hip along with radiation therapy, thoracic spine radiation, right hemipelvis and femoral radiation, prophylactic bilateral total shoulder replacements, and strontium therapy.

When the patient developed confusion, she was evaluated with a head CT scan. This suggested calvarial, but no definite brain, metastases (although the study was compromised by motion artifact). About 3 weeks later, the patient developed aphasia. A brain MRI showed extensive calvarial and dural metastases, with intraorbital extension, as well as parenchymal metastases (Figures 1, 2, and 3). Whole-brain radiation therapy was given, with marked improvement in the aphasia. The patient died a month later.

TEACHING POINTS

This case illustrates the predilection of breast cancer to involve multiple intracranial compartments (parenchyma, meninges, bone). This patient had known bone metastases for 4 years by the time she developed neurologic symptoms. Although there are brain parenchymal metastases, the

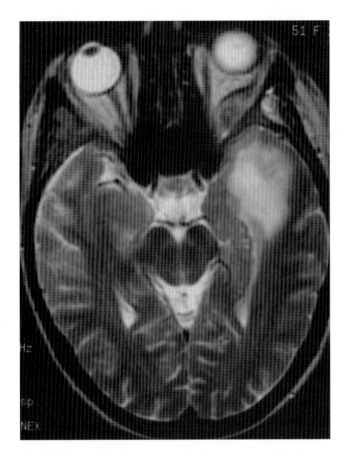

FIGURE 1. Axial T2-weighted MRI shows left temporal lobe edema. Abnormal hyperintense signal is seen within the left sphenoid bone. A heterogeneous mass extends into the left orbit.

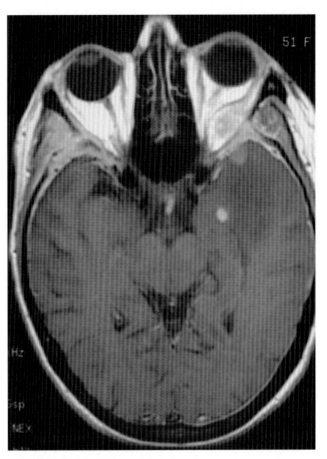

FIGURE 2. Axial T1-weighted enhanced MRI, at the same level, shows thickening and enhancement of the middle cranial fossa dura bilaterally. Abnormal enhancement is seen of both sphenoid bones, as well as of smoothly marginated masses on the left, which protrude into the orbit and the middle cranial fossa. Diffuse edema is seen of the left temporal lobe, and a separate small, enhancing metastasis is seen in the left temporal lobe.

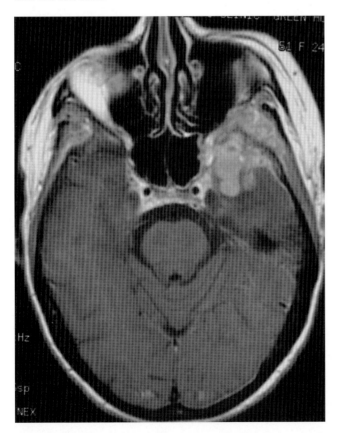

FIGURE 3. Axial T1-weighted enhanced MRI, inferior to Figure 2, shows enhancement and expansion of the replaced left sphenoid bone. Lesser changes are seen in the right sphenoid. A lobular left temporal lobe dural-based mass is associated with a "dural tail" of enhancement that extends posteriorly.

sphenoid-centered process, with encroachment on the middle cranial fossa and the secondary vasogenic edema, presumably is the culprit lesion.

CASE 7

Plaque-like dural metastases

A 47-year-old woman with metastatic breast cancer to bone, thorax, liver, and ovary developed vertigo and headache. The patient presented with stage IV disease 3.5 years earlier, with bone marrow involvement, as well as imaging evidence of bone, hilar, and pleural metastases. Her primary was a 6-cm infiltrating ductal carcinoma, estrogen receptor positive, with 12 of 13 lymph nodes involved. Prior treatments included right mastectomy, chemotherapy, high-dose chemotherapy with autologous stem cell support, breast cancer vaccine, radiation therapy to the spine, and most recently, paclitaxel (Taxol).

Brain MRI obtained to evaluate new symptoms of vertigo and headache showed two small adjacent enhancing cortical foci in the right posterior parietal lobe, with overlying dural thickening (Figures 1 and 2). This unifocal disease site was treated with gamma knife therapy.

Seven months later, the patient developed new expressive aphasia and recurrent headache, as well as mild right upper extremity tingling. An enhanced head CT showed new extra-axial enhancement on the left, with subjacent parenchymal edema and swelling and mild midline shift (Figure 3). A small, separate, round, enhancing metastasis was seen in the right cerebellum, near the transverse sinus. Contrast-enhanced brain MRI confirmed the findings, which were interpreted as extensive dural metastases, with a separate right cerebellar paren-

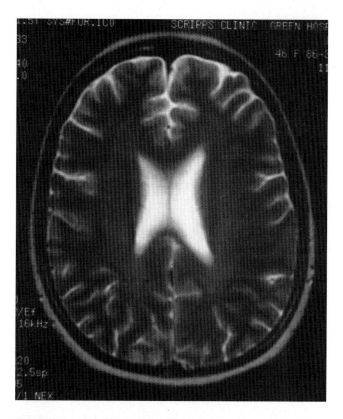

FIGURE 1. Axial enhanced, T1-weighted brain MRI shows adjacent foci of right posterior parietal cortical enhancement, with associated thickening and enhancement of the overlying dura (*arrow*). The patient was treated with gamma knife therapy for presumed brain metastases (no biopsy was performed). Note also the patchy enhancement in the diploic space, consistent with bone metastases.

FIGURE 2. Axial T2-weighted MRI, from the same study, at the same level as Figure 1, shows increased cortical signal at the same level as the enhancement seen in Figure 1. Note also the generalized white matter hyperintensity, attributable in this case to prior treatment with high-dose chemotherapy (see Case 9 in this chapter for another example).

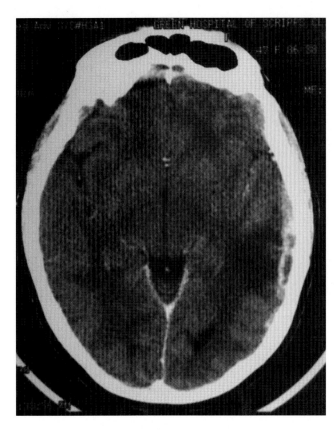

FIGURE 3. Seven months later, contrast-enhanced head CT shows new left posterior temporal extra-axial heterogeneous enhancement. Edema is noted in the subjacent brain parenchyma.

chymal metastasis and diffuse skull metastases (Figures 4 and 5). The patient was treated with high-dose dexamethasone (Decadron) and whole-brain radiation therapy, with nearly complete resolution of her expressive aphasia.

Repeat MRI was obtained 3 months later (2 months after whole-brain radiation) and showed improvement in the dural thickening, with resolution of the subjacent parenchymal edema (Figure 6).

Six months later, the patient developed jaundice, and progressive liver metastases were confirmed. She was referred to hospice, and died soon thereafter.

TEACHING POINTS

As is typical, this patient developed brain metastases late in the course of her disease. In this case, clinical symptoms of brain metastases developed 3.5 years after her initial diagnosis of breast cancer, which initially presented with stage IV disease, metastatic to thorax and bone. The median interval

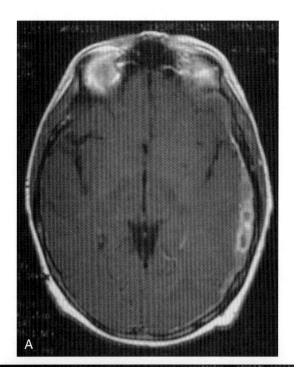

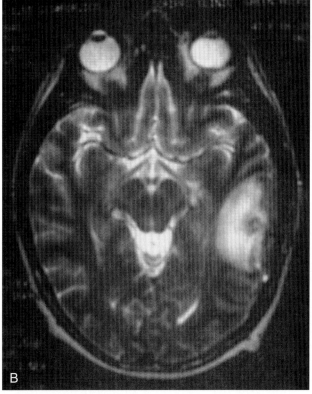

FIGURE 4. Axial brain MRIs at the same level as the CT scan in Figure 3 (**A,** enhanced T1-weighted; **B,** T2-weighted) show inhomogeneous extra-axial enhancement at the left temporoparietal level, with mass effect. The underlying edema is well seen on the T2-weighted image, and mass effect is seen as localized sulcal effacement and mild asymmetry of the sylvian fissure and lateral ventricular trigone. Skull metastases are seen as patchy areas of altered signal intensity in the diploic space, bright on T2 weighting and bright because of enhancement on T1-weighted, enhanced sequences.

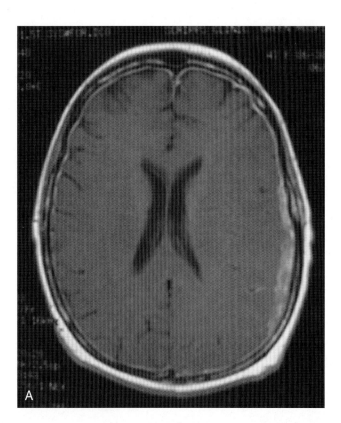
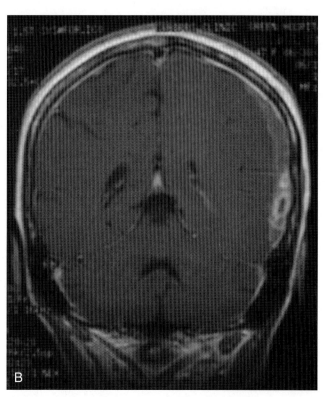

FIGURE 5. Additional axial (**A**) and coronal (**B**) enhanced, T1-weighted brain MR images show heterogeneous left extra-axial enhancement, compressing the subjacent brain. The sulci are effaced at the involved levels, and there is mild midline shift to the right. In addition to the localized dural thickening, there is generalized mild thickening and diffuse enhancement of the dura. Diffuse skull metastases are again noted.

between the diagnosis of breast cancer and brain metastases is 34 months.

This case is another illustration of the propensity of breast cancer, more than other tumors, to involve multiple intracranial compartments (parenchyma, meninges, bone) simultaneously. Although this patient had in the course of her disease at least one typical cerebellar parenchymal metastasis (not shown), most of her intracranial metastases manifested in less typical ways. Her presenting cerebral disease was unusual in appearance, not typical for parenchymal metastases, and unusually localized for leptomeningeal disease. This could be superficial parenchymal metastases, which secondarily involved the overlying dura, but more likely, this is leptomeningeal metastatic disease, or carcinomatous meningitis. Whatever its epicenter, this focus was suitable for local therapy with stereotactic radiosurgery (SRS). The lesion is small and localized, with no contraindications for SRS (<3 cm, minimal associated edema). SRS is noninvasive and delivers a high additive lethal radiation dose to a tumor by application of intersecting radiation beams to a target lesion. This largely spares the surrounding brain, which receives a considerably

smaller dose. It typically is administered as a single treatment, as an outpatient. Gamma knife therapy, which this patient received, is a form of SRS.

When this patient relapsed in the central nervous system (CNS) 7 months later, her intracranial disease again manifested in a relatively unusual but recognized manner, forming a plaque-like dural-based mass that locally compressed and invaded the underlying cerebrum, inducing vasogenic edema. Dural-based metastases may be mass-like and nodular, or flattened and plaque-like as this case illustrates, and can mimic meningiomas and subdural collections.

The more diffuse dural enhancement noted in this case could reflect diffuse dural metastatic disease or be reactive. The extent of the dural process and presence of edema were considered in the decision to treat with whole-brain radiation. After whole-brain radiation, the plaque-like dural-based mass decreased in thickness and much of the diffuse dural enhancement resolved. The vasogenic edema associated with the dural-based mass also resolved. The patient had an excellent clinical response, with nearly complete resolution of her presenting expressive aphasia. It is worth noting

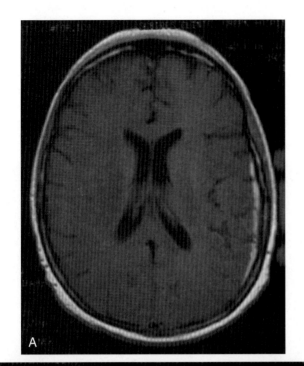

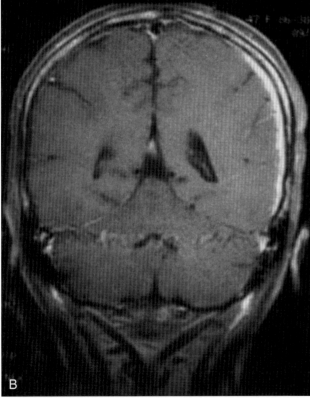

that administration of whole-brain radiation therapy decreases the incidence of subsequent CNS relapse and neurologic death.

CASE 8

Skull metastases with extracranial and intracranial extension

A 69-year-old woman with stage IV metastatic breast cancer developed new weakness of right upper and lower extremities, and a mild headache. The patient had known skull metastases with scalp and dural-based components. These had been identified on brain MRI 9 months earlier when she developed forgetfulness and slurring of words. At that time, she was evaluated for radiation therapy, but deferred because her measurable disease (scalp masses) appeared to be responding to systemic therapy, her symptoms were mild, and there was concern that scalp radiation could compromise future whole-brain radiation. The patient had known extensive bony metastatic disease

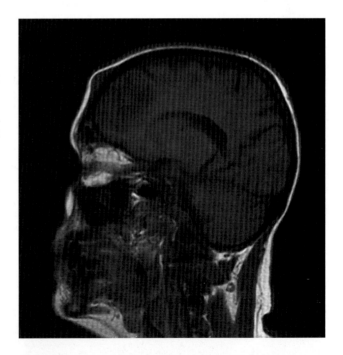

FIGURE 6. Repeat brain MRI (**A,** axial enhanced, T1-weighted; **B,** coronal fat-saturated, enhanced, T1-weighted), 3 months later (2 months after administration of whole-brain radiation), shows decreased generalized dural enhancement. The more localized left extra-axial thickening and enhancement show improvement as well. The mass effect has resolved. Note the diffuse bright signal in the diploic space on the fat-saturated coronal image, owing to enhancement of extensive skull metastases.

FIGURE 1. Sagittal, T1-weighted MRI shows diffuse hypointensity of the calvarium. At the right frontal level, there is edema as well as a subgaleal mass.

diagnosed 6 years earlier, and for which she had undergone palliative radiation to the pelvis and hips, as well as systemic treatment with samarium. Her original diagnosis of left breast cancer was 18 years before the onset of central nervous system (CNS) metastases. This was a T1cN1M0, left 1.9-cm infiltrating ductal carcinoma with 1 of 20 lymph nodes involved. She was treated with mastectomy as well as breast and regional lymphatic radiation.

When the patient developed symptoms of right-sided weakness, repeat brain MRI was obtained, which showed progression of metastases and increased mass effect and edema (Figures 1, 2, and 3). She was treated with dexamethasone and

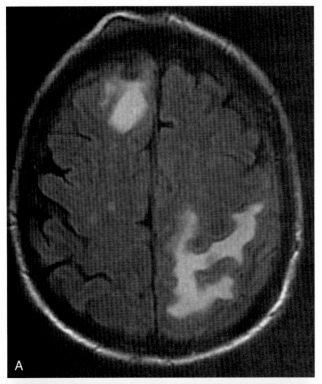

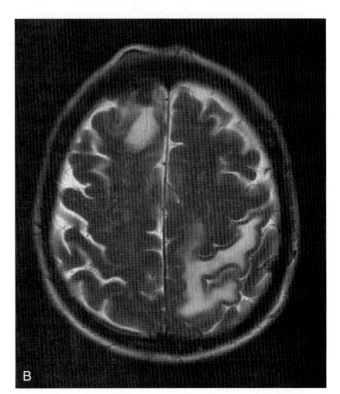

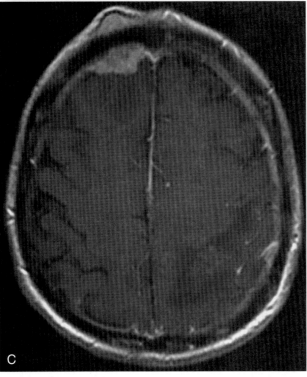

FIGURE 2. Axial brain MRIs from the same level (**A,** FLAIR; **B,** T2-weighted; **C,** enhanced, T1-weighted) shows a lobular, right frontal dural-based enhancing mass, with a similar-appearing subgaleal mass overlying the calvarium at the same level. The skull is extremely hypointense at this level, but patchy areas of enhancement are seen within the diploic space elsewhere. Edema accompanying the right frontal metastasis is seen on FLAIR and T2 weighting, as is edema at the left parietal level from another lesion (illustrated in Figure 3).

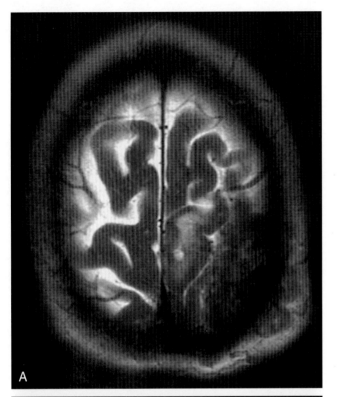

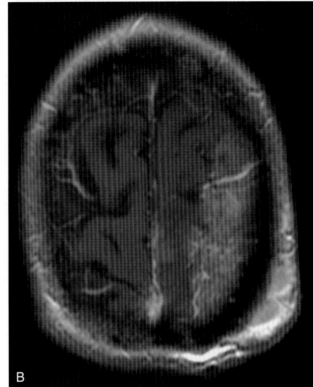

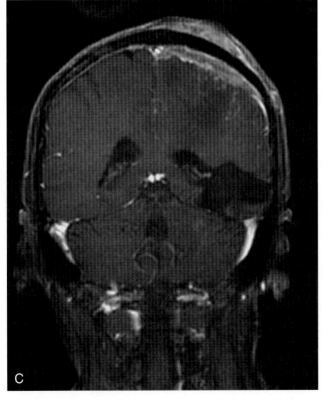

FIGURE 3. Brain MRIs showing the vertex (**A,** T2-weighted axial; **B,** enhanced, T1-weighted axial; **C,** fat-saturated, coronal, enhanced, T1-weighted) where a similar-appearing mass centered on the skull shows protruding extracranial (scalp) and intracranial (dural-based) components. The underlying brain is compressed and infiltrated. Left temporal cystic encephalomalacia seen in **C** was due to a remote and unrelated history of surgery for intracranial hemorrhage.

palliative whole-brain radiation therapy (WBRT) but had continued deterioration, with limited use of her right arm and inability to walk. Systemic therapy was discontinued in favor of hospice care.

TEACHING POINTS

Although the dural-based component of these metastases resembles Case 7, the epicenter of disease in this case is in the skull, from which expansile soft tissue components extend into the scalp and intracranially, infiltrating the dura and underlying brain. This patient had known extensive, refractory bone metastases for 6 years before developing CNS symptoms.

The timing of radiation therapy or other interventions for CNS metastases must take into account the patient's overall functional status as well as the level of control of her systemic disease. In this case, the patient had disease (palpable scalp masses) that could be monitored clinically to assess response to systemic therapy, and at initial presentation, she was minimally symptomatic. Because she appeared to be responding to systemic therapy with declining size of the scalp masses, radiation therapy to the scalp was deferred out of concern that it could compromise future whole-brain irradiation. When her symptoms progressed to the point at which radiation was necessary, she had little clinical response. These neurologic developments proved to be terminal for this patient.

CASE 9

Skull metastasis and chemotherapy-induced leukoencephalopathy

A 59-year-old woman with a history of premenopausal breast cancer presented for medical oncologic evaluation for possible metastatic disease. Her breast cancer history had been 10 years before, presenting as a large palpable left breast mass. She was treated with neoadjuvant chemotherapy (two cycles of Cytoxan, methotrexate, 5-fluorouracil (CMF), followed by one cycle of Cytoxan, Adriamycin, 5-fluorouracil (CAF) with clinical response,

followed by high-dose chemotherapy with cyclophosphamide (Cytoxan), cisplatin, and bischlorethylnitrosourea (BCNU), with stem cell rescue. Mastectomy and flap reconstruction were performed. The pathology specimen showed a 6-cm infiltrating lobular carcinoma (ILC), estrogen receptor positive, progesterone receptor negative. Six of 10 lymph nodes were involved. Chest wall radiation was performed. She declined tamoxifen therapy.

A month before presentation, the patient developed left back pain, radiating laterally and to the front of the chest. A bone scan was abnormal at multiple levels, including T5, T11, the skull, and right humerus.

Oncologic evaluation included tumor markers, which were elevated (CEA and CA 27.29). Positron emission tomography (PET) and CT imaging showed hypermetabolic mediastinal and hilar adenopathy and bone metastases (see Case 7 in Chapter 8). The patient had been noted to be hoarse on physical examination, and PET showed asymmetrical muscular activity of the vocal cords.

Fine-needle aspiration was performed of a mediastinal lymph node, confirming metastatic disease, which was estrogen receptor and progesterone receptor positive, *HER-2/neu* negative. Radiation therapy was begun to the spine for palliation of pain. The patient developed nausea during radiation therapy.

Brain MRI obtained to evaluate the nausea showed no focal intracranial lesions or enhancement to suggest brain parenchymal metastases. There was instead extensive, confluent, symmetrical white matter hyperintensity, or leukoencephalopathy, seen on fluid-sensitive sequences (Figure 1). Skull metastases were also seen, including the right frontal level (Figures 2, 3, and 4).

TEACHING POINTS

In cancer patients, the pattern of diffuse symmetrical white matter edema seen here most commonly reflects radiation therapy effects. However, this patient had never been treated with brain radiation. This pattern of leukoencephalopathy is also known to occur after high-dose chemotherapy, which this patient had previously received. A study reported by Brown and associates compared spectra obtained from advanced breast cancer patients with white matter changes after treatment with high-dose chemotherapy and bone marrow transplantation with age- and sex-matched controls. There was no significant difference in spectral ratios of *N*-acetyl aspartate (NAA) to either creatine

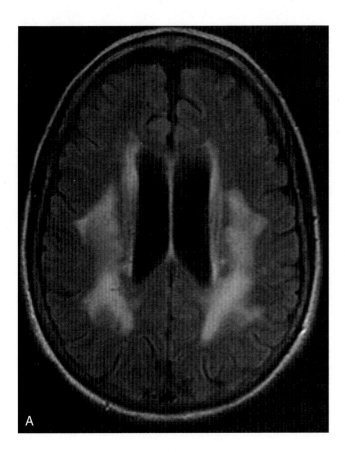
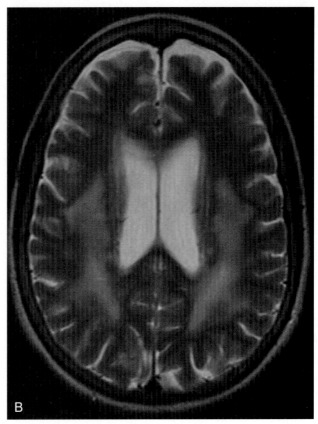

FIGURE 1. Axial FLAIR (**A**) and T2-weighted (**B**) sequences show extensive, confluent, symmetrical, white matter hyperintensity, or leukoencephalopathy, in a periventricular distribution. No enhancing parenchymal lesions were found on contrast-enhanced sequences.

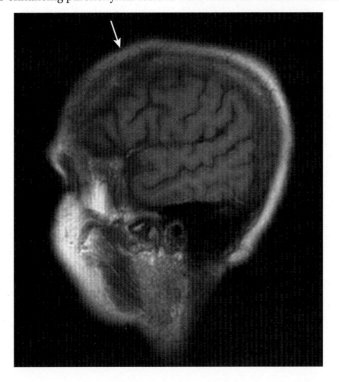

FIGURE 2. Sagittal T1-weighted MRI shows most of the diploic bone marrow signal to be bright, reflecting fatty marrow, as expected. A hypointense region of replacement of the normal bright signal is seen in the frontal region, suspicious for a metastasis (*arrow*).

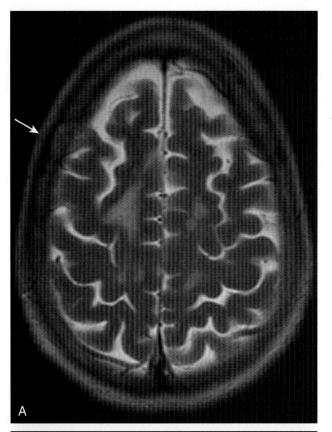

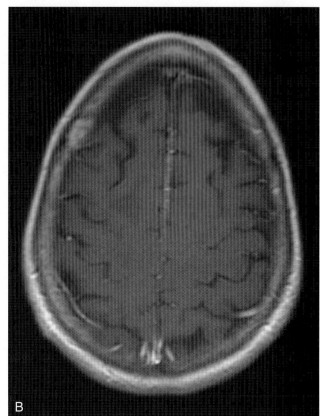

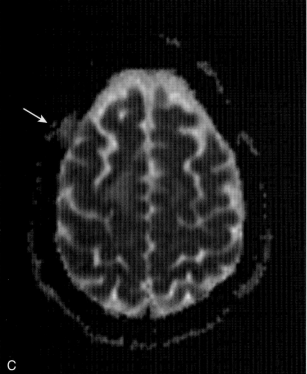

FIGURE 3. Axial brain images through the right frontal level in question (**A,** T2-weighted; **B,** enhanced, T1-weighted; **C,** diffusion) show the lesion (*arrows*) to be nearly isointense with marrow on T2 weighting. With contrast enhancement and T1 weighting, the enhancing metastasis becomes essentially isointense to normal fatty diploic marrow. The abnormality is seen relatively well on diffusion imaging. White matter hyperintensity can be seen on the T2-weighted and diffusion images.

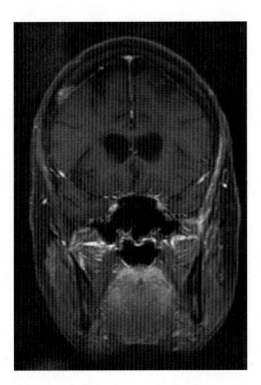

FIGURE 4. Coronal, contrast-enhanced, fat-saturated, T1-weighted image shows enhancement of the right frontal calvarial lesion, as expected with a metastasis. The lesion conspicuity is improved and the extent of enhancement better assessed with the use of fat saturation.

or choline in either short-echo or long-echo spectra. As NAA is considered to be reflective of neuronal structure and function, these results imply that the observed white matter changes do not reflect major neuronal or axonal injury and may reflect changes in free and bound water fraction resulting from chemotherapy. This result differs from spectroscopic studies of other white matter diseases, such as long-standing multiple sclerosis and adrenoleukodystrophy, in which significant decreases in NAA can be identified, presumably reflecting neuronal loss or dysfunction.

Typical findings of a skull metastasis on MRI are also demonstrated here. Osseous metastases are generally hypointense compared with normal fatty marrow on unenhanced, T1-weighted sequences. They are hyperintense on fluid-sensitive sequences, including T2-weighted sequences and STIR, but are most easily visualized when fat signal is mitigated (either fat-saturated proton density or T2-weighted, or STIR sequences). As well demonstrated here, metastases on contrast-enhanced, T1-weighted series may actually decrease in conspicuity if they enhance to isointensity with normal marrow. The addition of fat saturation to enhanced T1-weighted sequences allows enhancing focal lesions to stand out.

SUGGESTED READING

Brown MS, Simon JH, Stemmer SM, et al. MR and proton spectroscopy of white matter disease induced by high-dose chemotherapy with bone marrow transplant in advanced breast carcinoma. *Am J Neuroradiol* 1995; 16:2013–2020.

CASE 10

Recurrent brain metastasis; radiation-induced leukoencephalopathy

A 42-year-old woman with metastatic breast cancer to liver and brain developed recurrent headache. She had previously been treated with whole-brain radiation therapy (WBRT) 16 months before for multiple brain metastases, with resolution by MRI.

Her initial diagnosis of brain metastases occurred 2 years after her diagnosis at age 38 of a locally advanced breast cancer. This was a right breast, estrogen receptor– and progesterone receptor–positive, *HER-2/neu* positive, 2.7-cm infiltrating ductal carcinoma with an extensive intraductal component, with 10 of 12 metastatic lymph nodes, including a 3-cm lymph node with focal extra-capsular extension. She had been treated with mastectomy, four cycles of doxorubicin and cyclophosphamide, followed by four cycles of paclitaxel, as well as chest wall, supraclavicular, and axillary radiation.

The patient was diagnosed with liver metastases when she developed abdominal distention and increased fatigue a year after completing treatment for high-risk breast cancer.

Chemotherapy with carboplatin, docetaxel (Taxotere), and trastuzumab (Herceptin) was initiated, with good response by imaging. Later the same year, brain metastases were identified and treated with WBRT, with MRI resolution of lesions. Sixteen months later, a single recurrent left cerebellar metastasis was found on MRI, obtained to evaluate recurrent headache (Figures 1, 2, and 3). This was treated with gamma knife therapy.

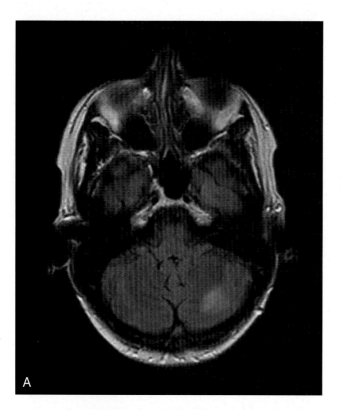
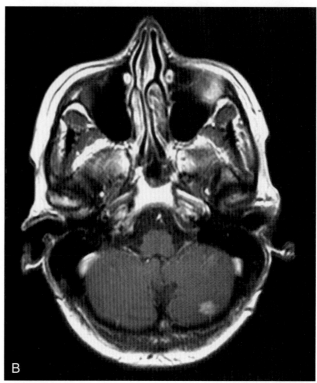

FIGURE 1. Axial MRIs through the posterior fossa (**A,** FLAIR; **B,** enhanced, T1-weighted) show a small, new enhancing nodule in the periphery of the left posterior cerebellum. The associate edema is well depicted on the FLAIR sequence.

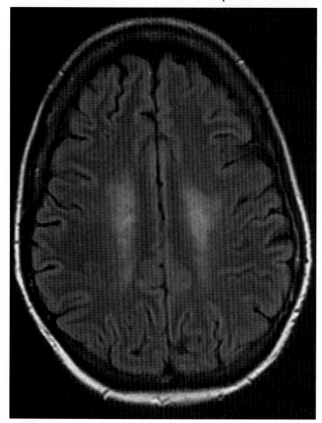

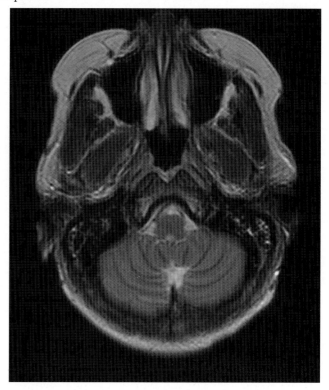

FIGURE 3. A follow-up study, obtained about 2 months after conclusion of WBRT, shows another frequently observed radiation effect. Fluid signal is seen in the mastoid air cells.

FIGURE 2. An axial FLAIR image through the centrum semiovale from the same study shows symmetrical white matter hyperintensity, which was unchanged from the first post-WBRT study obtained 14 months earlier.

TEACHING POINTS

Typical imaging findings from prior WBRT are demonstrated here. The white matter edema is diffuse and fairly symmetric. No mass effect or abnormal enhancement was seen supratentorially. In this case, the patient previously had a complete imaging response to WBRT for multiple brain metastases (not shown). The white matter findings were first seen on the first post-treatment MRI, obtained 2 months after the conclusion of radiation therapy. Similar findings can be seen after chemotherapy, particularly high-dose therapy (see Case 9 in this chapter). Fluid signal intensity is seen in the mastoid air cells after treatment, another commonly observed effect of radiation treatment.

When a patient such as this develops recurrent brain metastases, options for treatment include repeat WBRT versus local therapy with stereotactic radiosurgery (SRS). SRS is preferred to spare the normal brain. Repeat irradiation with WBRT can be considered for those patients with recurrent brain metastases that are too numerous.

CASE 11

Spinal leptomeningeal carcinomatosis

A 56-year-old woman presented for a second opinion on metastatic breast cancer. Her breast cancer had been diagnosed 1 year earlier. She was treated with a left modified radical mastectomy for a 3.5-cm infiltrating ductal carcinoma (IDC), 2 of 36 lymph nodes positive, estrogen receptor and progesterone receptor negative, HER-2/neu negative. Her mastectomy was performed 6 weeks after myocardial infarction. Her postoperative course was complicated by mastectomy site infection. The patient declined chemotherapy.

Six months later, the patient complained of back pain. A chest x-ray showed new lung nodules. These were confirmed on chest CT as consistent with lung metastases. No biopsy was performed, as the patient again declined chemotherapy.

Eight months later, brain CT and spine MRI showed bone and brain metastases and diffuse pial enhancement, consistent with leptomeningeal carcinomatosis (Figures 1, 2, and 3).

TEACHING POINTS

This case illustrates the typical CT features of intracranial metastases. Although MRI is the most sensitive modality for detection of CNS metastases, due to superior soft tissue contrast and higher sensitivity to contrast enhancement, at times it may be necessary to utilize CT primarily for the diagnosis and detection of brain metastases, such as in patients with MRI contraindications. CT scans of brain for suspected intracranial metastases should be performed with and without contrast enhancement. Unenhanced imaging is helpful to detect calcification and hemorrhage, findings which can influence decision making and differential diagnosis. As this case illustrates, brain metastases can be relatively subtle on unenhanced CT, and so contrast enhancement is an essential component of imaging for suspected neoplasia. The most common location of metastases, at the junction of the gray and white matter of the cerebral hemispheres, is also illustrated in this example.

More commonly than other tumors, breast cancer displays a propensity to involve multiple intracranial compartments, and can simultaneously involve parenchyma, meninges, and bone. This case illustrates concomitant bone metastases in the spine, spinal leptomeningeal carcinomatosis, and intracranial parenchymal metastases. Presumably, the central nervous system (CNS) was seeded by the brain parenchymal tumor, leading to the leptomeningeal involvement seen in the spine. Three possible mechanisms have been proposed for diffuse CNS tumor dissemination. Hematogenous metastases could rupture out of the subarachnoid space or pial vessels, or a metastasis to parenchyma could grow through the cortex or overlying pia to come into contact with cerebrospinal fluid (CSF), where the tumor might shed cells. The peripheral location of the metastasis illustrated here and the small adjacent tumor nodules on the surface of the brain suggest this latter mechanism. The third proposed mechanism is tumor growth within choroid plexus and subsequent seeding of the CSF.

This case nicely illustrates the role of contrast enhancement in evaluation of the spine for metastases. The high inherent soft tissue contrast of MRI is generally sufficient to detect bony metastases,

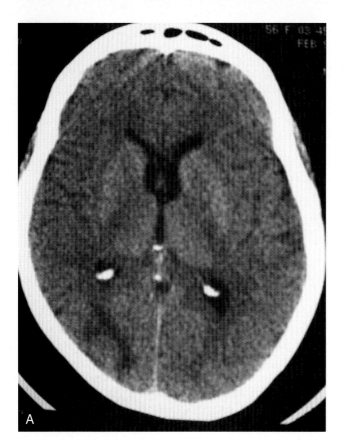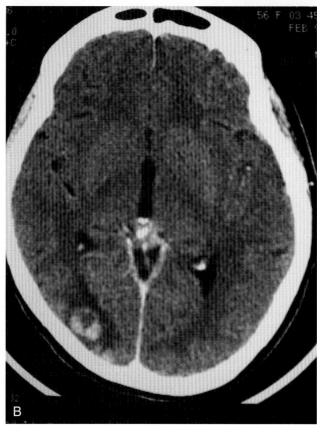

FIGURE 1. Head CT images (**A,** unenhanced; **B,** enhanced) show an enhancing mass in the right occipital lobe, with associated edema. The mass is isodense to parenchyma on noncontrast CT, and the adjacent white matter edema is subtle. Enhancement of the mass is heterogeneous, with a pattern suggesting central necrosis. Nodular enhancement is also seen near the surface of the brain posterior to this lesion. A separate lesion was seen in the left posterior parietal lobe (not shown).

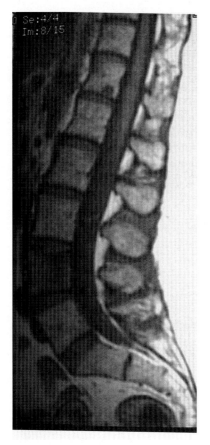

FIGURE 2. T1-weighted sagittal sequence through the midline of the lumbar spine shows replacement of the normal fatty marrow signal at the L4 vertebral body level. A focal hypointense signal alteration is also seen at the T12 level.

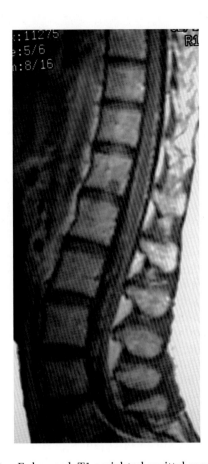

FIGURE 3. Enhanced, T1-weighted sagittal sequence through the lumbar spine shows enhancement of the L4 vertebral body metastasis, with loss of lesion conspicuity. The focal T12 lesion also shows enhancement, although visible. Irregular linear enhancement can now be seen on the surface of the thoracic cord and conus medullaris, as well as stippled, nodular enhancement of cauda equina. This pial enhancement is compatible with leptomeningeal tumor.

which generally does not require the use of contrast media. As shown here, contrast enhancement of bone metastases can result in a loss of lesion conspicuity, if enhancing metastases become isointense to the normal fatty marrow. For this reason, many centers utilize fat-saturated, T1-weighted, postcontrast sequences. Administration of contrast material, although not contributing much toward detecting bone metastases, can be helpful in assessing the activity of treated lesions and in assessing the extent of epidural tumor.

The use of contrast material is essential in the evaluation of intraspinal tumor, as seen here. Drop metastases and leptomeningeal tumor can be challenging to detect without contrast enhancement. This example is florid, but typical, with a nodular "sugar" coating of tumor on the surface of the cord and conus and studding the cauda equina.

CHAPTER 12

Multisystem Metastases and Assessment of Treatment Efficacy

A major focus in the management of cancer patients is the monitoring of response to treatment, whether chemotherapy, hormone therapy, or biologics. Two important issues are the accurate assessment of therapeutic efficacy and the provision of prognostic information. Clinical signs and symptoms can be subjective and difficult to evaluate because of the side effects of treatment. Serum tumor markers may lack sensitivity or specificity. Imaging offers an objective, and often quantifiable, method of measuring response. CT, MRI, positron emission tomography (PET), and bone scintigraphy have all demonstrated both advantages and disadvantages for patient monitoring and should be viewed as complementary modalities. Chemotherapeutic efficacy can be assessed in different contexts, such as neoadjuvant (i.e., presurgical) applications and in the setting of metastatic disease (measurable distant disease).

NEOADJUVANT

Neoadjuvant chemotherapy was initially applied to locally advanced breast cancer but has more recently been used in patients presenting with smaller, resectable breast cancers.[1] Studies identifying the amount of breast and axillary tumor after neoadjuvant chemotherapy have demonstrated prognostic value in predicting disease-free and overall survival.[2-5] In a study using fluorodeoxyglucose (FDG) PET, Bellon and coworkers found that internal mammary nodal involvement in patients with locally advanced breast cancer was predictive of regional or systemic failure.[6] Modalities with exquisite anatomic and localization capabilities, such as CT and MRI, rely on a change in lesion size to assess efficacy. It is well recognized that a change in size may lag for weeks or months. CT scans are not routinely used to monitor the efficacy of chemotherapy in the neoadjuvant setting, although they may be very helpful to investigate a new finding during this time period. MRI has shown promise, but early results require larger, confirmatory studies. Dynamic contrast-enhanced MRI allows analysis of both tumor size and contrast enhancement pattern. Although these parameters may ultimately prove to be of great value in separating responders from nonresponders, underestimation of residual tumor size, comparing baseline and follow-up studies, could produce false-negative results, especially in larger tumors.[7,8] In the neoadjuvant setting, imaging is used primarily to assess local response.

Metabolic imaging, specifically FDG PET, has shown encouraging results in the neoadjuvant setting.[9-12] PET can be assessed visually or semi-quantitatively. The most widely used quantitative method is measurement of the standardized uptake value (SUV) (Figure 1). This measures the amount of FDG uptake in a region of interest (i.e., tumor), divided by the injected dose corrected for patient weight. Many factors can affect this measurement, including lesion size, time interval between injection of FDG and time of imaging, and serum glucose level. Despite these and other variables, the SUV has proved useful for sequential assessment. Changes in SUV may be detected as early as after one cycle of chemotherapy. A significant fall in SUV separates responders from nonresponders and is also used prognostically. These data have been validated against histopathology.[11,13]

METASTATIC

Monitoring response to chemotherapy in the metastatic setting is also an evolving challenge for imaging. Supporting data from large, well-controlled, prospective studies are lacking for both soft tissue and bone metastases. Interest in this particular aspect of breast cancer treatment has been sparked by the continued development of new chemotherapeutic agents, as well as the significant potential toxicity of these drugs. As in the neoadjuvant setting, CT and MRI reliably provide data on lesion size changes. However, changes in size may not occur for months in patients who are

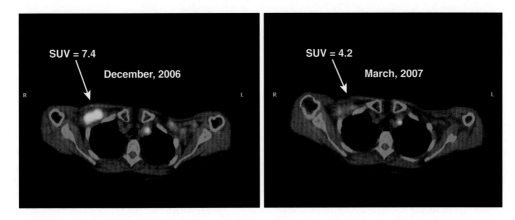

FIGURE 1. These images demonstrate the use of SUV measurements to assess response to therapy in an 83-year-old woman with nodal metastatic breast cancer. The image on the left shows metastatic foci in bilateral supraclavicular and left paratracheal regions. Note SUV of 7.4 (*arrow*). Four months later, following therapy, the repeat study shows a decline in SUV to 4.2 (*arrow*), without resolution of the uptake.

responding to treatment. Additionally, various cytostatic agents may never result in a decrease in size, even if efficacious in prolonging survival. Preliminary data on the use of FDG PET are encouraging, with some authors relying on a change in SUV to separate responders from nonresponders.[13–15] Significant differences have been shown between responders and nonresponders, with responders showing declining FDG uptake, as compared with minimal to no change in nonresponders. These changes have been demonstrated as early as after one cycle of chemotherapy. In the area of bone metastases, FDG PET appears to offer an advantage over conventional imaging (CI), including bone scintigraphy. Both CI and scintigraphy have difficulty assessing change in size of bone metastases; however, demonstration of significantly decreased or resolution of hypermetabolic activity on FDG PET provides valuable information.[16]

A possible caveat in the use of FDG PET to monitor response to therapy may be in patients treated with hormonal therapy. Initial studies have shown a transient increase in glucose use in responding patients, resulting in a "metabolic flare." This may be due to an initial agonist effect rather than an antagonist effect of therapy. In two reports, responders showed this early increase in FDG uptake, whereas nonresponders did not.[17,18]

Skeletal scintigraphy is covered in Chapter 8. Although whole-body bone scanning is a sensitive test for the identification of osteoblastic metastases, inherent problems with the physiologic basis for a positive study limit its utility for assessing efficacy of chemotherapy. As discussed previously, bone-seeking radiopharmaceuticals concentrate in large part owing to localized osteoblastic activity.

Even relatively small increases in osteoblastic activity result in focal hot spots, often weeks to months before these lesions become visible on plain radiography or CT. However, the healing response alone, even in the absence of viable tumor, typically elicits increased radiopharmaceutical uptake, indistinguishable from active metastases. The added issue of suboptimal specificity (i.e., inability to separate benign from malignant disease) limits the role of bone scintigraphy as a modality to assess chemotherapy response. Two exceptions would be the disappearance of previously identified bony metastases on scintiscan and the development of new sites while receiving treatment. Under these circumstances, more definitive statements can be made.

REFERENCES

1. Bonadonna G, Valagussa P, Zucali R, et al. Primary chemotherapy in surgically resectable breast cancer. *CA Cancer J Clin* 1995; 45:227–243.
2. Mankoff DA, Dunnwald LK. Changes in glucose metabolism and blood flow following chemotherapy for breast cancer. In Avril N (ed). PET Clinics, Vol. 1, No. 1. Philadelphia, WB Saunders, 2006, pp 71–81.
3. Machiavelli MR, Romero AD, Perez JE, et al. Prognostic significance of pathological response of primary tumor and metastatic axillary lymph nodes after neoadjuvant chemotherapy for locally advanced breast carcinoma. *Cancer J Sci Am* 1998; 4(2): 125–131.
4. Wolmark N, Wang J, Mamounas E, et al. Preoperative chemotherapy in patients with operable breast cancer: nine year results from national surgical adjuvant breast and bowel project B-18. *J Natl Cancer Inst Monog* 2001; 30:96–102.

5. McCready DR, Hortobagyi GN, Kau SW, et al. The prognostic significance of lymph node metastases after preoperative chemotherapy for locally advanced breast cancer. *Arch Surg* 1989; 124:21–25.

6. Bellon JR, Livingston RB, Eubank WB, et al. Evaluation of the internal mammary lymph nodes by FDG-PET in locally advanced breast cancer (LABC). *Am J Clin Oncol* 2004; 27(4):407–410.

7. Rieber A, Brambs HJ, Gabelmann A, et al. Breast MRI for monitoring response of primary breast cancer to neoadjuvant chemotherapy. *Eur Radiol* 2002; 12(7):1711–1719.

8. Martincich L, Montemurro F, De Rosa G, et al. Monitoring response to primary chemotherapy in breast cancer using dynamic contrast-enhanced magnetic resonance imaging. *Breast Cancer Res Treat* 2004; 83(1):67–76.

9. Wahl RL, Zasadny K, Helvie MA, et al. Metastatic monitoring of breast cancer chemohormonotherapy using positron emission tomography: initial evaluation. *J Clin Oncol* 1993; 11:2101–2111.

10. Bassa P, Kim EE, Inove T, et al. Evaluation of preoperative chemotherapy using PET with {fluorine-18} fluorodeoxyglucose in breast cancer. *J Nucl Med* 1996; 37:931–938.

11. Schelling M, Avril N, Nahrig J, et al. Positron emission tomography using [18F]-fluorodeoxyglucose for monitoring primary chemotherapy in breast cancer. *J Clin Oncol* 2000; 18:1689–1695.

12. Biersack HJ, Palmedo H. Locally advanced breast cancer: is PET useful for monitoring primary chemotherapy? *J Nucl Med* 2003; 44(11):1815–1817.

13. Jansson T, Westlin J, Ahlstrom H, et al. Positron emission tomography studies in patients with locally advanced and/or metastatic breast cancer: a method for early therapy evaluation? *J Clin Oncol* 1995; 13:1470–1477.

14. Gennari A, Donati S, Salvador, B, et al. Role of 2-[18F]–fluorodeoxyglucose (FDG) positron emission tomography (PET) in the early assessment of response to chemotherapy in metastatic breast cancer patients. *Clin Breast Cancer* 2002; 1:156–161, discussion 162–163.

15. Dose Schwartz J, Bader M, Jenicke L, et al. Early prediction of response to chemotherapy in metastatic breast cancer using sequential 18F-FDG-PET imaging. *J Nucl Med* 2005; 46(7):1144–1150.

16. Hoh CK, Schiepers C. 18-FDG imaging in breast cancer. *Semin Nucl Med* 1999; 29:49–56.

17. Dehdashti F, Flanagan FL, Mortimer JE, et al. Positron emission tomographic assessment of "metabolic flare" to predict response of metastatic breast cancer to antiestrogen therapy. *Eur J Nucl Med* 1999; 26:51–56.

18. Mortimer JE, Dehdashti F, Siegel BA, et al. Metabolic flare: indicator of hormone responsiveness in advanced breast cancer. *J Clin Oncol* 2001; 19:2797–2803.

Recurrent PET-positive activity in LABC and bone metastases with increased tumor markers

A 51-year-old woman presented with a greater than 1 year's history of a central, firm, and retracted left breast mass, involving the nipple, with fungation and spontaneous drainage. The patient had not sought medical attention, having a generalized aversion because of a history of multiple surgeries as a child for congenital orthopedic anomalies. When she developed hip pain, she saw her primary care physician, at which time the breast mass was noted. A palpation-guided biopsy confirmed poorly differentiated infiltrating ductal carcinoma. Surgical, oncologic, and imaging evaluations of her locally advanced breast cancer (LABC) showed a palpable, dominant lobulated and spiculated mass, with nipple retraction, skin thickening, malignant calcifications, and pathologic axillary adenopathy. Because of the patient's hip pain, a metastatic workup was performed, including bone scan; CT scans of the chest, abdomen, and pelvis; and positron emission tomography (PET)/CT imaging. Bone scan showed multiple abnormal sites of activity (Figure 1), consistent with metastatic disease, which corresponded to abnormal sites of hypermetabolism on PET/CT. CT images showed corresponding lytic lesions (Figure 2). Breast MRI showed multiple foci of abnormal signal intensity in bone (Figure 3). MRI showed the left breast to be extensively occupied by a massive neoplasm, with central necrosis, nipple extension and retraction, and skin thickening and enhancement. Abnormal enhancement and extension into the pectoral muscle was also noted.

The patient was started on chemotherapy for locally advanced and metastatic breast cancer. Clinically, the patient had an initial excellent response to chemotherapy (six cycles of trastuzumab [Herceptin], docetaxel [Taxotere], carboplatin, and zoledronic acid [Zometa]), with improved bone pain and partial regression of the dominant breast mass. PET scan hypermetabolism at both the breast and bony levels improved dramatically. The corresponding CT scans showed previously lytic bone lesions to convert to a sclerotic appearance, presumably a treatment response (Figure 4).

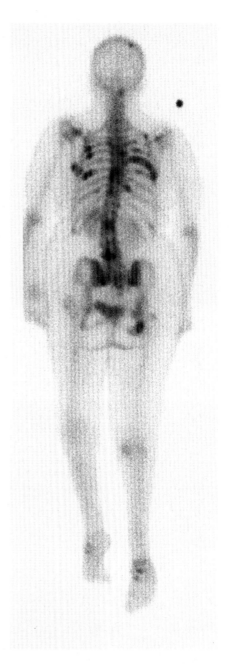

FIGURE 1. Posterior bone scan shows multiple foci of abnormally increased activity, in a pattern highly suspicious for bone metastases. Multiple sites of increased rib uptake include a long segment of activity on the right posteriorly. Multiple vertebral sites of abnormal uptake are seen, and small foci of increased activity are noted at the right calvarial vertex and at the right ischial level. The leg length discrepancy and unusual orientation of the left foot are accounted for by the known congenital anomalies.

She was maintained on a regimen of Herceptin, Zometa, and letrozole (Femara) every 3 weeks for nearly a year with continued clinical response, before her tumor markers were noted to rise, at which time she was reimaged with CT and PET.

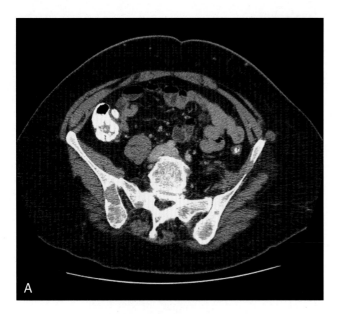 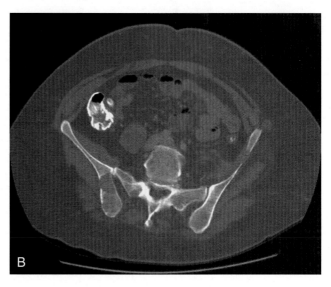

FIGURE 2.   Pelvis CT images (**A,** soft tissue window; **B,** bone window) through the same level show lytic bone metastases in the ilia bilaterally. There is frank soft tissue replacement of bone at these levels.

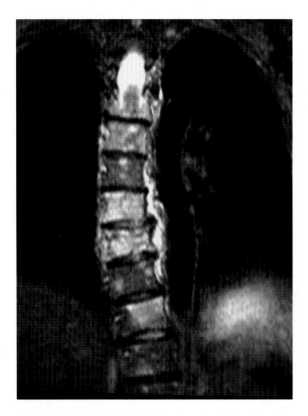

FIGURE 3.   Coronal short tau inversion recovery (STIR) image of the thoracic spine, obtained with the body coil in conjunction with breast MRI, shows diffuse, hyperintense, heterogeneous, altered bone marrow signal, consistent with extensive bone metastases.

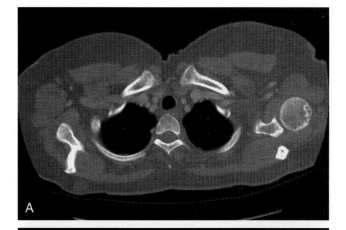

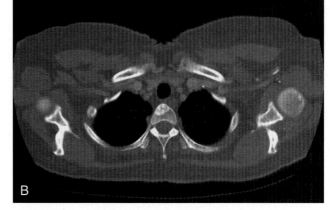

FIGURE 4.   **A** and **B**, Bone window images from chest CT scans through the same upper thoracic level, before and after chemotherapy, show a lytic lesion in the anterior vertebral centrum, converted to a blastic focus after chemotherapy.

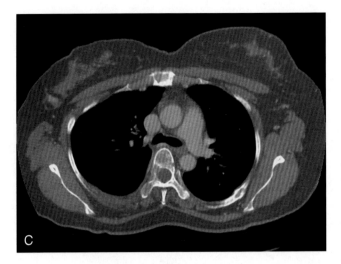
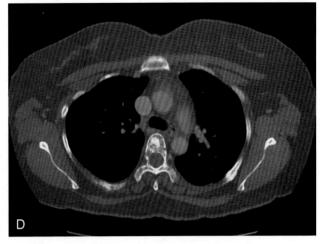

FIGURE 4, cont'd   **C** and **D,** Another level matched pair of chest CT images (bone windows) through the upper thorax show a lytic metastasis in the vertebral body, with a sclerotic reaction at the same level on reimaging while on chemotherapy. A pathologic left rib fracture deformity is partially demonstrated here. Examinations were performed three months apart.

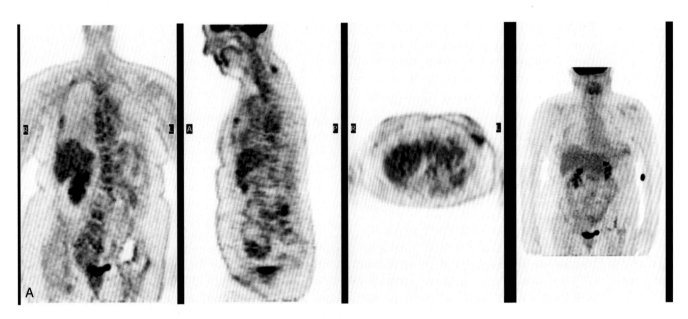

FIGURE 5.   **A** and **B,** Comparable images from PET scans, 7 months apart (*from left to right:* coronal, sagittal, and axial; *far right:* coronal volume projection image). The earlier PET scan (**A**) is obtained after the patient had been on chemotherapy for 5 months. The large, dominant breast mass (best seen on the axial view) shows persistent but decreased hypermetabolism. Residual findings of bone metastases are best seen at cervical spine, lumbar spine, and sternal levels on the sagittal view. Photopenia at the left hip level on the coronal image is due to a hip prosthesis.   (*Continued*)

Hypermetabolism in the index breast mass and in bone metastases on PET, which had markedly regressed on PET, now showed increased metabolic activity (Figure 5). The patient's hormonal therapy was stopped, and vinorelbine (Navelbine) chemotherapy was started.

TEACHING POINTS

This patient presented with a neglected breast cancer and extensive bone metastases. Bone scan, PET, CT, and MRI findings were all in agreement.

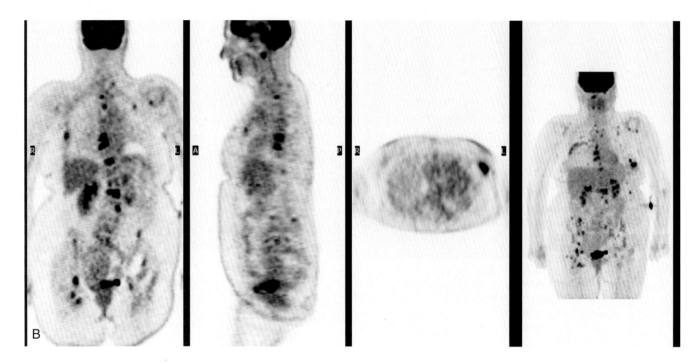

FIGURE 5, cont'd **B,** Repeat PET scan, 7 months later, when the patient's tumor markers were rising, shows increased metabolic activity of the left breast cancer and recurrence of innumerable hypermetabolic bone metastases. This PET scan bore a striking resemblance to the baseline, staging PET scan 1 year earlier.

With chemotherapy, the patient's bone pain, tumor markers, and PET scan findings markedly improved. The lesions on CT changed, showing sclerosis where previously there was lytic change. This indicated a healing response to the therapy. Of course, these patients are not cured per se; rather, their disease is held in check by chemotherapy or hormonal therapy. PET/CT is the most efficient whole-body means of evaluating such patients for relapse, which may be suspected based on increased tumor markers, as in this case, or by the development of new signs or symptoms.

CASE 2

Gastrointestinal metastases from breast cancer

A 77-year-old woman with a history of breast cancer presented with a near-syncopal episode, anemia, and GI bleeding, with melena and heme-positive stool. Upper endoscopy showed thickened, edematous, stiff gastric folds. An infiltrative process was suspected because the folds could not be effaced with insufflation of air. Superficial serpiginous gastric mucosal ulceration was noted along the greater curvature. Multiple biopsies were obtained. The specimens showed gastric mucosa heavily infiltrated with an invasive malignancy. Immunostains were positive for BRST-2, a breast marker, and tumor cells were also strongly estrogen receptor positive. The final interpretation was infiltrating carcinoma, with metastatic lobular carcinoma favored.

The patient's past history of breast cancer was that of lobular carcinoma, with 4 of 10 lymph nodes involved.

An abdominal and pelvic CT scan was subsequently obtained and showed the colon to be diffusely abnormal as well as the stomach. There were CT findings of a diffuse colitis with colonic wall thickening from cecum to rectum. The stomach also showed diffuse mural thickening. Colonoscopy showed markedly thickened transverse colonic mucosa. The colon was noted to be extremely rigid, and the endoscope could not be further advanced. Biopsies from the distal transverse colon showed a noncolorectal infiltrating

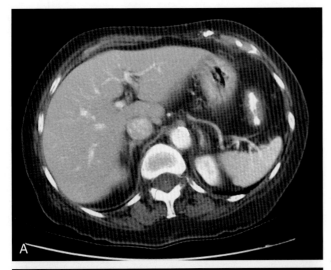

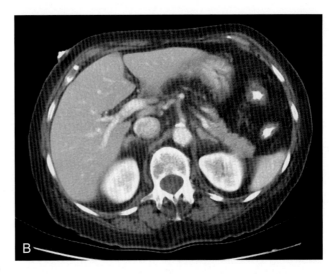

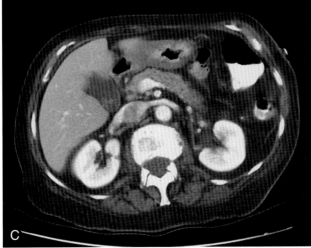

FIGURE 1. Enhanced abdominal CT images (**A** to **C**, above to below), with oral and intravenous contrast, show mural thickening of both the stomach and the visualized colon (splenic flexure). Gallstones are also seen in **C**.

carcinoma, compatible with metastatic breast primary (Figure 1).

TEACHING POINTS

This is a distinctly unusual case, with node-positive infiltrating lobular carcinoma (ILC) recurring as mucosal and intramural infiltration of both the stomach and colon. Although not a commonly recognized clinical manifestation of metastatic breast cancer, autopsy series estimate gastrointestinal (GI) metastases occur in 8% to 15% of patients who die from disseminated breast cancer. After melanoma, breast cancer is the second most common primary tumor type to metastasize to the GI tract. The most common breast cancer histology to manifest as GI metastatic disease is ILC. The most common type of involvement is illustrated in this case, with intramural stomach wall infiltration mimicking a scirrhous carcinoma, or linitis plastica. This is a recognized entity in the differential diagnosis of linitis plastica, along with primary gastric carcinoma, gastric lymphoma, and Crohn's disease.

In this case, the diagnosis was made by mucosal biopsies obtained at endoscopy, and superficial ulceration of the gastric mucosa was seen. Reports in the literature of similar cases indicate that at histology, breast carcinoma metastases occur most frequently in the deeper layers of the wall, including the submucosal, muscularis, and serosal layers, so that mucosal biopsies may be falsely negative.

SUGGESTED READINGS

Joffe N. Metastatic involvement of the stomach secondary to breast carcinoma. *AJR Am J Roentgenol* 1975; 123:512–521.

Trappen PV, Serreyn R, Elewaut AE, et al. Abdominal pain with anorexia in patients with breast carcinoma. *Ann Oncol* 1998; 9:1243–1245.

CASE 3

Peritoneal breast carcinomatosis

A 52-year-old woman with a history of treated breast cancer with a subsequent axillary recurrence presented with rising tumor markers and abdominal distention. Her original diagnosis of breast cancer was 14 years before, a left breast infiltrating ductal carcinoma with extensive ductal carcinoma in situ, which was treated with mastectomy, chemotherapy (six cycles of Cytoxan, methotrexate, 5-fluorouracil (CMF)) and radiation. Margins were close, and 0 of 12 lymph nodes were involved. Five years later, the patient developed a biopsy-proved axillary lymph node recurrence, which was surgically excised. She took tamoxifen for 8 years and was changed to letrozole (Femara) for rising tumor markers, without much response.

She was restaged with positron emission tomography (PET) and CT for rising tumor markers and abdominal distention and was found to have pleural effusions, ascites, and peritoneal tumor implants (Figures 1, 2, 3, 4, 5, 6, and 7). Analysis of pleural and peritoneal fluid confirmed adenocarcinoma, consistent with breast primary, estrogen receptor and progesterone receptor positive, *HER-2/neu* negative. The patient was begun on docetaxel (Taxotere) and gemcitabine (Gemzar), with improvement on repeat PET/CT 2 months later. Subsequent evaluations over the next year showed development of PET-positive retroperitoneal nodal disease and, later, a brain metastasis.

TEACHING POINTS

The lymphatic system is thought to be the dominant route of breast cancer spread to the thorax, rather than hematogenous. A seminal detailed

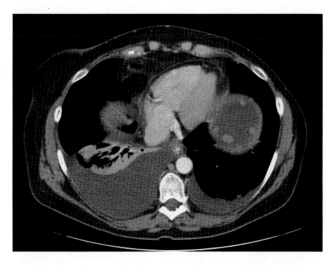

FIGURE 2. A more inferior enhanced slice again shows the pleural effusions. Volumetric effect of the larger right effusion is seen, with atelectasis and consolidation of the right lung base, with air bronchograms. Fluid is also seen below the diaphragm, on the left, with multiple soft tissue nodules outlined by the ascites.

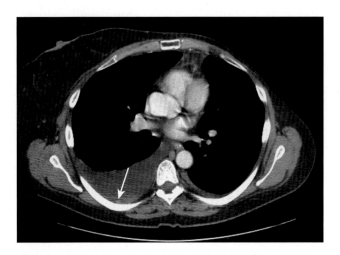

FIGURE 1. Enhanced chest CT image shows bilateral pleural effusions, right larger than left. A small soft tissue nodule is seen on the right, projecting into the pleural fluid (*arrow*). A strandy appearance of anterior mediastinal fat is seen. Post–left mastectomy changes are seen.

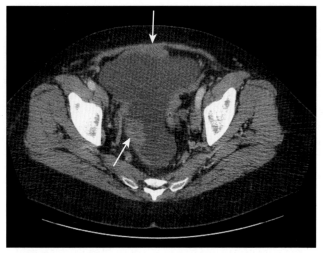

FIGURE 3. Contrast-enhanced pelvic CT image shows a large amount of ascites. Soft tissue nodules and conglomerate masses stud peritoneal surfaces, seen well anteriorly and on the right posterolaterally (*arrows*).

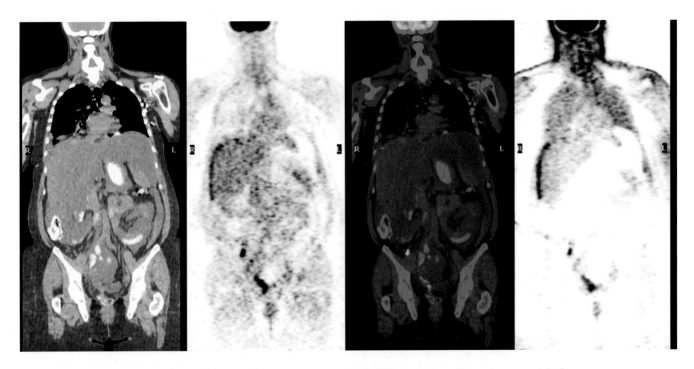

FIGURE 4. Coronal images from a concurrent PET/CT scan show linear hypermetabolism on the surface of the liver. Hypermetabolic foci are also evident in the right hemipelvis.

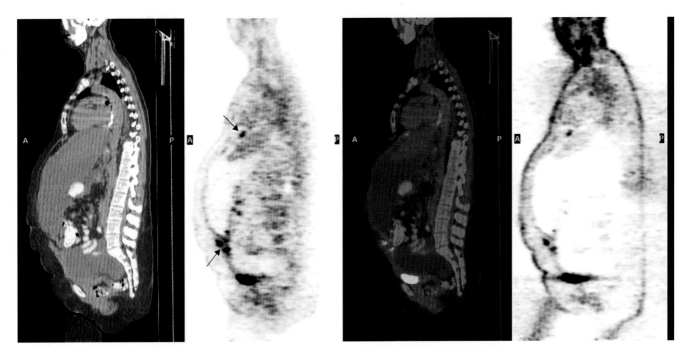

FIGURE 5. Sagittal PET/CT images show abdominal distention due to ascites. Scattered foci of hypermetabolic tumor studding peritoneal surfaces are seen, on the anterior surface of the liver and below the anterior abdominal wall, above the bladder (*arrows*).

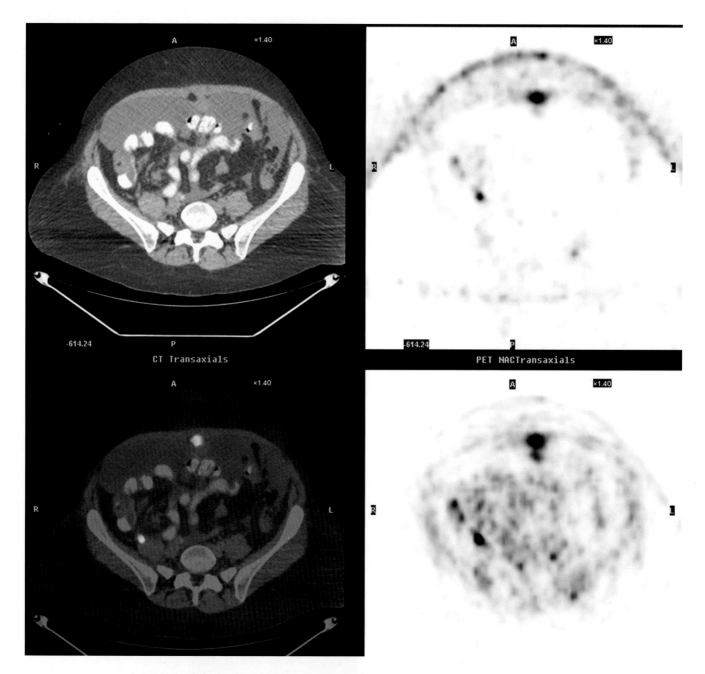

FIGURE 6. Axial PET/CT images through the lower abdomen show ascites and distention. Hypermetabolic soft tissue tumor foci stud peritoneal surfaces, seen here in the midline below the anterior abdominal wall, and on the right, anterolateral to the psoas muscle.

necropsy study published in 1979 by Thomas and colleagues of 26 patients who died of disseminated breast cancer looked at the frequency of tumor involvement of thoracic lymph node groups, lungs, pleura, and pericardium. Based on the findings of this study, spread from involved internal mammary nodes through lymphatic communications to intercommunicating nodal groups in the mediastinum and secondary lymphatic involvement of lung, pleura, and pericardium was implicated. The direction of spread to the lung would be centrifugal, from tracheobronchial lymph nodes peripherally. Lymphatics penetrating the diaphragm would be implicated in a case like this, with both pleural and peritoneal involvement. Potential routes include communications described between breast and liver through pericardial lymph nodes and superior liver surface drainage to inferior internal mammary lymph nodes. This can be characterized as an Internet-like system of collaterals extending

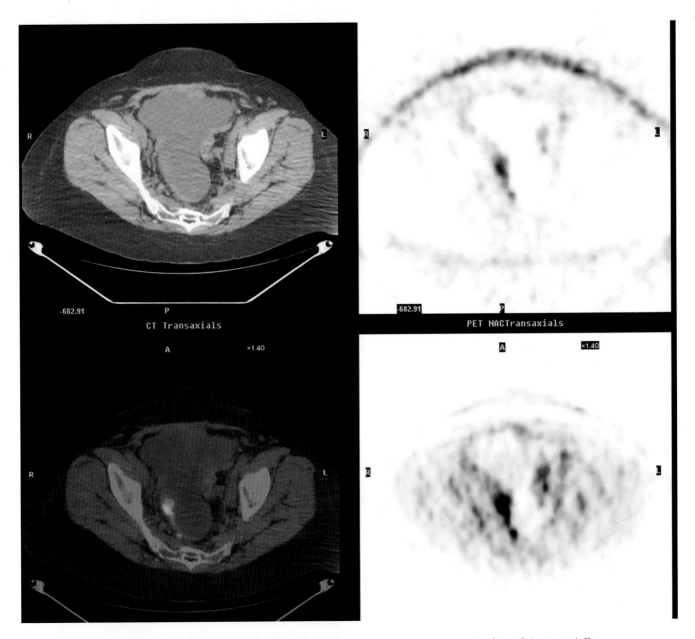

FIGURE 7. Additional findings of peritoneal carcinomatosis are seen in the pelvis, especially notable on the right posterolaterally (corresponding to Figure 3).

from scalp to inguinal nodes without valves, with distant lymphatic spread more likely to occur with bulky axillary tumor and with prior axillary surgery or radiation and with inflammatory carcinomas, namely conditions resulting in lymphatic obstruction.

SUGGESTED READING

Thomas JM, Redding WH, Sloane JP. The spread of breast cancer: importance of the intrathoracic lymphatic route and its relevance to treatment. *Br J Cancer* 1979; 40:540–547.

CASE 4

Bone, liver, pericardial, and ovarian metastases

A 48-year-old woman, who had been treated for breast cancer 6 years earlier with mastectomy, chemotherapy and chest wall radiation, presented with low back and progressive groin pain. The original tumor was detected on mammographic screening, and was a left breast, T1N1 (3 of 21 lymph nodes positive, with extracapsular extension), estrogen receptor–negative, progesterone receptor weakly positive, *HER-2/neu*-positive, 1.1-cm infiltrating ductal carcinoma (IDC) with an extensive intraductal component. Hormone therapy after chemotherapy had been refused.

Lumbar spine and pelvis MRI, obtained to evaluate complaints of back and pelvic pain, showed extensive bone metastases (Figures 1 and 2). The patient was restaged with CT and bone scans, which showed pleural and pericardial effusions (Figure 3), liver metastases (Figure 4), and the extensive bone metastases. The pericardial effusion was sizable, and echocardiographic evaluation suggested early tamponade. A pericardial window was created surgically, and 800 mL of serous fluid was drained. The pericardium appeared normal, and the histology was benign. The effusion was positive for metastatic adenocarcinoma, with cytologic features consistent with the patient's IDC. The patient was treated with chemotherapy, and her response was monitored by CT and positron emission tomography (PET)/CT scans (Figures 5, 6, 7, and 8).

TEACHING POINTS

This patient's metastatic breast cancer presented with skeletal symptoms, leading to imaging, which confirmed widespread metastases to bone, pericardial space, and liver. At first presentation of suspected recurrent breast cancer, it is desirable to confirm the diagnosis with histology. In this case, which site to sample was determined by the identification of a sizable pericardial effusion, initially seen on CT. Although findings suggesting tamponade can be seen on CT, assessment is generally made with echocardiography. In this case, echocardiography showed mild right atrial and right ventricular collapse in diastole, and lack of respiratory variation of the inferior vena cava, suggesting tamponade. This was treated with creation of a pericardial window, evacuating a large effusion with malignant cytology.

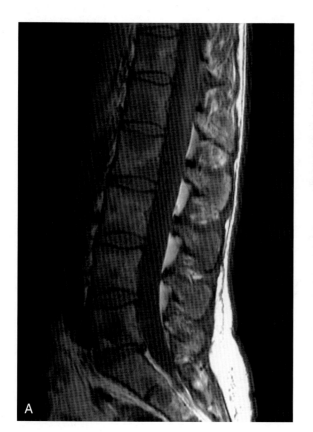 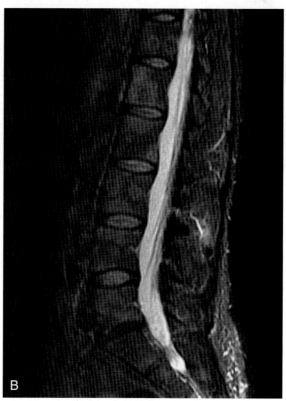

FIGURE 1. T1-weighted (**A**) and STIR (**B**) sagittal images of the lumbar spine show diffuse, patchy, abnormal marrow signal, hypointense on T1-weighted imaging and hyperintense on STIR.

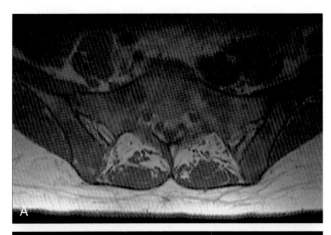

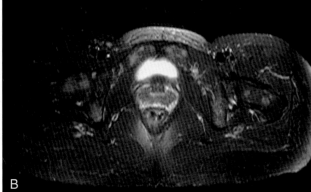

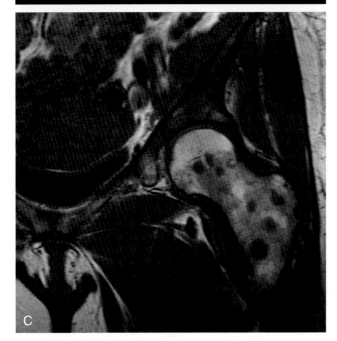

FIGURE 2. Images from a pelvis MRI (**A,** axial T1-weighted, through sacrum; **B,** fat-saturated, T2-weighted axial, through the hips; **C,** small-field-of-view, T1-weighted coronal view of the left hip) show extensive bone metastases. In the hip, spotty metastases contrast readily with bright fatty signal marrow, whereas disease in the ilium is nearly confluent.

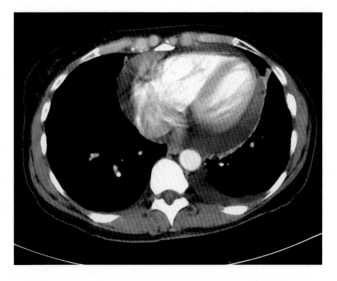

FIGURE 3. Contrast-enhanced chest CT shows a small left pleural effusion and large pericardial effusion. The straightening of the interventricular septum and enlargement of the right atrium suggest tamponade.

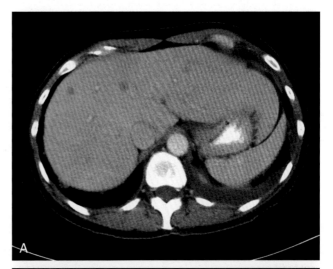

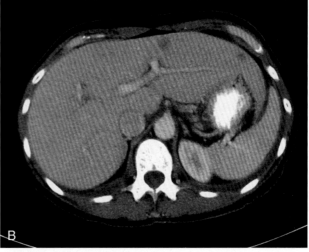

FIGURE 4. **A** and **B,** Portal venous (PV) phase, enhanced abdominal CT scans show periportal edema and multiple scattered hypovascular liver metastases. Note the smooth liver contours.

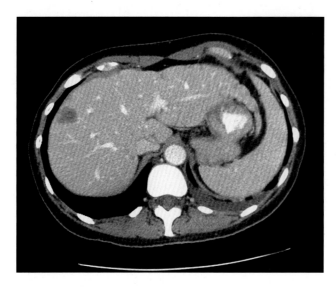

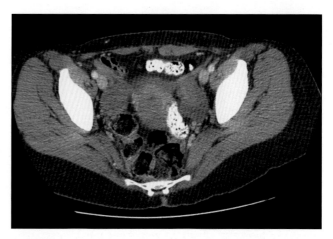

FIGURE 5. Repeat enhanced, PV phase abdominal CT scan shows a larger hypodense liver metastasis, with perilesional enhancement, in the right lobe. Note new nodularity of the liver contour, best seen in the left lobe (contrast with Figure 4, 1 year earlier). The localized capsular contraction coincides with sites of subjacent liver metastases.

FIGURE 6. Image from the pelvis from the same enhanced CT scan in Figure 5 shows bilateral ovarian enlargement, left greater than right.

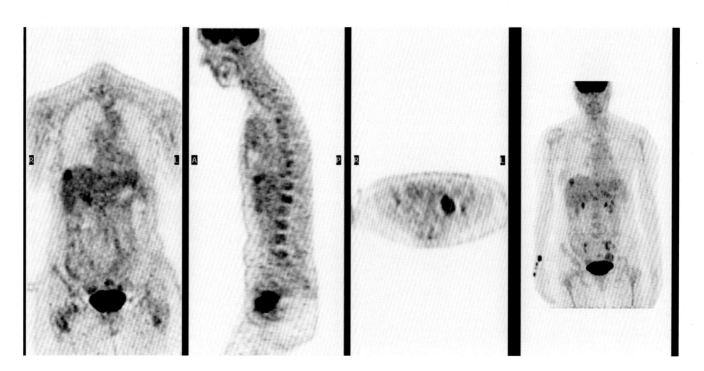

FIGURE 7. Concurrent PET scans (*left to right:* coronal, sagittal, axial, and coronal projection volume) show patchy bony hypermetabolism, best seen in the spine on the sagittal image. Hypermetabolic liver metastases are seen on the coronal and sagittal images, and the enlarged left ovary seen on the axial image is intensely hypermetabolic.

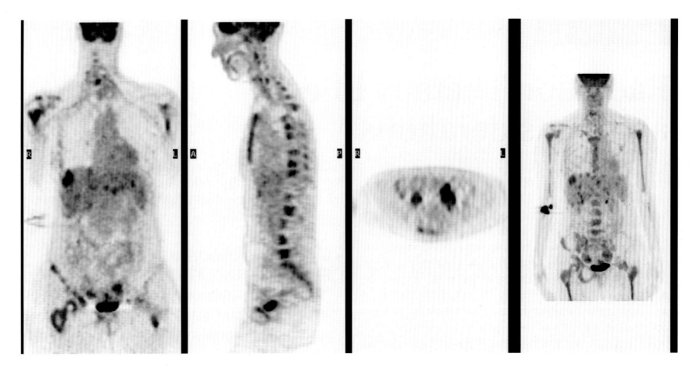

FIGURE 8. Repeat PET scan, 2 months later, shows diffusely increased and patchy bone marrow activity. Liver metastases are larger and more numerous. Hypermetabolism is seen in both ovaries on the axial view (left larger than right).

Once the diagnosis of metastatic breast cancer was established, the patient was begun on chemotherapy, and her response was monitored with periodic CT and PET/CT scans. The initial liver CT illustrated here showed liver metastases, and a comparable study a year later demonstrated evolving findings. Lesions seen on the first study were successfully treated, leaving behind areas of capsular contraction, imparting a nodular contour to the liver. This post-treatment appearance has been termed *pseudocirrhosis.* Unfortunately, these changes do not signify eradication of liver metastases, but rather local response and a degree of local control. More dramatic post-treatment changes (see Case 3 in Chapter 9) can be difficult to assess based solely on anatomic imaging modalities. Correlation with PET imaging can be very helpful in assessing the active tumor burden.

In a case like this, with multisystem metastatic disease, the whole-body capability of PET is most valuable. The adnexal activity seen here in the pelvis localizes to enlarged ovaries. The constellation of imaging findings in this context is most compatible with ovarian metastases. Although benign ovarian hypermetabolism can be seen in premenopausal patients because of corpus luteum cysts, the bilaterality and intensity of the activity seen here, as well as the abnormal size and appearance of the ovaries on the CT, strongly suggest metastatic involvement. See Case 17 in Chapter 3 for an example of benign pelvic PET activity due to a corpus luteum cyst.

SUGGESTED READINGS

Gupta AA, Kim DC, Krinsky GA, et al. CT and MRI of cirrhosis and its mimics. *Am J Roentgenol* 2004; 183: 1595–1601.

Nascimento AB, Mitchell DG, Rubin R, et al. Diffuse desmoplastic breast carcinoma metastases to the liver simulating cirrhosis at MR imaging: report of two cases. *Radiology,* Oct 2001; 221:117–121.

Young ST, Paulson EK, Washington K, et al. CT of the liver in patients with metastatic breast carcinoma treated by chemotherapy: findings simulating cirrhosis. *AJR Am J Roentgenol* 1994; 163:1385–1388.

Radiation Therapy Effects and Considerations

For more than 100 years, the treatment of breast cancer was exclusively surgical. The paradigm of breast malignancy management was eventually challenged by several landmark breast preservation trials, which led to the wide acceptance of treatment of most stage I and II breast cancer patients with whole-breast irradiation following tumor excision. In 1973, in Milan, Italy, women with clinically localized breast carcinoma were randomly assigned treatment with total mastectomy or breast conservation therapy (BCT) with partial mastectomy (quadrantectomy) and whole-breast irradiation. By 1980, a total of 701 patients were randomized and treated. In the United States, a similar trial was initiated in 1976. The National Surgical Adjuvant Breast Project B-06 (NSABP B-06) randomized 2163 women with T1–T2 and N0–N1 breast cancer to one of three treatments: total mastectomy, segmental mastectomy, or segmental mastectomy and radiation therapy (RT). In 2002, the results of both studies, with 20 years of follow-up, were published in the *New England Journal of Medicine*. The results of both trials supported the use of BCT as equally effective compared to mastectomy, in that disease-free survival and overall survival were not adversely affected by preserving the breast. The importance of the status of margins was stressed in NSABP B-06. These two studies and many subsequent international and multi-institutional trials led to a consensus statement by the National Cancer Institute in June 1990 recommending BCT as *preferable* to mastectomy in appropriately selected patients.[1–5]

PATIENT SELECTION FOR BREAST CONSERVATION THERAPY

Most women diagnosed with nonmetastatic, localized tumors are candidates for BCT. Contraindications for BCT include multicentricity, diffuse microcalcifications, pregnancy, prior chest radiation, and persistently positive margins after multiple re-excisions. Relative contraindications for BCT include collagen vascular disease (e.g., scleroderma) and large tumor size relative to the size of the breast. (Neoadjuvant chemotherapy may convert some initially ineligible patients into suitable BCT candidates.)

BREAST PRESERVING WHOLE-BREAST IRRADIATION (THREE-DIMENSIONAL NON-INTENSITY–MODULATED RADIATION THERAPY OR FORWARD PLANNING TECHNIQUE)

The patient is examined at consultation, paying special attention to the patient's breast size, location of the tumor, and any wound issues. Pathology and imaging studies are reviewed. Patients requiring chemotherapy often receive a full course of systemic treatment before radiation. Before RT starts, a mammogram of the involved breast may be obtained. This will serve as a baseline study for follow-up mammograms. Case 1 in this chapter is an illustration of the potential utility of preradiation mammography. Questionable abnormalities need to be worked up before initiation of RT.

Simulation Process

Imaging studies and pathology are reviewed in conjunction with design of the radiation fields. The requirement for reproducible positioning of the patient may involve the creation of custom immobilizing molds or breast or wing boards and the use of nets or other techniques. A treatment planning CT is performed. The entire breast, lung volumes, and heart (for left-sided tumors) are imaged. The surgical scars are wired and marked. The setup points are marked on the skin.

Treatment Planning

The computerized treatment planning process starts with the radiation oncologist outlining the volumes of interest (tumor bed, heart, lungs). The physicist or dosimetrist then creates an optimal arrangement of the tangential fields to cover the breast with a uniform isodose distribution (Figure 1). The dose-volume histograms are created, and the plan is reviewed and approved by the radiation oncologist. The patient is brought in for port films

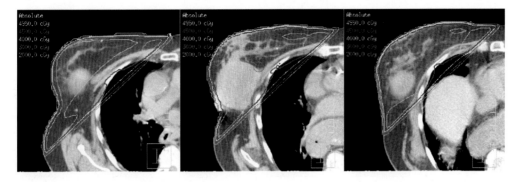

FIGURE 1. Isodose (indicated by the *colored outlines*) distribution diagram for a patient after lumpectomy for right breast cancer shows uniform distribution of the isodoses, avoiding hot spots and conforming to the chest wall contours, thus minimizing radiation exposure of the underlying lung. A large postoperative fluid collection can be seen in the lateral breast.

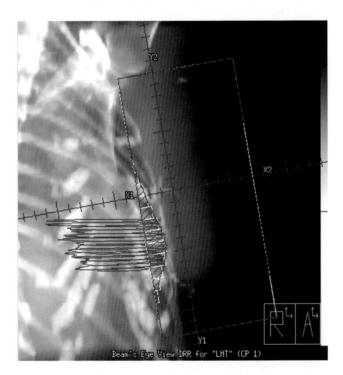

FIGURE 2. A weekly port film is obtained to verify the reproducibility of the setup (patient and breast positioning and radiation field coverage) and is checked by the radiation oncologist for quality assurance.

(Figure 2) and visual check of the fields on the skin to ensure a reproducible setup.

Daily Treatments

The typical course of treatment usually takes 6 to 7 weeks. Radiation treatments are given daily (5 days a week). At least once a week, port films are reviewed to ensure accuracy of the setup.

Tumor Bed Boost

Studies have shown that a boost dose of about 1600 cGy to the tumor bed improves local control.

Radiation oncologists use the findings on physical examination, as well as pretreatment imaging studies, and correlate these with the pathology and operative reports to design the volume of tissue to be included in the boost. The patient is placed on a simulation table in a position to even out the surface of the skin over the tumor bed. The volume is outlined and marked with a wire (Figure 3). Ultrasound or CT is obtained to verify the coverage of the tumor bed and to calculate the energy of the electron beam necessary to adequately treat the surgical bed. Once the coverage is approved by the radiation oncologist, a custom lead alloy cutout is created. The optimal energy of the electron beam is selected to adequately cover the depth of the postsurgical bed, without extending into underlying structures.[6–8]

WHOLE-BREAST IRRADIATION USING INTENSITY-MODULATED RADIATION THERAPY (IMRT) OR FORWARD TREATMENT PLANNING TECHNIQUE

The continuing search for improved delivery of the conformal dose of radiation to the breast, while protecting the underlying structures and minimizing exposure of the contralateral breast, led to development of treatment planning algorithms using IMRT. Based purely on dosimetry, the superiority of treatment plans created using IMRT or forward planning technique (without wedges, using multiple-shaped fields) over three-dimensional conformal opposed tangential fields (using wedges to compensate for uneven breast contours) is readily evident (Figure 4). The dose to the breast is more uniform, there is less of a "hot spot," and the isodose curves are concave,

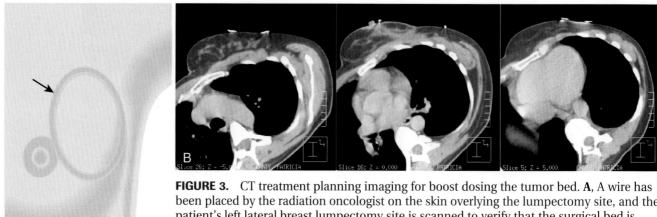

FIGURE 3.   CT treatment planning imaging for boost dosing the tumor bed. **A**, A wire has been placed by the radiation oncologist on the skin overlying the lumpectomy site, and the patient's left lateral breast lumpectomy site is scanned to verify that the surgical bed is encompassed by the wire (*arrow*), here depicted on a volume rendered view of the CT data. **B**, CT planning images, *from above to below*, with the wire in place on the skin overlying the lumpectomy bed, with the patient in a predetermined treatment position.

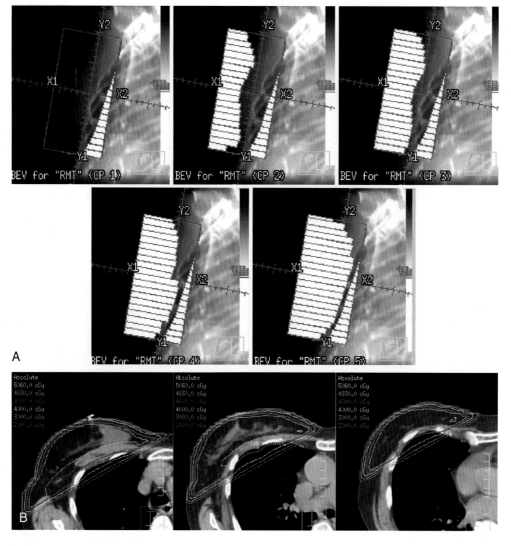

FIGURE 4.   **A**, IMRT process showing five different segments for a single tangential field. The dose is modified using multileaf collimation (indicated by *red and white shading*) to selectively expose areas to be treated or protect underlying structures. **B**, CT view of the resulting IMRT generated isodoses, showing better uniformity than achievable with traditional techniques. A postoperative fluid collection is seen in the medial breast.

conforming to the shape of the underlying chest wall. The dose to the ipsilateral lung can thus be reduced, and in cases of left breast treatment, the heart can be spared to a greater extent.

These dosimetric advantages are no longer just hypothetical, but are observed clinically. There is growing evidence suggesting that IMRT is the best technique available for treatment of the whole breast.

There are challenges associated with implementation of a breast cancer IMRT program on a routine basis. The planning and quality assurance processes are extensive, and the treatment time is longer (not an insignificant factor in a busy department). The patients tolerate treatment better, with less acute skin toxicity. Reduction in long-term toxicity is expected. Further efforts to improve the therapeutic index of RT (optimal dosing to the target volume and maximal protection of the surrounding tissues) involve alternative patient setup (prone), breath-hold and deep inspiration technique, and use of different fractionation. To further spare the surrounding tissues, techniques of partial-breast RT using IMRT have been developed. Partial-breast irradiation is being tested against whole-breast treatment in the ongoing NSABP B-39/Radiation Therapy Oncology Group (RTOG) 0413 study.[9–11]

TREATMENT OF LYMPH NODES

The optimal management of axillary and supraclavicular nodal basins is an area of ongoing research and debate. It is accepted and proven that involvement of more than three lymph nodes with metastases requires RT to the axilla and supraclavicular region. RT reduces axillary recurrence and improves survival. The Southwest Oncology Group (SWOG) S9927 (RTOG 99–15) study was designed to evaluate the benefit of axillary RT in patients with one to three positive lymph nodes. Unfortunately, the trial closed because of poor patient accrual. The decision whether to give RT to the regional lymphatics in patients with one to three involved lymph nodes must be individualized and based on careful weighing of the pathology and review of the risk-to-benefit relation issues with the patient.

The radiation of axillary lymph nodes can be achieved with either inclusion of the level I and II lymph nodes in the tangential fields (if the CT simulation confirms good coverage and if the lung and heart can be spared) or use of a separate oblique field matched inferiorly to the upper border of the tangential breast fields. Depending on the patient's anatomy, the use of an additional posterior axillary boost (PAB) field may be required. Coverage of the supraclavicular region depends on the available information delineating the exact location of the nodal basin and the brachial plexus (Figure 5).[12–14]

Internal Mammary Lymph Node Radiation Therapy

Primary lymphatic drainage into the internal mammary (IM) lymph nodes may occur in 17% to 25% of tumors located in medial, 29% in central, and 27% in lower outer quadrants of the breast. Information from lymphoscintigraphy or positron emission tomography (PET), CT, or MRI, if available, can help in localization of IM lymph nodes. Treatment of IM lymph nodes is individualized and dependent on many factors (Figure 6). Central, medial, or lower outer quadrant breast tumors with multiple positive axillary lymph nodes may require treatment of the IM lymph nodes. However, isolated IM failure is uncommon. The most commonly involved IM lymph nodes are in the second, third, and first interspaces, in that order. The potential for increased cardiopulmonary toxicity warrants caution. Published treatment guidelines give no definitive recommendation for routine treatment of IM lymph nodes and leave this decision to the discretion of the treating radiation oncologist.[15,16]

POST MASTECTOMY RADIATION THERAPY

Currently, postmastectomy RT is indicated in patients with large tumors (≥5 cm), involvement of four lymph nodes or more, close or positive margins, and sometimes multicentric tumors. A Danish study reported in the *New England Journal of Medicine* in 1997 on results of a trial in which 1708 women with stage II to III breast cancer were treated with mastectomy and then randomized to either eight cycles of Cytoxan, methotrexate, 5-fluorouracil (CMF) chemotherapy and chest wall and regional lymphatic RT, or nine cycles of CMF chemotherapy and no RT. After 114 months of median follow-up, the locoregional failure rate was 9% in the arm treated with RT, compared with 32% without RT. The 10-year overall survival rates were 54% and 45%, respectively. A Canadian study, also reported in the *New England Journal of Medicine* in 1997, reported results of a trial of 318 premenopausal node-positive patients after mastectomy who were randomized to undergo either CMF chemotherapy and RT or CMF chemotherapy alone. The arm treated with chemotherapy and RT received three cycles of CMF, followed by RT,

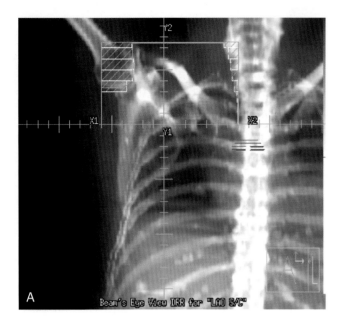 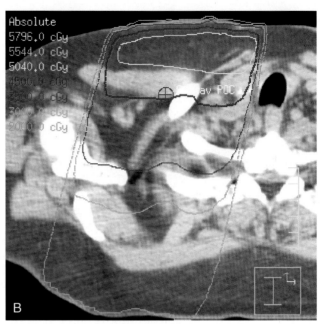

FIGURE 5. **A**, Supraclavicular and axillary field setup to cover the lymphatics, while protecting midline neck structures and the humeral head by use of oblique fields and blocks, here using multileaf collimation (indicated by the cross-hatched areas). **B**, CT view of left anterior oblique (LAO) field covering the right supraclavicular and axillary lymph node basins in the same patient, demonstrating sparing of midline structures (trachea, esophagus, cervical spine) while covering the lymphatic basins. Isodose depths can be modified with use of varying photon energies or opposed posterior axillary boost fields.

followed by another three cycles of CMF. After 150 months of median follow-up, there was a 33% reduction in recurrences, a 17% improvement in disease-free survival, and a 29% reduction in breast cancer–related mortality.

A more recent report reviewed data from five randomized studies, including NSABP B-15, B-16, B18, B-22 and B-25. A total of 5758 node-positive patients enrolled in these studies were treated with mastectomy and chemotherapy, with or without tamoxifen, but no RT. The median follow-up was 11.1 years. The cumulative incidence of isolated locoregional failure was 12.2%, compared with 19.8% for locoregional failure with or without distant failure and 43.3% for distant failure alone as a first event. The cumulative incidence rates of locoregional failure (with or without distant failure) increased with greater axillary nodal involvement, from 13% for one to three nodes involved, to 24.4% for four to nine involved nodes, to 31.9% for more than 10 involved nodes. Similarly, with increasing tumor size, the cumulative incidence rates of locoregional failure (with or without distant failure) increased from 14.9% for tumors smaller than 2 cm, to 21.3% for tumors 2.1 to 5 cm, and up to 24.6% for tumors larger than 5 cm.

These reports from Denmark and Canada and from review of the NSABP data indicate that postmastectomy RT improves local control, but, more importantly, also improves survival.

As the use of postmastectomy RT has increased, so have concerns regarding the effect of RT on reconstructive tissue, implants, and the overall cosmetic treatment outcome. The Therapeutic Index of Loco/Regional Treatment must first account for optimal tumor control, while resulting in the best cosmetic outcome. It is not just cosmesis that is at stake. Development of implant encapsulation can be painful. Fat necrosis can be difficult to differentiate from tumor recurrence and often leads to biopsy, causing patients anxiety. Development of infection or seromas in the reconstructed breast may lead to the removal of transplanted or implanted tissue. Although all these adverse outcomes can occur without use of RT, the incidence does increase with exposure of transplanted tissue or implanted devices to radiation. It is thus extremely important that any patient with even a remote possibility of needing postmastectomy RT be thoroughly evaluated by the whole team to select the best surgical option.[17–21]

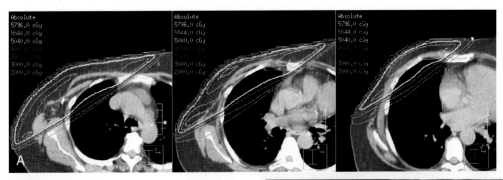

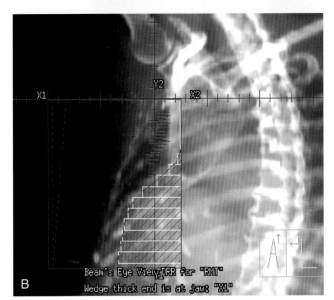

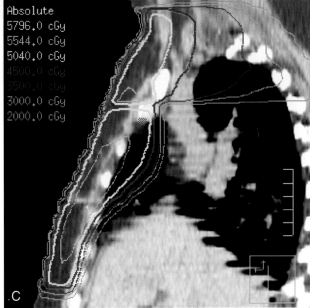

FIGURE 6. **A**, CT treatment planning images of a postmastectomy patient at high risk for internal mammary lymph node (IMLN) involvement, showing the position of the IMLN (*red dots* on left and middle images), which are covered by the isodoses, indicated by the *colored outlines*. **B**, Port film of same patient, showing the IMLN outlined (*red shaded area*). The lung protection afforded by multileaf collimation is outlined as well (*red and white shaded area*). **C**, Sagittal CT reconstruction of the same patient showing the isodose distributions from the supraclavicular, axillary, and chest wall–internal mammary contributions. The upper IMLN location is again designated by the *red shaded area*.

POSTMASTECTOMY RADIATION AND BREAST RECONSTRUCTION

Before mastectomy, patients should undergo an extensive consultation with review of the available reconstructive options. Clinically staged patients who are not expected to require postmastectomy RT are excellent candidates for immediate reconstruction. There are many factors that need to be taken into account while selecting the best surgical reconstruction option. Tumor-related considerations include the tumor size and location, multifocality or multicentricity, lymph node involvement, and chest wall fixation. Patient-related factors include body habitus, medical conditions affecting tissue healing (e.g., collagen vascular diseases), prior chest RT, the location of prior breast surgery scars, smoking history, and prior or planned chemotherapy. Patients with larger tumors (>5 cm), more than three lymph nodes involved, or close margins will require postmastectomy RT. Reconstructive surgery in this population of patients has to be planned carefully. Optimal approaches and timing of reconstruction are the subjects of ongoing discussion and continuing evolution. At many institutions, the anticipated need for postmastectomy RT is a relative contraindication to immediate breast reconstruction using implants. Delayed immediate reconstruction is a viable option in

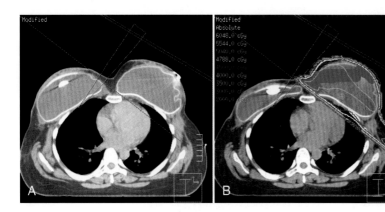

FIGURE 7. Illustration of the potential impact of immediate delayed reconstruction on the RT planning process. This patient had bilateral mastectomy with immediate delayed reconstruction, but needed RT on the left. **A**, Treatment planning was attempted, but the right expansion resulted in excessive exposure of the right chest wall. The patient was sent back to the plastic surgeon for right expander deflation, which resulted in a more desirable isodose distribution (**B**).

management of patients at high risk for needing postmastectomy RT. During mastectomy, tissue expanders are placed. While the patient is recovering from surgery and, if applicable, undergoing chemotherapy, tissue expansion is achieved by ongoing repetitive injections of saline. This process must be completed before the simulation and radiation treatment planning process can begin (Figure 7).[21]

Transverse rectus abdominis myocutaneous (TRAM) flap reconstruction surgery should be delayed if possible, until after completion of the full course of radiation. This allows for an optimal cosmetic outcome[22,23] and improved technical coverage with the radiation fields.[24,25]

LOCOREGIONAL TREATMENT OF BREAST CANCER IN THE ERA OF NEOADJUVANT CHEMOTHERAPY

Neoadjuvant chemotherapy was initially given in an effort to improve respectability, with planned subsequent mastectomy, to patients with bulky tumors and lymph nodes. Concerns that preoperative chemotherapy would increase postoperative complications and delay adjuvant RT and additional chemotherapy did not materialize.

Management of lymph nodes was and continues to be one of the major challenges of neoadjuvant chemotherapy. It has been demonstrated that the information from sentinel lymph node sampling and axillary dissection performed after completion of chemotherapy correlates well with overall prognosis. The role of sentinel lymph node sampling and axillary dissection in the postchemotherapy setting was reviewed in a meta-analysis, with an overall accuracy of 95%.

In an attempt to reduce false-negative sentinel lymph node findings after neoadjuvant chemo-

therapy, many surgeons favor routine sentinel lymph node sampling before initiation of chemotherapy. Positive sentinel lymph node biopsy would lead to completion axillary dissection, before or after chemotherapy. Pathology from prechemotherapy sentinel lymph node biopsy is used by the radiation oncologist to plan the extent of the radiation fields.[26,27]

NEOADJUVANT CHEMOTHERAPY TO ATTEMPT BREAST PRESERVATION

Once the safety and efficacy of neoadjuvant chemotherapy followed by mastectomy was established, its potential use in converting a mastectomy patient into a BCT candidate was tested. Randomized trials of neoadjuvant chemotherapy, followed by lumpectomy, were initiated. The largest study, NSABP B-18, reviewed results of 1523 patients with stage I to IIIB disease. The analysis showed equal median overall survival (69% versus 70%) and local recurrence rates (10.7% versus 7.6%) after preoperative and postoperative chemotherapy, respectively. Higher rates of BCT (68% versus 60%) were achieved in patients treated with neoadjuvant chemotherapy.

The increasing use of neoadjuvant chemotherapy for BCT necessitates even closer cooperation of the multidisciplinary team managing these patients. Unless there are obvious microcalcifications to mark the tumor, the lesion needs to be marked with a clip either before or within the first two cycles of chemotherapy. This is usually done with ultrasound or mammography guidance. In patients who reach clinical complete remission, these clips will guide the surgeon in planning the lumpectomy and the radiation oncologist in planning the extent of the tumor bed boost.[28]

RADIATION THERAPY IN THE MANAGEMENT OF DUCTAL CARCINOMA IN SITU

In the era of routine screening mammography, the diagnosis of ductal carcinoma in situ (DCIS) has become a frequent clinical presentation. Management with aggressive surgery has been largely replaced with breast preservation surgery, followed by RT to the breast. There is considerable confusion as to the optimal management, especially for the low-risk patient (low-grade, small tumors, negative margins). There are advocates of lumpectomy alone as a sole treatment.

Three randomized studies comparing tumor resection (with clear margins) with or without RT reported a strong beneficial effect of RT on local recurrence rates, but no effect on overall survival. Chemoprevention with tamoxifen further protects the involved, as well as the contralateral, breast. The technique of RT is the same as that for invasive tumors. There is no need for treatment of lymph nodes, although sentinel lymph node biopsy may be indicated in high-grade or large tumors.[29–31]

INFLAMMATORY BREAST CANCER

One of the most aggressive and dramatic presentations of breast malignancy is the clinically evident inflammatory breast carcinoma (IBC). The classic presentation leaves little doubt as to the diagnosis, and pathologic confirmation often is a formality. However, there are patients whose diagnosis of IBC is based on histology, rather than the clinical picture. Dermal lymphatic tumor invasion, the histologic hallmark of IBC, may or may not give rise to the clinically characteristic "inflammatory" presentation. Patients with less typical presentations usually undergo workup with mammography, ultrasound, MRI, and biopsy. Once the histologic diagnosis is made, further workup and management are directed toward excluding metastatic disease and initiating systemic chemotherapy as soon as possible. No attempt is made to preserve the breast in patients with IBC. A multimodality team approach to planning the treatment schedule allows for the most expeditious timing of the different components of treatment. The original tumor location is an important parameter in planning postchemotherapy and postmastectomy RT. Imaging studies obtained before and (if available) after chemotherapy assist the radiation oncologist in designing the optimal postmastectomy isodose distribution. Patients with IBC need RT to the regional lymph nodes as part of comprehensive treatment planning. Inclusion of IM lymph nodes is based on review of clinical, imaging, and pathologic information and on the technical feasibility of treatment with the patient's anatomy and scar location.

EVOLUTION OF RADIATION THERAPY IN BREAST CONSERVATION THERAPY

Until recently, BCT was synonymous with the use of whole-breast radiation, after primary tumor removal with lumpectomy, with clear resection margins. Partial-breast RT, in which lumpectomy is followed by less than whole-breast radiation, has been developed in recent years and parallels trends in breast cancer treatment toward less aggressive diagnostic and treatment methods (e.g., sentinel node sampling over axillary dissection, percutaneous over excisional biopsy for diagnosis). Partial-breast RT can be accomplished by brachytherapy, IMRT, and more recently, use of CyberKnife robotic radiosurgery.

Rationale and Options for Partial Breast Radiation

Numerous randomized trials[32–35] comparing whole-breast radiation after tumor excision to tumor excision alone have shown that most breast tumors recur in the tumor cavity. Additionally, these trials have shown that the risk for recurrence outside the tumor cavity is similar whether or not whole-breast radiation was given. This suggests that additional radiation given outside the tumor cavity may not be of additional benefit to patients.

Breast brachytherapy has been traditionally used to treat the lumpectomy cavity as a "boost" following external whole-breast RT. Many centers in recent years have adopted the use of accelerated partial breast RT, either with interstitial needle implants, balloon catheters, or even three-dimensional conformal external RT as the sole radiation treatment modality following breast-conserving surgery. By decreasing the volume of breast tissue that needed irradiation, higher radiation doses could be administered per fraction to the tumor bed. This shortened treatment times to 1 week, decreasing the burden for patients when compared with the need for daily travel for whole-breast radiation, which typically lasts 5 to 7 weeks.

Patients are potential candidates for accelerated partial breast RT if they have stage 0, I, or II tumors, a single tumor less than 3 cm in maximal dimension, minimal nodal involvement, and clear surgical margins. Typically, partial-breast radiation is delivered twice a day, with treatments given at least 6 hours apart, for a total of 10 fractions.

Interstitial breast brachytherapy alone has been successfully used at some U.S. centers for more than 10 years following breast-conserving surgery. A trial was started by Vicini and colleagues in 1993 using brachytherapy as the only radiation treatment modality for patients following breast-conserving surgery.[36,37] By 2001, 120 patients were enrolled in this trial. Four patients developed local recurrence at a median follow-up of 82 months. During 1997 to 2000, 100 patients were enrolled in an RTOG prospective phase I/II study of breast brachytherapy. At a median follow-up of 2.7 years, most patients experienced only mild treatment-related toxicities.[38]

In 2002, the U.S. Food and Drug Administration approved the Proxima Therapeutics MammoSite balloon catheter for intracavitary high-dose-rate breast brachytherapy (Figure 8). Seventy patients were initially enrolled in a prospective multicenter trial evaluating the safety of the MammoSite balloon catheter. Subsequent evaluation of 43 patients eligible for the therapy revealed only mild to moderate self-limited side effects.[39] Advantages of the balloon catheter are that it is easier to place in the cavity, placement is more reproducible, and patient comfort is improved. Only a single catheter needs to be temporarily placed in the lumpectomy cavity, as opposed to 10 to 20 catheters with traditional interstitial implants. However, the balloon needs to "conform" properly to the tumor cavity and optimal dosimetry could be problematic if a large air pocket develops along the periphery of the cavity. In addition, balloon catheters may not be appropriate for tumors near the skin surface. A more recent addition to the partial-breast RT armamentarium is the SAVI device, which allows a radiation oncologist to selectively direct radiation through up to 7 catheter channels, allowing more tailored manipulation of the isodose (Figure 9). The Contura multilumen balloon catheter combines features of these partial-breast RT devices, with multiple offset lumens around a balloon, also allowing dose-shaping opportunities to minimize skin and rib doses (Figure 10).

Three-dimensional conformal radiation technology has been developed and improved in recent years. This technique of accelerated partial breast radiation has the advantage of being noninvasive, eliminating an additional procedure and allowing many medical groups that do not perform brachytherapy to offer partial breast RT. No adverse side effects were seen in 28 patients treated with three-dimensional conformal radiation in a 1999 pilot study.[40] A potential disadvantage is that the breast is not a stationary target, and there is the potential for a geographic miss with external RT to a small target.

In 2005, the NSABP, along with the RTOG, activated a phase III randomized trial comparing whole-breast RT and partial-breast RT in women with stage 0, I, or II breast cancer. The trial is currently open and is expected to accrue 3000 patients over a period of about 2 years and 5 months. This trial will be comparing overall survival, recurrence-free survival, distant recurrence-free survival, and quality-of-life issues in women receiving whole-breast or partial-breast RT.[32–40]

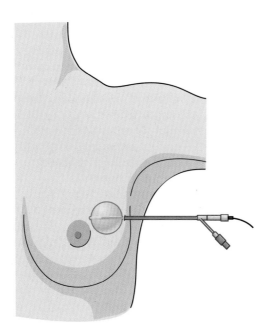

FIGURE 8. Drawing depicting MammoSite balloon catheter positioned within a lumpectomy cavity for performance of partial breast radiation. The balloon is expanded to fill the cavity, and the radiation point source is introduced through the attached silicone catheter. *Represented with permission of Cytyc Corporation, Marlborough, MA.*

RADIATION AFTER AUGMENTATION

Patients who develop breast cancer after they have undergone prior breast augmentation present additional challenges in designing their treatment to achieve optimal locoregional control and the best possible cosmetic outcome. With careful

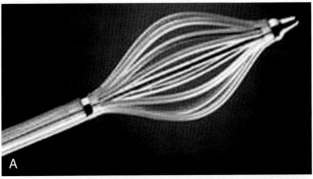

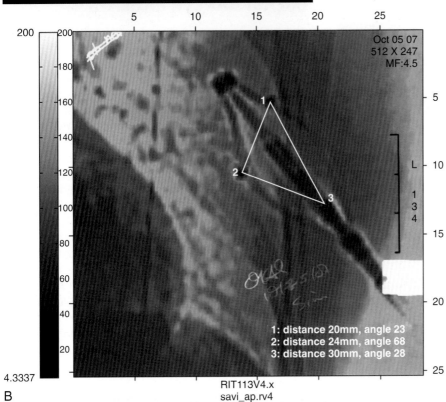

1: distance 20mm, angle 23
2: distance 24mm, angle 68
3: distance 30mm, angle 28

Oct 05 07
512 X 247
MF:4.5

RIT113V4.x
savi_ap.rv4

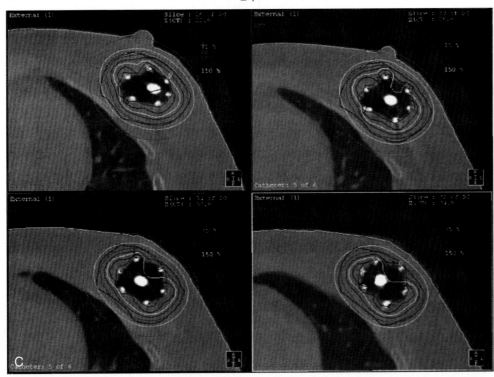

FIGURE 9. A newer, alternative device for partial breast radiation is the SAVI device. **A**, The SAVI device consists of a whisk-like arrangement of seven catheters. The device is expanded to fill the lumpectomy cavity. Radiation sources are selectively introduced into the channels to custom-design the desired isodose, enabling the skin, chest wall, and underlying lung to be more effectively spared. *Reproduced with permission of Cianna Medical, Inc., Aliso Viejo, CA.* **B**, Antero-posterior radiographic view of the SAVI device positioned within a left lumpectomy cavity. The triangle superimposed over the device outlines reference points, which are checked to ensure the device expansion and position are reproducible. **C**, CT isodose images of the same left breast, with the SAVI device in place. A larger central catheter channel is surrounded by six smaller catheters. The treatment area coverage can be customized by varying the degree of expansion of the device. Note the isodose distribution, which conforms well to the chest wall configuration, with little overlap with underlying lung. The flexibility of the device enables it to be used in patients who might not be able to undergo other forms of partial-breast RT, owing to lesion proximity to skin.

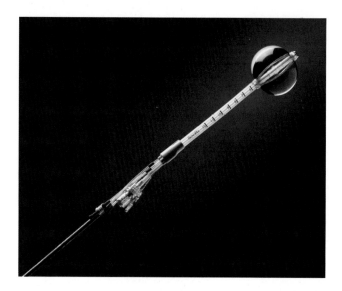

FIGURE 10. Another alternative for partial-breast RT is the Contura multilumen balloon catheter, which combines offset lumens for dose shaping with a balloon catheter. The balloon incorporates vacuum to remove fluid and air, which may also help to achieve more uniform dosing by better tissue conformance around the balloon. *Reproduced with permission of Seno Rx, Aliso Viejo, CA.*

dosimetry, using IMRT or three-dimensional treatment planning, breast tissue coverage with the desired isodose can be achieved, although there are technical challenges associated with the presence of the implanted device.[25,41]

A variety of factors influence the cosmetic outcome in patients with breast augmentation. Implant device factors include the age of the implant, the type of device (saline or silicone, smooth or textured), and what the status of the capsule is at presentation. Patient-related factors include the patient's desires and expectations, medical comorbidities (smoking, diabetes mellitus, collagen vascular disease), and *BRCA* gene status. Cancer-related considerations include tumor proximity to the implant capsule and the tumor grade and histology (e.g., IBC).

These patients should receive an extensive review of the expected effects of radiation on the augmented breast. They need to be evaluated by the radiation oncologist, breast surgeon, and plastic surgeon (if not the same) before the definitive cancer procedure is scheduled. Often the decision whether to retain, remove, or modify the existing augmentation device is patient driven. However, the patient has to be given appropriate information so that she can make an informed decision. One of the concerns frequently voiced by patients is the effectiveness of follow-up imaging. Cases illustrating the range of postoperative appearances

of a variety of reconstruction options, as well as manifestations of recurrences and treatment-related changes, are presented throughout this text, particularly in Chapter 6.[41]

IMAGING FOLLOW-UP OF RADIATION THERAPY–TREATED BREAST CANCER PATIENTS

BCT and RT induce readily visualized and potentially confusing changes in the treated breast on imaging, particularly on mammograms, CT scans, and breast MRI, with fewer effects generally noted on ultrasound and PET. Early postirradiation mammograms in particular can show variable degrees of skin thickening and a generalized increase in breast density and reticulation. These changes usually regress with time. In addition to routine follow-up imaging, clinically detected change should prompt imaging evaluation for possible recurrence. As with all breast imaging, mammography is the cornerstone modality for initial imaging, liberally supplemented with ultrasound. In cases in which there is persistent concern for possible recurrence, breast MRI can be very helpful, particularly more than 18 months after treatment, when little if any enhancement is seen in normal postoperative scars. Significantly enhancing scars older than 18 months should be further investigated, such as with biopsy, to exclude recurrent disease. A scar complicated by fat necrosis or fat necrosis developing in the treatment bed can at times perfectly mimic a local recurrence. Examples are presented in Chapters 6 and 7. A documented local recurrence should prompt systemic evaluation, to confirm that the recurrence is local only, before decision making on additional therapy. This is best accomplished with PET/CT and bone scan.

Chest CT scans (and thoracic MRI) can be expected to show changes of radiation pneumonitis in the tangential fields of patients treated with whole-breast radiation and apical changes in patients treated with RT to axillary and supraclavicular fields. Multiple examples are presented in this chapter.

Radiologic follow-up after reconstruction depends on the technique of reconstruction used and the clinical question. Detection of recurrences in implant and TRAM flap reconstruction patients has traditionally relied on physical examination, supplemented with imaging when questions arise, rather than on routine imaging surveillance with mammography. This has been advocated by some authors[42] as potentially enabling earlier diagnosis of recurrent disease than can be achieved by relying on physical examination. Familiarity with normal appearances of breast reconstructions is important to imagers interpreting these studies.[43–45]

RT COMPLICATIONS

Lymphedema

One of most dreaded complications of RT is arm lymphedema. The patients at highest risk for lymphedema have multiple positive lymph nodes, requiring lymph node dissection and RT to the lymphatics. The patients' overall health status and comorbidities such as diabetes, older age, obesity, and lifestyle may be contributory factors.

The diagnosis of lymphedema is a clinical one. Often, there is a discrepancy between the patient's perceptions and measurable arm swelling. It is important to have a baseline measurement of the arm diameter in a high-risk patient. The new onset of lymphedema, once documented (there are no universal parameters to determine the magnitude of lymphedema), needs to be followed by a clinical evaluation to rule out locoregional recurrence as an underlying cause of swelling of the arm. Imaging studies, such as ultrasound, CT, MRI, or PET, may be necessary to fully evaluate the lymphatics. Lymphedema is a difficult clinical problem and requires a lot of time and patience from the patient and managing physicians.

Rib Fracture

Tangential radiation fields covering the breast or chest wall deliver a portion of the prescribed dose to the underlying anterior ribs. This can lead to rib fracture. Fractures can be diagnosed clinically by typical symptoms or radiographically with x-rays or bone scan. These fractures typically heal without need for intervention.

Carcinogenesis: Radiation-Induced Sarcoma

A rare complication of radiation is a radiation-induced sarcoma. Primary sarcoma of the breast is very rare. Secondary sarcomas have been reported developing in breasts exposed to prior radiation or with chronic lymphedema from prior surgery. It is thought to be related to chronic changes in the breast resulting in prolonged edema (lymphedema). The most common histology is an angiosarcoma. This was initially described as Stewart-Treves syndrome and was first recognized in patients with long-standing extremity lymphedema. Clinically, it can present as a violaceous discoloration of the skin and a rapidly growing mass. Examples are Case 18 in Chapter 6 and Case 9 in this chapter.[46,47]

Carcinogenesis: Lung Cancer

A correlation has been suggested between RT to the breast and the eventual development of a lung malignancy. Patients who have been exposed to thoracic RT for treatment of breast cancer or Hodgkin's disease should be on heightened lung surveillance. Newer techniques of breast RT better protect the underlying lung, but there is still a small amount of lung parenchyma exposed, and the risk for lung carcinogenesis, even though markedly reduced, still exists.[48–50]

Carcinogenesis: Risk for Contralateral Breast Malignancy

An increased risk of contralateral breast cancer due to RT after BCT has also been suggested. Doses delivered to the contralateral breast from primary radiation could be a cause. There are several treatment techniques that can be used to minimize contralateral breast dose, such as elimination of a medial wedge. Nevertheless, the increased risk appears to be minimal, and there are conflicting reports about the patient subpopulations at risk (e.g., <45 years old versus >50 years old). Obviously, the patient with a previous diagnosis of breast malignancy is already at increased risk for a second breast cancer, independent of radiation treatment, and requires ongoing follow-up with mammography supplemented with ultrasound or MRI.[51–54]

Cardiotoxicity

One of the most important concerns in planning locoregional and systemic treatment of patients with breast cancer is the effect that treatment may have on the heart. There are a variety of potentially contributory factors for cardiotoxicity, including the patient's cardiac health status before the initiation of treatment.

Systemic therapy often includes known cardiotoxic drugs, such as doxorubicin (Adriamycin) and trastuzumab (Herceptin). Radiation therapy for left-sided breast cancers (either to the breast or chest wall) or treatment of left-sided tumors requiring RT to the axilla or supraclavicular region will overlap the heart, as will tumors of either breast that require RT to IM lymph nodes.

Long-term follow-up data on patients treated with RT in the 1960s and 1970s showed that even though the use of RT resulted in decreased breast cancer–specific deaths, overall survival suffered as a result of long-term cardiac toxicity associated with RT. This effect has been steadily diminishing with the implementation of modern techniques. More recent data suggest little increase in cardiac death rates due to RT, even with left breast tumors (without IM lymph node RT). Additionally, radiation doses delivered to the heart could be significantly reduced or virtually eliminated with newer treatment techniques such as forward planning IMRT or partial-breast irradiation. However, an increased risk for coronary artery disease in patients treated with radiation for left breast tumors has been suggested.[55–57]

REFERENCES

1. Fisher B, Anderson S, Bryant J, et al. Twenty-year follow-up of a randomized trial comparing total mastectomy, lumpectomy, and lumpectomy plus irradiation for the treatment of invasive breast cancer. *N Engl J Med* 2002; 347(16):1233–1241.

2. Veronesi U, Marubini E, Mariani L, et al. Radiotherapy after breast-conserving surgery in small breast carcinoma: long-term results of a randomized trial. *Ann Oncol* 2001; 12:997–1003.

3. Holli K, Saaristo R, Isalo J, et al. Lumpectomy with or without postoperative radiotherapy for breast cancer with favorable prognostic features: results of a randomized study. *Br J Cancer* 2001; 84:164–169.

4. Clark RM, Whalen T, Levine M, et al. Randomized clinical trial of breast irradiation following lumpectomy and axillary dissection for node-negative breast cancer: an update. Ontario Clinical Oncology Group. *J Natl Cancer Inst* 1996; 88:1659–1664.

5. NIH Office of the Director: NIH Consensus Statement. Nov 1–3, 2000; 17(4).

6. Bartelink H, Collette L, Fourquet A, et al. Impact of a boost dose of 16 Gy on the local control and cosmesis in patients with early breast cancer: The EORTC 'boost versus no boost' trial. *Int J Radiat Oncol Biol Phys* 2000; 48(3)111, abstract 1.

7. Romestaing P, Lehingue Y, Delaunay D, et al. Role of a 10-Gy boost in the conservation treatment of early breast cancer: results of randomized clinical trial in Lyon, France. *Int J Radiat Oncol Biol Phys* 2001; 51(3), abstract 1.

8. Horst KC, Goffinet DR. 10 Gy vs 16 Gy electron beam boost dose in breast conservation therapy for early breast cancer: a decision analysis. *Int J Radiat Oncol Biol Phys* 2002; 54(2):307.

9. Vicini FA, Sharpe MB, Kestin LL, et al. Optimizing breast cancer treatment efficacy with intensity-modulated radiotherapy. *Int J Radiat Oncol Biol Phys* 2002; 54(5):1336–1344.

10. Remouchamps VM, Vicini FA, Sharpe MB, et al. Significant reduction in heart and lung doses using deep inspiration breath hold with active breathing control and intensity-modulated radiation therapy for patients treated with locoregional breast radiation. *Int J Radiat Oncol Biol Phys* 2003; 55(2): 392–406.

11. Hurkmans CW, Cho BCJ, Damen E, et al. Reduction of cardiac and lung complication probabilities after breast irradiation using conformal radiotherapy with or without intensity modulation. *Radiother Oncol* 2002; 62(2):163–171.

12. Veronesi U, Rilke F, Luini A, et al. Distribution of axillary node metastases by level of Invasion. *Cancer* 1987; 59:682.

13. Fisher B, Wolmark N, Bauer M, et al. The accuracy of clinical nodal staging and of limited axillary dissection as a determinant of histologic nodal status in carcinoma of the breast. *Surg Gynecol Obstet* 1981; 152:765.

14. Dewar JA, Sarrazin D, Benhamou E, et al. Management of the axilla in conservatively treated breast cancer: 592 patients treated at Institut Gustave-Roussey. *Int J Radiat Oncol Biol Phys* 1987; 13:375.

15. Byrd DR, Dunnwald LK, Mankoff DA, et al. Internal mammary lymph node drainage patterns in patients with breast cancer documented by breast lymphoscintigraphy. *Ann Surg Oncol* 2001; 8(3):234–240.

16. Recht A, Edge SB, Solin LJ, et al. Postmastectomy radiotherapy: clinical practice guidelines of the American Society of Clinical Oncology. *J Clin Oncol* 2001; 19(5):1539–1569.

17. Overgaard M, Jensen MB, Overgaard J, et al. Postoperative radiotherapy in high risk premenopausal women with breast cancer who receive adjuvant chemotherapy. *N Engl J Med* 1997; 337:949–954.

18. Ragaz J, Jackson SM, Ne N, et al. Adjuvant radiotherapy and chemotherapy in node positive premenopausal women with breast cancer. *N Engl J Med* 1997; 337:956–962.

19. Recht A, Edge SB, Solin LJ, et al: Postmastectomy radiotherapy: clinical practice guidelines of the American Society of Clinical Oncology. *J Clin Oncol* 2001; 19(5):1539–1569.

20. Pierce L: The use of radiotherapy after mastectomy: a review of the literature. *J Clin Oncol* 2003; 23(8):1706–1717.

21. Taghian A, Jeong J-H, Mamounas E, et al. Patterns of locoregional failure in patients with operable breast cancer treated by mastectomy and adjuvant chemotherapy with or without tamoxifen and without radiotherapy: results from five National Surgical Adjuvant Breast and Bowel Project randomized clinical trials. *J Clin Oncol* 2004; 22: 4247–4254.

22. Barreau-Pouhear I, Le MG, Rietjens M, et al. Risk factors for failure of immediate breast reconstruction with prosthesis after total mastectomy for breast cancer. *Cancer* 1992; 70:1145–1151.

23. Pomahac B, Recht A, May JW, et al. New trends in breast cancer management: is the era of immediate breast reconstruction changing? *Ann Surg* 2006; 244(2):282–288.

24. Javaid M, Song F, Leinster S, et al. Radiation effects on the cosmetic outcomes of immediate and delayed autologous breast reconstruction: an argument about timing. *J Plast Reconstr Aesthet Surg* 2006; 59(1):16–26.

25. Motwani SB, Strom EA, Schechter NR, et al. The impact of immediate breast reconstruction on the technical delivery of postmastectomy radiotherapy. *Int J Radiat Oncol Biol Phys* 2006; 66(1):76–82.

26. Danforth DN Jr, Lippman ME, McDonald H, et al. Effect of pre-operative chemotherapy on mastectomy for locally advanced breast cancer. *Am Surg* 1990; 56:6–11.

27. Xing Y, Ding M, Ross M, et al. Metaanalysis of sentinel lymph node biopsy following pre operative chemotherapy in patients with operable breast cancer. ASCO Ann Meeting 2004; abstract 561.

28. Wolmark N, Wang J, Mamounas E, et al. Preoperative chemotherapy in patients with operable breast cancer: nine year results from National Surgical Adjuvant Breast and Bowel Project B-18. *Natl Cancer Inst Monogr* 2001; 96–102.

29. Fisher B, Dignam J, Wolmark N, et al. Lumpectomy and radiation therapy for the treatment of intraductal breast cancer. Findings from National Surgical Adjuvant Breast and Bowel Project B-17. *J Clin Oncol* 1998; 16:441–452.

30. Julien JP, Bijker N, Fentiman IS, et al: Radiotherapy in breast conserving treatment for ductal carcinoma in situ: first results of the EORTC randomized phase III trial 10853. *Lancet* 2000; 355:528–533.

31. Houghton J, George WD, Cuzick J, et al. Radiotherapy and tamoxifen in women with completely excised ductal carcinoma in situ of the breast in the UK, Australia and New Zealand: randomised controlled trial. *Lancet* 2003; 362:95–102.

32. Fisher B, Anderson S, Bryant J, et al. Twenty-year follow-up of a randomized trial comparing total mastectomy, lumpectomy, and lumpectomy plus irradiation for the treatment of invasive breast cancer. *N Engl J Med* 2002; 347:1233–1241.

33. Veronesi U, Marubini E, Mariani L, et al. Radiotherapy after breast-conserving surgery in small breast carcinoma: long-term results of a randomized trial. *Ann Oncol* 2001; 12:997–1003.

34. Holli K, Saaristo R, Isalo J, et al. Lumpectomy with or without postoperative radiotherapy for breast cancer with favorable prognostic features: results of a randomized study. *Br J Cancer* 2001; 84:164–169.

35. Clark RM, Whalen T, Levine M, et al. Randomized clinical trial of breast irradiation following lumpectomy and axillary dissection for node-negative breast cancer: an update. Ontario Clinical Oncology Group. *J Natl Cancer Inst* 1996; 88:1659–1664.

36. Vicini F, Baglan K, Kestin L, et al. Accelerated treatment of breast cancer. *J Clin Oncol* 2001; 19: 1993–2001.

37. Vicini F, Kini V, Chen P, et al. Irradiation of the tumor bed alone after lumpectomy in selected patients with early-stage breast cancer treated with breast conserving therapy. *J Surg Oncol* 1999; 70:33–40.

38. Kuske R, Winter K, Arthur D, et al. A phase I/II trial of brachytherapy alone following lumpectomy for select breast cancer: toxicity analysis of Radiation Therapy Oncology Group 95-17. *Int J Radiat Oncol Biol Phys* 2002; 54:87.

39. Keisch M, Vicini F, Kuske R, et al. Two-year cosmetic outcome with the MammoSite® breast brachytherapy applicator: technical factors associated with optimal results when performing partial breast irradiation. Proceedings of the 45th Annual Meeting of the American Society for Therapeutic Radiology and Oncology, Salt Lake City, Utah, October 2003.

40. Vicini F, Remouchamps V, Wallace M, et al. Ongoing clinical experience utilizing 3D conformal external beam radiotherapy to deliver partial-breast irradiation in patients with early-stage breast cancer treated with breast-conserving therapy. *Int J Radiat Oncol Biol Phys* 2003; 57:1247–1253.

41. Schechter NR, Strom EA, Perkins GH, et al. Immediate breast reconstruction can impact postmastectomy irradiation. *Am J Clin Oncol* 2005; 28:485.

42. Helvie MA, Bailey JE, Roubidoux MA, et al. Mammographic screening of TRAM flap breast reconstructions for detection of nonpalpable recurrent cancer. *Radiology* 2002; 224:211–216.

43. Kim SM, Park JM. Mammographic and ultrasonographic features after autogenous myocutaneous flap reconstruction mammoplasty. *J Ultrasound Med* 2004; 23(2):275–282.

44. LePage MA, Kazerooni EA, Helvie MA, Wilkins EG. Breast reconstruction with TRAM flaps: normal and abnormal appearance at CT. *RadioGraphics* 1999; 19:1593–1603.

45. Devon RK, Rosen MA, Mies C, et al. Breast reconstruction with a transverse rectus abdominis myocutaneous flap: spectrum of normal and abnormal MR imaging findings. *RadioGraphics* 2004; 24(5): 1287–1299.

46. Monroe AT, Feigenberg SJ, Mendenhall NP. Angiosarcoma after breast-conserving therapy. *Cancer* 2003; 97(8):1832–1840.

47. Stokkel MP, Peterse HL. Angiosarcoma of the breast after lumpectomy and radiation therapy for adenocarcinoma. *Cancer* 1992; 69(12):2965–2968.

48. Neugut AI, Robinson E, Lee WC, et al: Lung cancer after radiation therapy for breast cancer. *Cancer* 1993; 71(10):3054–3057.

49. Ford MB, Sigurdson AJ, Petrulis ES, et al. Effects of smoking and radiotherapy on lung carcinoma in breast carcinoma survivors. *Cancer* 2003; 98:1457–1464.

50. Scanlon EF, Suh O, Murthy SM, et al. Influence of smoking on the development of lung metastases from breast cancer. *Cancer* 1995; 75(11):2693–2699.

51. Clarke M, Collins R, Darby S, et al. Effects of radiotherapy and of differences in the extent of surgery for early breast cancer on local recurrence and 15-year survival: an overview of the randomised trials. *Lancet* 2005; 366:2087–2106.

52. Boice JD, Harvey EB, Blettneret M, et al. Cancer in the contralateral breast after radiotherapy for breast cancer. *N Engl J Med* 1992; 326(12):781–785.

53. Obedian E, Fischer DB, Haffty BG. Second malignancies after treatment of early-stage breast cancer: lumpectomy and radiation therapy versus mastectomy. *J Clin Oncol* 2000; 18(12):2406–2412.

54. Kelly CA, Wang XY, Chu JC, et al. Dose to the contralateral breast: a comparison of four primary breast irradiation techniques. *Int J Radiat Oncol Biol Phys* 1996; 34(3):727–732.

55. Early Breast Cancer Trialists' Collaborative Group. Favourable and unfavourable effects on long-term survival of radiotherapy for early breast cancer: an overview of the randomized trials. *Lancet* 2000; 355:1757–1770.

56. Early Breast Cancer Trialists' Collaborative Group. Effects of radiotherapy and of differences in the extent of surgery for early breast cancer on local recurrence and 15 years survival: an overview of randomized trials. *Lancet* 2005; 366:2087–2106.

57. Harris EER, Correa C, Hwang WT, et al. Late cardiac mortality and morbidity in early-stage breast cancer patients after breast-conservation treatment. *J Clin Oncol* 2006; 24(25):4100–4106.

CASE 1

Utility of preradiation mammography

A 39-year-old woman with limited ability to communicate was brought in by her family after the patient pointed to a breast lump. The patient had a variety of severe congenital impairments, including blindness, deafness, spasticity, ataxia, and mental retardation. A palpable, 2-cm left upper inner quadrant mass was confirmed on physical examination by her primary care physician. Mammography confirmed a lobular, dense mass with ductal extension at the site of the palpable lump (Figure 1). Extending anteriorly toward the nipple from the dominant mass was a wide expanse of pleomorphic microcalcifications over an additional 4 cm. Ultrasound identified the lobular mass and served as guidance for performance of core biopsy, confirming mucinous carcinoma (Figure 2).

Discussions with the family about the surgical options yielded a decision to have the patient undergo lumpectomy with radiation therapy, rather than mastectomy. This was motivated by a fear that the patient would have difficulty comprehending the loss of the breast. Surgical consultation noted that with the calcifications, there would be a high likelihood of positive margins with lumpectomy.

Lumpectomy was performed with palpation guidance, and no specimen radiograph was sent. The pathology confirmed a 2.2-cm grade 9/9 mucinous adenocarcinoma, estrogen receptor– and progesterone receptor–positive, *HER-2/neu* positive, node-negative tumor, with negative margins. No ductal carcinoma in situ (DCIS) was identified in the specimen. The patient underwent radiation therapy as planned, and was placed on tamoxifen.

On her first post-treatment mammogram, obtained 3 months after completing radiation therapy, it became apparent that although the dominant mass was excised, the suspicious, pleomorphic microcalcifications remained. These were sampled with stereotactic technique, confirming DCIS.

Chemotherapy had been declined, and the patient was placed on tamoxifen after the initial diagnosis of mucinous carcinoma. Mastectomy was declined by the family after the identification of DCIS because of concern for the patient's psychological well-being.

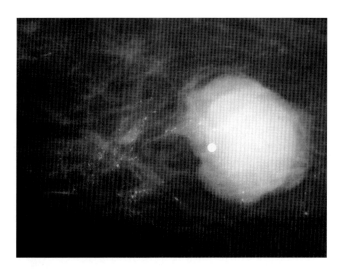

FIGURE 1. Detail view from the diagnostic mammogram shows a dominant mass with lobular margins, with a tail of ductal extension toward the nipple and with microcalcifications. Extending from the mass toward the nipple is a 4-cm expanse of pleomorphic, suspicious microcalcifications. The calcifications vary in size, shape, and density from one another, and many are linear in shape.

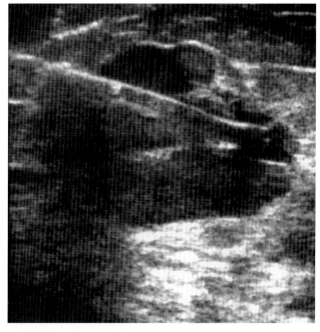

FIGURE 2. Ultrasound of the dominant, palpable mass shows lobular, relatively circumscribed margins. This image was obtained during ultrasound-guided core biopsy and shows the needle within the mass, entering from the left.

TEACHING POINTS

How did it happen that this patient's suspicious DCIS calcifications were not excised at the time of her lumpectomy? Quality control happens at many different levels, and perhaps with additional checks in the system, these calcifications might not have "slipped through the cracks." The initial interpretation clearly indicated that the microcalcifications were extensive and suspicious. The palpable lump corresponded to the dominant mass. One problem was the use of palpation guidance for localization of the abnormality in surgery. This proved effective for excision of the dominant mass, but made no provision for excision of the calcifications. In retrospect, they probably should have been needle-localized to guide more complete surgical excision.

If there had been a universal specimen radiograph policy, this omission might have been recognized earlier. But this is far from a universal practice. Most sites routinely utilize specimen radiography for needle-localized mammographic abnormalities, but do not routinely perform specimen x-rays of palpation or ultrasound-guided abnormalities. The use of postexcision, preradiation therapy mammograms is also generally on a case-by-case basis, usually when there is a question of completeness of excision of microcalcifications. Review of the pathology and assessment of the concordance (or lack thereof) of the findings with the results was another opportunity to recognize this problem. The dominant mass proved to be a 2.2-cm mucinous carcinoma, but the clear margins misled the entire team taking care of this patient into thinking the excision was complete. In retrospect, the pathologic results, with no evidence of DCIS, are not concordant with the overall imaging findings. It is surprising that the margins were clear, given the proximity on mammography of the proven mucinous carcinoma mass to the subsequently proven DCIS calcifications. The preoperative expectation was that the margins would likely be positive in light of the imaging findings.

This case also is a nice illustration of the relatively benign appearance certain cancers, like the mucinous histology here, can have. The margins are predominantly lobular, but the lobulations are too numerous and not gentle enough (with three or fewer lobulations) to be considered probably benign criteria, per the criteria of Stavros. In addition, although most of the margins appear circumscribed and lobular, a mass must always be judged by its worst-looking feature. On mammography, a tail-like focus of ductal extension is seen extending from the mass into the calcifications, both of which are features of malignancy.

SUGGESTED READING

Stavros AT, Thickman D, Rapp CL, et al. Solid breast nodules: use of sonography to distinguish between benign and malignant lesions. *Radiology* 1995; 196: 123–134.

CASE 2

Dramatic breast radiation therapy changes on mammography and MRI

A 64-year-old woman underwent routine bilateral screening mammography, which showed a left lower inner quadrant (LIQ) irregular mass. Bilateral increased microcalcifications were also noted. Workup with spot compression showed a 2×1 cm spiculated, bilobed mass, which on ultrasound measured 1.2 cm. Left breast ultrasound-guided biopsy confirmed infiltrating ductal carcinoma (IDC).

Bilateral stereotactic biopsies of microcalcifications were performed. Right upper outer quadrant (UOQ) microcalcifications proved to be intermediate-grade ductal carcinoma in situ (DCIS). Bilateral lumpectomies were performed, as well as left axillary lymph node dissection (no sentinel lymph node was identified). No axillary sampling was performed on the right because only noninvasive disease was known.

The left breast pathology showed a stage IIIA, T1N2, 1.7-cm, left breast IDC with intermediate-grade DCIS, estrogen receptor and progesterone receptor positive, *HER-2/neu* negative, with 7 of 10 positive lymph nodes.

The right lumpectomy removed a 1.5-cm right UOQ IDC with intermediate grade DCIS, also estrogen receptor and progesterone receptor positive and *HER-2/neu* negative.

The patient was treated with four cycles of dose-dense doxorubicin (Adriamycin) plus cyclophosphamide (Cytoxan) (AC) chemotherapy, but refused subsequent additional planned chemotherapy and was placed on anastrozole (Arimidex).

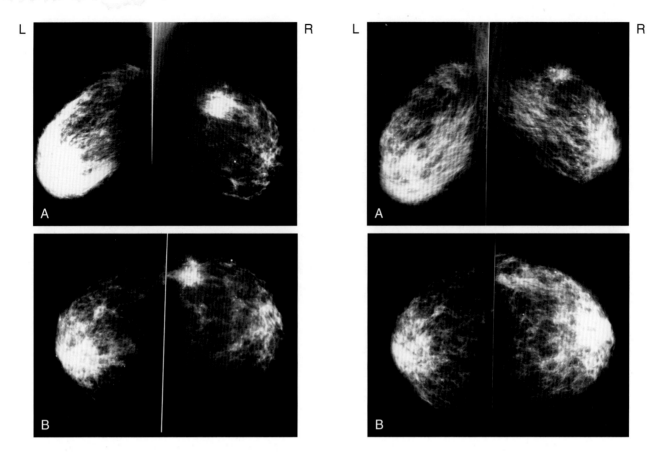

FIGURE 1. Mediolateral oblique (MLO) (**A**) and cranial-caudal (CC) (**B**) bilateral mammography 3 months after bilateral lumpectomies and left axillary lymph node dissection and four cycles of AC chemotherapy, before starting radiation therapy, shows a right UOQ spiculated lumpectomy scar. The left breast shows marked increased density in the retroareolar region and LIQ, at the site of the lumpectomy. There is generalized increased density and trabeculation of the left breast compared with the right.

Bilateral breast and peripheral lymphatic radiation therapy was given. The right regional lymphatics were treated because there was no axillary sampling. Radiation therapy was poorly tolerated with skin desquamation and fatigue.

Both breasts were treated to doses of 50.40 Gy. The left lumpectomy cavity was boosted to 60.40 Gy. Planned right lumpectomy boost was not completed because of patient intolerance, and received a dose of 54.40. Mammograms were obtained before starting radiation therapy (Figure 1) and 4 months after completing radiation therapy (Figure 2).

Breast MRI obtained for surveillance 4 months after completing radiation therapy shows marked bilateral changes of radiation therapy (Figure 3).

FIGURE 2. MLO (**A**) and CC (**B**) bilateral mammography 6 months later and 4 months after completing bilateral radiation therapy shows dramatic radiation therapy changes. There is diffuse increased density and trabeculation of both breasts. The right UOQ scar and ill-defined density associated with the left LIQ scar have regressed.

TEACHING POINTS

This is a dramatic example of radiation therapy changes that can be seen on mammograms and MRI after treatment. Skin thickening and edema and diffuse increased edema, density, and trabeculation of breast parenchyma are typical changes of radiation therapy. The degree to which these changes are visualized varies from patient to patient, and timing of studies after completion of radiation also influences the appearance of these changes. They can be expected to regress with time, although they may not resolve completely. The imaging differential for these changes includes inflammatory breast cancer, lymphedema, systemic causes of anasarca (such as congestive heart failure), and mastitis.

One curious finding in this case is the preradiation mammographic appearance of the left breast,

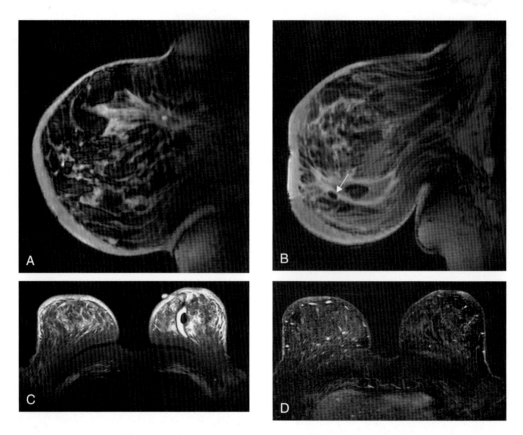

FIGURE 3. Breast MRI, concurrent with the mammogram in Figure 2, obtained 4 months after completing bilateral radiation therapy and 9 months after bilateral lumpectomies, shows dramatic radiation therapy changes. **A**, Unenhanced sagittal, T1-weighted, fat-saturated gradient echo image through the right lateral breast shows the UOQ scar. Architectural distortion surrounds a small fluid collection, which contains a small hyperintense focus of blood (methemoglobin). Note the marked skin thickening. **B**, Unenhanced sagittal, T1-weighted, fat-saturated gradient echo image through the left medial breast shows the LIQ scar as a fluid collection with surrounding distortion and scarring, containing a hypointense focus of clot (*arrow*). Note the marked skin thickening. **C**, Axial short tau inversion recovery (STIR) MRI of both breasts, through the left LIQ scar, shows hyperintense fluid outlining hypointense clot in the left scar. The skin is markedly thickened and edematous. Increased edema signal and increased trabeculation are seen throughout both breasts. Increased edema signal is also seen in the chest wall bilaterally. **D**, Despite the above changes, there is no notable enhancement on subtracted, enhanced, T1-weighted, gradient echo imaging, obtained at the same level as C. No enhancement outlines the left LIQ lumpectomy cavity. Only minimal enhancement of the lateral breast skin is seen bilaterally.

seen in Figure 1, which strongly mimics radiation effects in appearance. This was 3 months after lumpectomy and axillary lymph node dissection, with 7 of 10 lymph nodes involved. This preradiation appearance was most likely due to lymphedema, given the extent of her axillary involvement and the recent surgery.

CASE 3

Two-month-old radiation therapy effects on lung (CT and PET)

A 50-year-old woman developed right breast swelling and skin changes. The prior year, she had been treated with breast conservation for a high-risk,

4.7-cm left breast cancer, estrogen receptor positive, progesterone receptor negative, unknown *HER-2/neu*, with angiolymphatic invasion and 10 of 11 lymph nodes involved and with focal extracapsular extension. She had been treated with chemotherapy with doxorubicin (Adriamycin), cyclophosphamide (Cytoxan), and paclitaxel (Taxol), completed 3 months before, and started tamoxifen. Radiation therapy was concluded less than 2 months before she presented with the new right breast symptoms. Physical examination showed a dominant, mobile, irregular, hard mass in the right upper breast with peau d'orange changes and periareolar erythema.

Breast imaging showed a right upper outer quadrant, 4-cm mass, best seen on ultrasound. Enlarged axillary lymph nodes were noted. Palpation-guided biopsy by the surgeon confirmed infiltrating ductal carcinoma, estrogen receptor and progesterone receptor negative, *HER-2/neu* negative. Punch skin biopsies were initially negative, but a repeat skin punch biopsy 3 months later confirmed infiltrating ductal carcinoma (IDC) with dermal lymphatic involvement. Axillary fine-needle aspiration (FNA) confirmed axillary nodal disease.

Staging for the clinically suspected inflammatory breast cancer was performed with positron emission tomography (PET)/CT. The dominant right breast cancer was intensely hypermetabolic, as were multiple right axillary lymph nodes (Figure 1). The right breast skin was thickened and increased in metabolic activity, supporting the suspected

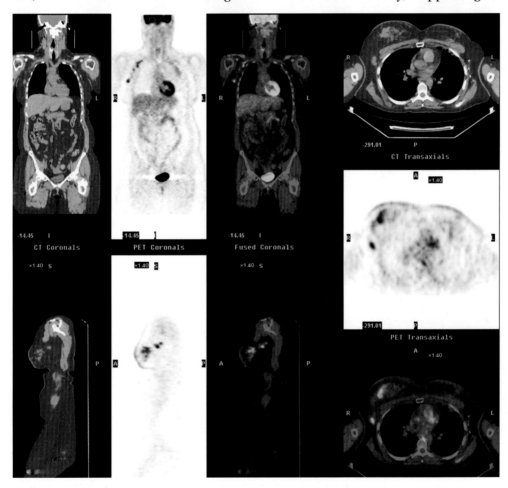

FIGURE 1. PET/CT images in coronal (*upper left*), sagittal (*lower left*), and axial (*right*) projections. There is intense hypermetabolism focally in the right lateral breast, seen on sagittal and axial images, accompanied by multiple hypermetabolic right axillary lymph nodes, seen in all three planes. The skin of the right breast is thickened and shows increased activity, as can be seen on the sagittal and axial images. This is suspicious with the clinical findings for an inflammatory component, which was subsequently confirmed by skin biopsy. On the left, there also is thickening and increased activity of the breast skin. This is accompanied by low-level peripheral left upper lung activity, seen on the coronal and axial images. These left-sided findings are due to radiation therapy, which had been completed 2 months before.

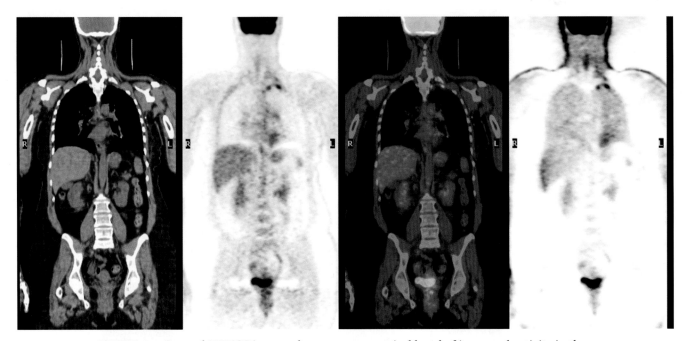

FIGURE 2.   Coronal PET/CT images show an asymmetrical band of increased activity in the left lung apex from recent radiation therapy, completed 2 months before.

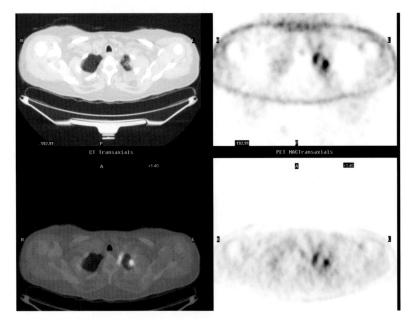

FIGURE 3.   Axial PET/CT images through the lung apices show the asymmetrical consolidation of the lung parenchyma on CT (*left*), and the corresponding increased PET activity from recently completed radiation therapy for left breast cancer.

diagnosis of inflammatory cancer (subsequently confirmed by skin biopsy). In the left lung, moderately intense linear apical and subpleural parenchymal activity was seen, commensurate with recent radiation therapy (Figures 2, 3, 4, and 5). There was no evidence of distant metastases.

The patient was treated with four cycles of chemotherapy using docetaxel (Taxotere) and capecitabine (Xeloda), with clinical improvement in the right palpable breast cancer. She was restaged with PET/CT, with improvement noted, with decreased activity of the index breast cancer and axillary nodes. The PET scan showed no evidence of other disease, but a concurrent CT showed two new small hypodense liver lesions.

The patient was re-evaluated for surgery. However, persistent skin changes were noted, and so repeat skin punch biopsy was performed. This confirmed dermal lymphatic involvement.

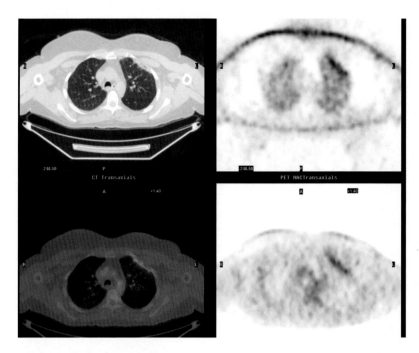

FIGURE 4. A more inferior axial PET/CT image shows a left anterior subpleural band of lung consolidation and fibrosis, which is moderately active on PET. The linear configuration and distribution of the activity are characteristic changes resulting from left breast and chest wall external-beam radiation therapy. The intensity of the activity is compatible with the time course of the treatment, being only 2 months old.

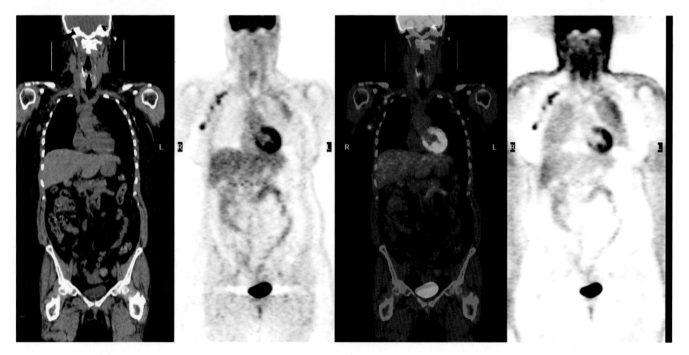

FIGURE 5. Coronal PET/CT images show multiple hypermetabolic (seven on this slice) right axillary lymph nodes extending in a line high into the axilla. Low-level peripheral linear left upper lung activity from radiation therapy is also seen on this slice.

The patient's chemotherapy regimen was changed to Taxol and bevacizumab (Avastin). After two cycles, her response was assessed with repeat PET/CT. These studies confirmed liver metastases, with growth of the previously seen lesions, and development of multiple, new, PET-positive liver masses. Development of right superior mediastinal and supraclavicular nodal foci of activity was also noted. The patient's regimen was changed to gemcitabine.

TEACHING POINTS

This is an unusual case of an aggressive inflammatory breast cancer developing on the heels of a

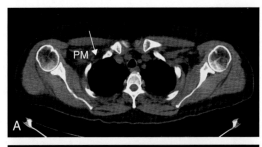

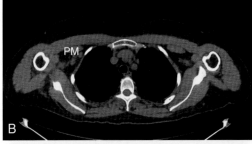

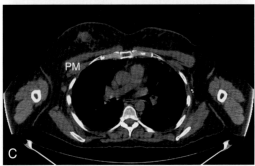

FIGURE 6. Axial unenhanced chest CT images for correlation with figure 5 (**A** to **C**, from above to below). **A**, A cluster of five mildly enlarged right axillary level III lymph nodes is seen medial to the pectoralis minor muscle (PM) (*arrow*). **B**, Two enlarged right axillary level II lymph nodes are seen deep to the PM. **C**, Two enlarged right axillary level I lymph nodes are seen lateral to the PM. A portion of the patient's right IDC can be seen on this section. Surgical clips can be seen on the left at axillary level I from prior lymph node dissection.

high-risk contralateral breast cancer. From an imaging point of view, it provides several take-off points for discussion. The significance and implications of breast skin activity and thickening are completely different between the two sides, emphasizing the importance of accurate clinical history and correlation. On the right, the skin changes reinforced the clinical suspicion of an inflammatory breast cancer, and dermal lymphatic involvement was subsequently confirmed by skin biopsy. On the left, the skin activity and thickening are entirely commensurate with the fact that external-beam radiation to this breast concluded only 2 months before. The distribution of the left lung changes on CT are typical of radiation fibrosis, and the accompanying activity on PET is commensurate with the time course since treatment and

would be expected to decline in intensity on subsequent follow-ups.

Axillary nodal involvement on the right was suspected both clinically and by imaging with ultrasound, and confirmed by FNA. However, the combination of PET and CT provides the best noninvasive estimate of the extent of involvement. In this case, we see evidence of involvement of axillary levels I, II, and III. On coronal PET/CT, we see a line of hypermetabolic right axillary lymph nodes ascending high into the axilla (Figure 5). Correlation with axial CT images allows us to localize these lymph nodes more precisely, with axillary lymph nodes lateral to the pectoralis minor designated level I, under the muscle level II, and those medial to it level III (Figure 6).

CASE 4

Breast cancer radiation–induced lung changes on CT and PET

A 55-year-old woman with a large, locally advanced palpable left upper outer quadrant (UOQ) mass was treated for biopsy-proven infiltrating ductal carcinoma (IDC) with dermal lymphatic carcinoma. Clinically, the manifestations of inflammatory carcinoma were subtle at presentation, with faint periareolar erythema extending into the lower quadrants. She underwent four cycles of doxorubicin (Adriamycin) and cyclophosphamide (Cytoxan) (AC) neoadjuvant chemotherapy, followed by modified radical mastectomy, radiation to the chest wall, supraclavicular region, and posterior axilla (Figure 1).

Details of the radiation therapy include treatment of supraclavicular and axillary nodes with a right anterior oblique (RAO) field, delivering 180 cGy per day to a depth of 3 cm. A total dose of 5040 cGy in 28 fractions was given. The posterior axillary boost (PAB) brought the mid-axilla dose to 44.7 Gy. Chest wall tangential fields delivered 180 cGy daily for a total of 5040 cGy. Six-megavolt photons were used in all fields. The chest wall was treated with a 0.5-cm bolus for the first 22 fractions. On the lateral tangential field, a 60-degree wedge was used daily. The scar was boosted with 9-MeV electron beam with 5-mm bolus. The scar was treated with medial and lateral fields, receiving 14.4- and 16.2-cGy boost doses, respectively.

After completion of radiation therapy, additional chemotherapy was given with four cycles of docetaxel (Taxotere). Margins of the mastectomy specimen were positive for both IDC and ductal carcinoma in situ (DCIS). The tumor was a 7- to 8-cm IDC with a 3.5-cm region of intermediate-grade DCIS, with extensive angiolymphatic invasion. Seven of 16 lymph nodes were involved. Final stage was stage IIIB, T4N2Mx, left breast inflammatory carcinoma, estrogen receptor and progesterone receptor positive, *HER-2/neu* negative.

Imaging with PET/CT 4 months after the conclusion of radiation therapy showed characteristic changes of early radiation fibrosis of the underlying lung on both CT and PET (Figures 2, 3, and 4).

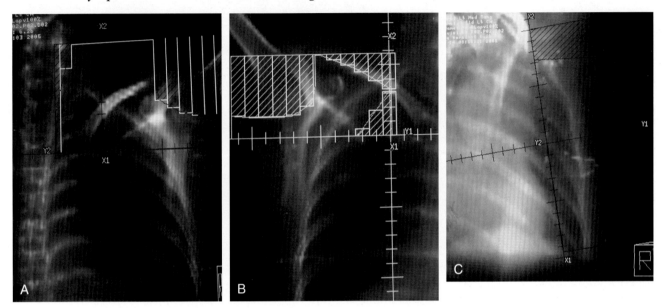

FIGURE 1.   Radiation therapy port films. **A,** Right anterior oblique planning film for left supraclavicular fossa (SCF) and upper axillary lymph node coverage overlaps the lung apex. The humerus will be excluded from the field, as diagrammed on the film. **B,** A posterior view of the left axilla for planning of the posterior axillary boost (PAB) dose, necessary for complete radiation treatment of the axilla. Areas to be excluded are indicated by the *cross-hatches*, including the humeral head. A portion of the superolateral lung apex is included in the field. **C,** Medial tangential field for chest wall irradiation of this postmastectomy patient encompasses a band of underlying lung, as outlined by the grid. Depending on a patient's anatomy, up to 3 cm of the underlying lung may be included in the field. Treatment of left-sided breast cancers may also encompass some of the heart, increasing the patient's subsequent risk for coronary artery disease.

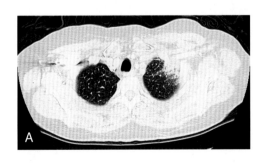
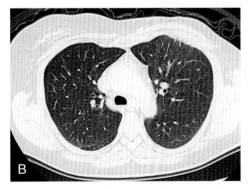

FIGURE 2.   Chest CT images (lung windows, *from above to below,* **A** to **D**) from a study obtained 4 months after conclusion of left chest wall, supraclavicular, and posterior axillary radiation therapy already show peripheral lung consolidative changes. The straight edge in the periphery of the anterolateral lung is a characteristic clue to the iatrogenic nature of these findings. The changes are more rounded in the apex and inferiorly but can be assumed to be the same process in this context. *(Continued)*

FIGURE 2, cont'd

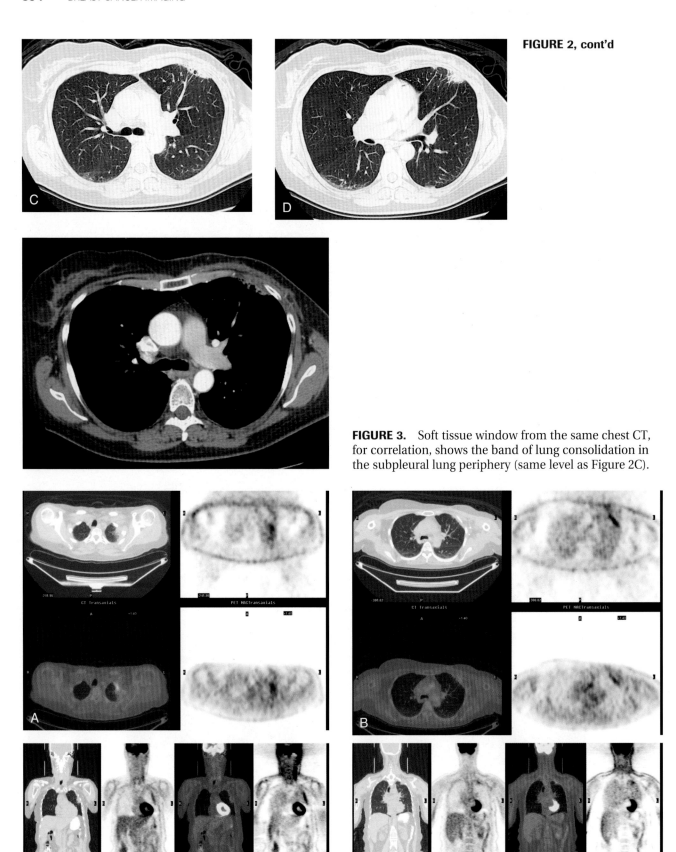

FIGURE 3. Soft tissue window from the same chest CT, for correlation, shows the band of lung consolidation in the subpleural lung periphery (same level as Figure 2C).

FIGURE 4. Corresponding PET/CT images show the changes to be hypermetabolic, with a sharply demarcated, linear configuration. **A**, Axial, through the lung apices. **B**, Axial, more inferior. **C**, Coronal. **D**, Coronal, more posterior, through the apices.

TEACHING POINTS

The radiation-induced changes of the lung parenchyma seen in this case delineate the most typical radiation portals utilized in breast cancer patients. The chest wall is radiated using tangential beams, which overlap with the underlying lung up to 3 cm. Administration of radiation to the supraclavicular fossa and posterior axillary boost doses include the lung apex. The most typical early lung changes visualized immediately after radiation therapy (in the first 3 months) are ground-glass opacity (see Case 8 in Chapter 6 for an example). The changes seen here show more dense lung consolidation. Lucencies within the band of consolidated lung are air bronchograms. These changes are typical of radiation-induced lung fibrosis, which is most commonly seen after 6 months or so. This may be progressive, but generally stabilizes by 2 years after treatment. Both radiation pneumonitis and fibrosis can be metabolically active on PET. The more recent the treatment, the higher the activity level can be, and for this reason, it is desirable when possible to delay PET imaging until 2 to 3 months after conclusion of radiation.

CASE 5

Typical apical changes from supraclavicular radiation therapy on CT, MRI, and PET

A 57-year-old woman, previously treated for a high-risk right breast cancer, is followed with periodic breast MRI. Her tumor was a stage IIIA, T2N2M0, 2.2-cm infiltrating ductal carcinoma, grade 9/9, with angiolymphatic invasion, estrogen receptor and progesterone receptor negative, and *HER-2/ neu* negative, with 19 of 26 lymph nodes positive for metastatic disease. She was treated 5 years before with lumpectomy, lymph node dissection, and radiation to the breast, axillary, and supraclavicular nodal basins. Systemic treatment was chemotherapy (four cycles of doxorubicin [Adriamycin] and cyclophosphamide [Cytoxan] [AC] and four cycles of paclitaxel [Taxol]).

Details of her radiation therapy were as follows: Radiation fields covered the right supraclavicular

fossa (SCF) and the upper axillary lymph nodes with a left anterior oblique field (Figure 1). Radiation dose of 180 cGy was given daily. After 28 fractions, the SCF received 5040 cGy. In order to bring the deeper tissue of the mid-axilla to a full dose, a daily posterior axillary boost (PAB) dose of 27 cGy was used (Figure 2). The breast was treated with

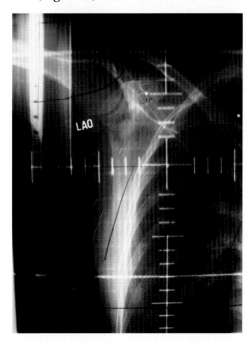

FIGURE 1. Left anterior oblique (LAO) projection right supraclavicular field radiation planning film. The humerus will be coned out, as drawn on the film.

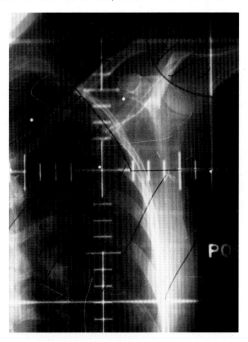

FIGURE 2. Right posterior axillary boost (PAB) radiation therapy planning film. The intended coverage area has been mapped out on the film.

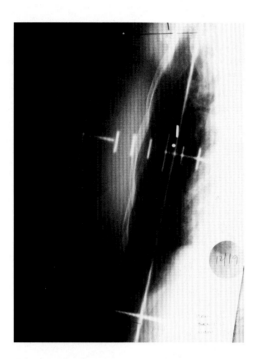

FIGURE 3.   Medial tangential coverage of the right breast, showing that several centimeters of the underlying lung will be overlapped.

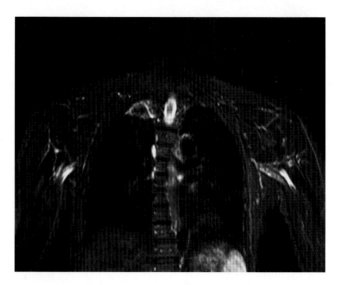

FIGURE 4.   Coronal STIR image of the thorax, obtained with the body coil, shows increased parenchymal signal at the right lung apex. Note the sharp line at the inferior margin of the altered signal, suggesting its iatrogenic etiology.

non-coplanar tangential fields (Figure 3) delivering a daily dose of 180 cGy. The whole breast received 5040 cGy. The breast and regional lymphatics were treated with 9-MV photons. Technical details of the setup included use of half-beam block, wedges, table kick-out, and non-coplanar tangential orientation.

A coronal STIR sequence of the thorax (obtained in conjunction with the breast MRI) was interpreted as showing abnormal right apical signal intensity of uncertain significance (Figure 4), and a chest CT was recommended for further evaluation. As it happened, the patient had been previously evaluated with positron emission tomography (PET) and CT the year before for an unexplained rise in CA 27.29. No evidence of metastatic disease or recurrence was found at the time, and the tumor marker had subsequently normalized without treatment. Correlation with these studies showed stable findings of right apical radiation fibrosis (Figures 5, 6, 7, and 8).

TEACHING POINTS

Patients treated with breast-conserving surgery generally also undergo radiation therapy. Radiation effects will often be noted on subsequent imaging, and so it is important for imagers to be familiar with the typical resulting findings. Tangential fields used in breast or chest wall radiation include up to 3 cm of the underlying peripheral lung, which may develop changes that can be visualized on chest x-ray or, more commonly, on CT. Early changes, with hazy opacity, can be seen within a month after radiation therapy (range, 1 to 3 months). This may evolve to coalescent consolidation, which may subsequently dissipate or may progress to a relatively sharply demarcated zone of lung fibrosis over a period of 6 months to 2 years. The typical anterolateral peripheral lung location of tangential beam radiation changes is well illustrated by Figure 8.

The apical lung parenchymal changes depicted in Figures 4 to 7, with a sharp inferior linear edge, delineate the inferior extent of a supraclavicular port, which generally will be at the first or second intercostal space level. Mature effects such as these generally develop by 2 years after treatment and remain stable thereafter. The low-level apical cap of activity seen on PET is also typical and may persist for years or indefinitely.

Patients such as this, previously treated with lumpectomy for a high-risk tumor and with breast implants, are more difficult to image with mammography. Mammography is still useful, but postsurgical distortion and implants can limit its utility. The imaging surveillance of difficult-to-image patients such as this can be supplemented with ultrasound and MRI. MRI in particular overcomes limitations of breast density, postsurgical alterations, and the presence of implants. It is the most

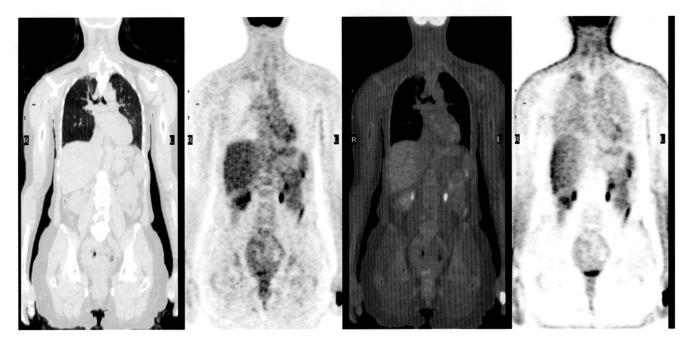

FIGURE 5. Coronal PET/CT images (*from left to right:* CT, PET, fused PET/CT, non-attenuation-corrected PET) show a right apical cap of very modest activity, corresponding to the MRI findings and quite characteristic of radiation therapy changes.

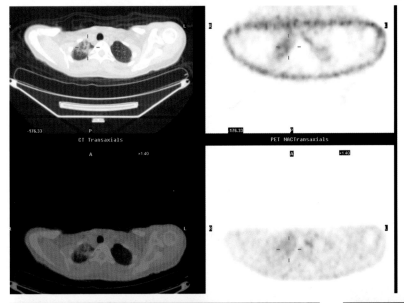

FIGURE 6. Axial PET/CT findings at the same level show the asymmetrical right apical lung consolidation, with only minimal associated increased metabolic activity (*cursors*).

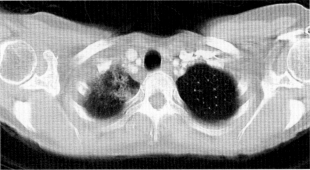

FIGURE 7. Lung window from a contrast-enhanced chest CT through the same level as Figure 6 better shows the apical consolidation.

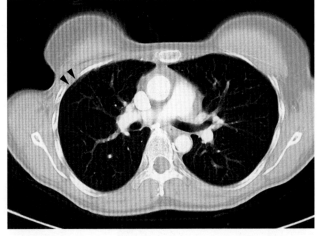

FIGURE 8. A more inferior chest CT section shows a more subtle right anterior subpleural band of increased lung parenchymal density from the breast irradiation (*arrowheads*).

sensitive modality for the detection of occult breast malignancies.

SUGGESTED READINGS

Davis SD, Yankelevitz DF, Henschke CI. Radiation effects on the lung: clinical features, pathology, and imaging findings. *AJR Am J Roentgenol* 1992; 159:1157–1164.

Jung JI, Kim HH, Park SH, et al. Thoracic manifestations of breast cancer and its therapy. *RadioGraphics* 2004; 24:1269–1285.

CASE 6

Mass-like radiation fibrosis

A 47-year-old woman with recurrent left chest wall infiltrating lobular carcinoma (ILC) underwent CT and PET scans while being restaged. She presented with a tender palpable lump at the superior aspect of her left breast implant. She also complained of chronic left chest wall pain, between the reconstructed breast and the axilla, in a region of clinically dense fixation.

Her original diagnosis of ILC was 10 years before, at age 37, a 2-cm, T2N0M0 lesion, estrogen receptor and progesterone receptor positive, *HER-2/neu* negative, treated with mastectomy. The margins were close, and so she underwent chest wall

(5040 cGy) and supraclavicular (4500 cGy) radiation, as well as six cycles of Cytoxan, methotrexate, 5-fluorouracil (CMF) chemotherapy. Subsequently, she was on tamoxifen for 3 years before developing a left axillary recurrence. This was excised, confirming metastatic breast cancer and treated with left axillary radiation. Additional staging workup at the time showed ovarian cysts. Bilateral oophorectomy was negative for malignancy, and the patient had been on anastrozole (Arimidex) since.

CT scans obtained at the time of the current left chest wall recurrence (same patient as Case 11 in Chapter 10) showed a spiculated, mass-like finding in the left lung apex (Figure 1). This was associated with only minimal, linear, low-level positron emission tomography (PET) scan activity (Figures 2 and 3) and correlated with the history of

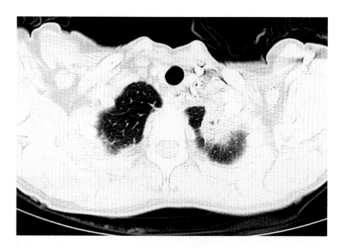

FIGURE 1.   Lung window from chest CT shows a spiculated, mass-like focus in the left lung apex.

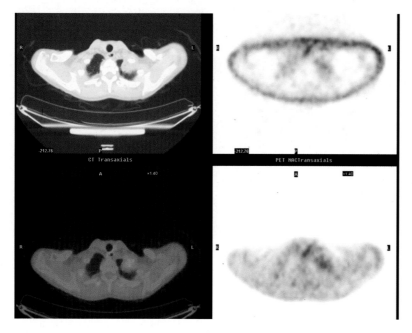

FIGURE 2.   Axial PET/CT images at the corresponding level show only low-level activity in the left apex.

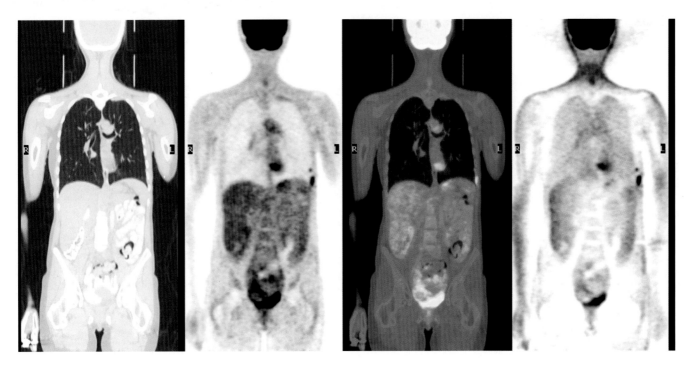

FIGURE 3. Coronal PET/CT images show only a low-level linear band of activity in the left lung apex. More intense activity is seen at the left lower chest wall level from the patient's concurrent recurrence (see Case 11 in Chapter 10 for additional delineation of the chest wall recurrence).

supraclavicular radiation therapy 10 years before, as well as axillary radiation 7 years before. Review of the patient's prior records identified a prior CT scan with similar findings 3 years before, at which time she had undergone a biopsy, with no malignancy obtained.

TEACHING POINTS

Not everything that is rounded and mass-like is a mass. In this case, the left apical finding appears this way only in the axial projection. Its true nature, with a sharply delineated inferior border belying its iatrogenic etiology, is better appreciated in other planes. Especially in the coronal plane, where it can be easily compared with the untreated side, the finding appears much more benign. This represents a relatively mass-like appearance of radiation fibrosis, which in this case is at least 7 years old. The low level of PET scan activity is also typical and may persist indefinitely.

CASE 7

Early postradiation changes on breast MRI

A 53-year-old perimenopausal woman underwent lumpectomy for a stage I, T1N0, 1.2-cm left infiltrating ductal carcinoma (IDC), which was estrogen receptor and progesterone receptor positive and *HER-2/neu* negative. One sentinel lymph node was negative. Breast MRI was obtained during her preoperative evaluation because of extreme breast density (Figures 1 and 2). Extensive stippled fibrocystic type foci of enhancement made the evaluation of the opposite breast difficult, for which repeat breast MRI was recommended in 6 months. In the meantime, the patient underwent surgery on the left for the known IDC and completed radiation therapy 3 months before returning for repeat breast MRI (Figure 3).

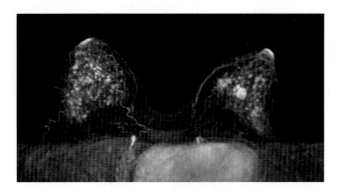

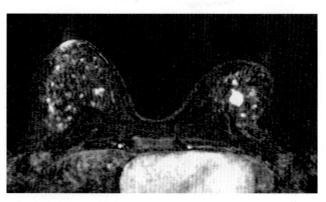

FIGURE 1.   Enhanced, subtracted, axial maximal intensity projection (MIP) view of both breasts (obtained at initial staging for left breast IDC) shows bilateral, diffuse, scattered, punctate foci of enhancement. The patient was perimenopausal, with very dense breast tissue and many cysts. The diffuse background pattern of enhancement is compatible with fibrocystic change and hormonal effects. Even against this background with MIP projection, the patient's central left IDC can be appreciated.

FIGURE 2.   A single slice from early in the enhanced, subtracted, dynamic axial series shows the central known left IDC mass. Both breasts show scattered, stippled, punctate foci of enhancement, and normal variant nipple activity is seen on the right on this section.

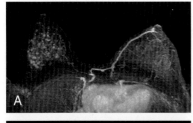

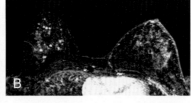

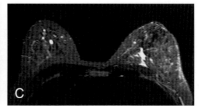

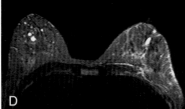

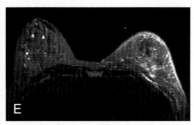

FIGURE 3.   Repeat breast MRI, 6 months later, obtained to follow up the right breast, because of concern at the time of the first MRI that the extensive enhancement could be obscuring an abnormality. The patient had finished radiation therapy to the left breast 3 months before this study, and multiple post-treatment findings are seen as follows: **A**, Enhanced, subtracted, axial MIP view of both breasts shows a similar pattern of diffuse punctate foci of enhancement on the right. The pattern has changed considerably on the left. The dominant mass has been resected and is no longer seen. The enhancement is lower level, diffuse, and subdued (compare with Figure 1). **B**, A single slice from early in the enhanced, subtracted, dynamic axial series of this follow-up breast MRI shows new left breast skin thickening and mild enhancement, secondary to the radiation therapy. There also is new, linear enhancement of the left chest wall. **C** to **E**, Axial STIR images, *from above to below* show a postsurgical fluid collection on the left centrally, which tracks posteriorly to the pectoral muscle level. Radiation therapy effects are evident, with diffuse edema and reticulation of the left breast. Thickening and edema are noted of the left breast skin, particularly laterally. Increased signal from edema is also noted within the left pectoral and chest wall musculature. On the right side, scattered tiny breast cysts are seen. **F**, Enhanced, subtracted, sagittal view of the left breast, obtained about 5 minutes after contrast administration, shows the scar as architectural distortion in the retroareolar area (*arrow*), which enhances to the same degree as the breast parenchyma. Surgery was performed 6 months before this study.

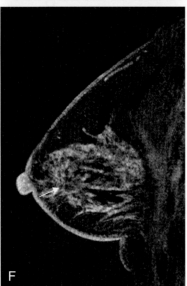

TEACHING POINTS

In general, treatment effects from prior surgery and radiation are readily identifiable and generally do not significantly hamper breast MRI interpretation. That said, it is important to have accurate clinical information about the location of prior surgeries and the time course since interventions like surgery or radiation therapy. Breast MRI technologists should mark with vitamin E capsules or another suitable marker the locations of any palpable lumps that the patient can identify, as well as the locations of surgical scars or biopsy sites. The interpreter needs to bear in mind that if prior biopsies were image-guided, marker placements at the skin entry site may correspond in location only generally to the actual sites of underlying lesions.

Radiation therapy findings on breast MRI depend on the time course since treatment. Early reports of the use of breast MRI after radiation therapy suggested that radiation therapy effects and enhancement hampered the diagnostic utility of breast MRI for up to 18 months after treatment. However, that has not been our experience, and a study by Morakkabati and colleagues of 116 breast MRIs performed in 72 patients in the first year after breast conservation and radiation found that the changes due to radiation were less severe than previously reported and did not impair the diagnostic performance of breast MRI in detecting clinically relevant residual disease.

Findings attributable to radiation therapy are most evident in the first 3 to 6 months after treatment. They include skin thickening, edema, and enhancement, as well as parenchymal edema and reticulation. These findings, best seen on fluid-sensitive sequences (STIR, T2-weighted, or fat-saturated T2-weighted), peak at 3 to 6 months. Mild generalized increased parenchymal enhancement compared with the untreated opposite side can be detected in the first 3 months after treatment. This low level of enhancement is not sufficiently intense to interfere with detection of clinically relevant disease. These changes are the result of acute tissue reaction to the ionizing radiation.

After about 6 months, the process of scarring begins, with some degree of retraction of the tissues and thickening of the skin. The changes seen on imaging studies done immediately after completion of radiation therapy will regress.

One late effect of radiation therapy that we have observed on a number of occasions is demonstrated here but has not been well documented in the literature. Radiated breasts often have marked reduction of their baseline "stippled" pattern of enhancement after treatment. Presumably, this is due to the diffuse tissue and vascular damage induced by radiation to the treated field. The processes underlying radiation injury of tissues are still being delineated. Depletion of certain target cells, leading to fewer source cells for repopulation during post-treatment recovery, appears to be implicated. See also Case 8 for another example.

SUGGESTED READINGS

Morakkabati N, Leutner CC, Schmiedel A, et al. Breast MR Imaging during or soon after radiation therapy. *Radiology* 2003; 229:893–901.

Withers HR. The dose-survival relationship for irradiation of epithelial cells of mouse skin. *Br J Radiol* 1967; 40:187.

CASE 8

Late postradiation changes on breast MRI

A pregnant 37-year-old patient was evaluated with breast MRI because of a past history of treatment 6 years before for a left T1N0 poorly differentiated infiltrating ductal carcinoma, estrogen receptor and progesterone receptor positive, with 15 negative lymph nodes. She had undergone a lumpectomy and axillary lymph node dissection, as well as chemotherapy (four cycles of doxorubicin [Adriamycin] plus cyclophosphamide [Cytoxan] [AC]) and radiation therapy. She had been able to tolerate tamoxifen for only 6 weeks. At the time of breast MRI, the patient was 4 months pregnant and had undergone surgery on the right for a lactating adenoma.

Breast MRI showed striking asymmetry between the two sides in enhancement (Figure 1). The right side showed the expected pregnancy-induced hormonal effects, with intense, diffuse enhancement, making it difficult to exclude a breast cancer. The previously radiated left side was smaller and showed diffuse but subdued enhancement compared with the untreated side (Figures 2 and 3).

Repeat breast MRI, obtained a year later (8 months postpartum), showed persistent asymmetry between sides, but both sides showed

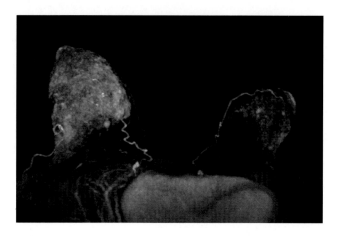

FIGURE 1. Subtracted, enhanced axial maximal intensity projection image (MIP), obtained when the patient was 4 months pregnant, shows the untreated right side to be enhancing diffusely and intensely. The previously treated left side is smaller because of prior surgery. It also shows diffuse enhancement, but much lower in intensity than the opposite side.

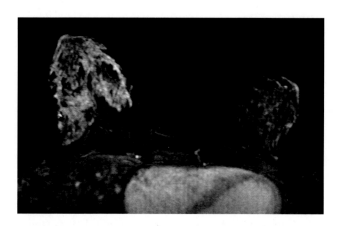

FIGURE 2. A representative section from the enhanced, subtracted dynamic series shows the intense diffuse parenchymal enhancement of pregnancy-induced hormonal effects on the right, with similar, but much dampened findings on the previously radiated left side.

marked interval regression of the pregnancy-related hormonal effects and enhancement (Figures 4 and 5).

TEACHING POINTS

Breast imaging during pregnancy is difficult. Hormonal changes of pregnancy result in growth of the breasts, which double in weight, and blood flow increases dramatically (180%). When a patient who has previously been treated for breast cancer becomes pregnant, her physicians may request

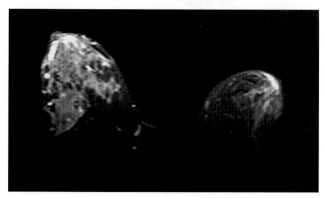

FIGURE 3. Axial STIR image of the breasts from the same study, for correlation, shows the parenchyma of both breasts to be very fluid in signal intensity. Again, the hormonal effects are much more pronounced on the untreated right side.

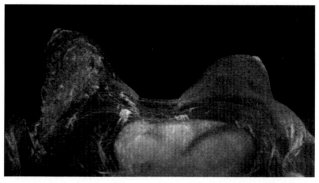

FIGURE 4. Axial MIP from a follow-up study, 1 year later and 8 months postpartum, shows persistent asymmetry between sides, with both sides showing marked regression of the pregnancy-induced enhancement. Compare with Figure 1.

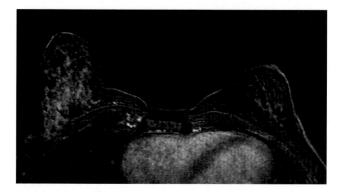

FIGURE 5. A representative image from the enhanced, subtracted dynamic series, for comparison with Figure 2, shows markedly decreased diffuse enhancement compared with the study obtained during pregnancy.

imaging "clearance" of the breasts. Two-view film screen mammography with abdominal shielding results in a fetal dose estimated to be 500 µGy, which is considered acceptable. Of course, in a patient as young as this, mammography during pregnancy may well be limited because of breast density. There are data to suggest that mammographic density does not significantly change during pregnancy from baseline.

Screening whole-breast ultrasound may be considered as a higher sensitivity alternative. The most sensitive modality, breast MRI, may also be considered to screen for occult breast cancer in such higher-risk patients. Even though breast density is not considered a limitation of breast MRI, the ramped-up hormonal status of pregnant patients may make breast MRI difficult to interpret, as demonstrated by this case.

This case also provides an interesting view of presumed late effects of radiation therapy on a previously treated breast. Radiation therapy results in diffuse tissue and microvascular damage. Tissues exposed to radiation are less likely to enlarge under hormonal influence (e.g., pregnancy) or even weight gain. The previously treated breast generally does not undergo the expected pregnancy hormone-induced growth. The field effect seen here on the previously treated side is presumably the result of prior radiation therapy. Both sides show hormonal effects of pregnancy, which later regress, as can be seen on the follow-up examination. Presumably, radiation-induced tissue injury limits how much response to pregnancy hormones the treated breast can muster.

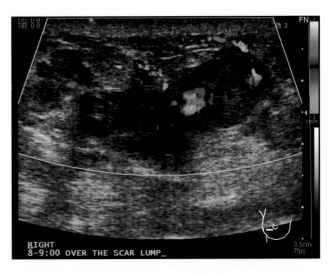

FIGURE 1. Breast sonogram shows a dominant, hypoechoic, solid, highly vascular mass with irregular borders at the level of the patient's lumpectomy scar. Smaller, similar-appearing sites of apparent multifocal disease were also seen (not shown).

CASE 9

Radiation-induced angiosarcoma

An 86-year-old woman noted new right breast changes, with burning pain, nodularity, and firmness. She had been treated for stage II, T1N1, right breast cancer 19 years before, with partial mastectomy and axillary dissection and radiation therapy with interstitial implant boost. Three of 13 lymph nodes were involved. No chemotherapy was given, but she had taken tamoxifen for 9 years, stopping 10 years before.

Imaging evaluations were highly suspicious for a multifocal recurrence. Ultrasound showed a highly irregular and very vascular dominant mass (Figure 1), with smaller additional sites of involvement suggested as well by ultrasound. Ultrasound-guided core needle biopsy confirmed a high-grade angiosarcoma.

The patient underwent mastectomy, with pathology showing a high-grade, multifocal angiosarcoma, with subareolar and dermal-subcutaneous involvement. Marked radiation change was also noted in the specimen.

Postoperative evaluations for right rib pain and headaches suggested rib and brain metastases. Radiation oncology was consulted. The patient was noted to be frail and weak, with poor appetite, nausea, recent weight loss, blurry vision, and headache.

Right posterior ribs were radiated, with relief of her pain. Initial brain MRI suggested a left occipital metastasis, with a tiny additional left frontal lesion. On high-resolution repeat brain MRI before gamma knife therapy, additional lesions were seen. Two occipital lesions were treated to address the patient's visual symptoms.

Whole-brain radiation therapy was then planned. However, it was subsequently declined. The patient died in hospice care 3 months after her initial diagnosis of radiation-induced breast angiosarcoma.

TEACHING POINTS

This case represents a late, rare complication of breast radiation therapy, with induction of an angiosarcoma. Breast angiosarcoma is rare, accounting for 0.04% of all breast malignancies. Breast angiosarcomas may be primary or secondary; secondary angiosarcoma occurs in patients previously treated for breast cancer with radiation therapy or complicated by lymphedema. Primary angiosarcomas tend to occur in younger women (second to fourth decades of life) than secondary angiosarcomas, which generally occur in women after the age of 50 years, with a latency period after treatment of 4 to 7 years.

The most common clinical presentation is with a palpable mass; diffuse breast enlargement has been reported as well. Violaceous discoloration of the skin is a relatively specific sign that can be seen in 17% to 35% of breast angiosarcomas.

Because angiosarcomas spread hematogenously, the surgical treatment of breast angiosarcoma differs from that of other primary breast malignancies. Axillary lymph nodes are not usually involved, and so axillary dissection is not indicated in the surgical treatment of these patients. Mastectomy is usually necessary to achieve negative margins.

The prognosis is uniformly poor for patients such as this with high-grade disease.

SUGGESTED READINGS

Liberman L, Dershaw DD, Kaufman RJ, et al. Angiosarcoma of the breast. *Radiology* 1992; 183:649. (Retrospective review of 29 cases of primary angiosarcoma of the breast.)

Marchant LK, Orel SG, Perez-Jaffe LA, et al. Bilateral angiosarcoma of the breast on MR imaging. *AJR Am J Roentgenol* 1997; 169:1009–1010. (Case report of bilateral primary angiosarcoma appearance on breast MRI.)

Index

Note: Page numbers followed by f indicate figures; page numbers followed by t indicate tables.